LIPPINCOTT'S
VISUAL ENCYCLOPEDIA OF CLINICAL SKILLS

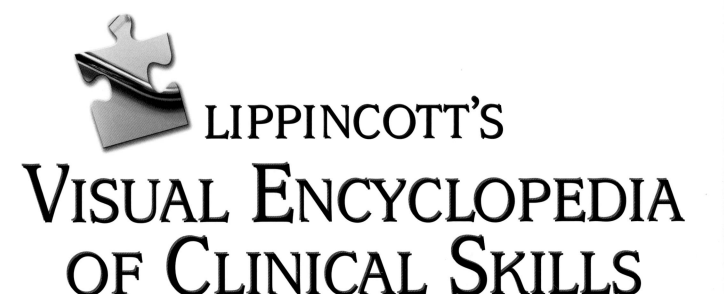

LIPPINCOTT'S
VISUAL ENCYCLOPEDIA
OF CLINICAL SKILLS

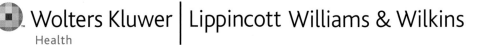

Wolters Kluwer | Lippincott Williams & Wilkins
Health

Philadelphia • Baltimore • New York • London
Buenos Aires • Hong Kong • Sydney • Tokyo

STAFF

Executive Publisher
Judith A. Schilling McCann, RN, MSN

Editorial Director
H. Nancy Holmes

Clinical Director
Joan M. Robinson, RN, MSN

Art Director
Mary Ludwicki

Editorial Project Manager
Ann Houska

Clinical Project Manager
Jennifer Meyering, RN, BSN, MS, CCRN

Editors
Rita Doyle, Jennifer Kowalak

Copy Editors
Kimberly Bilotta (supervisor), Leslie
Dworkin, Linda Hager, Pamela Wingrod

Designer
Arlene Putterman

Digital Composition Services
Diane Paluba (manager),
Joyce Rossi Biletz, Donna S. Morris

Associate Manufacturing Manager
Beth J. Welsh

Editorial Assistants
Karen J. Kirk, Jeri O'Shea, Linda K. Ruhf

Design Assistant
Kate Zulak

Indexer
Barbara Hodgson

*Library of Congress
Cataloging-in-Publication Data*

Lippincott's visual encyclopedia of clinical skills.
        p. ; cm.
    Includes bibliographical references and index.
    1. Nursing—Encyclopedias. 2. Nursing—
Atlases. I. Lippincott Williams & Wilkins.
II. Title: Visual encyclopedia of clinical skills.
    [DNLM: 1. Nursing Care—methods—Encyclopedias—English. 2. Clinical Competence—Encyclopedias—English. WY 13 L7655 2009]
    RT21.L57 2009
    610.7303—dc22
                                        2008023519
    ISBN-13: 978-0-7817-9832-7 (alk. paper)
    ISBN-10: 0-7817-9832-9 (alk. paper)

CONTENTS

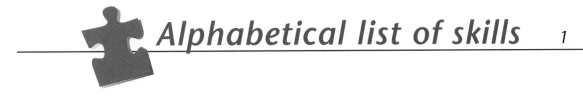

CONTRIBUTORS AND CONSULTANTS

Deborah H. Allen, *RN, MSN, FNP, APRN,BC, AOCNP*
Neuro-Oncology Nurse Practitioner, Duke University Medical Center
Durham, N.C.

Laura Kierol Andrews, *RN, PhD, APRN, ACNP*
Acute Care Nurse Practitioner, Manager of Medical Rapid Response Team
Department of Critical Care Medicine, The Hospital of Central Connecticut
New Britain General Campus

Rosemary Ashby, *ARNP-C, BSN, MS, CGRN*
Nurse Practitioner, Gastroenterology and Hepatology
James A. Haley Veteran's Hospital
Tampa, Fla.

Leslie A. Atkins, *RN, PhD*
Staff Nurse, Intensive Care Unit
Norman (Okla.) Regional Hospital

Debbie Berry, *RN, MSN, CPHQ*
Internal Consultant, Resource Management, MedStar Health
Lutherville, Md.

Cheryl L. Brady, *RN, MSN*
Assistant Professor, Kent State University
Salem, Ohio

Denise Brehmer, *RN, MSN*
Visiting Lecturer
Indiana University Kokomo

Tamara Capik-Zupanc, *RN, BSN, CCRN*
Critical Care Nurse Educator, St. Joseph Hospital—Ministry Health Care
Marshfield, Wisc.

Kathy Cochran, *RN, MSN*
Division Chair Health Technologies/Director and Instructor
Coosa Valley Technical College
Rome, Ga.

Cathy Conner, *RN, ADN*
Practical Nursing Instructor, Concorde Career College
Jacksonville, Fla.

Claire Cottrell, *RN, MSN*
Nursing Instructor, Mississippi Gulf Coast Community College
Perkinston

Lillian Craig, *RN, MSN, FNP-C*
Adjunct Faculty, Oklahoma Panhandle State University
Goodwell

Sherry Currie, *RN, BSN, MN*
Lead Instructor, Butler Community College
El Dorado, Kans.

Michelle Deligencia, *RN, MSN, CNOR*
Clinical Consultant
San Diego

Louise Diehl-Oplinger, *RN, MSN, CCRN, APRN-BC, NP-C*
Nurse Practitioner, Practice Owner
Lehigh Valley Wellness Center
Phillipsburg, N.J.

Jennifer E. DiMedio, *CRNP, MSN, FNP*
Family Nurse Practitioner
University of Pennsylvania—West Chester

Laurie Donaghy, *RN, CEN*
Staff Nurse, Temple University Health System
Philadelphia

David Dunham, *RN, MS, CRNI*
Assistant Professor of Nursing, Hawaii Pacific University
Kaneohe

Shelba Durston, *RN, MSN, CCRN*
Nursing Instructor, San Joaquin Delta College
Stockton, Calif.

Patricia Eisenbraun, *RN, ADN, ONC*
Research Coordinator—Cardiovascular Area
North Central Heart Institute
Sioux Falls, S.D.

Judith Faust, *RN, MSN*
Assistant Professor, Ivy Tech Community College of Indiana
Lafayette

Emilie M. Fedorov, *RN, MSN, CS, CNRN*
Neuroscience/Surgical ICU Director, St. Mary's Hospital
Madison, Wisc.

Vivian Gamblian, RN, MSN
Nursing Faculty, Baylor University, Louise Herrington School of Nursing
Dallas

Stephen Gilliam, RN, PhD, APRN-BC
Assistant Professor, Medical College of Georgia, School of Nursing
Athens

Margaret M. Gingrich, RN, MSN
Professor
Harrisburg (Pa.) Area Community College

Catherine Grant, MSN, CRNP
Instructor, Carlow University
Pittsburgh

Kim Graves, RN, MSN
Critical Care Nurse, Jewish Hospital
Cincinnati

Sandra Hamilton, RN, BSN, MEd, CRNI
Faculty, Great Basin College
Hospice Nurse, Nathan Adelson Hospice
Pahrump, Nev.

Allen Hanberg, RN, MSN
Assistant Professor of Nursing, Weber State University
Ogden, Utah

Donna Headrick, RN, MSN, FNP
Instructor, Taft (Calif.) Community College
Family Nurse Practitioner, Advanced Cosmetic Dermatology
Bakersfield, Calif.

Joy L. Herzog, RN
Director of Nursing Services, LifeQuest Nursing Center
Quakertown, Pa.

Timothy L. Hudson, RN, PhD (ABD), MEd, CCRN, FACHE
Joint Theater Trauma Nurse Coordinator-Afghanistan
U.S. Army Institute of Surgical Research
Ft. Sam Houston, Tex.

Angela R. Irvin, RN, MSN, ARNP, NP-C
Assistant Professor of Nursing. Western Kentucky University
Bowling Green

Pamela L. Isbell, RN, MSN, CEN
Staff Nurse, Orlando (Fla.) Regional Medical Center

Anna L. Jarrett, APRN,BC, PhD, ACNP, CNS
Advanced Practice Nurse—Rapid Response Team
Central Arkansas Veterans Health Systems
Little Rock

Fiona Johnson, *RN, MSN, CCRN*
Clinical Education Specialist/MedSurg Residency Coordinator
Memorial Health University Medical Center
Savannah, Ga.

Karla Jones, *RN, MS*
Associate Professor, School of Nursing
University of Alaska Anchorage

Christine Kennedy, *RN, MSN*
Staff Nurse—Specialty Clinics Area, VA Connecticut Healthcare System
Adjunct Nursing Faculty, Excelsior College
West Haven

Susan M. Kilroy, *RN, MS*
Clinical Nurse Specialist, Massachusetts General Hospital
Boston

Carol T. Lemay, *RN, ADN*
Consultant
Brattleboro, Vt.

Grace G. Lewis, *RN, MS, BC*
Assistant Professor of Nursing, Georgia Baptist College of Nursing of Mercer University
Atlanta

Patricia J. McBride, *RN, MSN, CIC*
Infection Control Manager
Bryn Mawr (Pa.) Hospital

Pamela Moody, *CRNP, MSN, PhD*
Nurse Administrator Public Health—Area 3, Alabama Department of Public Health
Tuscaloosa

Jill Morsbach, *RNC, MSN*
Staff Nurse
St. Joseph Medical Center
Kansas City, Mo.

Beverly J. Murphy, *RN, BSN, MS, APN, CRNA*
Certified Registered Nurse Anesthetist, Anesthesia Associates of Northeast Illinois
Tinley Park
Adjunct Faculty, University of St. Francis
Joliet, Ill.

William J. Pawlyshyn, *RN, BSN, MS, MN, APRN,BC, MDiv*
Nurse Practitioner, Mid and Upper Cape Community Health Center
Hyannis, Mass.

Noel C. Piano, *RN, MS*
Instructor/Coordinator, Lafayette School of Practical Nursing
Williamsburg, Va.
Adjunct Faculty, Thomas Nelson Community College
Hampton, Va.

Jacqueline Regennitter, ADN
Gerontological Nurse
Staff Nurse
Loring Care Center
Sac City, Iowa

Lauren R. Roach, LPN, HCS-D
Nurse Support Coordinator, Good Samaritan Home Care Services, LLC
Vincennes, Ind.

Tracy A. Robinson, RN, BSN, CWOCN
Home Health Care
MacNeal Hospital
Berwyn, Ill.

Catherine Shields, RN, BSN
Nurse Educator, Ocean County Vocational School
Toms River, N.J.

Concha Carrillo Sitter, APN, MS, CGRN, FNP-BC
Gastroenterology Nurse Practitioner, Sterling Rock Falls Clinic
Sterling, Ill.

Allison J. Terry, RN, MSN, PhD
Director, Center for Nursing
Alabama Board of Nursing
Montgomery

Mary E. Walker, RN, MSN, CCRN, CCNS
Clinical Instructor, Department of Chronic Nursing Care
University of Texas Health Science Center at San Antonio

Marsha Wamsley, RN, MSN
Associate Professor, Sinclair Community College
Dayton, Ohio

Kelly Witter, RN, MSN
Director, Great Oaks School of Practical Nursing
Cincinnati

Evelyn Yeaw, RN, PhD
Professor, University of Rhode Island College of Nursing
Kingston

Dawn M. Zwick, RN, MSN, CRNP
Lecturer, Kent State University
Nurse Practitioner, Cleveland Clinic Foundation
Kent, Ohio

HOW TO USE THIS BOOK

Throughout *Lippincott's Visual Encyclopedia of Clinical Skills,* you'll find bold initials in the form of icons, after heads, paragraphs, sentences, or bullets. These icons represent evidence-based data and their supporting research reports, and the professional organizations, health care organizations, and government groups whose standards, protocols, guidelines, and mandates underlie and dictate the very best in clinical health care practice today. Use this list to identify the organizations that the icons represent.

AABB	American Association of Blood Banks	ANNA	American Nephrology Nurses Association	INS	Infusion Nurses Society
AACN	American Association of Critical Care Nurses	AOA	American Optometric Association	ISMP	Institute for Safe Medication Practices
AACT	American Academy of Clinical Toxicology	AORN	Association of Operating Room Nurses	JC	The Joint Commission
AANN	American Association of Neuroscience Nurses	ASA	American Society of Anesthesiologists	MFR	Manufacturer's Recommendation
				NAON	National Association of Orthopaedic Nurses
AAO	American Academy of Otolaryngology—Head & Neck Surgery	ASIPP	American Society of Interventional Pain Physicians	NIDCD	National Institute on Deafness and other Communication Disorders
		ASPEN	American Society for Parenteral and Enteral Nutrition		
AARC	American Association for Respiratory Care	ASPMN	American Society of Pain Management Nurses	NPUAP	National Pressure Ulcer Advisory Panel
ABA	American Burn Association			ONS	Oncology Nursing Society
ACC	American College of Cardiology	ASPN	American Society of PeriAnesthesia Nurses	OSHA	Occupation Safety and Health Administration
ACCP	American College of Chest Physicians	CAP	College of American Pathologists	SUNA	Society of Urologic Nurses and Associates
		CDC	Centers for Disease Control and Prevention		
ACSC	American College of Surgeons Committee			WHO	World Health Organization
		CMS	Centers for Medicare and Medicaid Standards	WOCN	Wound, Ostomy, and Continence Nurses Society
ADA	American Diabetes Association				
AHA	American Heart Association	CS	Clinical Study		

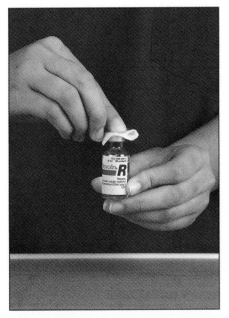

A

Admixture of drugs in a syringe

Combining two drugs in one syringe avoids the discomfort of two injections. It can be done in one of the following four ways: from two multidose vials (for example, regular and long-acting insulin), from one multidose vial and one ampule, from two ampules, or from a cartridge-injection system combined with either a multidose vial or an ampule.

Such combinations are contraindicated when the drugs aren't compatible and when the combined doses exceed the amount of solution that can be absorbed from a single injection site.

Equipment

Prescribed medications ◆ patient's medication record and chart ◆ alcohol pads ◆ syringe and needle ◆ filter needle as needed ◆ optional: cartridge-injection system.

The type and size of the syringe and needle depend on the prescribed medications, patient's body build, and route of administration. Medications that come in prefilled cartridges require a cartridge-injection system. (See *Cartridge-injection system,* page 2.)

Implementation

▶ Verify that the drugs to be administered agree with the patient's medication record and the practitioner's orders. **JC** **ISMP**
▶ Calculate the dose to be given.
▶ Wash your hands.

Mixing drugs from two multidose vials

▶ Using an alcohol pad, wipe the rubber stopper on the first vial (as shown at right).

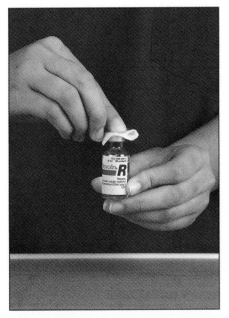

▶ Pull back the syringe plunger until the volume of air drawn into the syringe equals the volume to be withdrawn from the drug vial.
▶ Without inverting the vial, insert the needle into the top of the vial, making sure that the needle's bevel tip doesn't touch the solution. Inject the air into the vial and withdraw the needle. This replaces air in the vial, thus preventing

creation of a partial vacuum upon withdrawal of the drug.

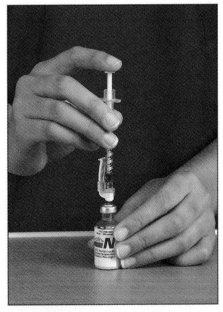

▶ Repeat the steps above for the second vial. Then, after injecting the air into the second vial, invert the vial, withdraw the prescribed dose, and then withdraw the needle (as shown at the top of the next page).

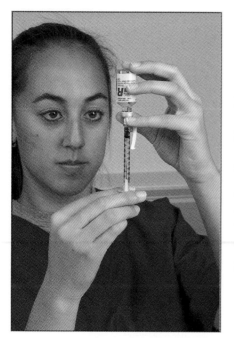

▶ Wipe the rubber stopper of the first vial again and insert the needle, taking care not to depress the plunger. Invert the vial, withdraw the prescribed dose, and then withdraw the needle (as shown at the top of the next column).

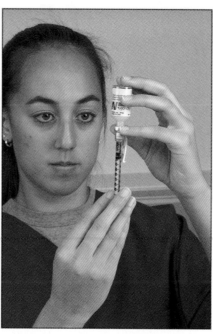

Mixing drugs from a multidose vial and an ampule

▶ Using an alcohol pad, clean the vial's rubber stopper.

▶ Pull back on the syringe plunger until the volume of air drawn into the syringe equals the volume to be withdrawn from the drug vial.

▶ Insert the needle into the top of the vial and inject the air. Then invert the vial and keep the needle's bevel tip below the level of the solution as you withdraw the prescribed dose. Put the sterile needle cover over the needle.

▶ Tap the stem of the ampule to move any medication from the stem into the body of the ampule.

▶ Wrap a sterile gauze pad or an alcohol pad around the ampule's neck to protect yourself from injury in case the glass splinters. Break open the ampule, directing the force away from you.

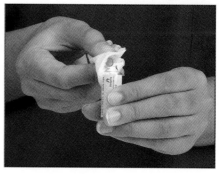

▶ Switch to the filter needle at this point to filter out glass splinters. **INS** **CS**

Cartridge-injection system

A cartridge-injection system, such as Tubex or Carpuject, is a convenient, easy-to-use method of injection that facilitates accuracy and sterility. The device consists of a plastic cartridge-holder syringe and a prefilled medication cartridge with needle attached.

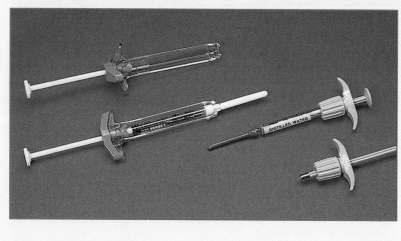

The medication in the cartridge is premixed and premeasured, which saves time and helps ensure an exact dose. The medication remains sealed in the cartridge and sterile until the injection is administered to the patient.

The disadvantage of this system is that not all drugs are available in cartridge form. However, compatible drugs can be added to partially filled cartridges.

▶ Insert the needle into the ampule. Be careful not to touch the outside of the ampule with the needle. Draw the correct dose into the syringe.

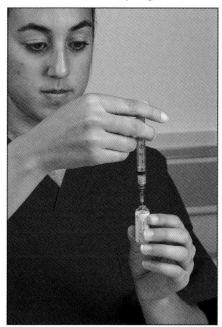

▶ Change back to a regular needle to administer the injection.

Mixing drugs from two ampules
▶ Tap the stem of the ampule to move medication from the stem into the body of the ampule.
▶ Open both ampules; wrap a small gauze pad or alcohol pad around the neck of the ampule and quickly snap off the top along the scored line at the neck. Snap the neck away from your body.
▶ Insert a syringe—with the filter needle attached—into the ampule without allowing the needle to come in contact with the rim of the ampule.
▶ Withdraw the amount ordered from the first ampule and remove the needle from the solution.
▶ Change the needle, if necessary, and repeat with the second ampule.
▶ Discard the used equipment appropriately.

Special considerations

▶ Insert a needle through the vial's rubber stopper at a slight angle, bevel up, and exert slight lateral pressure. This way you won't cut a piece of rubber out of the stopper, which can then be pushed into the vial.
▶ When withdrawing the medication from an ampule, place the ampule upright on a flat surface and insert the needle into the solution. Then withdraw the ordered amount. Alternatively, after the needle is in the solution, you can invert the ampule, keeping the needle centered and in the solution to withdraw the ordered amount. Fluid is held in place in the inverted ampule by surface tension.

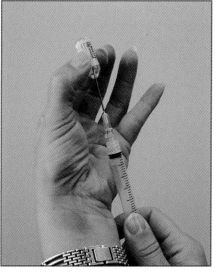

▶ When mixing drugs from multidose vials, be careful not to contaminate one drug with the other. Ideally, the needle should be changed after drawing the first medication into the syringe. This isn't always possible because many disposable syringes don't have removable needles.

▶ Some medications are compatible for only a brief time after being combined and should be administered within 10 minutes after mixing. After this time, environmental factors, such as temperature, exposure to light, and humidity, may alter compatibility.
▶ To reduce the risk of contamination, most facilities dispense parenteral medications in single-dose vials. However, insulin is one of the few drugs still packaged in multidose vials. So, when mixing regular and long-acting insulin, be sure to draw up the regular insulin first to avoid contamination by the long-acting suspension. (If a minute amount of the regular insulin is accidentally mixed with the long-acting insulin, it won't appreciably change the effect of the long-acting insulin.) Check your facility's policy before mixing different types of insulin.
▶ When you combine a cartridge-injection system and a multidose vial, use a separate needle and syringe to inject air into the multidose vial. This prevents contamination of the multidose vial by the cartridge-injection system.

References

The Joint Commission. *Comprehensive Accreditation Manual for Hospitals: The Official Handbook*. Standard MM.1.10. Oakbrook Terrace, Ill.: The Joint Commission, 2007.

The Joint Commission. *Comprehensive Accreditation Manual for Hospitals: The Official Handbook*. Standard MM.2.10. Oakbrook Terrace, Ill.: The Joint Commission, 2007.

The Joint Commission. *Comprehensive Accreditation Manual for Hospitals: The Official Handbook*. Standard MM.3.10. Oakbrook Terrace, Ill.: The Joint Commission, 2007.

The Joint Commission. *Comprehensive Accreditation Manual for Hospitals: The Official Handbook*. Standard MM.4.10. Oakbrook Terrace, Ill.: The Joint Commission, 2007.

The Joint Commission. *Comprehensive Accreditation Manual for Hospitals: The Official Handbook*. Standard MM.4.20. Oakbrook Terrace, Ill.: The Joint Commission, 2007.

The Joint Commission. *Comprehensive Accreditation Manual for Hospitals: The Official Handbook*. Standard MM.5.10. Oakbrook Terrace, Ill.: The Joint Commission, 2007.

The Joint Commission. *Comprehensive Accreditation Manual for Hospitals: The Official Handbook*. Standard MM.6.10. Oakbrook Terrace, Ill.: The Joint Commission, 2007.

The Joint Commission. *Comprehensive Accreditation Manual for Hospitals: The Official Handbook*. Standard MM.6.20. Oakbrook Terrace, Ill.: The Joint Commission, 2007.

The Joint Commission. *Comprehensive Accreditation Manual for Hospitals: The Official Handbook*. Standard MM.7.10. Oakbrook Terrace, Ill.: The Joint Commission, 2007.

Preston, S.T., and Hegadoren, K. "Glass Contamination in Parenterally Administered Medication," *Journal of Advanced Nursing* 48(3):266-70, November 2004. CS

"Standard 32. Filters. Infusion Nursing Standards of Practice," *Journal of Infusion Nursing* 29(1S):S33-34, January-February 2006.

Taylor, C., et al. *Fundamentals of Nursing: The Art and Science of Nursing Care,* 6th ed. Philadelphia: Lippincott Williams & Wilkins, 2008.

Antiembolism stockings

Elastic antiembolism stockings help prevent deep vein thrombosis (DVT) and pulmonary embolism by compressing superficial leg veins. Such compression increases venous return by forcing blood into the deep venous system rather than allowing it to pool in the legs and form clots.

Antiembolism stockings can provide equal pressure over the entire leg or a graded pressure that's greatest at the ankle and decreases over the length of the leg. Usually indicated for postoperative, bedridden, elderly, or other patients at risk for DVT, these stockings shouldn't be used on patients with dermatoses or open skin lesions, gangrene, severe arteriosclerosis or other ischemic vascular diseases, pulmonary or massive edema, recent vein ligation, or vascular or skin grafts. **AORN** For patients with chronic venous problems, intermittent pneumatic compression stockings may be ordered during surgery and postoperatively.

Equipment

Tape measure ◆ antiembolism stockings of correct size and length ◆ talcum powder.

Implementation

▶ Check the practitioner's order.
▶ Confirm the patient's identity using two patient identifiers according to your facility's policy. **JC**
▶ Assess the patient's condition. If his legs are cold or cyanotic, notify the practitioner before proceeding.
▶ Obtain the correct size of stocking according to the manufacturer's specifications. Before applying the stocking, however, measure the patient. (See *Measuring for antiembolism stockings,* page 6.) If the patient's measurements are outside the range indicated by the manufacturer or if his legs are deformed or edematous, ask the practitioner if he wants to order custom-made stockings.
▶ Explain the procedure to the patient, provide privacy, and wash your hands thoroughly.
▶ Have the patient lie down. Then dust his ankle with talcum powder to ease application.

Applying a knee-length stocking
▶ Insert your hand into the stocking from the top, and grasp the heel pocket from the inside. Holding the heel, turn the stocking inside out so that the foot is inside the stocking leg.

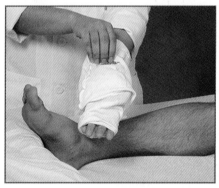

▶ With the heel pocket down, hook the index and middle fingers of both your hands into the foot section. Facing the patient, ease the stocking over the toes, stretching it sideways as you move it up the foot.

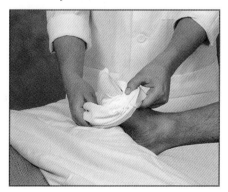

▶ Support the patient's ankle with one hand, and use the other hand to pull the heel pocket under the heel. Then center the heel in the pocket.
▶ Gather the loose portion of the stocking at the toe, and pull only this section over the heel. Gather the loose material at the ankle, and slide the rest of the stocking up over the heel with short pulls, alternating front and back.
▶ Insert your index and middle fingers into the gathered stocking at the ankle, and ease the fabric up the leg to the knee.

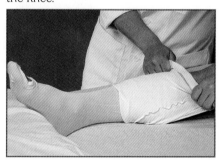

▶ Supporting the patient's ankle with one hand, use your other hand to stretch the stocking toward the knee, front and back, to distribute the material evenly. The stocking top should be 1″ to 2″ (2.5 to 5 cm) below the bottom of the patella.
▶ Gently snap the fabric around the ankle to ensure a tight fit and to eliminate gaps that could reduce pressure.

Measuring for antiembolism stockings

Measure the patient carefully to make sure that his antiembolism stockings provide enough compression for adequate venous return.

To choose the correct *knee-length* stocking, measure the circumference of the calf at its widest point (top left) and the leg length from the bottom of the heel to the back of the knee (bottom left).

To choose a *thigh-length* stocking, measure the calf as for a knee-length stocking and the thigh at its widest point (below). Then measure leg length from the bottom of the heel to the gluteal fold.

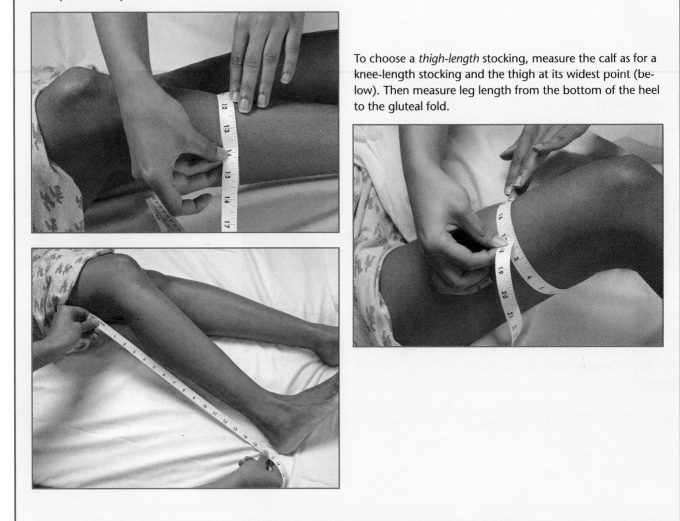

▶ Adjust the foot section for fabric smoothness and toe comfort by tugging on the toe section. Properly position the toe window, if any.
▶ Repeat the procedure for the second stocking, if ordered.

Applying a thigh-length stocking
▶ Follow the procedure for applying a knee-length stocking, taking care to distribute the fabric evenly below the knee before continuing the procedure.
▶ With the patient's leg extended, stretch the rest of the stocking over the knee.

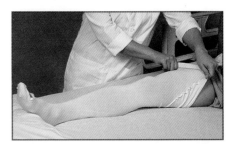

▶ Flex the patient's knee, and pull the stocking over the thigh until the top is 1″ to 3″ (2.5 to 7.5 cm) below the gluteal fold.

▶ Stretch the stocking from the top, front and back, to distribute the fabric evenly over the thigh.

▶ Gently snap the fabric behind the knee to eliminate gaps that could reduce pressure.

Applying a waist-length stocking

▶ Follow the procedure for applying knee-length and thigh-length stockings, and extend the stocking top to the gluteal fold.

▶ Fit the patient with the adjustable belt that accompanies the stockings. Make sure the waistband and the fabric don't interfere with any incision, drainage tube, catheter, or other device.

Special considerations

▶ Apply the stockings in the morning, if possible, before edema develops. If the patient has been ambulating, ask him to lie down and elevate his legs for 15 to 30 minutes before applying the stockings to facilitate venous return.

▶ Don't allow the stockings to roll or turn down at the top or toe because the excess pressure could cause venous strangulation. Have the patient wear the stockings in bed and during ambulation to provide continuous protection against thrombosis.

▶ Check the patient's toes at least once every 4 hours—more often in the patient with a faint pulse or edema. Note skin color and temperature, sensation, swelling, and ability to move. Obstruction of arterial blood flow—characterized by cold and bluish toes, dusky toenail beds, decreased or absent pedal pulses, and leg pain or cramps—can result from application of antiembolism stockings.

▶ Be alert for an allergic reaction because some patients can't tolerate the sizing in new stockings. Laundering the stockings before applying them reduces the risk of an allergic reaction. Remove the stockings at least once daily to bathe the skin and observe for irritation and breakdown.

▶ Using warm water and mild soap, wash the stockings when soiled. Keep a second pair handy for the patient to wear while the other pair is being laundered.

References

Howard, A., et al. "Randomized Clinical Trial of Low Molecular Weight Heparin with Thigh-length or Knee-length Antiembolism Stockings for Patients Undergoing Surgery," *British Journal of Surgery* 91(7):842-47, July 2004.

Ingram, J.E., et al. "A Review of Thigh-length vs. Knee-length Antiembolism Stockings," *British Journal of Nursing* 12(14):845-51, July-August 2003.

Segal, J.B., et al. "Management of Venous Thromboembolism: A Systematic Review for a Practice Guideline," *Annals of Internal Medicine* 146(3):211-22, February 2007.

Snow, V., et al. "Management of Venous Thromboembolism: A Clinical Practice Guideline from the American College of Physicians and the American Academy of Family Physicians," *Annals of Internal Medicine* 146(3):204-10, February 2006.

Arterial and venous sheath removal

Endovascular procedures performed by cardiologists and vascular surgeons have dramatically increased in the past decade. Following these procedures, arterial sheaths, venous sheaths, or both may be left in place. Upon sheath removal, patient comfort may be improved and the amount of bed rest required may be shortened, thus leading to positive patient outcomes. However, sheath removal is not without risk, and nurses must be appropriately trained.

There are several methods available to control bleeding following sheath removal, including manual compression (used alone or with a hemostasis pad), mechanical compression devices, collagen plug devices, and percutaneous suture-mediated closure devices. (See *Products to use with sheath removal,* page 9.) Manual compression can cause fatigue and injury, which can result in carpal tunnel problems for nurses. Mechanical compression techniques are effective for preventing hematoma formation; however, the prevalence of bleeding doesn't differ significantly for different methods of compression. If a plug-type or suture-mediated closure device is used, sheaths can be immediately removed at the end of a case, regardless of the coagulation status of the patient.

Equipment

Nonsterile gloves ◆ gown ◆ goggles or face shield with mask ◆ cardiac monitor ◆ indelible marker ◆ antiseptic solution ◆ sterile gauze ◆ sterile gloves ◆ suture removal kit (if sheath is sutured in place) ◆ hypoallergenic tape ◆ linen-saver pad ◆ sterile saline (if using noninvasive hemostasis pad) ◆ transparent dressing (if using noninvasive hemostasis pad) ◆ optional: mechanical hemostasis device, noninvasive hemostasis pad.

Implementation

▶ Verify the order for sheath removal in the patient's chart.
▶ Confirm the patient's identity using two patient identifiers according to your facility's policy. **JC**
▶ Wash your hands and bring the equipment to the patient's bedside.
▶ Using sterile technique, open the suture removal kit and gauze packages and place them within reach. If a hemostasis pad is being used, open it using sterile technique and open the normal saline solution.

Preparing for sheath removal

▶ Explain the procedure to the patient. Include activity restrictions, discomfort caused by pressure to the site, and signs and symptoms to report following the procedure.
▶ Before sheath removal, assess for bleeding disorders and check the patient's platelet count, prothrombin time, International Normalized Ratio, partial thromboplastin time, complete blood count, and activated clotting time.
▶ Take the patient's vital signs and check the electrocardiogram to establish a baseline. Check that the systolic blood pressure is less than 150 mm Hg to facilitate hemostasis.
▶ Assess the patient's neurovascular status in the extremity distal to the sheath insertion site to establish a baseline.
▶ Mark the pulses distal to the sheath insertion site using an indelible marker to facilitate finding the pulses.
▶ Administer an analgesic 20 to 30 minutes before the procedure.
▶ Confirm that the patient has patent I.V. access in case emergency fluids or medications are required.
▶ Position the patient with the head of the bed flat.

▶ Place the linen-saver pad underneath the affected extremity.
▶ If a mechanical compression device is being used, place it under the patient before sheath removal to reduce patient movement and the risk of bleeding after the sheath is removed.
▶ Wash your hands and put on goggles, a mask, gloves, and a gown.
▶ Carefully remove the dressing covering the sheath insertion site.
▶ Clean the insertion site with antiseptic solution.
▶ Remove the nonsterile gloves and put on sterile gloves.
▶ Remove sutures, if present.

Arterial sheath removal using manual or mechanical compression

▶ Locate the femoral pulse proximal to the insertion site so that compression (manual or mechanical) can be properly positioned ½″ to ¾″ (1 to 2 cm) above the insertion site.
▶ Hold the sheath with one hand while applying manual or mechanical pressure over the femoral artery with the other hand to reduce bleeding.
▶ Remove the sheath slowly while the patient exhales to prevent Valsalva's maneuver and while continuing to ap-

ply pressure manually or with the mechanical device.

Arterial sheath removal using a noninvasive hemostasis pad with manual compression

▶ Moisten the pad with sterile saline to activate the hemostatic system.

▶ Apply pressure $1/2''$ to $3/4''$ proximal to the insertion site.

▶ Apply a sterile gauze pad over the insertion site, and then place the moistened pad over the gauze and apply pressure.

▶ Gently remove the sheath as described earlier.

▶ Slowly let up on applying pressure proximal to the insertion site after 3 to 4 minutes while continuing to apply pressure to the insertion site for no less than 10 minutes.

▶ Apply another sterile gauze pad over the hemostasis pad, and cover the site with a transparent dressing. **MFR**

Products to use with sheath removal

There are several products and methods that can be used when removing an arterial or venous sheath. Products include manual compression devices (such as the FemoStop), noninvasive hemostasis pads (such as the Syvek Patch), collagen plug devices (such as the Angio-Seal closure device), and percutaneous suture-mediated closure devices (such as the Perclose).

FemoStop

Syvek Patch

Angio-Seal closure device

Perclose

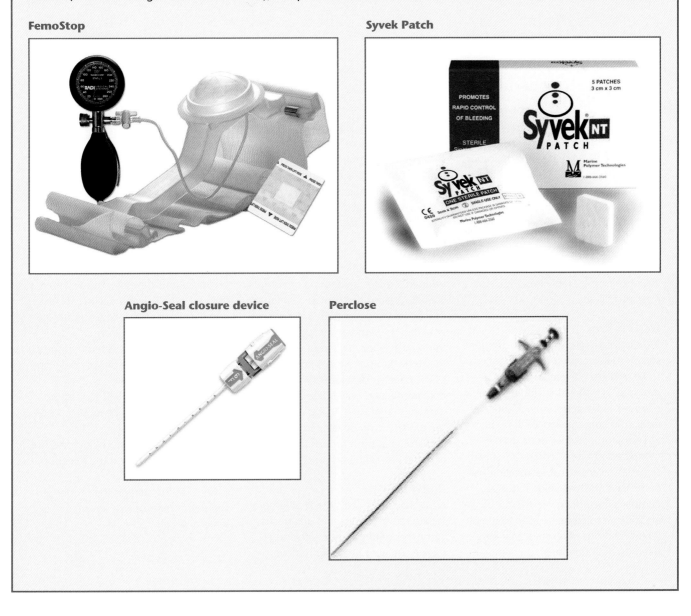

▶ Leave the hemostasis pad in place for 24 hours.

Venous sheath removal

▶ Remove the venous sheath, if present, no less than 10 minutes after removal of the arterial sheath because pressure at the arterial site needs to be maintained for a longer time.

▶ Apply pressure over the venous and arterial sites for 10 more minutes or until bleeding has stopped.

▶ If a hemostasis pad is used, follow the directions for its use.

Post–sheath removal care

▶ Apply a sterile dressing to the arterial and venous insertion sites to keep the area clean and to reduce the risk of infection.

▶ Assess the patient's neurovascular status, his vital signs, and the insertion site in the affected limb every 15 minutes for 1 hour, every 30 minutes for 1 hour, and then every hour for 4 hours to ensure adequate circulation and neurologic function.

▶ Tell the patient not to elevate the head of the bed greater than 30 degrees to reduce the risk of disrupting

hemostasis and to relieve back discomfort. **CS**

▶ Instruct the patient to report bleeding from the site, if the dressing becomes saturated, or feelings of wetness and warmth on his groin or leg.

▶ Tell the patient to report coolness, numbness, tingling, or pain in the affected extremity.

▶ Keep the patient on bed rest for 2 to 6 hours, or per your facility's policy, when applying manual or mechanical pressure after arterial sheath removal to reduce complications of bed rest and back discomfort.

EVIDENCE-BASED RESEARCH

Safety of nurses removing femoral sheaths

Liew, R., et al. "Very Low Complication Rates with a Manual, Nurse-Led Protocol for Femoral Sheath Removal Following Coronary Angiography," *European Journal of Cardiovascular Nursing* 6(4):303-307, December 2007.

Level VI
Evidence from a single descriptive or qualitative study

Description
After coronary angioplasty, the femoral sheath that was used for access needs to be removed. There are several methods of removal, including manual compression, arteriotomy closure devices, and compression devices (such as Fem-Stop). Studies done on the complication rate after femoral sheath removal in cardiac catheterization patients have shown a wide range of complications. However, these studies are difficult to compare, due to the different methods of removal that have been used. In this study, the femoral

sheaths were removed using manual compression by cardiac nurses with special training in sheath removal. There were a total of 516 patients that were followed in the study.

Findings
None of the patients in the study developed a major hematoma or complication. A minor hematoma developed in 1.6% of the patients. In 416 patients who had the femoral sheath removed using an arteriotomy closure device, the same findings were reported: none of the patients developed a major hematoma, and only 0.8% developed a minor hematoma. It was noted that the patients who developed a minor hematoma in both groups had a higher mean arterial blood pressure.

Conclusions
A manual, nurse-led system of femoral sheath removal following diagnostic coronary angiography is safe and effective. Training nurses to remove

femoral sheaths manually after angiography doesn't result in an increase in complications.

Nursing practice implications
Nurses should be trained in the proper way to manually remove femoral sheaths, and what to look for when complications develop. This will help minimize the risk and occurrence of complications. The following practice implications are important:

▶ Monitor the patient's femoral sheath site for increased bleeding or development of a hematoma.

▶ Encourage the patient to keep his affected leg as still as possible to minimize bleeding.

▶ Monitor the patient's blood pressure, and notify the doctor if the patient become hypertensive.

▶ Educate the staff on the proper procedure for manually removing a femoral sheath.

▶ Keep the patient on bed rest for 1 to 4 hours, or per your facility's policy, when achieving hemostasis through percutaneous suture-mediated closure and hemostasis pads.

▶ Keep the patient on bed rest for no more than 4 hours, or per your facility's policy, following venous sheath removal.

Special considerations

▶ If the patient is obese, a second person may be required to help hold back skin and abdominal folds.

▶ Pressure may need to be applied for a longer period to ensure hemostasis in the patient with hypertension.

▶ Make sure to read the manufacturer's instructions and your facility's policy and procedure for correct use of mechanical compression devices. Tissue damage can occur if the device is used incorrectly. **MFR**

▶ The compression time required to control bleeding depends on several factors, including the size of the sheath, whether or not the patient received heparin and antiplatelets, and blood coagulation levels.

▶ The most common complication following sheath removal is bleeding, which occurs most frequently at the femoral artery access site. Retroperitoneal bleeding may also occur. Vascular complications include hematoma, pseudoaneurysm, arteriovenous fistula formation, embolus, and thrombus. Sensory or motor impairment may occur in the affected limb. Vasovagal complications may also occur.

References

Benson, L.M., et al. "Determining Best Practice: Comparison of Three Methods of Femoral Sheath Removal after Cardiac Interventional Procedures," *Heart Lung* 34(2):115-21, March-April 2005.

Chlan, L.L., et al. "Effects of Three Groin Compression Methods on Patient Discomfort, Distress, and Vascular Complications Following a Percutaneous Coronary Intervention Procedure," *Nursing Research* 54(6):391-98, November-December 2005.

Galli, A., and Palatnik, A. "What Is the Proper Activated Clotting Time (ACT) at Which to Remove a Femoral Sheath after PCI? What Are the Best 'Protocols' for Sheath Removal?" *Critical Care Nurse* 25(2):88-95, April 2005.

Jones, T., and McCutcheon, H. "A Randomised Controlled Trial Comparing the Use of Manual Versus Mechanical Compression to Obtain Haemostasis following Coronary Angiography," *Intensive & Critical Care Nursing* 19(1):11-20, February 2003.

Jones, T., and McCutcheon, H. "Effectiveness of Mechanical Compression Devices in Attaining Hemostasis after Femoral Sheath Removal," *American Journal of Critical Care* 11(2):155-62, March 2002.

Lynn-McHale Wiegand, D.J., and Carlson, K.K., eds. *AACN Procedure Manual for Critical Care,* 5th ed. Philadelphia: W.B. Saunders Co., 2005.

Mlekusch, W., et al. "Arterial Puncture Site Management after Percutaneous Transluminal Procedures Using a Hemostatic Wound Dressing (Clo-Sur P.A.D.) versus Conventional Manual Compression: A Randomized Controlled Trial," *Journal of Endovascular Therapy* 13(1):23-31, February 2006.

Niederstadt, J.A. "Frequency and Timing of Activated Clotting Time Levels for Sheath Removal," *Journal of Nursing Care Quality* 19(1):34-38, January-March 2004.

Sluzbach, L.M., et al. "A Randomized Clinical Trial of the Effect of Bed Position after PTCA," *American Journal of Critical Care* 4(3):221-26, May 1995. **CS**

Tagney, J., and Lackie, D. "Bed-rest Post-femoral Arterial Sheath Removal— What Is Safe Practice? A Clinical Audit," *Nursing in Critical Care* 10(4):167-73, July-August 2005.

Arterial pressure monitoring

Direct arterial pressure monitoring permits continuous measurement of systolic, diastolic, and mean pressures and allows arterial blood sampling. Because direct measurement reflects systemic vascular resistance as well as blood flow, it's generally more accurate than indirect methods (such as palpation and auscultation of Korotkoff, or audible pulse, sounds), which are based on blood flow.

Direct monitoring is indicated when highly accurate or frequent blood pressure measurements are required—for example, in patients with low cardiac output and high systemic vascular resistance. It may also be used for hospitalized patients who are obese or who have severe edema—if these conditions make indirect measurement hard to perform. In addition, it may be used for patients who are receiving titrated doses of vasoactive drugs or who need frequent blood sampling.

An arterial pressure monitoring system can be open or closed. An *open* system is one in which you attach a syringe to the stopcock and withdraw 5 to 10 ml of blood for waste, which is then discarded and not returned to the patient. A *closed* system has an attached reservoir in which you can withdraw the waste. When you're finished drawing the blood samples, you can return the blood in the reservoir to the patient.

Equipment

For catheter insertion: Gloves ◆ gown ◆ mask ◆ protective eyewear ◆ sterile gloves ◆ 16G to 20G catheter (type and length depend on the insertion site, patient's size, and other anticipated uses of the line) ◆ preassembled preparation kit (if available) ◆ sterile drapes ◆ sheet protector ◆ sterile towels ◆ prepared pressure transducer system ◆ ordered local anesthetic ◆ sutures ◆ syringe and needle (21G to 25G, 1″) ◆ I.V. pole ◆ tubing and medication labels ◆ site care kit (containing sterile dressing and hypoallergenic tape) ◆ arm board ◆ soft limb restraint as needed ◆ optional: electric clipper (for femoral artery insertion).

For blood sample collection: If an *open system* is in place: gloves ◆ gown ◆ mask ◆ sterile 4″ × 4″ gauze pads ◆ protective eyewear ◆ sheet protector ◆ 5- or 10-ml syringe for discard sample ◆ needleless Vacutainer luerlock adapter needle ◆ appropriate blood specimen collection tubes ◆ sterile dead-end cap ◆ laboratory request forms and labels ◆ Vacutainers.

If a *closed system* is in place: gloves ◆ gown ◆ mask ◆ protective eyewear ◆ closed system cannula ◆ appropriate blood specimen collection tubes ◆ syringes of appropriate size and number for ordered laboratory tests ◆ laboratory request forms and labels ◆ alcohol swabs ◆ blood transfer unit.

For arterial line tubing changes: Gloves ◆ gown ◆ mask ◆ protective eyewear ◆ sheet protector ◆ preassembled arterial pressure tubing with flush device and disposable pressure transducer ◆ sterile gloves ◆ 500-ml bag of I.V. flush solution (usually normal saline solution) ◆ 500 or 1,000 units of heparin ◆ syringe and needle (21G to 25G, 1″) ◆ alcohol swabs ◆ medication label ◆ pressure bag ◆ site care kit ◆ tubing labels.

For arterial catheter removal: Gloves ◆ mask ◆ gown ◆ protective eyewear ◆ two sterile 4″ × 4″ gauze pads ◆ sheet protector ◆ sterile suture removal set ◆ dressing ◆ alcohol swabs ◆ hypoallergenic tape ◆ sterile container (if catheter-tip culture is ordered).

Implementation

▶ Confirm the patient's identity using two patient identifiers according to your facility's policy. **JC**

▶ Before setting up and priming the monitoring system, wash your hands thoroughly.

▶ Explain the procedure to the patient and his family, including the purpose of arterial pressure monitoring and the anticipated duration of catheter placement. Make sure the patient signs a consent form. If he can't sign, ask a responsible family member to give written consent.

▶ Check the patient's history for an allergy or a hypersensitivity to iodine, heparin, or the ordered local anesthetic.

▶ Maintain asepsis by wearing personal protective equipment throughout preparation. (For instructions on setting up and priming the monitoring system, see "Transducer system setup," page 556.)

▶ Label all medications, medication containers, and other solutions on and off the sterile field. **JC**

▶ When you have completed equipment preparation, set the alarms on the bedside monitor according to your facility's policy. **JC**

▶ Continue to maintain asepsis by wearing personal protective equipment throughout all procedures described below.

▶ Position the patient for easy access to the catheter insertion site. Place a sheet protector under the site.

▶ If the catheter will be inserted into the radial artery, perform Allen's test to assess collateral circulation in the hand.

Inserting an arterial catheter

▶ Using a preassembled preparation kit, the practitioner prepares and anesthetizes the insertion site. He covers the surrounding area with either sterile drapes or towels. The catheter is then inserted into the artery and attached to the fluid-filled pressure tubing.

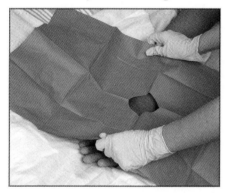

▶ While the practitioner holds the catheter in place, activate the fast-flush release to flush blood from the catheter. After each fast-flush operation, observe the drip chamber to verify that the continuous flush rate is as desired. A waveform should appear on the bedside monitor. (See *Square wave test,* page 14.)

▶ The practitioner may suture the catheter in place, or you may secure it with hypoallergenic tape. Cover the insertion site with a dressing, as specified by your facility's policy.

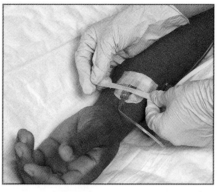

▶ Immobilize the insertion site. With a radial or brachial site, use an arm board and soft wrist restraint (if the patient's condition requires). With a femoral site, assess the need for an ankle restraint; maintain the patient on bed rest, with the head of the bed raised no more than 15 to 30 degrees, to prevent the catheter from kinking. Level the zeroing stopcock of the transducer with the phlebostatic axis. Then zero the system to atmospheric pressure.

▶ Activate monitor alarms, as appropriate. **JC**

Obtaining a blood sample from an open system

▶ Assemble the equipment, taking care not to contaminate the nonvented cap, stopcock, and syringes.

▶ Attach the needleless luerlock adapter needle to the Vacutainer. Turn off, or temporarily silence, the monitor alarms, depending on your facility's policy. (However, some facilities require that alarms be left on.)

▶ Locate the blood sampling port nearest the patient. Remove the dead-end cap from the stopcock, (as shown at the top of the next column).

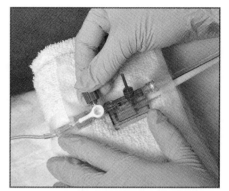

▶ Connect the needleless adapter of the Vacutainer into the sampling port of the stopcock and turn the stopcock off to the flush solution. Attach a blood specimen collection tube for the discard sample into the stopcock. Follow your facility's policy on how much discard blood to collect. In most cases, you'll withdraw 5 to 10 ml.

▶ Remove the discard specimen blood collection tube from the Vacutainer.

▶ Attach each blood specimen collection tube into the Vacutainer, keeping the stopcock turned off to the flush solution. If the practitioner has ordered coagulation tests, obtain blood for this sample from the final syringe to prevent dilution from the flush device.

▶ After you've obtained blood for the final sample, turn the stopcock off to the sampling port and activate the fast-flush release.

▶ Turn the stopcock off to the patient and attach an empty blood specimen collection tube, or place a sterile 4″ × 4″ gauze pad beneath the sampling port of the stopcock and activate the fast-flush release to clear the stopcock port of any remaining blood.

▶ Turn the stopcock off to the stopcock port, and remove the Vacutainer. Place a new sterile dead-end cap on the blood sampling port. Reactivate the monitor alarms.

Square wave test CS AACN

When using a pressure monitoring system, you must ensure and document the system's accuracy. Along with leveling and zeroing the system to atmospheric pressure at the phlebostatic axis and interpreting waveforms, you can ensure accuracy by performing the square wave test (or dynamic response test). To perform the test, implement the following:

When using a pressure monitoring system, you must ensure and document the system's accuracy. Along with leveling and zeroing the system to atmospheric pressure at the phlebostatic axis and interpreting waveforms, you can ensure accuracy by performing the square wave test (or dynamic response test). To perform the test, implement the following:

▶ Activate the fast-flush device for 1 second, and then release. Obtain a graphic printout.

▶ Observe for the desired response: the pressure wave rises rapidly, squares off, and is followed by a series of oscillations. (See illustration below.)

▶ Know that these oscillations should have an initial downstroke, which extends below the baseline and just 1 to 2 oscillations after the initial downstroke. Usually, but not always, the first upstroke is about one-third the height of the initial downstroke.

▶ Be aware that the intervals between oscillations should be no more than 0.04 to 0.08 second (1 to 2 small boxes).

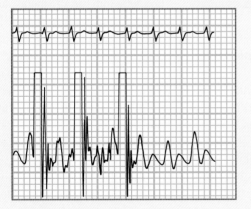

Underdamped square wave

If you observe extra oscillations after the initial downstroke or more than 0.08 second between oscillations, the waveform is underdamped. (See illustration at top of next column.) This can cause falsely high pressure readings and artifact in the waveforms. It can be corrected by:

▶ removing excess tubing or extra stopcocks from the system

▶ inserting a damping device (available from pressure tubing companies)

▶ dampening the wave by inserting a small air bubble at the transducer stopcock.

Repeat the square wave test, read the pressure waveform, and then remove the small air bubble.

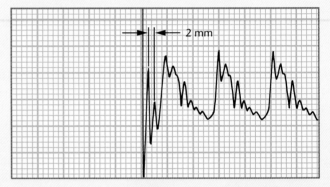

Overdamped square wave

If you observe a slurred upstroke at the beginning of the square wave and a loss of oscillations after the initial downstroke, the waveform is overdamped. (See illustration below.) This can cause falsely low pressure readings, and you can lose the sharpness of waveform peaks and the dicrotic notch. It can be corrected by:

▶ clearing the line of blood or air

▶ making sure there are no kinks or obstructions in the line

▶ ensuring that you're using short, low-compliance tubing.

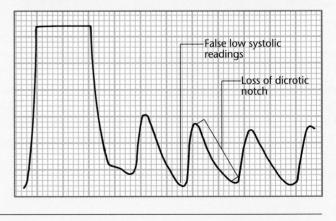

Adapted with permission from Quaal, S.J. "Improving the Accuracy of Pulmonary Artery Catheter Measurements," *Journal of Cardiovascular Nursing* 15(2):71-82, January 2001. © 2001 Aspen Publishers.

Understanding the arterial waveform

Normal arterial blood pressure produces a characteristic waveform, representing ventricular systole and diastole. The waveform has five distinct components: anacrotic limb, systolic peak, dicrotic limb, dicrotic notch, and end diastole.

The *anacrotic limb* marks the waveform's initial upstroke, which results as blood is rapidly ejected from the ventricle through the open aortic valve into the aorta. The rapid ejection causes a sharp rise in arterial pressure, which appears as the waveform's highest point. This is called the *systolic peak*.

As blood continues into the peripheral vessels, arterial pressure falls and the waveform begins a downward trend. This part is called the *dicrotic limb*. Arterial pressure usually will continue to fall until pressure in the ventricle is less than pressure in the aortic root. When this occurs, the aortic valve closes. This event appears as a small notch (the *dicrotic notch*) on the waveform's downside. When the aortic valve closes, diastole begins, progressing until the aortic root pressure gradually descends to its lowest point. On the waveform, this is known as *end diastole*.

Normal arterial waveform

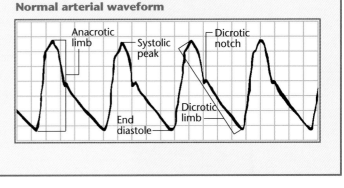

▶ Label all blood specimen collection tubes with correct labels. Send all samples to the laboratory with appropriate documentation.

▶ Check the monitor for return of the arterial waveform and pressure reading. (See *Understanding the arterial waveform*.)

Obtaining a blood sample from a closed system

▶ Assemble the equipment, maintaining sterile technique. Locate the closed-system reservoir and blood sampling site.

▶ Deactivate, or temporarily silence, monitor alarms. (However, some facilities require that alarms be left on.)

▶ Holding the reservoir upright, grasp the flexures and slowly fill the reservoir with blood over a 3- to 5-second period. (This blood serves as discard blood.) If you feel resistance, reposition the affected extremity, and check the catheter site for obvious problems (such as kinking). Then resume blood withdrawal.

▶ Turn the one-way valve off to the reservoir by turning the handle perpendicular to the tubing. Clean the sampling site with an alcohol pad. Using a syringe with attached cannula, insert the cannula into the sampling site. (Make sure the plunger is depressed to the bottom of the syringe barrel.) Slowly fill the syringe. Then grasp the cannula near the sampling site, and remove the syringe and cannula as one unit. Repeat the procedure, as needed, to fill the required number of syringes. If the practitioner has ordered coagulation tests, obtain blood for those tests from the final syringe to prevent dilution from the flush solution. **AACN** **CDC**

▶ After filling the syringes, turn the one-way valve to its original position, parallel to the tubing. Smoothly and evenly push down on the plunger until the flexures lock in place in the fully closed position and all fluid has been reinfused. The fluid should be reinfused over a 3- to 5-second period. Then activate the fast-flush release to clear blood from the tubing and reservoir.

▶ Clean the sampling site with an alcohol swab. Reactivate the monitor alarms. Using the blood transfer unit, transfer blood samples to the appropriate Vacutainers, labeling them according to your facility's policy. Send all samples to the laboratory with appropriate documentation.

Changing arterial line tubing

▶ Wash your hands and follow standard precautions. Assemble the new pressure monitoring system.

▶ Consult your facility's policy and procedure manual to determine how much tubing length to change.

▶ Position the patient for easy access to the catheter site. Place a sheet protector under the site.

▶ Inflate the pressure bag to 300 mm Hg, and check it for air leaks. Then release the pressure.

▶ Prepare the I.V. flush solution, and prime the pressure tubing and transducer system. At this time, add medication and tubing labels. Apply 300 mm Hg of pressure to the system. Then hang the I.V. bag on a pole.

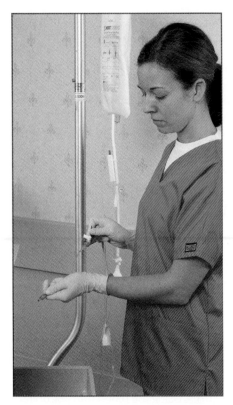

▶ Remove the dressing from the catheter insertion site, taking care not to dislodge the catheter or cause vessel trauma. Turn off, or temporarily silence, monitor alarms. (However, some facilities require that alarms be left on.)

▶ Turn off the flow clamp of the tubing segment that you'll change. Disconnect the tubing from the catheter hub, taking care not to dislodge the catheter. Immediately insert new tubing into the catheter hub. Secure the tubing, and then activate the fast-flush release to clear it.

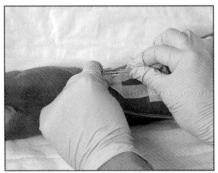

▶ Reactivate the monitor alarms. Apply an appropriate dressing.

▶ Level the zeroing stopcock of the transducer with the phlebostatic axis, and zero the system to atmospheric pressure.

Removing an arterial line

▶ Consult your facility's policy to determine whether you're permitted to perform this procedure.

▶ Check the patient's coagulation studies before removing the catheter to determine whether pressure needs to be held for a longer time to achieve hemostasis.

▶ Explain the procedure to the patient.

▶ Assemble all equipment. Wash your hands. Observe standard precautions, including wearing personal protective equipment, for this procedure.

▶ Record the patient's systolic, diastolic, and mean blood pressures. If a manual, indirect blood pressure hasn't been assessed recently, obtain one now to establish a new baseline.

▶ Turn off the monitor alarms. Then turn off the flow clamp to the flush solution.

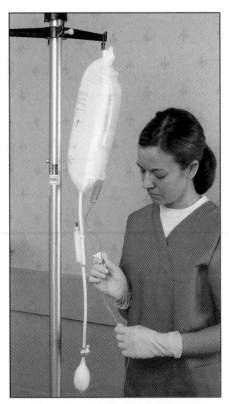

▶ Carefully remove the dressing over the insertion site. Remove any sutures, using the suture removal kit, and then carefully check that all sutures have been removed.

▶ Withdraw the catheter using a gentle, steady motion. Keep the catheter parallel to the artery during withdrawal to reduce the risk of traumatic injury.

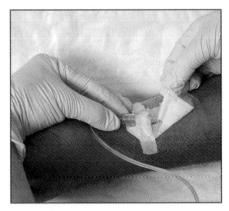

▶ Immediately after withdrawing the catheter, apply pressure to the site with a sterile 4″ × 4″ gauze pad. Maintain pressure for at least 5 minutes (longer if bleeding or oozing persists). Apply additional pressure to a femoral site or if the patient has coagulopathy or is receiving anticoagulants. In some facilities, a compression device may be used to apply pressure to the femoral site.

▶ Apply a pressure dressing to the site to help prevent rebleeding.

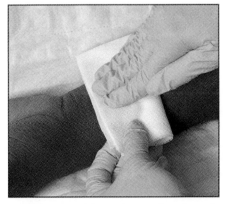

▶ If the practitioner has ordered a culture of the catheter tip (to diagnose a suspected infection), gently place the catheter tip on a 4″ × 4″ sterile gauze pad. When the bleeding is under control, hold the catheter over the sterile container. Using sterile scissors, cut the tip so it falls into the sterile container. Label the specimen and send it to the laboratory.

▶ Observe the site for bleeding. Assess circulation in the extremity distal to the site by evaluating color, pulses, and sensation. Repeat this assessment every 15 minutes for the first 4 hours, every 30 minutes for the next 2 hours, and then hourly for the next 6 hours.

Special considerations

▶ Observing the pressure waveform on the monitor can enhance assessment of arterial pressure. An abnormal waveform may reflect an arrhythmia (such as atrial fibrillation) or other cardiovascular problems, such as aortic stenosis, aortic insufficiency, pulsus alternans, or pulsus paradoxus.

▶ Assess the site for signs of infection, such as redness and swelling. Notify the practitioner if you see such signs.

▶ Change the pressure tubing every 96 hours, or according to your facility's policy. Change the dressing at the catheter site at intervals specified by your facility's policy. **CDC** **INS** **AACN**

▶ Be aware that erroneous pressure readings may result from a catheter that's clotted or positional, loose connections, addition of extra stopcocks or extension tubing, inadvertent entry of air into the system, or improper calibrating, leveling, or zeroing of the monitoring system. If the catheter lumen clots, the flush system may be improperly pressurized. Regularly assess the amount of flush solution in the I.V. bag, and maintain 300 mm Hg of pressure in the pressure bag.

▶ Complications of direct arterial pressure monitoring include arterial bleeding, infection, air embolism, arterial spasm, or thrombosis.

References

Centers for Disease Control and Prevention. "Guidelines for the Prevention of Intravascular Catheter-related Infections," *MMWR* 51(RR-10):1-26, August 2002.

Giuliano, K.K., and Kleinpell, R. "The Use of Common Continuous Monitoring Parameters: A Quality Indicator for Critically Ill Patients with Sepsis," *AACN Clinical Issues* 16(2):140-48, April-June 2005.

Lynn-McHale Wiegand, D.J., and Carlson, K.K., eds. *AACN Procedure Manual for Critical Care,* 5th ed. Philadelphia: W.B. Saunders Co., 2005.

Murphy, G.S., et al. "Retrograde Air Embolization during Routine Radial Artery Catheter Flushing in Adult Cardiac Surgical Patients: An Ultrasound Study," *Anesthesiology* 101(3):614-19, September 2004.

Quaal, S.J. "Improving the Accuracy of Pulmonary Artery Catheter Measurements," *Journal of Cardiovascular Nursing* 15(2):71–82. January 2001. **CS**

"Standard 48. Administration Set Change. Infusion Nursing Standards of Practice," *Journal of Infusion Nursing* 29(1S):S48-51, January-February 2006.

Task Force of the American College of Critical Care Medicine, Society of Critical Medicine. "Practice Parameters for Hemodynamic Support of Sepsis in Adult Patients: 2004 Update," *Critical Care Medicine* 32(9):1928-948, September 2004.

Arterial puncture for blood gas analysis

Obtaining an arterial blood sample requires percutaneous puncture of the brachial, radial, or femoral artery or withdrawal of a sample from an arterial line. After it has been collected, the sample can be analyzed to determine arterial blood gas (ABG) values.

ABG analysis evaluates ventilation by measuring blood pH and the partial pressures of arterial oxygen and carbon dioxide. Blood pH measurement reveals the blood's acid-base balance. ABG samples can also be analyzed for oxygen content and saturation and for bicarbonate values.

Typically, ABG analysis is ordered for patients who have chronic obstructive pulmonary disease, pulmonary edema, acute respiratory distress syndrome, myocardial infarction, or pneumonia. It's also performed during episodes of shock and after coronary artery bypass surgery, resuscitation from cardiac arrest, changes in respiratory therapy or status, and prolonged anesthesia.

Most ABG samples can be collected by a respiratory technician or specially trained nurse. Collection from the femoral artery, however, is usually performed by a physician or as your facility's policy indicates. Before attempting a radial puncture, Allen's test should be performed. (See *Performing Allen's test.*)

Equipment

Preheparanized syringe or 10-ml syringe specially made for drawing blood for ABG analysis ◆ 20G 1¼" needle ◆ 22G 1" needle ◆ glove ◆ alcohol pad ◆ two 2" × 2" gauze pads ◆ rubber cap for syringe hub ◆ ice-filled plastic bag ◆ label ◆ laboratory request form ◆ bandage ◆ optional: 1% lidocaine solution.

Many health care facilities use a commercial ABG analysis kit that contains most of the equipment listed above.

Implementation

▶ Confirm the patient's identity using two patient identifiers according to your facility's policy. **JC**
▶ Tell the patient you need to collect an arterial blood sample, and explain the procedure to help ease anxiety and promote cooperation. Tell him that the needle stick will cause some discomfort but that he must remain still during the procedure.
▶ Wash your hands, and put on gloves.

▶ Open the ABG analysis kit, and remove the sample label and plastic bag. Record on the label the patient's name, room number, body temperature, the date and collection time, the flow rate and delivery method of oxygen (if present), and the practitioner's name. Fill the plastic bag with ice and set it aside.
▶ Place a rolled towel under the patient's wrist for support. Locate the artery, and palpate it for a strong pulse.
▶ Clean the puncture site with an alcohol pad, starting in the center of the site and spiraling outward in a circular motion for 30 seconds or until the pad comes away clean.
▶ Allow the skin to dry.
▶ Palpate the artery with the index and middle fingers of one hand while holding the syringe over the puncture site with the other hand. **AARC**
▶ When puncturing the radial artery, hold the needle bevel up at a 30- to 45-degree angle. When puncturing the brachial artery, hold the needle at a 60-degree angle. (See *Arterial puncture technique.*)

▶ Puncture the skin and arterial wall in one motion, following the path of the artery.
▶ Watch for blood backflow in the syringe. Don't pull back on the plunger because arterial blood should enter the syringe automatically. Fill the syringe to the 5-ml mark.
▶ After collecting the sample, press a gauze pad firmly over the puncture site until the bleeding stops—at least 5 minutes. If the patient is receiving anti-coagulant therapy or has a blood dyscrasia, apply pressure for 10 to 15 minutes; if necessary, ask a coworker to hold the gauze pad in place while you prepare the sample for transport to the laboratory. Don't ask the patient to hold the pad because if he fails to apply sufficient pressure, a large, painful hematoma may form, hindering future arterial punctures at that site.
▶ Check the syringe for air bubbles. If any appear, remove them by holding the syringe upright and slowly ejecting some of the blood onto a 2" x 2" gauze pad.
▶ Remove the needle, and place a rubber cap directly on the syringe tip to

Performing Allen's test

Rest the patient's arm on the mattress or bedside stand, and support his wrist with a rolled towel. Have him clench his fist. Then, using your index and middle fingers, press on the radial and ulnar arteries. Hold this position for a few seconds.

Without removing your fingers from the patient's arteries, ask him to unclench his fist and hold his hand in a relaxed position. The palm will be blanched because pressure from your fingers has impaired normal blood flow.

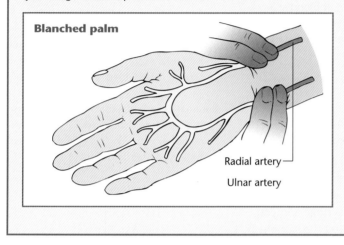

Blanched palm

Radial artery

Ulnar artery

Release pressure on the patient's ulnar artery. If the hand becomes flushed, which indicates blood filling the vessels, you can safely proceed with the radial artery puncture. If the hand doesn't become flushed, perform the test on the other arm.

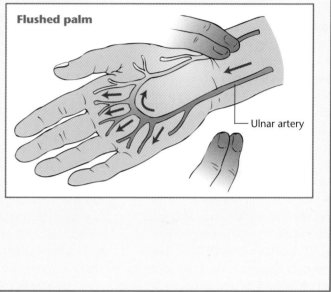

Flushed palm

Ulnar artery

prevent the sample from leaking and to keep air out of the syringe.
▶ Put the labeled sample into the ice-filled plastic bag. Attach a properly completed laboratory request form, and send the sample to the laboratory immediately.

▶ When bleeding stops, apply a small adhesive bandage to the site.
▶ Monitor the patient's vital signs, and observe for signs of circulatory impair-

Arterial puncture technique

The angle of needle penetration in arterial blood gas sampling depends on which artery will be sampled. For the radial artery, which is used most often, the needle should enter bevel up at a 30- to 45-degree angle over the radial artery.

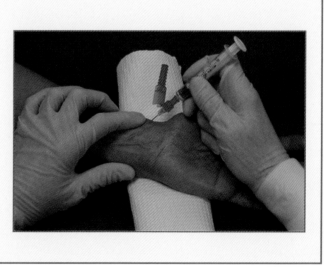

ment, such as swelling, discoloration, pain, numbness, or tingling in the bandaged arm or leg. Watch for bleeding at the puncture site.

Special considerations

▶ If the patient is receiving oxygen, make sure that his therapy has been under way for at least 15 minutes before collecting an arterial blood sample.

▶ Unless ordered, don't turn off existing oxygen therapy before collecting arterial blood samples. Be sure to indicate on the laboratory request form the amount and type of oxygen therapy the patient is receiving.

▶ If the patient isn't receiving oxygen, indicate that he's breathing room air.

▶ If the patient has just received a nebulizer treatment, wait about 20 minutes before collecting the sample.

▶ If necessary, you can anesthetize the puncture site with 1% lidocaine solution or 0.9% benzyl alcohol according to your facility's policy. Consider the use of lidocaine carefully because it delays the procedure, the patient may be allergic to the drug, or the resulting vasoconstriction may prevent successful puncture.

CLINICAL ALERT

If you use too much force when attempting to puncture the artery, the needle may touch the periosteum of the bone, causing the patient considerable pain, or you may advance the needle through the opposite wall of the artery. If this happens, slowly pull the needle back a short distance, and check to see whether you obtain a blood return. If blood still fails to enter the syringe, withdraw the needle completely and start with a fresh syringe.

▶ Don't make more than two attempts to withdraw blood from the same site. Probing the artery may injure it and the radial nerve. Also, hemolysis will alter test results.

▶ If arterial spasm occurs, blood won't flow into the syringe and you won't be able to collect the sample. If this happens, replace the needle with a smaller one and try the puncture again. A smaller-bore needle is less likely to cause arterial spasm.

References

American Association for Respiratory Care. "AARC Clinical Guidelines: Blood Gas Analysis and Hemoximetry. 2001 Revision and Update," *Respiratory Care* 46(5):498-505, May 2001.

Crawford, A. "An Audit of the Patient's Experience of Arterial Blood Gas Testing," *British Journal of Nursing* 13(9):529-32, May 2004.

Hudson, T.L., et al. "Use of Local Anesthesia for Arterial Punctures," *American Journal of Critical Care* 15(6):595-66, November 2006.

Lynn-McHale Wiegand, D.J., and Carlson, K.K., eds. *AACN Procedure Manual for Critical Care,* 5th ed. Philadelphia: W.B. Saunders Co., 2005.

National Committee for Clinical Laboratory Standards. *Procedures for the Collection of Arterial Blood Specimens,* 4th ed. Approved Standard H11-A4, 2004.

Assessment techniques

To perform physical assessment, a nurse uses four basic techniques: inspection, palpation, percussion, and auscultation. Performing these techniques correctly helps elicit valuable information about the patient's condition.

Inspection requires the use of vision, hearing, touch, and smell. Special lighting and various equipment—such as an otoscope, a tongue blade, or an ophthalmoscope—may be used to enhance vision or examine an otherwise hidden area. Inspection begins during the first patient contact and continues throughout the assessment.

Palpation usually follows inspection, except when examining the abdomen or assessing infants and children. Palpation involves touching the body to determine the size, shape, and position of structures; to detect and evaluate temperature, pulsations, and other movement; and to elicit tenderness.

The four palpation techniques include light palpation, deep palpation, light ballottement, and deep ballottement. Ballottement is the technique used to evaluate a flowing or movable structure. The nurse gently bounces the structure being assessed by applying pressure against it and then waits to feel it rebound. This technique may be used, for example, to check the position of an organ or a fetus.

Percussion uses quick, sharp tapping of the fingers or hands against body surfaces to produce sounds, detect tenderness, or assess reflexes. Percussing for sound helps locate organ borders, identify organ shape and position, and determine whether an organ is solid or filled with fluid or gas.

Organs and tissues produce sounds of varying loudness, pitch, and duration, depending on their density. For example, air-filled cavities, such as the lungs, produce markedly different sounds from those produced by the liver and other dense organs and tissues. Percussion techniques include indirect percussion, direct percussion, and blunt percussion.

Auscultation involves listening to various sounds of the body—particularly those produced by the heart, lungs, vessels, stomach, and intestines. Most auscultated sounds result from the movement of air or fluid through these structures.

Usually, the nurse auscultates after performing the other assessment techniques. When examining the abdomen, however, auscultation should occur after inspection but before percussion and palpation. This way, bowel sounds can be heard before palpation disrupts them. Auscultation is most successful when performed in a quiet environment with a properly fitted stethoscope.

Equipment

Flashlight or gooseneck lamp, as appropriate ◆ patient drape ◆ ophthalmoscope ◆ otoscope ◆ stethoscope.

Implementation

▶ Confirm the patient's identity using two patient identifiers according to your facility's policy. **JC**
▶ Explain the procedure to the patient, have him undress, and drape him appropriately.
▶ Make sure the room is warm and adequately lit to make the patient comfortable and to aid visual inspection.
▶ Warm your hands and the stethoscope.

Inspection

▶ Focus on areas related to the patient's chief complaint. Use your eyes, ears, and sense of smell to observe the patient.
▶ To inspect a specific body area, first make sure the area is sufficiently exposed and adequately lit. Then survey the entire area, noting key landmarks and checking its overall condition. Next, focus on specifics—color, shape, texture, size, and movement. Note unusual findings as well as predictable ones.

Palpation

▶ Explain the procedure to the patient, and tell him what to expect, such as occasional discomfort as pressure is applied. Encourage him to relax because muscle tension or guarding can interfere with the performance and results of palpation.

Identifying percussion sounds

Percussion produces sounds that vary according to the tissue being percussed. This table lists important percussion sounds along with their characteristics and typical sources.

SOUND	INTENSITY	PITCH	DURATION	QUALITY	SOURCE
Resonance	Moderate to loud	Low	Long	Hollow	Normal lung
Tympany	Loud	High	Moderate	Drumlike	Gastric air bubble, intestinal air
Dullness	Soft to moderate	High	Moderate	Thudlike	Liver, full bladder, pregnant uterus
Hyperresonance	Very loud	Very low	Long	Booming	Hyperinflated lung (as in emphysema)
Flatness	Soft	High	Short	Flat	Muscle

▶ Use the flattened fingerpads for palpating tender tissues, feeling for crepitus (crackling) at the joints, and lightly probing the abdomen. Use the thumb and index finger for assessing hair texture, grasping tissues, and feeling for lymph node enlargement. Use the back, or dorsal, surface of the hand when feeling for warmth.

▶ Provide just enough pressure to assess the tissue beneath one or both hands. Then release pressure and gently move to the next area, systematically covering the entire surface to be assessed.

▶ To perform light palpation, depress the skin, indenting ½" to ¾" (1 to 2 cm). Use the lightest touch possible because excessive pressure blunts your sensitivity.

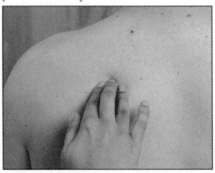

▶ If the patient tolerates light palpation and you need to assess deeper structures, palpate deeply by increasing your fingertip pressure, indenting the skin about 1½" (4 cm). Place your other hand on top of the palpating hand to control and guide your movements.

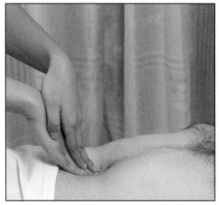

▶ To perform light ballottement, apply light, rapid pressure from quadrant to quadrant on the patient's abdomen. Keep your hand on the skin to detect tissue rebound (as shown at the top of the next column).

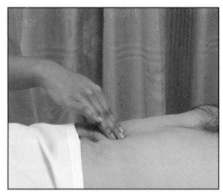

▶ To perform deeper ballottement, apply abrupt, deep pressure and then release it. Maintain fingertip contact.

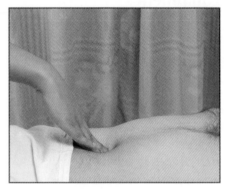

▶ Use both hands (bimanual palpation) to trap a deep, underlying, hard-to-palpate organ (such as the kidney or spleen) or to fix or stabilize an organ (such as the uterus) with one hand while you palpate it with the other.

Percussion

▶ First, decide which of the percussion techniques best suits your assessment needs. Indirect percussion helps reveal the size and density of underlying thoracic and abdominal organs and tissues. Direct percussion helps assess an adult's sinuses for tenderness and elicits sounds in a child's thorax. Blunt percussion aims to elicit tenderness over organs, such as the kidneys, gallbladder, or liver. When percussing, note the characteristic sounds produced. (See *Identifying percussion sounds*.)

▶ To perform indirect percussion, place one hand on the patient and tap the middle finger with the middle finger of the other hand. (See *Performing indirect percussion*.)

▶ To perform direct percussion, tap your hand or fingertip directly against the body surface.

▶ To perform blunt percussion, strike the ulnar surface of your fist against the body surface. Or, place the palm of one hand against the body, make a fist with the other hand, and strike the back of the first hand.

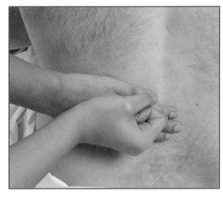

Auscultation

▶ First, determine whether to use the diaphragm or bell of your stethoscope. Use the diaphragm to detect high-pitched sounds, such as breath and bowel sounds. Use the bell to detect lower-pitched sounds, such as heart and vascular sounds.

▶ Place the diaphragm or bell of the stethoscope over the appropriate area of the patient's body. Place the ear-pieces in your ears, listen intently to individual sounds, and try to identify their characteristics. Determine the intensity, pitch, and duration of each sound, and check the frequency of recurring sounds.

AGE FACTOR

Auscultation is best performed first on infants and young children, who may start to cry when palpated or percussed.

Special considerations

▶ Avoid palpating or percussing an area of the body known to be tender at the start of your examination. Instead, work around the area; then gently palpate or percuss it at the end of the examination. This progression minimizes the patient's discomfort and apprehension.

▶ To assess the abdomen, inspect it visually first. Then auscultate bowel

Performing indirect percussion

To perform indirect percussion, use the middle finger of your nondominant hand as the pleximeter (the mediating device used to receive the taps) and the middle finger of your dominant hand as the plexor (the device used to tap the pleximeter). Place the pleximeter finger firmly against a body surface such as the upper back.

With your wrist flexed loosely, use the tip of your plexor finger to deliver a crisp blow just beneath the distal joint of the pleximeter. Be sure to hold the plexor perpendicular to the pleximeter.

Tap lightly and quickly, removing the plexor as soon as you have delivered each blow.

Move your nondominant hand to cover the entire area to be percussed.

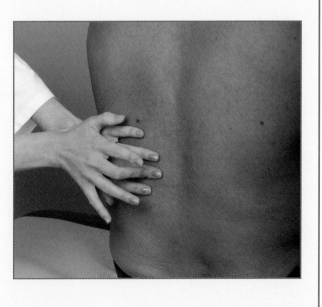

sounds before palpation and percussion, which alter these sounds.

▶ To pinpoint an inflamed area deep within the patient's body, perform a variation on deep palpation: Press firmly with one hand over the area you suspect is involved, and then lift your hand away quickly. If the patient reports that pain increases when you release the pressure, then you've identified rebound tenderness. Suspect peritonitis if you elicit rebound tenderness when examining the abdomen.

▶ If you can't palpate because the patient fears pain, try distracting him with conversation. Then perform auscultation and gently press your stethoscope into the affected area to try to elicit tenderness.

CLINICAL ALERT

Palpation may cause an enlarged spleen or infected appendix to rupture.

References

Bickley, L.S. *Bates' Guide to Physical Examination and History Taking,* 9th ed. Philadelphia: Lippincott Williams & Wilkins, 2008.

Craven, R.F., and Hirnle, C.J. *Fundamentals of Nursing: Human Health and Function,* 5th ed. Philadelphia: Lippincott Williams & Wilkins, 2006.

Jevon, P. "Chest Examination Part 1—Chest Palpation," *Nursing Times* 102(44):26-27, October-November 2006.

Jevon, P. "Chest Examination Part 2—Chest Percussion," *Nursing Times* 102(45):26-27, November 2006.

Jevon, P., and Cunnington, A. "Chest Examination Part 3—Chest Auscultation," *Nursing Times* 102(46):26-27, November 2006.

Automated external defibrillation

Automated external defibrillators (AEDs) are commonly used today to meet the need for early defibrillation, which is currently considered the most effective treatment for ventricular fibrillation. Some facilities now require an AED in every noncritical care unit. Their use is also common in such public places as shopping malls, sports stadiums, and airplanes. Instruction in using the AED is required as part of basic life support (BLS) and advanced cardiac life support (ACLS) training.

AEDs provide early defibrillation—even when no health care provider is present. The AED interprets the victim's cardiac rhythm and gives the operator step-by-step directions on how to proceed. (See *Understanding an AED*.)

Equipment

AED ◆ two prepackaged electrodes.

Implementation

▶ After discovering that your patient is unresponsive to your questions, pulseless, and apneic, follow BLS and ACLS protocols. Then ask a colleague to bring the AED into the patient's room and set it up before the code team arrives.

▶ Open the foil packets containing the two electrode pads. Attach the white electrode cable connector to one pad and the red electrode cable connector to the other. The electrode pads aren't site-specific. **MFR**

▶ Expose the patient's chest. Remove the plastic backing film from the electrode pads, and place the electrode pad attached to the white cable connector on the right upper portion of the patient's chest, just beneath his clavicle.

▶ Place the pad attached to the red cable connector to the left of the heart's apex. To help remember where to place the pads, think "white—right, red—ribs."

▶ Firmly press the device's ON button, and wait while the machine performs a brief self-test. Most AEDs signal their readiness by a computerized voice that says "Stand clear" or by emitting a series of loud beeps. (If the AED isn't functioning properly, it will convey the message "Don't use the AED. Remove and continue cardiopulmonary resuscitation [CPR].") Remember to report AED malfunctions in accordance with your facility's procedure.

Understanding an AED

Most automatic external defibrillators (AEDs) have a "quick-look" feature that allows the paddles to visualize the rhythm before electrodes are connected.

The AED is equipped with a microcomputer that senses and analyzes a patient's heart rhythm at the push of a button. Then it audibly or visually prompts you to deliver a shock.

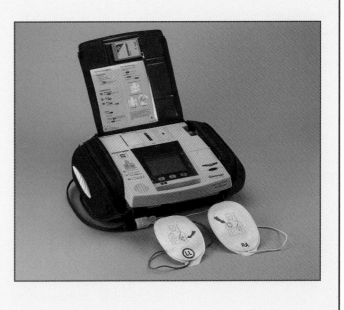

▶ Now the machine is ready to analyze the patient's heart rhythm. Ask everyone to stand clear, and press the ANALYZE button when the machine prompts you. Be careful not to touch or move the patient while the AED is in analysis mode. (If you get the message "Check electrodes," make sure the electrodes are correctly placed and the patient cable is securely attached; then press the ANALYZE button again.)

▶ In 15 to 30 seconds, the AED will analyze the patient's rhythm. When the patient needs a shock, the AED will display a "Stand clear" message and emit a beep that changes into a steady tone as it's charging.

▶ When the AED is fully charged and ready to deliver a shock, it will prompt you to press the SHOCK button. (Some fully automatic AED models automatically deliver a shock within 15 seconds after analyzing the patient's rhythm. If a shock isn't needed, the AED will display "No shock indicated" and prompt you to "Check patient.")

▶ Make sure no one is touching the patient or his bed, and call out "Stand clear." Then press the SHOCK button on the AED.

▶ After the first shock, continue CPR, beginning with five cycles of chest compressions for about 2 minutes. Don't delay compressions to recheck the patient's rhythm or pulse. After five cycles of CPR, the AED should analyze the rhythm and deliver another shock, if indicated. **AHA**

▶ If a nonshockable rhythm is detected, the AED should instruct you to resume CPR. Then continue the algorithm sequence until the code team leader arrives. **AHA**

▶ After the code, remove and transcribe the AED's computer memory module or tape, or prompt the AED to print a rhythm strip with code data. Follow your facility's policy for analyzing and storing code data.

Special considerations

▶ Defibrillators vary among manufacturers, so be sure to familiarize yourself with your facility's equipment. **MFR**

▶ Defibrillator operation should be checked at least every 8 hours and after each use. **JC**

▶ Defibrillation can cause accidental electric shock to those providing care. Using an insufficient amount of conduction medium can lead to skin burns.

References

American Heart Association. "2005 American Heart Association Guidelines for Cardiopulmonary Resuscitation and Emergency Cardiovascular Care: International Consensus on Science," *Circulation* 112(22 Suppl):IV-1-IV-221, November 2005.

American Heart Association. "Highlights of the 2005 American Heart Association Guidelines for Cardiopulmonary Resuscitation and Emergency Cardiovascular Care," *Currents* 16(4):1-27, Winter 2005-2006.

Hazinski, M.F., et al. "Lay Rescuer Automated External Defibrillator ("Public Access Defibrillation") Programs: Lessons Learned from an International Multicenter Trial," *Circulation* 111(24):3336-340, June 2005.

Sanna, T., et al. "Home Defibrillation: A Feasibility Study in Myocardial Infarction Survivors at Intermediate Risk of Sudden Death," *American Heart Journal* 152(4):685, e1-7, October 2006.

Valenzuela, T.D., et al. "Interruptions of Chest Compressions during Emergency Medical Systems Resuscitation," *Circulation* 112(9):1259-265, August 2005.

B

Back care

Regular bathing and massage of the neck, back, buttocks, and upper arms promotes patient relaxation and allows assessment of skin condition. Particularly important for the bedridden patient, massage causes cutaneous vasodilation, helping to prevent pressure ulcers caused by prolonged pressure on bony prominences or by perspiration. Gentle back massage can be performed after myocardial infarction but may be contraindicated in patients with rib fractures, surgical incisions, or other recent traumatic injury to the back.

Equipment

Basin ◆ soap ◆ bath blanket ◆ bath towel ◆ washcloth ◆ back lotion with lanolin base ◆ gloves, if the patient has open lesions or has been incontinent.

Implementation

▶ Assemble the equipment at the patient's bedside.

▶ Explain the procedure to the patient, and provide privacy. Ask him to tell you if you're applying too much or too little pressure.

▶ Fill the basin two-thirds full with warm water, and place the lotion bottle in the basin. Application of warmed lotion won't startle the patient and will also help to reduce muscle tension and vasoconstriction.

▶ Adjust the bed to a comfortable working height, and lower the head of the bed, if allowed. Wash your hands, and put on gloves, if applicable.

▶ Place the patient in the prone position, if possible, or on his side. Position him along the edge of the bed nearest you to prevent back strain.

▶ Untie the patient's gown, and expose his back, shoulders, and buttocks. Then drape the patient with a bath blanket to prevent chills and minimize exposure. Place a bath towel next to or under the patient's side to protect bed linens from moisture.

▶ Fold the washcloth around your hand to form a mitt. Then work up a lather with soap. (See *Making a washcloth mitt,* page 28.)

▶ Using long, firm strokes, bathe the patient's back, beginning at the neck and shoulders and moving downward to the buttocks. Rinse and dry well because moisture trapped between the buttocks can cause chafing and predispose the patient to the formation of pressure ulcers. While giving back care, closely examine the patient's skin—especially the bony prominences of the shoulders, the scapulae, and the coccyx—for redness or abrasions. **NPUAP**

▶ Remove the warmed lotion bottle from the basin, and pour a small amount of lotion into your palm. Rub your hands together to distribute the lotion. Then apply the lotion to the patient's back, using long, firm strokes.

▶ Massage the patient's back, beginning at the base of the spine and moving upward to the shoulders. For a relaxing effect, massage slowly; for a stimulating effect, massage quickly. Alternate the three basic strokes: effleurage, friction, and petrissage. (See *How to give a back massage,* page 28.) Add lotion, as needed, keeping one hand on the patient's back to avoid interrupting the massage.

▶ Compress, squeeze, and lift the trapezius muscle to help relax the patient.

▶ Finish the massage by using long, firm strokes, and blot any excess lotion from the patient's back with a towel. Then retie the patient's gown, and straighten or change the bed linens as necessary.

▶ Return the bed to its original position, and make the patient comfortable. Empty and clean the basin. Dispose of gloves, if used, and return equipment to the appropriate storage area.

Making a washcloth mitt

To make a washcloth mitt, take a clean, dry washcloth and fold it in thirds lengthwise around your hand. Fold the top of the washcloth down, and tuck it in the bottom of the mitt.

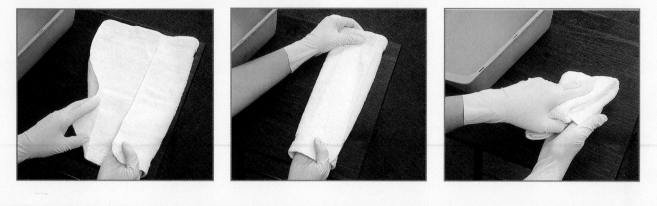

How to give a back massage

Effleurage, friction, and petrissage are the three strokes used commonly when giving a back massage. Start with effleurage, go on to friction, and then to petrissage. Perform each stroke at least six times before moving on to the next, and then repeat the whole series, if desired.

When performing effleurage and friction, keep your hands parallel to the vertebrae to avoid tickling the patient. For all three strokes, maintain a regular rhythm and steady contact with the patient's back to help him relax.

Effleurage
Using your palm, stroke from the buttocks up to the shoulders, over the upper arms, and back to the buttocks (as shown below). Use slightly less pressure on the downward strokes.

Friction
Use circular thumb strokes to move from buttocks to shoulders; then, using a smooth stroke, return to the buttocks (as shown below).

Petrissage
Using your thumb to oppose your fingers, knead and stroke half the back and upper arms, starting at the buttocks and moving toward the shoulder (as shown below). Then knead and stroke the other half of the back, rhythmically alternating your hands.

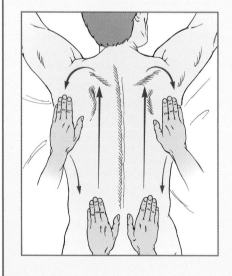

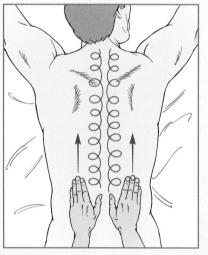

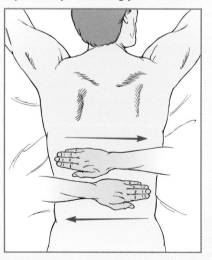

Special considerations

▶ Before giving back care, assess the patient's body structure and skin condition and tailor the duration and intensity of the massage accordingly. If you're giving back care at bedtime, have the patient ready for bed beforehand, so the massage can help him fall asleep.

▶ When massaging the patient's back, stand with one foot slightly forward and your knees slightly bent to allow effective use of your arm and shoulder muscles.

▶ Give special attention to bony prominences because these areas are predisposed to the formation of pressure ulcers. Don't massage the patient's legs, unless ordered, because reddened legs can signal clot formation and massage can dislodge the clot, causing an embolus. Develop a turning schedule, and give back care at each position change.

References

Craven, R.F., and Hirnle, C.J. *Fundamentals of Nursing: Human Health and Function,* 6th ed. Philadelphia: Lippincott Williams & Wilkins, 2009.

Robinson, S.B., et al. "The Sh-h-h-h Project: Nonpharmacological Interventions," *Holistic Nursing Practice* 19(6):263-66, November-December 2005.

Bariatric beds

Typical hospital beds are designed to hold patients weighing up to 450 lb (204 kg) and who don't have a wide abdominal girth. Bariatric beds are a recent addition to hospital equipment designed to accommodate patients who are considered obese. Several bariatric beds are available, ranging from simply being a larger version of a standard bed to a low-air-loss mattress that provides pressure relief.

Use of a bariatric bed provides more comfort for obese patients than a standard-size bed. It preserves self-esteem by providing these patients with a bed that easily fits their larger body size as well as special side rails that help them turn and reposition themselves. Bariatric beds also allow caregivers to perform routine care, such as boosting, turning, and transferring in and out of bed, with greater ease and less risk of injury. Most bariatric beds also have a built-in scale that allows the nurse to more easily weigh the patient. Some bariatric beds easily convert to a cardiac chair. (See *A bariatric bed*.)

Equipment

Bariatric bed ◆ optional: overhead trapeze, special sheets.

Implementation

▶ Discuss the need for a specialized bed with the patient so that he understands its benefits and therapeutic effects.

▶ Consult with other health care team members, such as the practitioner, surgical team, physical therapy, occupational therapy, wound care, and respiratory therapy, to choose the appropriate type of bed and mattress for the patient's needs. A company representative may be involved in the patient assessment to ensure that the appropriate type and size of bed are provided.

▶ Verify the practitioner's order for the bariatric bed.

▶ Obtain the bariatric bed from central supply, or contact the company representative to have the bed delivered, according to facility protocol.

▶ Prepare the bed according to the manufacturer's guidelines. Specialized sheets may be necessary. Attach an overhead trapeze, if indicated.

▶ If the bed is rented, ask the company representative for an in-service so that all health care team members understand its use and can provide safe care.

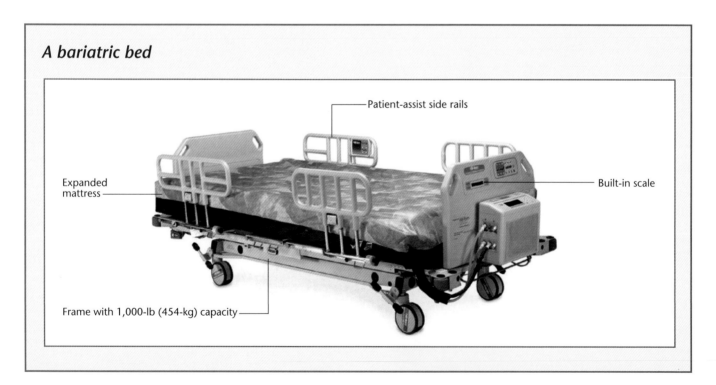

A bariatric bed

Patient-assist side rails

Expanded mattress

Built-in scale

Frame with 1,000-lb (454-kg) capacity

► Make sure that written instructions come with the bed, and keep them at the bedside.

► Provide the patient with any product information, and instruct him in the use of the bed's functions and controls so that he understands its features and safe use.

Special considerations

► Provide for other bariatric equipment, such as hospital gowns, commodes, wheelchairs, lifts, scales, and stretchers, for patient comfort and safety.

► Before sending the patient to other departments, call ahead to make sure they can accommodate a larger bed and are familiar with its use.

References

Arzouman, J., et al. "Developing a Comprehensive Bariatric Protocol: A Template for Improving Patient Care," *MedSurg Nursing* 15(1):21-26, February 2006.

Barth, M.M., and Jensen, C.E. "Postoperative Nursing Care of Gastric Bypass Patients," *American Journal of Critical Care* 15(4):378-87, July 2006.

Grindel, M.E., and Grindel, C.G. "Nursing Care of the Person Having Bariatric Surgery," *MedSurg Nursing* 15(3):129-45, June 2006.

National Institutes of Health. Clinical Guidelines on the Identification, Evaluation, and Treatment of Overweight and Obesity in Adults—Executive Summary: Evidence-based Guidelines. Available at *www.nhlbi.nih.gov/guidelines/obesity/sum_evid.htm.*

Wright, W., and Bauer, C. "Meeting Bariatric Patient Care Needs. Procedures and Protocol Development," *Journal of Wound, Ostomy, and Continence Nursing* 32(6):402-405, November-December 2005.

Basic sterile technique

Sterile technique, also referred to as *aseptic technique,* is used for any procedure that requires the absence of microorganisms. Sterile technique should be followed any time the patient's skin is intentionally perforated, during procedures that involve entry into a sterile body cavity, or when coming into contact with nonintact skin resulting from trauma or surgery.

Sterile technique is used in conjunction with other procedures—it isn't a procedure in itself. Procedures requiring sterile technique include I.V. catheter insertion, any type of injection, urinary catheter insertion, and dressing changes. Patients with a compromised immune system (such as those with burns, those following organ transplant, and those receiving chemotherapy or radiation therapy) also require sterile technique, even for some procedures that would normally require only clean technique.

Equipment

Sterile gloves ◆ personal protective equipment ◆ sterile supplies, as required by the procedure to be performed ◆ optional: sterile bowl, sterile normal saline solution, sterile drape.

Many procedures have commercially prepared kits, which provide all of the necessary components.

Implementation

▶ Verify the practitioner's order.
▶ Confirm the patient's identity using two patient identifiers according to your facility's policy. **JC**
▶ Explain the procedure to the patient and his family to relieve anxiety and ensure understanding and cooperation.
▶ Assess the patient's level of pain, and administer analgesics 20 to 30 minutes before the procedure to promote patient comfort.
▶ Wash your hands thoroughly to reduce the risk of transmission of microorganisms. (See "Hand hygiene," page 225.) **CDC AORN**
▶ Follow standard precautions by putting on the necessary personal protective equipment for the procedure.
▶ Assemble all of the equipment in the patient's room. Check each package carefully, and discard any with a

hole or tear or that's wet. Note the expiration date, and discard any package that's beyond the date. Make sure that the sterilization tape has turned the appropriate color (see your facility's policy; color will depend on the product used and the sterilization method). Prepare a clean surface to set up the equipment for the sterile procedure.

Opening sterile kits

▶ Remove the plastic outer wrapper from the procedure kit, if one is present.
▶ Place the inner wrapped kit on a clean, dry, flat surface because moisture on the table could be absorbed through the wrapper and contaminate the sterile supplies.
▶ Position the kit so that the tip of the triangle-pointed wrapper is toward you—this way you won't have to reach over the sterile contents after the other flaps are opened.
▶ Grasp the outer portion of the outermost flap to avoid contaminating the sterile field.
▶ Open the flap away from the body, keeping the arm outstretched to the side so it doesn't cross over the sterile field (as shown at the top of the next column).

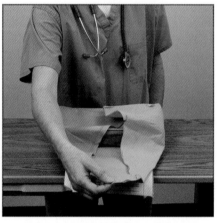

▶ Grasp the outer surface of the first side flap with the hand on the same side as the flap to avoid crossing over the sterile field. Be sure to open the flap fully to avoid allowing the wrapper to spring back.

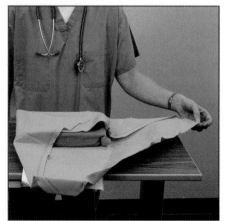

▶ Grasp the outer surface of the second side flap, and open it with the hand on the same side.

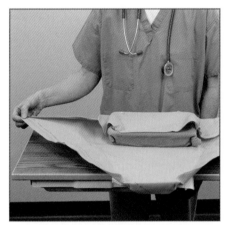

▶ Grasp the outer surface of the innermost flap, and open it toward your body.

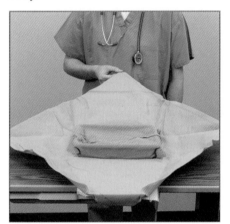

Opening peel pack containers or pouches

▶ Grasp the unsealed corner of the wrapper, and pull it toward you.

▶ If the item is light, it can be dropped onto the sterile field. Heavy items should be carefully set onto the sterile field. **AORN**

▶ Open a peel pack pouch (such as gloves and syringes) by grasping each side of the unsealed edge with the thumb side of each hand parallel to the seal and pulling it apart gently (as shown at the top of the next column).

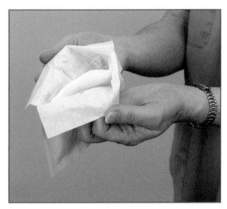

▶ Hold the sides back so the wrap covers your hands and exposes the sterile item.

▶ Don't allow the item to slide across the package side when dropping the item onto the sterile field.

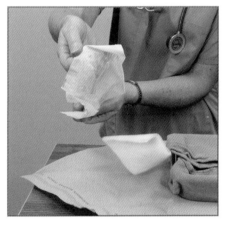

Pouring sterile solutions

▶ Open the wrapped package containing the sterile cup, as described above, to avoid contaminating the sterile field.

▶ Place the cup on the edge of the sterile field but inside of the 1″ (2.5-cm) safety margin so that solution can be poured without reaching across the sterile field.

▶ Unwrap the seal on the sterile normal saline solution bottle.

▶ Unscrew the cap without touching the edges of the bottle.

▶ Place the inverted cap on a nonsterile surface to keep the inside of the cap from touching contaminated surfaces.

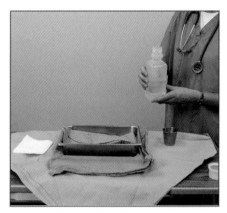

▶ Pour the solution into the cup without reaching over the sterile field and from a distance of about 6″ (15 cm) above the cup to reduce the risk of touching sterile surfaces.

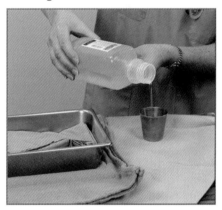

▶ Pour the solution slowly to avoid splashing onto the drape and contaminating the sterile field.

▶ Discard unused solution or recap the container, and label the bottle with the date, time, and your initials to be used within 24 hours, depending on your facility's policy.

Opening and putting on sterile gloves

▶ Open the package containing the sterile gloves following the above procedures. Touch only the outer side of the glove wrapper.

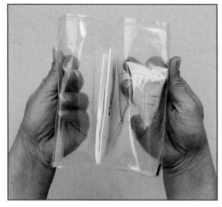

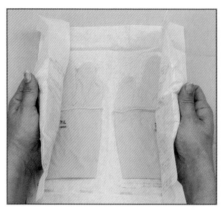

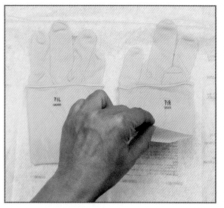

▶ Grasp the paper glove wrapper and place it on a clean, dry, flat surface.
▶ Open the package, touching only the outer edges of the wrapper.

▶ Use the thumb and fingers of the nondominant hand to grasp the folded inner surface portion of the glove for the dominant hand, touching only the inner portion of the glove.

▶ Lift the glove up, and insert the dominant hand into the glove, palm side up (as shown at the top of the next column).

Removing contaminated gloves

Proper removal techniques are essential for preventing the spread of pathogens from gloves to your skin surface. Follow these steps carefully.

1. Using your left hand, pinch the right glove near the top. Avoid allowing the glove's outer surface to buckle inward against your wrist.

Pull downward, allowing the glove to turn inside out as it comes off. Keep the right glove in your left hand after removing it.

2. Now insert the first two fingers of your ungloved right hand under the edge of the left glove. Avoid touching the glove's outer surface or folding it against your left wrist.

3. Pull downward so that the glove turns inside out as it comes off. Continue pulling until the left glove completely encloses the right one and its uncontaminated inner surface is facing out.

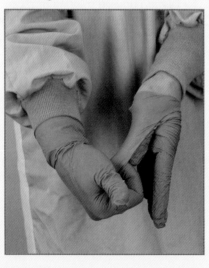

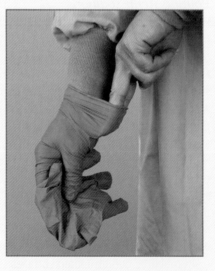

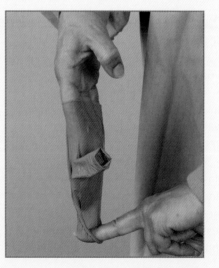

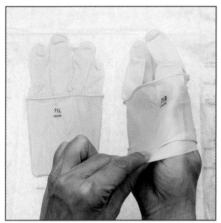

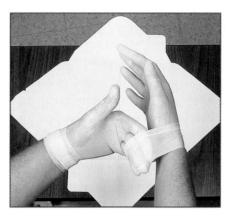

▶ Pull the cuff down by touching only the inner surface of the glove.

▶ Insert the four fingers of the dominant gloved hand into the sterile outer cuff of the other glove, keeping the thumb pulled back out of the way.

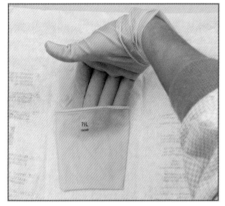

▶ Lift the glove up, and insert the nondominant hand into the glove. Allow the cuff to come uncuffed as you finish putting it on, but don't touch the skin of the arm with the gloved hand.

▶ After both hands are gloved, adjust the fingers as necessary.

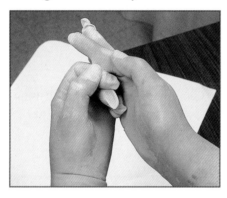

Special considerations

▶ When removing sterile gloves, take care not to spread organisms or other infectious material. (See *Removing contaminated gloves*).

▶ If additional sterile supplies need to be added to a sterile field, open the sterile packages as described above. Be sure to open them away from the already set up sterile field to avoid contaminating the field. Hold the opened additional supplies above the sterile field, and drop them onto the field.
AORN

References

Association of Perioperative Registered Nurses. *Standards, Recommended Practices, and Guidelines.* Denver: AORN, Inc., 2006.

Craven, R.F., and Hirnle, C.J. *Fundamentals of Nursing: Human Health and Function,* 6th ed. Philadelphia: Lippincott Williams & Wilkins, 2009.

Occupational Safety and Health Administration. Personal Protective Equipment Standard 1910.132.

Bedside hemoglobin testing

Nurses monitor hemoglobin level at the patient's bedside because the fast, accurate results obtained this way allow for immediate intervention, if necessary. In contrast to traditional monitoring methods, blood samples must be sent to the laboratory for interpretation. Numerous testing systems are available for bedside monitoring. Bedside systems are also convenient for the patient's home use.

One such system, the HemoCue photometer, gives accurate results without having to pipette, dispense, or mix blood and reagents to obtain readings. Thus, it eliminates the risk of leakage, broken tubes, and splattered blood. A plastic, disposable microcuvette functions as a combination pipette, test tube, and measuring vessel. It contains a reagent that produces a precise chemical reaction as soon as it comes into contact with blood. The photometer is a handheld device that recharges its battery and downloads data at a docking station. (See *Using a bedside hemoglobin monitor*.)

Normal hemoglobin values range from 12.5 to 15 g/dl. A below-normal hemoglobin value may indicate anemia, recent hemorrhage, or fluid retention, causing hemodilution. An elevated hemoglobin value suggests hemoconcentration from polycythemia or dehydration.

Equipment

Lancet ◆ microcuvette ◆ photometer ◆ gloves ◆ alcohol pads ◆ gauze pads.

Implementation

▶ Confirm the patient's identity using two patient identifiers according to your facility's policy. **JC**

▶ Take the equipment to the patient's bedside, and explain the purpose of the test to him. Tell him that he'll feel a pinprick in his finger during blood sampling.

Using a bedside hemoglobin monitor

Monitoring hemoglobin level at the patient's bedside is a straightforward procedure. A photometer, such as the HemoCue analyzer featured here, relies on capillary action to draw blood into a disposable microcuvette.

This method of obtaining blood minimizes a health care worker's exposure to the patient's blood and decreases the risk of cross-contamination. Follow the steps shown here when using the HemoCue system.

After you pierce the skin, the microcuvette draws blood automatically.

Next, place the microcuvette in the photometer. The photometer screen displays the patient's hemoglobin level.

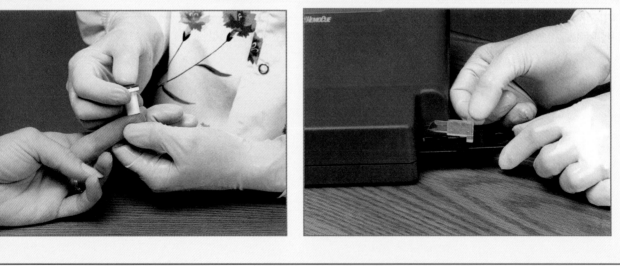

▶ Turn the photometer on. If it hasn't been used recently, insert the control cuvette to make sure that the photometer is working properly. **MFR**

▶ Wash your hands and put on gloves. **CDC**

▶ Select an appropriate puncture site. You'll usually use a fingertip for an adult. The middle and fourth fingers are the best choices. The second finger is usually the most sensitive, and the thumb may have thickened skin or calluses. Blood should circulate freely in the finger from which you're collecting blood, so avoid using a ring-bearing finger.

AGE FACTOR

For an infant, use the heel or great toe.

▶ Keep the patient's finger straight, and ask him to relax it. Holding his finger between the thumb and index finger of your nondominant hand, gently rock the patient's finger as you move your fingers from his top knuckle to his fingertip. This causes blood to flow to the sampling point.

▶ Use an alcohol pad to clean the puncture site, wiping in a circular motion from the center of the site outward. Dry the site thoroughly with a gauze pad.

▶ Pierce the skin quickly and sharply with the lancet, and apply the microcuvette, which automatically collects a precise amount of blood (about 5 µl).

▶ Wipe excess blood from the sides of the microcuvette to obtain the most accurate reading.

▶ Place the microcuvette into the photometer. Results will appear on the photometer screen within 1 minute.

▶ Place a gauze pad over the puncture site until bleeding stops.

▶ Dispose of the lancet and microcuvette according to your facility's policy. Remove your gloves and wash your hands. Notify the practitioner if the test result is outside the expected parameters.

Special considerations

▶ Before using a microcuvette, note its expiration date.

▶ Before collecting a blood sample, operate the photometer with the control cuvette to check for proper function. **MFR**

▶ To ensure an adequate blood sample, don't use a cold, cyanotic, or swollen area as the puncture site.

▶ When performing bedside hemoglobin testing, follow your facility's policy for point-of-care testing.

References

Diesel, D., et al. "Point-of-care Testing (POCT): Key Factors to Ensure Efficiency and High Quality," *International Journal of Clinical Chemistry,* May 2004. Available at *www.cli-online.com/uploads/tx_ttproducts/datasheet/point-of-care-testing-(poct)—key-factors-to-ensure-efficiency-and-high-quality.pdf.*

Bladder ultrasonography

Urine retention, a potentially life-threatening condition, may result from neurologic or psychological disorders or the obstruction of urine flow. Such medications as anticholinergics, antihistamines, and antidepressants may also cause urine retention. Urinary catheterization, while a traditional diagnostic method for measuring urine volume in the bladder, places the patient at risk for infection. **CDC** Bladder ultrasonography, however, is a noninvasive tool and provides an equally accurate assessment of urine volume.

Equipment

BladderScan (ultrasound) unit with scanhead ◆ ultrasonic transmission gel ◆ alcohol pad ◆ washcloth ◆ gloves.

Implementation

▶ Confirm the patient's identity using two patient identifiers according to your facility's policy. **JC**
▶ Bring the ultrasound unit to the bedside. Explain the procedure to the patient to help reduce his anxiety. Wash your hands.
▶ Provide privacy. If this is a postvoiding scan, ask the patient to void and assist him, if necessary. Help the patient into a supine position.
▶ Put on gloves, and clean the rounded end of the scanhead with an alcohol pad.

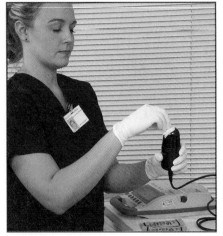

▶ Expose the patient's suprapubic area.

▶ Turn on the ultrasound by pressing the button (designated by a dot within a circle) on the far left, and press SCAN.
▶ Tell the patient that the gel will feel cold when placed on the abdomen. Placing ultrasonic gel on the patient promotes an airtight seal for optimal sound wave transmission.

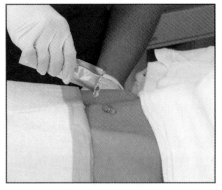

▶ Locate the icon (a rough figure of a patient) on the probe, and make sure the head of the icon points toward the head of the patient.
▶ Locate the symphysis pubis, and place the scanhead about 1″ (2.5 cm) superior to the symphysis pubis.

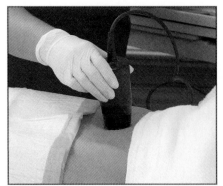

▶ Press the scanhead button marked with a sound wave pattern to activate the scan. Hold the scanhead steady until you hear the beep.
▶ Look at the aiming icon and screen, which displays the bladder position and volume.
▶ Reposition the probe, and scan until the bladder is centered in the aiming screen. The largest measurement will be saved.
▶ Press DONE when finished.
▶ The ultrasound will display the measured urine volume and the longitudinal and horizontal axis scans.
▶ Press PRINT to obtain a hard copy of your results.
▶ Turn off the ultrasound. Use an alcohol pad to clean the gel off the scanhead.
▶ Using a washcloth, clean the gel from the patient's skin.

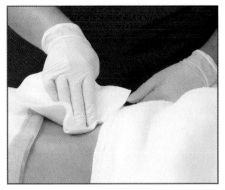

▶ Remove your gloves and wash your hands.

Special considerations

▶ Some scanners include an option that requires you to choose the sex of the patient. (*Note:* If the patient has had a hysterectomy, you would choose male.)

References

Addison, R. "Assessing Continence with Bladder Ultrasound," *Nursing Times* 103(19):44-45, May 2007.

Graf, J. "Efficient Bladder Ultrasonography," *Pediatrics* 116(3):797, September 2005.

Oh-Oka, H., and Fujisawa, M. "Study of Low Bladder Volume Measurement Using 3-dimensional Ultrasound Scanning Device: Improvement in Measurement Accuracy through Training When Bladder Volume Is 150 ml or Less," *Journal of Urology* 177(2):595-99, February 2007.

Taylor, C., et al. *Fundamentals of Nursing: The Art and Science of Nursing Care,* 6th ed. Philadelphia: Lippincott Williams & Wilkins, 2008.

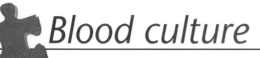

Blood culture

Normally bacteria-free, blood is susceptible to infection through infusion lines as well as from thrombophlebitis, infected shunts, and bacterial endocarditis due to prosthetic heart valve replacements. Bacteria may also invade the vascular system (from local tissue infections) through the lymphatic system and thoracic duct.

Blood cultures are performed to detect bacterial invasion (bacteremia) and the systemic spread of such an infection (septicemia) through the bloodstream. In this procedure, a venous blood sample is collected by venipuncture at the patient's bedside and then transferred into two bottles—one containing an anaerobic medium and the other, an aerobic medium. The bottles are then incubated, encouraging any organisms that are present in the sample to grow in the media. Blood cultures allow for identification of about 67% of pathogens within 24 hours and up to 90% within 72 hours. Two sets of blood cultures should be drawn, with no waiting time between the sets. Central venous access devices shouldn't be used to draw the blood cultures unless there's no peripheral venous access available.

Equipment

Tourniquet ◆ gloves ◆ alcohol ◆ chlorhexidine scrub ◆ 20-ml syringe for an adult; 6-ml syringe for a child ◆ three or four 20G 1″ needles ◆ two or three blood culture bottles (50-ml bottles for adults; 20-ml bottles for infants and children) with sodium polyethanol sulfonate added (one aerobic bottle containing a suitable medium, such as Trypticase soy broth with 10% carbon dioxide atmosphere; one anaerobic bottle with prereduced medium; and, possibly, one hyperosmotic bottle with 10% sucrose medium) ◆ laboratory request form and laboratory biohazard transport bags ◆ 2″ × 2″ gauze pads ◆ small adhesive bandages ◆ labels.

Implementation

▶ Confirm the patient's identity using two patient identifiers according to your facility's policy. **JC**

▶ Tell the patient that you need to collect a series of blood samples to check for infection. Explain the procedure to ease his anxiety and promote cooperation. Explain that the procedure usually requires two blood samples collected at different times.

▶ Check the expiration dates on the culture bottles, and replace outdated bottles.

▶ Wash your hands and put on gloves. **CDC**

▶ Tie a tourniquet 2″ (5 cm) proximal to the area chosen. (See "Venipuncture," page 592.)

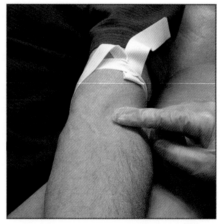

▶ Clean the venipuncture site with an alcohol pad.

▶ Scrub the area with chlorhexidine with a side-to-side motion for 30 seconds. Wait 30 to 60 seconds for the skin to dry. **CDC**

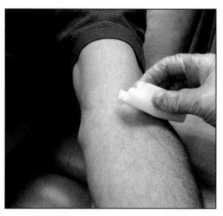

▶ Clean the tops of the blood culture bottles with an alcohol pad, and then leave the alcohol pad on top of the bottle to keep the top of the bottle free from contaminants.

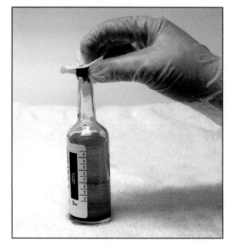

▶ Perform a venipuncture, drawing 10 ml of blood from an adult.

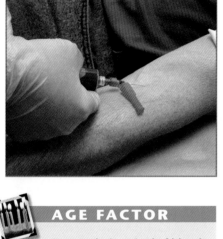

AGE FACTOR

Draw only 2 to 6 ml of blood from a child.

▶ Change the needle on the syringe used to draw the blood.

▶ Inject 10 ml of blood into each bottle or 2 ml into each 20-ml pediatric culture bottle. **CAP**

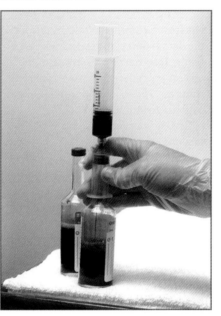

▶ Remove the tourniquet. Apply pressure to the venipuncture site using a

2″ × 2″ dressing. Then cover the site with a small adhesive bandage.

▶ Label the culture bottles with the patient's name and identification number, practitioner's name, and date and time of collection. Indicate the suspected diagnosis and the patient's temperature, and note on the laboratory request form any recent antibiotic therapy. Place the samples in the laboratory biohazard transport bag. Send the samples to the laboratory immediately.

▶ Discard syringes, needles, and gloves in the appropriate containers.

Special considerations

▶ Obtain each set of cultures from a different site.

▶ Avoid using existing blood lines for cultures unless the sample is drawn when the line is inserted or if catheter sepsis is suspected. **CAP**

EVIDENCE-BASED RESEARCH

Drawing enough blood for a culture

Donnino, M.W., Goyal, N., et al. "Inadequate Blood Volume Collected for Culture: A Survey of Health Care Professionals," *Mayo Clinic Proceedings* 82(9):1069-1072, September 2007.

Level VI
Evidence from a single descriptive or qualitative study

Description
Blood cultures are commonly drawn on hospitalized patients to determine the presence of bacteremia. The results of the blood culture typically serve as an important factor in making therapeutic decisions. Having enough blood to culture is the most important factor

in the process of drawing blood cultures. National guidelines currently state that at least 10 ml of blood per culture per bottle should be drawn. A study was done to determine whether nurses and other health care professionals who draw blood cultures know the correct amount of blood to draw for an adequate sample. A questionnaire was distributed to nurses, physicians, technicians, and other personnel who were qualified to draw blood cultures. The questionnaire asked the job title, workplace, years of experience, and what volume of blood should be collected in one bottle for a blood culture. The questionnaire was collected anonymously.

Findings
Of the 360 questionnaires, 355 were returned with usable responses. A total of 79% of the health care personnel answered that less than 10 ml of blood was needed for a blood culture. Approximately 90% of nurses answered incorrectly; the answers ranged from more than 10 ml to less than 1 ml was needed. Nurses with more than 10 years of experience answered incorrectly at a rate of 53%, whereas nurses with less than 10 years of experience answered incorrectly at a rate of 41%.

Conclusions
Many nurses working today aren't aware of the amount of blood that's

(continued)

Drawing enough blood for a culture *(continued)*

recommended for an accurate blood culture. Because blood culture volume is still the most important factor for determining yield of organism, these findings raise an important quality assurance issue. Future educational and quality assurance initiatives should be considered for proper collection of volume for blood cultures.

Nursing practice implications
Nurses are commonly responsible for drawing blood cultures on their patients. They need to be aware of the correct procedure for drawing blood cultures. The following practice implications are important:
► Review your facility's policy on drawing blood cultures.

► Make sure to draw a minimum of 10 ml of blood per bottle when drawing a blood culture.
► Monitor staff drawing blood cultures to make sure the correct amount of blood is being drawn.
► Educate staff on the proper procedure for drawing blood cultures.

References

Bekeris, B., et al. "Trends in Blood Culture Contamination: A College of American Pathologists Q-tracks Study of 356 Institutions," *Archives of Pathology and Laboratory Medicine* 129(10):1222-225, October 2005.

Clinical Laboratory Standards. "Principles and Procedures for Blood Cultures." Approved Guidelines MH7-A, 2007.

College of American Pathologists. "Drawing Blood for a Valid Culture." Accessed August 2007 at *www.cap.org/apps/docs/ newspath/spring_2004/0404_Laboratory_Report_Drawing_Blood_for_a_Valid_ Culture.doc.*

Craven, R.F., and Hirnle, C.J. *Fundamentals of Nursing: Human Health and Function,* 5th ed. Philadelphia: Lippincott Williams & Wilkins, 2007.

Fischbach, F.T. *A Manual of Laboratory and Diagnostic Tests,* 7th ed. Philadelphia: Lippincott Williams & Wilkins, 2003.

Rushing, J. "Drawing Blood Culture Specimens for Reliable Results," *Nursing* 34(12):20, December 2004.

Blood glucose tests

Blood glucose monitors measure blood glucose concentration. A drop of whole blood is placed on a blood glucose test strip before or after the strip is inserted into the monitor. A portable blood glucose meter provides quantitative measurements that compare in accuracy with other laboratory tests. Some meters store successive test results electronically to help determine glucose patterns.

Equipment

Portable blood glucose meter ◆ alcohol pads ◆ gauze pads ◆ disposable lancets or mechanical blood-letting devices ◆ blood glucose test strips ◆ optional: small adhesive bandage.

Implementation

▶ When using a blood glucose meter, calibrate it and run it with a quality control test to ensure accurate test results. Follow the manufacturer's instructions for calibration. If appropriate, ensure that the code strip number on the test strip matches the code number on the meter. **MFR**

▶ Confirm the patient's identity using two patient identifiers according to your facility's policy. **JC**

▶ Explain the procedure to the patient or to a child's parents.

▶ Next, select the puncture site—usually the fingertip or earlobe for an adult or a child.

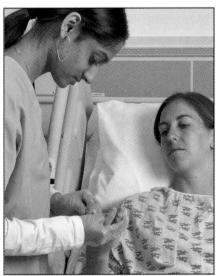

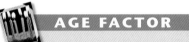
AGE FACTOR

Select the heel or great toe for an infant.

▶ Wash your hands and put on gloves.

▶ If necessary, dilate the capillaries by applying warm, moist compresses to the area for about 10 minutes.

▶ Wipe the puncture site with an alcohol pad, and allow to dry completely.

▶ Turn on the monitor.

▶ To collect a sample from the fingertip with a disposable lancet (smaller than 2 mm), position the lancet on the side of the patient's fingertip, perpendicular to the lines of the fingerprints. Pierce the skin sharply and quickly to minimize the patient's anxiety and pain and to increase blood flow. Alternatively, you can use a mechanical blood-letting device, which uses a spring-loaded lancet.

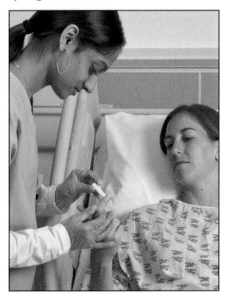

▶ After puncturing the fingertip, don't squeeze the puncture site, to avoid diluting the sample with tissue fluid.

▶ Touch a drop of blood to the test area of the test strip.

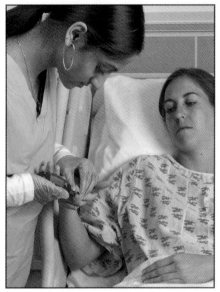

▶ After collecting the blood sample, briefly apply pressure to the puncture site to prevent painful extravasation of blood into subcutaneous tissues. Ask the adult patient to hold a gauze pad firmly over the puncture site until bleeding stops.

▶ Insert the test strip into the blood glucose meter according to the manufacturer's instructions.

▶ Read the digital display when the alarm sounds.

▶ Remove the test strip and dispose of it according to your facility's policy.

▶ After bleeding has stopped, you may apply a small adhesive bandage to the puncture site (as shown at the top of the next page).

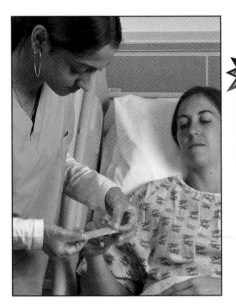

▶ Remove your gloves and wash your hands.

CLINICAL ALERT

If you get an extremely low or high blood glucose reading, obtain a serum blood glucose level immediately to confirm the result.

▶ Clean the blood glucose monitor when it becomes contaminated with blood, at intervals recommended by the manufacturer, or according to your facility's policy **MFR**

Special considerations

▶ Follow your facility's policy for bedside point-of-care testing.
▶ Avoid selecting cold, cyanotic, or swollen puncture sites to ensure an adequate blood sample. If you can't obtain a capillary sample, perform venipuncture and place a large drop of venous blood on the reagent strip. If you want to test blood from a refrigerated sample, allow the blood to return to room temperature before testing it.
▶ To help detect abnormal glucose metabolism and to diagnose diabetes mellitus, the practitioner may order

---

EVIDENCE-BASED RESEARCH

Glucose control in the intensive care unit

Holzinger, U.L., et al. "Improvement of Glucose Control in the Intensive Care Unit: An Interdisciplinary Collaboration Study," *American Journal of Critical Care* 17(2):150-58, March 2008.

Level VI
Evidence from a single descriptive or qualitative study

Description
Many patients in the intensive care unit (ICU) have an increased metabolic response because of stress and other pathologic processes. One characteristic of this increased metabolic response is increased gluconeogenesis and peripheral insulin resistance. This in turn leads to hyperglycemia, which has a proven link to higher mortality and morbidity in ICU patients. Many nurses are unaware of the risks related to continued hyperglycemia in ICU patients. A prospective observation study was done in an ICU that involved de-

veloping and implementing a glucose control protocol with a nurse-managed insulin therapy algorithm. Every measured blood glucose value and hourly and daily insulin dose were documented in 36 patients before and 44 patients after implementing the protocol.

Findings
After the glucose control protocol was implemented, the median blood glucose level decreased from 133 mg/dl to 110 mg/dl. The median amount of insulin used each day increased from 28 units to 35 units. Overall, diabetic patients continued to have higher blood glucose levels than nondiabetic patients, despite an increase in insulin use.

Conclusions
Glucose control protocols help decrease glucose levels for patients in the ICU. Along with the development of glucose control protocols, staff mem-

bers should also undergo education about the protocols and the need for increased glucose control in ICUs.

Nursing practice implications
Nurses are responsible for monitoring blood glucose levels and administering insulin therapy to patients in the ICU. The following practice implications are important for helping patients achieve their optimum glucose levels:
▶ Monitor blood glucose levels in patients frequently to help keep a tighter control on glucose levels.
▶ Notify physicians about abnormal glucose levels in a timely manner.
▶ Administer insulin as scheduled to help decrease fluctuations in glucose levels.
▶ Be aware of medications that may increase glucose levels, such as corticosteroids.

other blood glucose tests such as an oral or I.V. glucose tolerance test. **ADA**

▶ Some blood glucose meters require smaller amounts of blood; the puncture may be done on the patient's arm instead of his finger.

References

American Diabetes Association. "Clinical Practice Recommendations 2008," *Diabetes Care* 31(Supplement 1): S1-S108, January 2008.

Clinical Laboratories Standards Institute. "Point-of-care Blood Glucose Testing in Acute and Chronic Care Facilities," Approved Guideline, 2nd ed. C30-A2, 2002.

Dale, L. "Make a Point about Alternate Site Blood Glucose Sampling," *Nursing* 36(2):52-53, February 2006.

Miller, C. "Using Standards of Care to Drive Evidence-based Clinical Practice and Outcomes for Diabetes Mellitus," *Home Healthcare Nurse* 24(5):307-12, May 2006.

Rizvi, A.A., and Sanders, M.B. "Assessment and Monitoring of Glycemic Control in Primary Diabetes Care: Monitoring Techniques, Record Keeping, Meter Downloads, Tests of Average Glycemia, and Point-of-care Evaluation," *Journal of American Academy of Nurse Practitioners* 18(1):11-21, January 2006.

Scovell, C. "Using Audit to Change Practice for Routine Glucochecks," *Nursing Times* 102(39):33-34, September-October 2006.

Seley, J.J., and Zaldivar, A. "Read That Meter! Getting the Most Out of Blood Glucose Monitoring," *Advance for Nurse Practitioners* 14(4):55-56, April 2006.

Blood pressure assessment

Defined as the lateral force exerted by blood on the arterial walls, blood pressure depends on the force of ventricular contractions, arterial wall elasticity, peripheral vascular resistance, and blood volume and viscosity. Systolic, or maximum, pressure occurs during left ventricular contraction and reflects the integrity of the heart, arteries, and arterioles. Diastolic, or minimum, pressure occurs during left ventricular relaxation and directly indicates blood vessel resistance.

Frequent blood pressure measurement is critical after serious injury, surgery, or anesthesia and during an illness or condition that threatens cardiovascular stability. (Frequent measurement may be done with an automated vital signs monitor.) Regular measurement is indicated for patients with a history of hypertension or hypotension, and yearly screening is recommended for all adults.

Equipment

Mercury or aneroid sphygmomanometer ◆ stethoscope ◆ alcohol pad ◆ automated vital signs monitor (if available).

The sphygmomanometer consists of an inflatable compression cuff linked to a manual air pump and a mercury manometer or an aneroid gauge. The mercury sphygmomanometer is recommended because it's more accurate and requires calibration less frequently than the aneroid model. **CS1** However, a recently calibrated aneroid manometer may be used. To obtain an accurate reading from a mercury sphygmomanometer, you must rest its gauge on a level surface and view the meniscus at eye level; you can rest an aneroid gauge in any position but must view it directly from the front.

Cuffs come in sizes ranging from neonate to extra-large adult. Disposable cuffs and thigh cuffs are available.

The automated vital signs monitor is a noninvasive device that measures pulse rate, systolic and diastolic pressures, and mean arterial pressure at preset intervals. (See *Using an electronic vital signs monitor*.)

Implementation

▶ Confirm the patient's identity using two patient identifiers according to your facility's policy. **JC**
▶ Tell the patient that you're going to take his blood pressure.
▶ Have the patient rest for at least 5 minutes before measuring his blood pressure. Make sure that he hasn't had caffeine or smoked for at least 30 minutes.
▶ Carefully choose a cuff of appropriate size for the patient; the bladder should encircle at least 80% of the upper arm. An excessively narrow cuff may cause a false-high pressure reading; an excessively wide one, a false-low reading.
▶ If you aren't using your own stethoscope, disinfect the earpieces with an alcohol pad before placing them in your ears to avoid cross-contamination.
▶ The patient can lie supine or sit erect during blood pressure measurement. If the patient is sitting erect, make sure that he has both feet flat on the floor because crossing the legs may elevate blood pressure. His arm should be extended at heart level and be well supported. If the artery is below heart level, you may get a false-high reading. Make sure the patient is relaxed and comfortable when you take his blood pressure so it stays at its normal level. **CS2**

▶ Wrap the deflated cuff snugly around the upper arm. (See *Positioning the blood pressure cuff*, page 48.)
▶ If the arm is very large or misshapen and the conventional cuff won't fit properly, take a leg or forearm measurement.
▶ To obtain a thigh blood pressure, apply the appropriate-size cuff to the thigh, and auscultate the pulsations over the popliteal artery. To obtain a forearm blood pressure, apply the appropriate-size cuff to the forearm 5″ (12.7 cm) below the elbow.

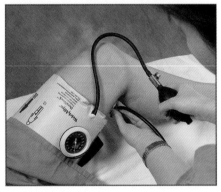

▶ If necessary, connect the appropriate tube to the rubber bulb of the air pump and the other tube to the manometer. Then insert the stethoscope earpieces into your ears.
▶ To determine how high to pump the blood pressure cuff, first estimate the systolic blood pressure by palpation. As you feel the radial artery with the fingers of one hand, inflate the cuff with

Using an electronic vital signs monitor

An electronic vital signs monitor allows you to track a patient's vital signs continually, without having to reapply a blood pressure cuff each time. In addition, the patient won't need an invasive arterial line to gather similar data.

Some automated vital signs monitors are lightweight and battery-operated and can be attached to an I.V. pole for continual monitoring, even during patient transfers. Some models can also display patient temperature and pulse oximetry as well as blood pressure. A built-in printer is also available on certain models. Make sure that you know the capacity of the monitor's battery, and plug the machine in whenever possible to keep it charged. Regularly calibrate the monitor to ensure accurate readings.

Before using any monitor, check its accuracy. Determine the patient's pulse rate and blood pressure manually, using the same arm you'll use for the monitor cuff. Compare your results when you get initial readings from the monitor. If the results differ, call your supply department or the manufacturer's representative.

Check the manufacturer's guidelines because most automated monitoring devices are intended for serial monitoring only and may be inaccurate for a onetime measurement. **MFR**

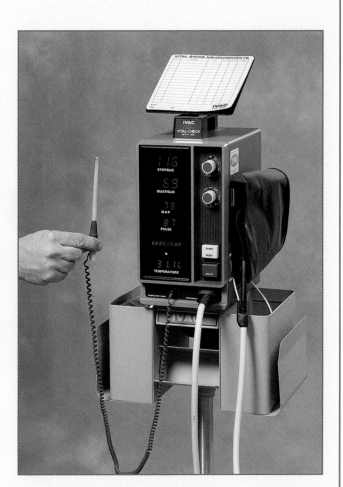

Preparing the device

▶ Explain the procedure to the patient. Describe the alarm system so he won't be frightened if it's triggered.
▶ Make sure that the power switch is off. Then plug the monitor into a properly grounded wall outlet. Secure the dual air hose to the front of the monitor.
▶ Connect the pressure cuff's tubing into the other ends of the dual air hose, and tighten the connections to prevent air leaks. Keep the air hose away from the patient to avoid accidental dislodgment.
▶ Squeeze all air from the cuff, and wrap the cuff loosely around the patient's arm—about 1″ (2.5 cm) above the antecubital fossa. Never apply the cuff to a limb that has an I.V. catheter in place. Position the cuff's "artery" arrow over the palpated brachial artery. Then secure the cuff for a snug fit.

Selecting parameters

▶ When you turn on the monitor, it will default to a manual mode. (In this mode, you can obtain vital signs yourself before switching to the automatic mode.) Press the AUTO/MANUAL button to select the automatic mode. The monitor will give you baseline data for the pulse rate, systolic and diastolic pressures, and mean arterial pressure.

▶ Compare your previous manual results with these baseline data. If they match, you're ready to set the alarm parameters. Press the SELECT button to blank out all displays except systolic pressure.
▶ Use the HIGH and LOW limit buttons to set the specific parameters for systolic pressure. (These limits range from a high of 240 to a low of 0.) You'll also do this three more times for mean arterial pressure, pulse rate, and diastolic pressure. After you've set the parameters for diastolic pressure, press the SELECT button again to display all current data. Even if you forget to do this last step, the monitor will automatically display current data 10 seconds after you set the last parameters. **JC**

Collecting data

▶ You also need to tell the monitor how often to obtain data. Press the SET button until you reach the desired time interval in minutes. If you've chosen the automatic mode,

(continued)

Using an electronic vital signs monitor (continued)

the monitor will display a default cycle time of 3 minutes. You can override the default cycle time to set the interval you prefer.

▶ You can obtain a set of vital signs at any time by pressing the START button. Also, pressing the CANCEL button will stop the interval and deflate the cuff. You can retrieve stored data by pressing the PRIOR DATA button. The monitor will display the last data obtained along with the time elapsed since then. Scrolling backward, you can retrieve data from the previous 99 minutes. Make sure that the patient's vital signs are documented frequently on a vital signs assessment sheet.

your other hand until the radial pulse disappears. Read this pressure on the manometer, and add 30 mm Hg to it. Use this sum as the target inflation to prevent discomfort from overinflation. Deflate the cuff and wait at least 2 minutes.

▶ Locate the brachial artery by palpation. Center the diaphragm or bell of the stethoscope over the part of the artery where you detect the strongest beats, and hold it in place with one hand. The bell of the stethoscope transmits low-pitched arterial blood sounds more effectively than the diaphragm.

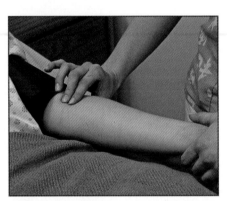

▶ Using the thumb and index finger of your other hand, turn the thumbscrew on the rubber bulb of the air pump clockwise to close the valve.

▶ Pump up the cuff to the predetermined level.

▶ Carefully open the valve of the air pump, and then slowly deflate the cuff—no faster than 2 to 3 mm Hg per second. While releasing air, watch the mercury column or aneroid gauge and auscultate for the sound over the artery.

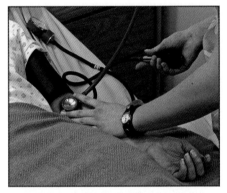

▶ When you hear the first beat or a clear tapping sound, note the pressure on the column or gauge. This is the systolic pressure. (The beat or tapping sound is the first of five Korotkoff sounds. The second sound resembles a murmur or swish; the third sound, crisp tapping; the fourth sound, a soft, muffled tone; and the fifth, the last sound heard.)

▶ Continue to release air gradually while auscultating for the sound over the artery.

▶ Note the pressure where the sound disappears. This is the diastolic pressure—the fifth Korotkoff sound.

▶ After you hear the last Korotkoff sound, deflate the cuff slowly for at least another 10 mm Hg to ensure that no further sounds are audible.

Positioning the blood pressure cuff

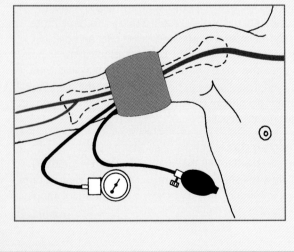

Palpate the brachial artery. Position the cuff 1″ (2.5 cm) above the site of pulsation, center the bladder above the artery with the cuff fully deflated, and wrap the cuff evenly and snugly around the upper arm.

▶ Rapidly deflate the cuff. Record the pressure, wait 2 minutes, and then repeat the procedure. If the average of the readings is greater than 5 mm Hg, take the average of two more readings. After doing so, remove and fold the cuff and return it to storage. **AHA**

▶ Document the blood pressure results.

Special considerations

▶ If you can't auscultate blood pressure, you may estimate systolic pressure. To do this, first palpate the brachial or radial pulse. Then inflate the cuff until you no longer detect the pulse. Slowly deflate the cuff and, when you detect the pulse again, record the pressure as the palpated systolic pressure.

▶ Palpation of systolic blood pressure may also be important to avoid underestimating blood pressure in patients with an auscultatory gap. This gap is a loss of sound between the first and second Korotkoff sounds that may be as great as 40 mm Hg. You may find this in patients with venous congestion or hypotension.

▶ Another alternative to auscultating with a stethoscope is to use Doppler ultrasound to hear Korotkoff sounds. This is useful when the blood pressure is diminished or when the pulse is nonpalpable.

▶ If the patient is crying or anxious, delay blood pressure measurement, if possible, until he becomes calm, to avoid falsely elevated readings.

▶ Remember that malfunction in an aneroid sphygmomanometer can be identified only by checking it against a mercury manometer of known accuracy. Be sure to check your aneroid manometer this way periodically. Malfunction in a mercury manometer is evident in abnormal behavior of the mercury column. Don't attempt to repair either type yourself; instead, send it to the appropriate service department.

▶ Occasionally, blood pressure must be measured in both arms or with the patient in two different positions (such as lying and standing or sitting and standing). In such cases, observe and record a significant difference between the two readings and record blood pressure and the extremity and position used.

▶ Measure the blood pressure of a patient taking antihypertensive medication while he's sitting to ensure accurate measurements.

▶ Don't take blood pressure in the arm on the affected side of a mastectomy patient because it may decrease already compromised lymphatic circulation, worsen edema, and damage the arm. Likewise, don't take blood pressure on an arm with an arteriovenous fistula or hemodialysis shunt because blood flow through the vascular device may be compromised.

References

Craven, R.F., and Hirnle, C.J. *Fundamentals of Nursing: Human Health and Function,* 6th ed. Philadelphia: Lippincott Williams & Wilkins, 2009.

Eser, I. "The Effect of Different Body Positions on Blood Pressure," *Journal of Clinical Nursing* 16(1):137-40, January 2007.

Keele-Smith, R., and Price-Daniel, C. "Effects of Crossing Legs on Blood Pressure Measurement," *Clinical Nursing Research* 10(2):202-13, May 2001. **CS2**

O'Rourke, M.F., and Seward, J.B. "Central Arterial Pressure and Arterial Pressure Pulse: New Views Entering the Second Century after Korotkoff," *Mayo Clinic Proceedings* 81(8):1057-68, August 2006.

Schell, K.A. "Evidence-based Practice: Noninvasive Blood Pressure Measurement in Children," *Pediatric Nursing* 32(3):263-67, May-June 2006.

The Seventh Report of the Joint National Committee on Prevention, Detection, and Treatment of High Blood Pressure. NIH Publication No. 03-5233. Bethesda, Md.: National Institutes of Health; National Heart, Lung, and Blood Institute; National High Blood Pressure Education Program. December 2003. Available at *www.nhlbi.nih.gov/guidelines/hypertension/express.pdf.* **CS1**

Body mechanics

Body mechanics is the term used to describe the efficient, coordinated, and safe use of muscle groups to maintain balance, reduce fatigue, reduce energy requirements, and decrease the risk of injury while moving objects and carrying out activities of daily living. It involves the concepts of center of gravity, line of gravity, and base of support in relation to body alignment and balance.

The best practice for body mechanics can be summed up in three principles. First, keep a low center of gravity by flexing the hips and knees instead of bending at the waist. This position distributes weight evenly between the upper and lower body, helps maintain balance, and decreases the load on the back muscles by transferring the weight to the stronger leg muscles. Second, create a wide base of support by spreading the feet apart. This tactic provides lateral stability and lowers the body's center of gravity. Finally, maintain proper body alignment—spine straight, head in neutral position, and all extremities in functional position—and keep the center of gravity directly over the base of support by moving the feet rather than twisting and bending at the waist.

Many patient care activities require the nurse to push, pull, lift, and carry. Application of proper body mechanics enables her to use the appropriate muscle groups when performing nursing care and can prevent musculoskeletal injury and fatigue and reduce the risk of injuring patients.

Implementation

Follow the directions below to push, pull, stoop, lift, and carry correctly.

Pushing and pulling correctly

▶ Stand close to the object, and place one foot slightly ahead of the other, as in a walking position. Tighten the leg muscles and set the pelvis by simultaneously contracting the abdominal and gluteal muscles.

▶ To push, place your hands on the object and flex your elbows. Lean into the object by shifting weight from the back leg to the front leg, and apply smooth, continuous pressure, using your leg muscles (as shown at right).

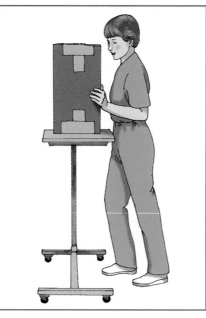

▶ To pull, grasp the object and flex your elbows. Lean away from the object by shifting weight from the front leg to the back leg. Pull smoothly, avoiding sudden, jerky movements.

▶ After you've started to move the object, keep it in motion; stopping and starting uses more energy.

Stooping correctly

▶ Stand with your feet 10″ to 12″ (25 to 30.5 cm) apart and with one foot slightly ahead of the other to widen the base of support.

▶ Lower yourself by flexing your knees, and place more weight on the front foot than on the back foot. Keep the upper body straight by not bending at the waist (as shown below).

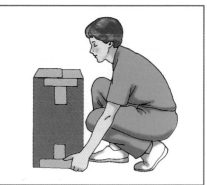

▶ To stand up again, straighten the knees and keep the back straight.

Lifting and carrying correctly

▶ Assume the stooping position directly in front of the object to minimize back flexion and avoid spinal rotation when lifting.

▶ Grasp the object, and tighten your abdominal muscles.

▶ Stand up by straightening the knees, using the leg and hip muscles. Always keep your back straight to maintain a fixed center of gravity (as shown below).

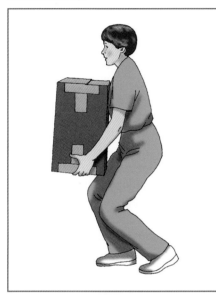

▶ Carry the object close to your body at waist height—near the body's center of gravity—to avoid straining the back muscles.

Special considerations

▶ Wear shoes with low heels, flexible nonslip soles, and closed backs to promote correct body alignment, facilitate proper body mechanics, and prevent accidents.

▶ When possible, pull rather than push an object because the elbow flexors are stronger than the extensors. Pulling an object allows the use of hip and leg muscles and avoids the use of lower back muscles.

▶ When doing heavy lifting or moving, remember to use assistive or mechanical devices, if available, or obtain assistance from coworkers; know your limitations and use sound judgment.

▶ Mechanical and other assistive devices have been shown to significantly decrease incidences of lower back injury in nursing personnel. **CS1** **CS2**

References

Collins, J., and Owen, B. "NIOSH Research Initiatives to Prevent Back Injuries to Nursing Assistants, Aides, and Orderlies in Nursing Homes," *American Journal of Industrial Medicine* 29(4):421-24, April 1996. **CS1**

Craven, R.F., and Hirnle, C.J. *Fundamentals of Nursing: Human Health and Function,* 6th ed. Philadelphia: Lippincott Williams & Wilkins, 2009.

Nelson, A., and Baptiste, A.S. "Evidence-based Practices for Safe Patient Handling and Movement," *Online Journal of Issues in Nursing* 9(3):4, September 2004.

Pellino, T.A., et al. "The Evaluation of Mechanical Devices for Lateral Transfers on Perceived Exertion and Patient Comfort," *Orthopaedic Nursing* 25(1): 4-10, January-February 2006.

Viera, E.R., et al. "Low Back Problems and Possible Improvements in Nursing Jobs," *Journal for Advanced Nursing* 55(1):79-89, July 2006. **CS2**

Bone marrow aspiration and biopsy

A specimen of bone marrow—the major site of blood cell formation—may be obtained by aspiration or needle biopsy. The procedure allows evaluation of overall blood composition by studying blood elements and precursor cells as well as abnormal or malignant cells. (See *Obtaining a bone marrow specimen.*) Both procedures are usually performed by a physician, but some facilities authorize specially trained chemotherapy nurses or nurse clinicians to perform them with an assistant.

Aspiration aids in diagnosing various disorders and cancers, such as oat cell carcinoma, leukemia, and lymphomas such as Hodgkin's disease. Biopsy is commonly performed simultaneously to stage the disease and monitor response to treatment. Bone marrow biopsy is contraindicated in patients with severe bleeding disorders.

Equipment

For aspiration: Mask ◆ gown ◆ nonsterile gloves ◆ prepackaged bone marrow set, which includes antiseptic pads ◆ two sterile drapes (one fenestrated, one plain) ◆ ten 4″ × 4″ gauze pads ◆ ten 2″ × 2″ gauze pads ◆ two 12-ml syringes ◆ 22G 1″ or 2″ needle ◆ scalpel ◆ sedative ◆ specimen containers ◆ bone marrow needle ◆ 70% isopropyl alcohol ◆ 1% lidocaine (unopened bottle) ◆ 26G or 27G ½″ or ⅝″ needle ◆ adhesive tape ◆ sterile gloves ◆ glass slides and coverglass ◆ labels and laboratory biohazard transport bags.

For biopsy: All equipment listed above ◆ biopsy needle ◆ Zenker's fixative.

Implementation

▶ Confirm the patient's identity using two patient identifiers according to your facility's policy. **JC**
▶ Tell the patient that the physician will collect a bone marrow specimen, and explain the procedure to ease his anxiety and ensure cooperation. Make sure the patient or a responsible family member understands the procedure and signs a consent form obtained by the practitioner.
▶ Inform the patient that the procedure normally takes about 20 minutes, that test results usually are available in 1 to 3 days, and that more than one marrow specimen may be required.
▶ Check the patient's history for hypersensitivity to the local anesthetic. Tell him which bone—sternum or posterior superior or anterior iliac crest—will be sampled. Inform him that he will receive a local anesthetic and will feel heavy pressure from insertion of the biopsy or aspiration needle as well as a brief, pulling sensation.
▶ If the patient has osteoporosis, tell him that the needle pressure may be minimal; if he has osteopetrosis, inform him that a drill may be needed.
▶ Provide a sedative, as ordered, before the test. **AORN**
▶ Position the patient according to the selected puncture site. (See *Common sites for bone marrow aspiration and biopsy,* page 54.)
▶ Label all medications, medication containers, and other solutions on and off the sterile field. **JC**
▶ Using sterile technique, the puncture site is cleaned with antiseptic pads and allowed to dry; then the area is draped.
▶ To anesthetize the site, the practitioner infiltrates it with 1% lidocaine, using a 26G or 27G ½″ or ⅝″ needle to inject a small amount intradermally and then a larger 22G 1″ or 2″ needle to anesthetize the tissue down to the bone.
▶ When the needle tip reaches the bone, the practitioner anesthetizes the periosteum by injecting a small amount of lidocaine in a circular area about ¾″ (2 cm) in diameter. The needle should be withdrawn from the periosteum after each injection.
▶ After allowing about 1 minute for the lidocaine to take effect, a scalpel may be used to make a small stab incision in the patient's skin to accommodate the bone marrow needle.

Bone marrow aspiration

▶ The practitoner inserts the bone marrow needle and lodges it firmly in the bone cortex. If the patient feels sharp pain instead of pressure when the needle first touches bone, the needle was probably inserted outside the anesthetized area. If this happens, the needle should be withdrawn slightly and moved to the anesthetized area.
▶ The needle is advanced by applying an even, downward force with the heel of the hand or the palm, while twisting it back and forth slightly. A crackling sensation means that the needle has entered the marrow cavity.
▶ Next, the practitoner removes the inner cannula, attaches the syringe to the needle, aspirates the required specimen, and withdraws the needle.

Obtaining a bone marrow specimen

Aspiration removes cells through a needle inserted into the marrow cavity of the bone; a biopsy removes a small, solid core of marrow tissue through the needle. The illustration below shows the removal of bone marrow from the posterior iliac crest.

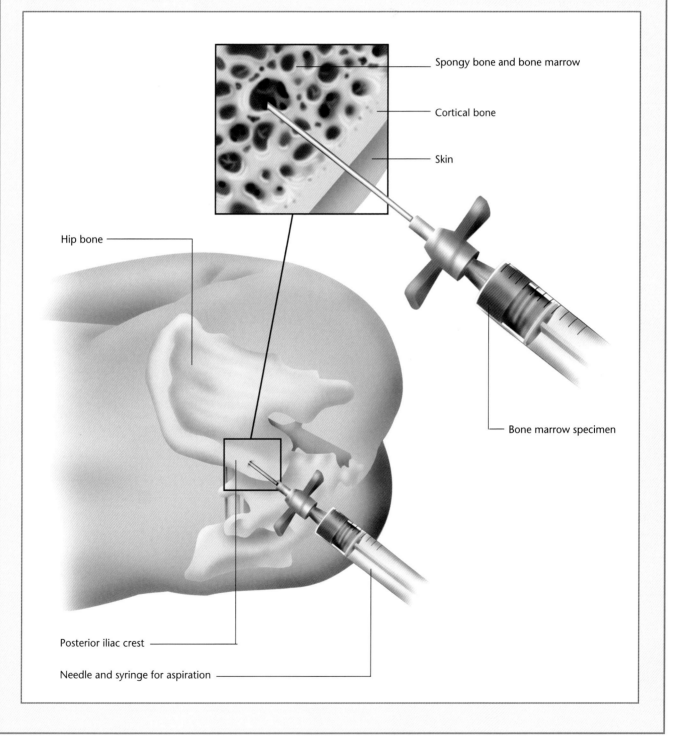

Spongy bone and bone marrow

Cortical bone

Skin

Bone marrow specimen

Hip bone

Posterior iliac crest

Needle and syringe for aspiration

Common sites for bone marrow aspiration and biopsy

The posterior superior iliac crest is the preferred site for bone marrow aspiration because no vital organs or vessels are nearby. The patient is placed either in the lateral position with one leg flexed or in the prone position. The anterior iliac crest may be used with a patient who can't lie in a prone position.

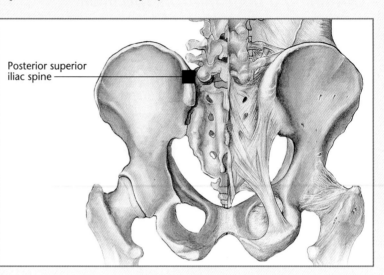

Posterior superior iliac spine

Aspiration from the sternum involves the greatest risk but may be used because the site is near the surface, the cortical bone is thin, and the marrow cavity contains numerous cells and relatively little fat or supporting bone. The patient is placed in a supine position. This site is seldom used for biopsy.

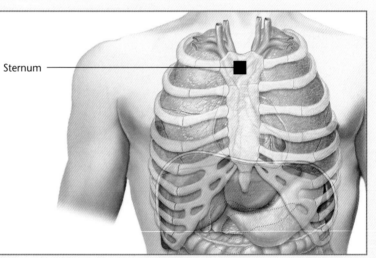

Sternum

The spinous process of the third or fourth lumbar vertebra is the preferred site if multiple punctures are necessary or if marrow is absent at other sites. The patient sits on the edge of the bed, leaning over the bedside stand.

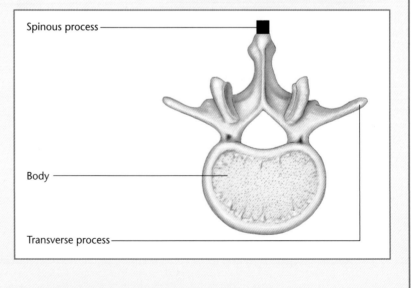

Spinous process

Body

Transverse process

▶ The nurse puts on gloves and applies pressure to the aspiration site with a gauze pad for 5 minutes to control bleeding while an assistant prepares the marrow slides. The area is then cleaned with alcohol to remove the antiseptic, the skin is dried thoroughly with a 4″ × 4″ gauze pad, and a sterile pressure dressing is applied. Specimens are labeled appropriately, placed in laboratory biohazard transport bags, and sent to the laboratory.

Bone marrow biopsy

▶ The practitioner inserts the biopsy needle into the periosteum and advances it steadily until the outer needle passes into the marrow cavity.

▶ The biopsy needle is directed into the marrow cavity by alternately rotating the inner needle clockwise and counterclockwise. Then a plug of tissue is removed, the needle assembly is withdrawn, and the marrow specimen is expelled into a properly labeled specimen bottle containing Zenker's fixative or formaldehyde. It's then placed in the laboratory biohazard transport bag and sent to the laboratory.

▶ The nurse puts on gloves, cleans the area around the biopsy site with alcohol to remove the antiseptic solution, firmly presses a sterile 2″ × 2″ gauze pad against the incision to control bleeding, and applies a sterile pressure dressing.

Special considerations

▶ Faulty needle placement may yield too little aspirate. If no specimen is produced, the needle must be withdrawn from the bone (but not from the overlying soft tissue), the stylet replaced, and the needle inserted into a second site within the anesthetized field.

▶ Bone marrow specimens shouldn't be collected from irradiated areas because radiation may have altered or destroyed the marrow.

▶ Bleeding and infection are potentially life-threatening complications of aspiration or biopsy at any site.

▶ Complications of sternal needle puncture are uncommon but include puncture of the heart and major vessels, causing severe hemorrhage; puncture of the mediastinum, causing mediastinitis or pneumomediastinum; and puncture of the lung, causing pneumothorax.

References

Christensen, J., and Fatchett, D. "Promoting Parental Use of Distraction and Relaxation in Pediatric Oncology Patients during Invasive Procedures," *Journal of Pediatric Oncology Nursing* 19(4):127-32, July-August 2002.

Islam, A. "Bone Marrow Aspiration before Bone Marrow Core Biopsy Using the Same Bone Marrow Biopsy Needle: A Good or Bad Practice?" *Journal of Clinical Pathology* 60(2):212-15, February 2007.

Rushing, J. "Assisting with Bone Marrow Aspiration and Biopsy," *Nursing* 36(3):68, March 2006.

Buccal, sublingual, and translingual drugs

Certain drugs are given buccally, sublingually, or translingually to prevent their destruction or transformation in the stomach or small intestine. These drugs act quickly because the oral mucosa's thin epithelium and abundant vasculature allow direct absorption into the bloodstream.

Drugs given buccally include nitroglycerin and methyltestosterone; drugs given sublingually include ergotamine tartrate, isosorbide dinitrate, and nitroglycerin. Translingual drugs, which are sprayed onto the tongue, include nitrate preparations for patients with chronic angina.

Equipment

Patient's medication record and chart ◆ prescribed medication ◆ medication cup.

Implementation

▶ Verify the order on the patient's medication record by checking it against the practitioner's order on his chart. **JC** **ISMP**

▶ Wash your hands with warm water and soap. Explain the procedure to the patient if he's never taken a drug buccally, sublingually, or translingually before.

▶ Check the label on the medication before administering it to make sure you'll be giving the prescribed medication. Verify the expiration date of all medications, especially nitroglycerin. **JC** **ISMP**

▶ Confirm the patient's identity using two patient identifiers according to your facility's policy. **JC**

▶ If your facility utilizes a bar code scanning system, be sure to scan your ID badge, the patient's ID bracelet, and the medication's bar code. **JC** **ISMP**

Placing drugs in the oral mucosa

Buccal and sublingual administration routes allow some drugs, such as nitroglycerin and methyltestosterone, to enter the bloodstream rapidly without being degraded in the GI tract.

To give a drug buccally, insert it between the patient's cheek and teeth (as shown below). Ask her to close her mouth and hold the tablet against her cheek until the tablet is absorbed.

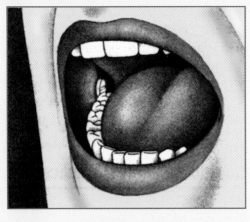

To give a drug sublingually, place it under the patient's tongue (as shown below) and ask her to leave it there until it dissolves.

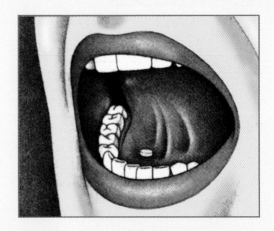

Buccal and sublingual administration

▶ For buccal administration, place the tablet in the buccal pouch, between the cheek and gum. For sublingual administration, place the tablet under the patient's tongue. (See *Placing drugs in the oral mucosa.*)

▶ Instruct the patient to keep the medication in place until it dissolves completely to ensure absorption.

▶ Caution him against chewing the tablet or touching it with his tongue to prevent accidental swallowing.

▶ If the patient smokes, tell him not to do so before the drug has dissolved because nicotine's vasoconstrictive effects slow absorption.

Translingual administration

▶ To administer a translingual drug, tell the patient to hold the medication canister vertically, with the valve head at the top and the spray orifice as close to his mouth as possible.

▶ Instruct him to spray the dose onto his tongue by pressing the button firmly.

▶ Remind the patient using a translingual aerosol form that he shouldn't inhale the spray but should release it under his tongue. Also tell him to wait 10 seconds or so before swallowing.

Special considerations

▶ Don't give liquids to a patient receiving buccal medication because some buccal tablets can take up to 1 hour to be absorbed. Tell the patient not to rinse his mouth until the tablet has been absorbed.

▶ Tell the angina patient to wet the nitroglycerin tablet with saliva and to keep it under his tongue until it has been fully absorbed.

▶ Alternate sides of the mouth for repeat doses to prevent continuous irritation of the same site.

References

Ferguson, A. "Administration of Oral Medication," *Nursing Times* 101(45):24-25, November 2005.

Finn, A., et al. "Bioavailability and Metabolism of Prochlorperazine Administered via the Buccal or Oral Delivery Route," *Journal of Clinical Pharmacology* 45(12):1383-390, December 2005.

The Joint Commission. *Comprehensive Accreditation Manual for Hospitals: The Official Handbook.* Standard MM.1.10. Oakbrook Terrace, Ill.: The Joint Commission, 2007.

The Joint Commission. *Comprehensive Accreditation Manual for Hospitals: The Official Handbook.* Standard MM.3.10. Oakbrook Terrace, Ill.: The Joint Commission, 2007.

The Joint Commission. *Comprehensive Accreditation Manual for Hospitals: The Official Handbook.* Standard MM.4.10. Oakbrook Terrace, Ill.: The Joint Commission, 2007.

The Joint Commission. *Comprehensive Accreditation Manual for Hospitals: The Official Handbook.* Standard MM.4.20. Oakbrook Terrace, Ill.: The Joint Commission, 2007.

The Joint Commission. *Comprehensive Accreditation Manual for Hospitals: The Official Handbook.* Standard MM.4.30. Oakbrook Terrace, Ill.: The Joint Commission, 2007.

The Joint Commission. *Comprehensive Accreditation Manual for Hospitals: The Official Handbook.* Standard MM.5.10. Oakbrook Terrace, Ill.: The Joint Commission, 2007.

The Joint Commission. *Comprehensive Accreditation Manual for Hospitals: The Official Handbook.* Standard MM.6.10. Oakbrook Terrace, Ill.: The Joint Commission, 2007.

The Joint Commission. *Comprehensive Accreditation Manual for Hospitals: The Official Handbook.* Standard MM.6.20. Oakbrook Terrace, Ill.: The Joint Commission, 2007.

The Joint Commission. *Comprehensive Accreditation Manual for Hospitals: The Official Handbook.* Standard MM.7.10. Oakbrook Terrace, Ill.: The Joint Commission, 2007.

Smart, J.D. "Buccal Drug Delivery," *Expert Opinion on Drug Delivery* 2(3):507-17, May 2005.

Taylor, C., et al. *Fundamentals of Nursing: The Art and Science of Nursing Care,* 6th ed. Philadelphia: Lippincott Williams & Wilkins, 2008.

Burn care

The goals of burn care are to maintain the patient's physiologic stability, repair skin integrity, prevent infection, and promote maximal functioning and psychosocial health. Competent care immediately after a burn occurs can dramatically improve the success of overall treatment.

All burn victims should be evaluated initially as trauma patients following the systematic approach developed by the American College of Surgeons Committee. The primary survey focuses mainly on maintaining the patient's airway, breathing, and circulation. When the burn is caused by a chemical agent, the priority is to remove the offending agent and institute water lavage to the affected area. The secondary survey focuses on a head-to-toe assessment, followed by efforts to stop the burn and extension of the injury. Specific elements of the survey should include burn severity, which is determined by the depth and extent of the burn; determination of a possible inhalation injury; and other factors, such as age, complications, coexisting illnesses, and the possibility of abuse. (See *Estimating burn surfaces in adults and children*. See also *Evaluating burn severity,* page 61.) **ACSC**

Early postburn positioning is extremely important to prevent contractures. Careful positioning and regular exercise for burned extremities help maintain joint function and minimize deformity. When the extremities aren't being exercised, they should be maintained in maximal extension, using splints, if necessary. Pay particular attention to the hands and neck because they're the most prone to rapid contracture. **ABA**

Skin integrity is repaired through aggressive wound debridement, followed by maintenance of a clean wound bed until the wound heals or is covered with a skin graft.

Early excision and debridement of the wound in the first 48 hours has been shown to decrease blood loss and reduce hospital stay; however, this procedure should be used only on wounds that are clearly full-thickness burns. Surgery takes place as soon as possible after fluid resuscitation. Most wounds are managed with twice-daily dressing changes using topical antibiotics. Burn dressings encourage healing by barring germ entry and by removing exudate, eschar, and other debris that host infection. After thorough wound cleaning, topical antibacterial agents are applied, and the wound is covered with absorptive, coarse mesh gauze. Roller gauze typically tops the dressing and is secured with elastic netting or tape.

Equipment

Normal saline solution ◆ bowl ◆ scissors ◆ tissue forceps ◆ ordered topical medication ◆ burn gauze ◆ roller gauze ◆ elastic netting or tape ◆ fine mesh gauze ◆ cotton-tipped applicators ◆ ordered pain medication ◆ three pairs of gloves ◆ cotton bath blanket ◆ 4″ × 4″ gauze pads ◆ gown ◆ mask ◆ surgical cap ◆ heat lamps ◆ impervious plastic trash bag.

A sterile field is required; all equipment and supplies used to clean and dress the wound should be sterile.

Implementation

▶ Confirm the patient's identity using two patient identifiers according to your facility's policy. **JC**

▶ Administer the ordered pain medication about 20 minutes before beginning wound care to maximize patient comfort and cooperation.

▶ Explain the procedure to the patient, and provide privacy.

▶ Warm normal saline solution by immersing unopened bottles in warm water.

▶ Assemble equipment on the dressing table. Make sure the treatment area has adequate light to allow accurate wound assessment.

▶ Open equipment packages using sterile technique. Arrange supplies on a sterile field in order of use.

▶ To prevent cross-contamination, plan to dress the cleanest areas first and the dirtiest or most contaminated areas last. To help prevent excessive pain or cross-contamination, you may need to perform the dressing in stages to avoid exposing all wounds at the same time.

▶ Turn on overhead heat lamps to keep the patient warm. Make sure they don't overheat the patient.

▶ Pour warmed normal saline solution into the sterile bowl in the sterile field.

▶ Wash your hands.

Removing a dressing without hydrotherapy

▶ Put on a gown, a mask, and sterile gloves. **CDC** **ABA**

▶ Remove dressing layers down to the innermost layer by cutting the outer dressings with sterile blunt scissors. Lay open the dressings.

▶ If the inner layer appears dry, soak it with warm normal saline solution to ease removal.

▶ Remove the inner dressing with sterile tissue forceps or your gloved hand.

▶ Because soiled dressings harbor infectious microorganisms, dispose of the dressings carefully in the impervious plastic trash bag according to your facility's policy. Dispose of your gloves, and wash your hands.

▶ Put on a new pair of sterile gloves. Using gauze pads moistened with normal saline solution, gently remove exudate and old topical medication.

Estimating burn surfaces in adults and children

You need to use different formulas to compute burned body surface area (BSA) in adults and children because the proportion of BSA varies with growth.

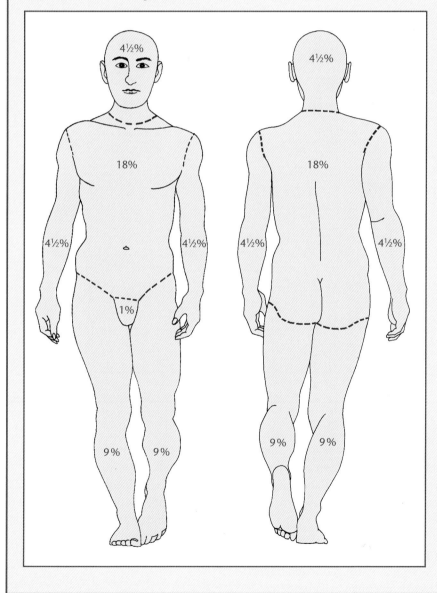

Rule of Nines

You can quickly estimate the extent of an adult patient's burn by using the "Rule of Nines." This method quantifies BSA in percentages either in fractions of nine or in multiples of nine. To use this method, mentally assess your patient's burns by the body chart shown at left. Add the corresponding percentages for each body section burned. Use the total—a rough estimate of burn extent—to calculate initial fluid replacement needs.

(continued)

Estimating burn surfaces in adults and children *(continued)*

Lund-Browder chart

The Rule of Nines isn't accurate for infants and children because their body shapes differ from those of adults. An infant's head, for example, accounts for about 17% of his total BSA, compared with 7% for an adult. Instead, use the Lund-Browder chart shown here.

	AT BIRTH	0 TO 1 YEAR	1 TO 4 YEARS	5 TO 9 YEARS	10 TO 15 YEARS	ADULT
A: Half of head						
	9½%	8½%	6½%	5½%	4½%	3½%
B: Half of one thigh						
	2¾%	3¼%	4%	4¼%	4½%	4¾%
C: Half of one leg						
	2½%	2½%	2¾%	3%	3¼%	3½%

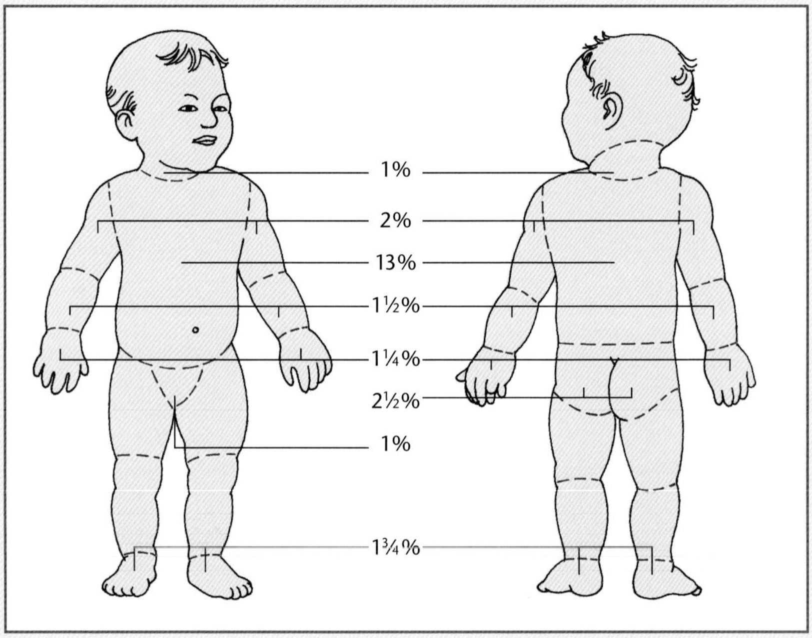

▶ Carefully remove all loose eschar with sterile forceps and scissors, if ordered. (See "Mechanical debridement," page 315.) **ABA**

▶ Assess wound condition. The wound should appear clean, with no debris, loose tissue, purulence, inflammation, or darkened margins.

▶ Before applying a new dressing, remove your gown, gloves, and mask. Discard them properly, and put on a clean mask, surgical cap, gown, and sterile gloves.

Applying a wet dressing

▶ Soak fine-mesh gauze and the elastic gauze dressing in a large sterile basin containing the ordered solution (for example, silver nitrate).

▶ Wring out the fine-mesh gauze until it's moist but not dripping, and apply it to the wound. Warn the patient that he may feel transient pain when you apply the dressing.

Evaluating burn severity ABA

To judge a burn's severity, assess its depth and extent as well as the presence of other factors.

Superficial partial-thickness burn

Does the burned area appear pink or red with minimal edema? Is the area sensitive to touch and temperature changes? If so, your patient most likely has a superficial partial-thickness, or first-degree, burn, affecting only the epidermal skin layer.

Deep partial-thickness burn

Does the burned area appear pink or red, with a mottled appearance? Do red areas blanch when you touch them? Does the skin have large, thick-walled blisters with subcutaneous edema? Does touching the burn cause severe pain? Is the hair still present? If so, your patient most likely has a deep partial-thickness, or second-degree, burn, affecting the epidermal and dermal layers.

Full-thickness burn

Does the burned area appear red, waxy white, brown, or black? Does red skin remain red with no blanching when you touch it? Is the skin leathery with extensive subcutaneous edema? Is the skin insensitive to touch? Does the hair fall out easily? If so, your patient most likely has a full-thickness, or third-degree, burn, affecting all skin layers.

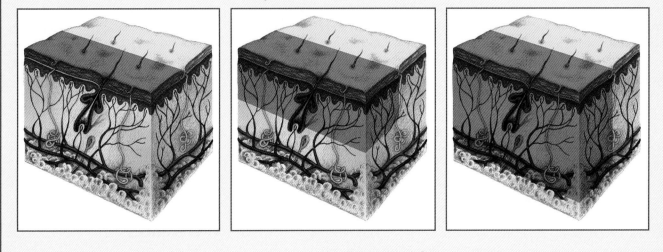

▶ Wring out the elastic gauze dressing, and position it to hold the fine-mesh gauze in place.

▶ Roll an elastic gauze dressing over these two dressings to keep them intact.

▶ Cover the patient with a cotton bath blanket to prevent chills. Change the blanket if it becomes damp. Use an overhead heat lamp, if necessary.

▶ Change the dressings frequently, as ordered, to keep the wound moist, especially if you're using silver nitrate. Silver nitrate becomes ineffective, and the silver ions may damage tissue, if the dressings become dry. (To maintain moisture, some protocols call for irrigating the dressing with solution at least every 4 hours through small slits cut into the outer dressing.) ABA

Applying a dry dressing with a topical medication

▶ Remove old dressings and clean the wound (as described previously).

▶ Apply the ordered medication to the wound in a thin layer (about 2 to 4 mm thick) with your sterile gloved hand. Then apply several layers of burn gauze over the wound to contain the medication but allow exudate to escape.

▶ Remember to cut the dry dressing to fit only the wound areas; don't cover unburned areas.

▶ Cover the entire dressing with roller gauze, and secure it with elastic netting or tape.

Providing arm and leg care

▶ Apply the dressings from the distal to the proximal area to stimulate circulation and prevent constriction. Wrap the burn gauze once around the arm or leg so the edges overlap slightly. Continue wrapping in this way until the gauze covers the wound. ABA

▶ Apply a dry roller gauze dressing to hold the bottom layers in place. Secure with elastic netting or tape.

Providing hand and foot care

▶ Wrap each finger separately with a single layer of a 4″ × 4″ sterile gauze pad to allow the patient to use his hands and to prevent webbing contractures.

▶ Place the hand in a functional position, and secure this position using a dressing. Apply splints, if ordered.

▶ Put gauze between each toe, as appropriate, to prevent webbing contractures.

Providing chest, abdomen, and back care

▶ Apply the ordered medication to the wound in a thin layer. Then cover the entire burned area with sheets of burn gauze.

▶ Wrap the area with roller gauze or apply a specialty vest dressing to hold the burn gauze in place.

▶ Secure the dressing with elastic netting or tape. Make sure the dressing doesn't restrict respiratory motion, especially in very young or elderly patients or in those with circumferential injuries.

Providing facial care

▶ If the patient has scalp burns, clip the hair around the burn, as ordered. Clip other hair until it's about 2″ (5 cm) long to prevent contamination of burned scalp areas.

▶ Shave facial hair if it comes in contact with burned areas.

▶ Typically, facial burns are managed with milder topical agents (such as triple antibiotic ointment) and are left open to air. If dressings are required, make sure they don't cover the eyes, nostrils, or mouth.

Providing ear care

▶ Clip hair around the affected ear.

▶ Remove exudate and crusts with cotton-tipped applicators dipped in normal saline solution.

▶ Place a 4″ × 4″ layer of gauze behind the auricle to prevent webbing.

▶ Apply the ordered medication to 4″ × 4″ gauze pads, and place the pads over the burned area. Before securing the dressing with a roller bandage, position the patient's ears normally to avoid damaging the auricular cartilage. **ABA**

▶ Assess patient's hearing ability. **ABA**

Providing eye care

▶ Clean the eye and eyelid area with a cotton-tipped applicator and normal saline solution every 4 to 6 hours, or as needed, to remove crusts and drainage.

▶ Administer ordered eye ointments or drops.

▶ If the eyes can't be closed, apply lubricating ointments or drops, as ordered.

▶ Be sure to close the patient's eyes before applying eye pads to prevent corneal abrasion.

Providing nasal care

▶ Check the nostrils for inhalation injury: inflamed mucosa, singed vibrissae, and soot.

▶ Clean the nostrils with cotton-tipped applicators dipped in normal saline solution. Remove crusts.

▶ Apply the ordered ointments.

▶ If the patient has a nasogastric tube, use tracheostomy ties to secure the tube. Be sure to check the ties frequently for tightness resulting from swelling of facial tissue. Clean the area around the tube every 4 to 6 hours. **ABA**

Special considerations

▶ Thorough assessment and documentation of the wound's appearance are essential to detect infection and other complications. A purulent wound or green-gray exudate indicates infection, an overly dry wound suggests dehydration, and a wound with a swollen, red edge suggests cellulitis. Suspect a fungal infection if the wound is white and powdery. Healthy granulation tissue appears clean, pinkish, faintly shiny, and free from exudate.

▶ Because blisters protect underlying tissue, leave them intact unless they impede joint motion, become infected, or cause patient discomfort.

▶ Keep in mind that the patient with healing burns has increased nutritional needs. He'll require extra protein and carbohydrates to accommodate an almost doubled basal metabolism.

▶ If you must manage a burn with topical medications, exposure to air, and no dressing, watch for such problems as wound adherence to bed linens, poor drainage control, and partial loss of topical medications.

References

ABA. "Practice Guidelines for Burn Care," *Journal of Burn Care and Rehabilitation* 22(3 Suppl), May-June 2001.

Hemington-Gorse, S.J. "Colloid or Crystalloid for Resuscitation of Major Burns," *Journal of Wound Care* 14(6):256-58, June 2005.

Lipley, N. "New Guidelines for Managing Patients with Burns," *Emergency Nurse* 14(10):3, March 2007.

Mendez-Eastman, S. "Burn Injuries," *Plastic Surgical Nursing* 25(3):133-39, July-September 2005.

Tenqvall, O.M., et al. "Differences in Pain Patterns for Infected and Non-infected Patients with Burn Injuries," *Pain Management Nursing* 7(4):176-82, December 2006.

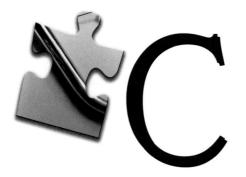

C

Canes

Indicated for the patient with one-sided weakness or injury, occasional loss of balance, or increased joint pressure, a cane provides balance and support for walking and reduces fatigue and strain on weight-bearing joints. Available in various sizes, the cane should extend from the greater trochanter to the floor and have a rubber tip to prevent slipping. Canes are contraindicated for the patient with bilateral weakness—such a patient should use crutches or a walker.

Equipment

Rubber-tipped cane ◆ optional: walking belt.

Although wooden canes are available, three types of aluminum canes are used most frequently. The standard aluminum cane (used by the patient who needs only slight assistance with walking) provides the least support; its half-circle handle allows it to be hooked over chairs. The T-handle cane (used by the patient with hand weakness) has a straight-shaped handle with grips and a bent shaft. It provides greater stability than the standard cane. Three- or four-pronged (quad) canes are used by the patient with poor balance or one-sided weakness and an inability to hold onto a walker with both hands. The base of these types of canes splits into three or four short, splayed legs and provides greater stability than a standard cane but considerably less than a walker.

Implementation

▶ Explain the mechanics of cane walking to the patient. Demonstrate the technique; then have the patient return the demonstration. Coordinate practice sessions in the physical therapy department, if necessary.
▶ Ask the patient to hold the cane on the uninvolved side 6″ (15 cm) from the base of the little toe. Adjust the height until the handle of the cane is level with the greater trochanter and allows about 30-degree flexion at the elbow.
▶ Tell the patient to hold the cane on the uninvolved side to promote a reciprocal gait pattern and to distribute weight away from the involved side.
▶ Instruct the patient to hold the cane close to his body to prevent leaning and to simultaneously move the cane and the involved leg forward 4″ to 8″ (10 to 20 cm), followed by the uninvolved leg.
▶ Encourage the patient to keep the stride length of each leg and the timing of each step (cadence) equal.

Negotiating stairs
▶ Instruct the patient to always use a railing, if present, when going up or down stairs. Tell him to hold the cane with the other hand or to keep it in the hand grasping the railing. To ascend stairs, the patient should lead with the uninvolved leg and follow with the involved leg; to descend, he should lead with the involved leg and follow with the uninvolved leg. Help the patient remember by telling him to use this mnemonic device: "The good goes up; the bad goes down."

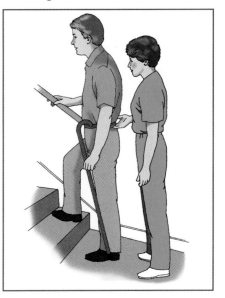

▶ To negotiate stairs without a railing, the patient should use the walking technique to ascend and descend the stairs, but should move the cane just before the involved leg. Thus, to ascend stairs, the patient should hold the cane on the uninvolved side, step with the uninvolved leg, advance the cane, and then move the involved leg. To descend, he should hold the cane on the uninvolved side, lead with the cane, advance the involved leg, and then, finally, move the uninvolved leg.

Using a chair

▶ To teach the patient to sit down, stand by his affected side, and tell him to place the backs of his legs against the edge of the chair seat. Then tell him to move the cane out from his side and to reach back with both hands to grasp the chair's armrests. Supporting his weight on the armrests, he can then lower himself onto the seat. While he's seated, he should keep the cane hooked on the armrest or the chair.

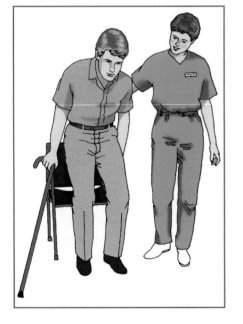

▶ To teach the patient to get up, stand by his affected side, and tell him to unhook the cane from the chair and hold it in his stronger hand as he grasps the armrests. Then tell him to move his uninvolved foot slightly forward, to lean slightly forward, and to push against the armrests to raise himself upright.

▶ Instruct the patient not to lean on the cane when sitting or rising from the chair to prevent falls.

▶ Supervise the patient each time he gets in or out of a chair until you're both certain he can do it alone.

Special considerations

To prevent falls during the learning period, guard the patient carefully by standing behind him slightly to his stronger side and putting one foot between his feet and your other foot to the outside of the uninvolved leg. If necessary, use a walking belt.

References

Bateni, H., and Maki, B.E. "Assistive Devices for Balance and Mobility: Benefits, Demands, and Adverse Consequences," *Archives of Physical Medicine and Rehabilitation* 86(1):134-45, January 2005.

Craven, R.F., and Hirnle, C.J. *Fundamentals of Nursing Human Health and Function,* 6th ed. Philadelphia: Lippincott Williams & Wilkins, 2009.

Mincer, A.B. "Assistive Devices for the Adult Patient with Orthopedic Dysfunction. Why Physical Therapists Choose What They Do," *Orthopaedic Nursing* 26(4):226-31, July-August 2007.

Youdas, J.W., et al. "Partial Weight-Bearing Gait using Conventional Assistive Devices," *Archives of Physical Medicine and Rehabilitation* 86(3):394-98, March 2005.

Cardiac monitoring

Because it allows continuous observation of the heart's electrical activity, cardiac monitoring is used in patients with conduction disturbances and in those at risk for life-threatening arrhythmias. Like other forms of electrocardiography, cardiac monitoring uses electrodes placed on the patient's chest to transmit electrical signals that are converted into a tracing of cardiac rhythm on an oscilloscope.

Two types of monitoring may be performed: hardwire or telemetry. In *hardwire monitoring,* the patient is connected to a monitor at the bedside. The rhythm display appears at bedside, but it may also be transmitted to a console at a remote location. *Telemetry* uses a small transmitter connected to the ambulatory patient to send electrical signals to another location, where they're displayed on a monitor screen. Cardiac monitors can display the patient's heart rate and rhythm, produce a printed record of cardiac rhythm, and sound an alarm if the heart rate exceeds or falls below specified limits. Monitors also recognize and count abnormal heartbeats as well as changes. The lead that you should select to monitor the patient depends on what area of the heart you want to monitor. **AACN** (See *Lead selection.*)

Equipment

For hardwire monitoring: Cardiac monitor ◆ leadwires ◆ patient cable ◆ disposable pregelled electrodes (number of electrodes varies from three to five, depending on the monitoring system) ◆ 4″ × 4″ gauze pads ◆ washcloth ◆ optional: clippers, alcohol pads.

For telemetry monitoring: Transmitter ◆ transmitter pouch ◆ telemetry battery pack, leads, and electrodes.

Implementation

▶ Confirm the patient's identity using two patient identifiers according to your facility's policy. **JC**

For hardwire monitoring

▶ Plug the cardiac monitor into an electrical outlet and turn it on to warm up the unit while you prepare the equipment and the patient.

▶ Insert the cable into the appropriate socket in the monitor. Connect the leadwires to the cable, if necessary. Each leadwire should indicate the location for attachment to the patient: right arm (RA), left arm (LA), right leg (RL), left leg (LL), and ground (C or G).

Lead selection

Your patient's clinical condition determines the leads you'll monitor. Note: If the monitor can detect arrhythmias, know which leads perform this function. Even if you don't continuously monitor these leads, periodically check the quality of their waveforms because the arrhythmia detection algorithm will fail without adequate waveforms.

CLINICAL CONCERN	LEAD
Bundle-branch block	V_1 or V_6
Ischemia based on the area of infarction or site of percutaneous coronary intervention	
Anterior	V_3, V_4
Septal	V_1, V_2
Lateral	I, aV_L, V_5, V_6
Inferior	II, III, aV_F
Right ventricle	V_{4R}
Junctional rhythm with retrograde P waves	II
Optimal view of atrial activity	I, II, or Lewis lead
Ventricular ectopy, wide complex tachycardia	V_1 (may use V_6 along with V_1)
Ventricular pacing	V_1 or II

▶ Explain the procedure to the patient, provide privacy, and ask the patient to expose his chest. Wash your hands.

▶ Determine electrode positions on the patient's chest, based on which system and lead you're using. (See *Positioning monitoring leads*.)

▶ If necessary, clip the hair from an area about 4″ (10 cm) in diameter around each electrode site. Clean the area with soap and water and dry it.

Positioning monitoring leads

This chart shows the correct electrode positions for some of the monitoring leads you'll use most often. For each lead, you'll see electrode placement for a five-leadwire system, a three-leadwire system, and a telemetry system.

In the two hardwire systems, the electrode positions for one lead may be identical to the electrode positions for another lead. In this case, you simply change the lead selector switch to the setting that corresponds to the lead you want. In some cases, you'll need to reposition the electrodes.

In the telemetry system, you can create the same lead with two electrodes that you do with three, simply by eliminating the ground electrode.

These illustrations use these abbreviations: RA, right arm; LA, left arm; RL, right leg; LL, left leg; C, chest; and G, ground.

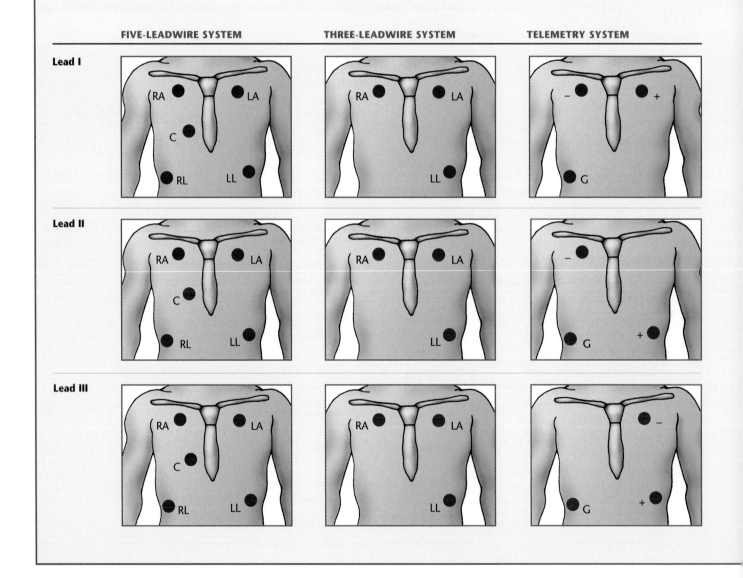

An alcohol pad may be used to completely to remove skin secretions that may interfere with electrode function. Gently abrade the dried area by rubbing it briskly until it reddens to remove dead skin cells and to promote better electrical contact with living cells. (Some electrodes have a small, rough patch for abrading the skin; otherwise, use a dry washcloth or a dry gauze pad.) CDC MFR AACN

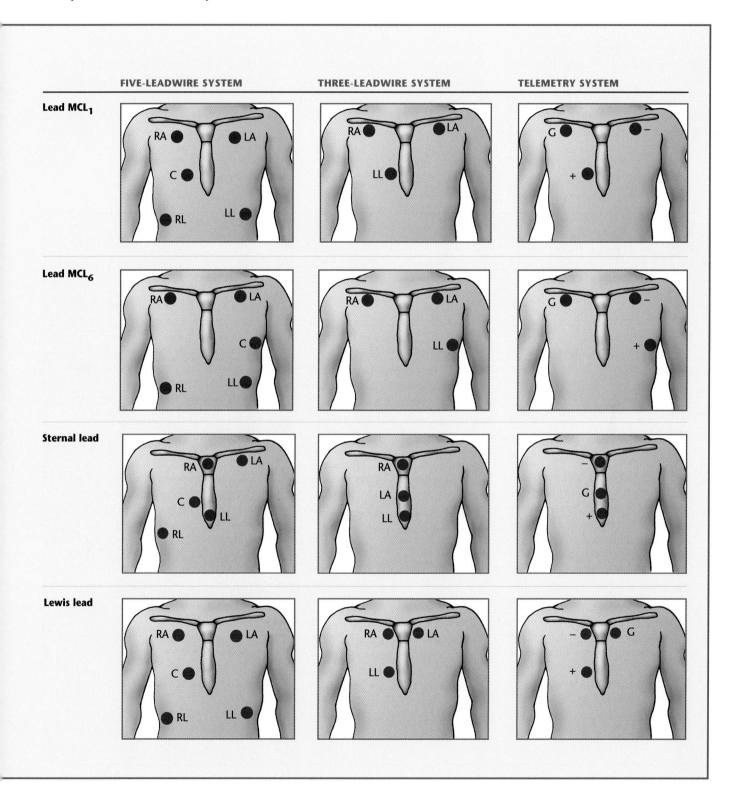

▶ Remove the backing from the pregelled electrode. Check the gel for moistness. If the gel is dry, discard it, and replace it with a fresh electrode.

▶ Attach the leadwires to the electrodes, then apply the electrode to the site, and press firmly to ensure a tight seal. Repeat with the remaining electrodes.

▶ When all the electrodes are in place, check for a tracing on the cardiac monitor. Assess the quality of the electrocardiogram (ECG).

▶ To verify that each beat is being detected by the monitor, compare the digital heart rate display with your count of the patient's heart rate.

▶ If necessary, use the gain control to adjust the size of the rhythm tracing, and use the position control to adjust the waveform position on the recording paper.

▶ Set the upper and lower limits of the heart rate alarm, based on unit policy. Turn the alarm on. **JC**

For telemetry monitoring

▶ Wash your hands. Explain the procedure to the patient, and provide privacy.

▶ Insert a new battery into the transmitter. By pressing the button at the top of the unit, test the battery's charge, and test the unit to ensure that the battery is operational. If the leadwires aren't permanently affixed to the telemetry unit, attach them securely. If they must be attached individually, be

EVIDENCE-BASED RESEARCH

Effectiveness of Clinical Alarms

Korniewicz, D., Clark, T., and David, Y. "A national online survey on the effectiveness of clinical alarms," *American Journal of Critical Care* 17(1):36-41, January 2008.

Level VI
Evidence from a single descriptive or qualitative study

Description
Alarms on clinical devices are to call to the attention of caregivers conditions of patients or devices that deviate from a predetermined normal status. The Joint Commission has accreditation requirements related to clinical alarms and patient safety. The American College of Clinical Engineers formed a foundation in 2002 and made addressing the issue of clinical alarms as one of its major initiatives. An online survey was developed to determine the reasons health care workers don't respond to clinical alarms. The survey was implemented online from August 15, 2005 until January 15, 2006.

Findings
A total of 1,327 persons responded to the survey; 94% worked in acute care hospitals. About 51% of the respondents were registered nurses, and 31% of respondents worked in a critical care unit. More than 90% agreed or strongly agreed with the statements covering the purpose of clinical alarms and the need for prioritized and easily differentiated audible and visual alarms. Likewise, many respondents identified nuisance alarms as problematic. Most (81%) agreed or strongly agreed that the alarms occur frequently, disrupt patient care (77%), and can reduce trust in alarms and cause caregivers to disable them (78%).

Conclusions
Effective management of clinical alarms relies on equipment designs that promote appropriate use, clinicians who actively learn how to use equipment safely, and hospitals that recognize the complexities of managing clinical alarms and devote the necessary resources to develop effective management schemes.

Nursing practice implications
Nurses continuously monitor patients' conditions. They are often the first line of defense for safety in the hospital environment. These practices are important:

▶ Make daily rounds to monitor safety of clinical alarms.

▶ Assure that devices have been configured to minimize nuisance alarms.

▶ Actively learn how to use equipment safely.

▶ Discuss adverse events associated with clinical alarms on a regular basis and develop action plans.

▶ Conduct an annual review of data associated with nuisance and nonnuisance clinical alarms

▶ Educate staff on proper use of clinical alarms.

sure to connect each one to the correct outlet. **MFR**

▶ Apply the electrode to the appropriate site by pressing one side of the electrode against the patient's skin, pulling gently, and then pressing the other side against the skin. Press your fingers in a circular motion around the electrode to fix the gel and stabilize the electrode. Repeat for each electrode.

▶ Attach an electrode to the end of each leadwire.

▶ Expose the patient's chest, and select the lead arrangement. Remove the backing from one of the gelled electrodes. Check the gel for moistness. If it's dry, discard the electrode, and obtain a new one.

▶ Place the transmitter in the pouch. Tie the pouch strings around the patient's neck and waist, making sure that the pouch fits snugly without causing him discomfort. If no pouch is available, place the transmitter in the patient's bathrobe pocket.

▶ Check the patient's waveform for clarity, position, and size. Adjust the gain and baseline, as needed. (If necessary, ask the patient to remain resting or sitting in his room while you locate his telemetry monitor at the central station.)

▶ To obtain a rhythm strip, press the RECORD key at the central station. Label the strip with the patient's name and room number as well as the date and time. Also identify the rhythm. Place the rhythm strip in the appropriate location in the patient's chart.

Special considerations

▶ Make sure all electrical equipment and outlets are grounded to avoid electric shock and interference (artifacts). Also ensure that the patient is clean and dry to prevent electric shock. **MFR**

▶ Avoid opening the electrode packages until just before using to prevent the gel from drying out.

▶ Avoid placing the electrodes on bony prominences, hairy locations, areas where defibrillator pads will be placed, or areas for chest compression.

▶ Have the patient breathe normally during the procedure. If his respirations distort the recording, ask him to hold his breath briefly to reduce baseline wander in the tracing.

▶ Assess skin integrity, and reposition the electrodes every 24 hours or as necessary.

▶ If the patient is being monitored by telemetry, show him how the transmitter works. If applicable, show him the button that will produce a recording of his ECG at the central station. Teach him how to push the button whenever he has symptoms. This causes the central console to print a rhythm strip. Tell the patient to remove the transmitter if he takes a shower or bath, but stress that he should let you know before he removes the unit.

References

American Association of Critical Care Nurses Practice Alert: "Dysrhythmia Monitoring." [Online] Available at: *http://www.aacn.org/AACN/practiceAlert.nsf/Files/DYS/$file/Dysrhythmia%20Monitoring%208-2004.pdf*

American Heart Association. "Practice Standard for Electrocardiographic Monitoring in Hospital Settings," *Circulation* 110(17):2721-746, October 2004.

Jevon, P. "Cardiac Monitoring. Part 1— Electrocardiography (ECG)," *Nursing Times* 103(1):26-27, January 2007.

Lynn-McHale Wiegand, D.J., and Carlson, K.K., eds. *AACN Procedure Manual for Critical Care*, 5th ed. Philadelphia: W.B. Saunders Co., 2005.

Cardiac output measurement

Cardiac output (CO)—the amount of blood ejected by the heart—helps evaluate cardiac function. Each ventricle has a CO of 4 to 6 L/minute. The most widely used method of calculating this measurement is the bolus thermodilution technique. Performed at the bedside, the thermodilution technique is the most practical method of evaluating the cardiac status of critically ill patients and those suspected of having cardiac disease. (See *A closer look at the thermodilution method.*)

To measure CO, a quantity of solution colder than the patient's blood is injected into the right atrium via a port on a pulmonary artery (PA) catheter. This indicator solution mixes with the blood as it travels through the right ventricle into the PA, and a thermistor on the catheter registers the change in temperature of the flowing blood. A computer then plots the temperature change over time as a curve and calculates flow based on the area under the curve. (See *Analyzing thermodilution curves.*)

Iced or room-temperature injectant may be used—the choice should be based on your facility's policy as well as the patient's status. The accuracy of the bolus thermodilution technique depends on the computer being able to differentiate the temperature change caused by the injectant in the pulmonary artery and the temperature changes in the pulmonary artery. Because iced injectant is colder than room-temperature injectant, it provides a stronger signal to be detected.

Typically, however, room-temperature injectant is more convenient and provides equally accurate measurements. Iced injectant may be more accurate in patients with high or low COs, hypothermic patients, or when smaller volumes of injectant must be used (3 to 5 ml), as in patients with volume restrictions or in children.

A closer look at the thermodilution method

This illustration shows the path of the injectant solution through the heart during thermodilution cardiac output monitoring.

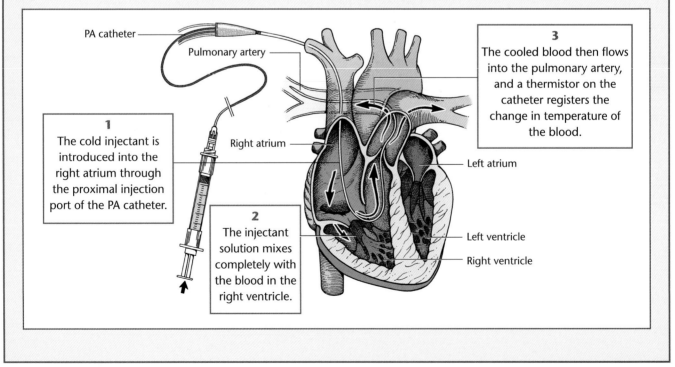

PA catheter

Pulmonary artery

1
The cold injectant is introduced into the right atrium through the proximal injection port of the PA catheter.

Right atrium

2
The injectant solution mixes completely with the blood in the right ventricle.

3
The cooled blood then flows into the pulmonary artery, and a thermistor on the catheter registers the change in temperature of the blood.

Left atrium

Left ventricle

Right ventricle

Analyzing thermodilution curves

The thermodilution curve provides valuable information about cardiac output (CO), injection technique, and equipment problems. When studying the curve, keep in mind that the area under the curve is inversely proportionate to CO: The smaller the area under the curve, the higher the CO; the larger the area under the curve, the lower the CO.

Besides providing a record of CO, the curve may indicate problems related to technique, such as erratic or slow injectant instillations, or other problems, such as respiratory variations or electrical interference. The curves below correspond to those typically seen in clinical practice.

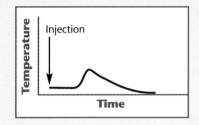

Normal thermodilution curve
With an accurate monitoring system and a patient who has adequate CO, the thermodilution curve begins with a smooth, rapid upstroke and is followed by a smooth, gradual downslope. The curve shown at left indicates that the injectant instillation time was within the recommended 4 seconds and that the temperature curve returned to baseline.

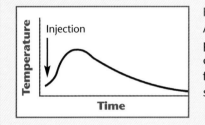

Low CO curve
A thermodilution curve representing low CO shows a rapid, smooth upstroke (from proper injection technique). However, because the heart is ejecting blood less efficiently from the ventricles, the injectant warms slowly and takes longer to be ejected from the ventricle. Consequently, the curve takes longer to return to baseline. This slow return produces a larger area under the curve, corresponding to low CO.

High CO curve
Again, the curve has a rapid, smooth upstroke from proper injection technique. However, because the ventricles are ejecting blood too forcefully, the injectant moves through the heart quickly and the curve returns to baseline more rapidly. The smaller area under the curve suggests higher CO.

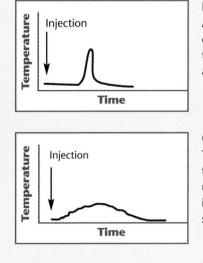

Curve reflecting poor technique
This curve results from an uneven and too slow (taking more than 4 seconds) administration of injectant. The uneven and slower than normal upstroke and the larger area under the curve erroneously indicate low CO. A kinked catheter, unsteady hands during the injection, or improper placement of the injectant lumen in the introducer sheath may also cause this type of curve.

Equipment

Thermodilution PA catheter in position ◆ output computer and cables (or a module for the bedside cardiac monitor) ◆ closed or open injectant delivery system ◆ 10-ml syringe ◆ 500-ml bag of dextrose 5% in water or normal saline solution ◆ crushed ice and water (if iced injectant is used).

Some bedside cardiac monitors measure CO continuously, using either an invasive or a noninvasive method. If your bedside monitor doesn't have this capability, you'll need a free-standing CO computer.

Cardiac output setup

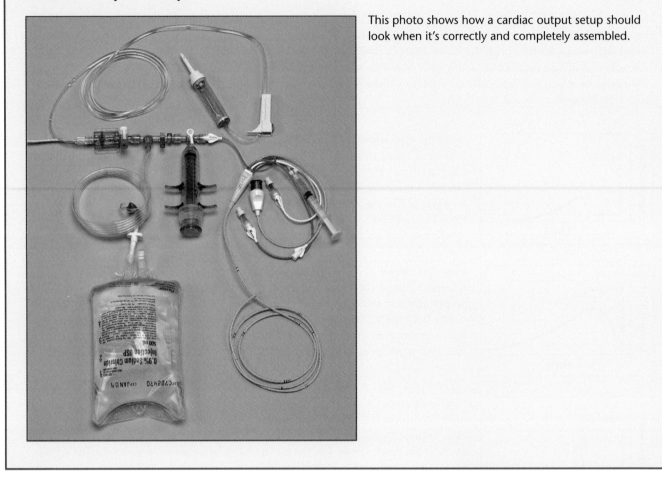

This photo shows how a cardiac output setup should look when it's correctly and completely assembled.

Implementation

▶ Wash your hands thoroughly, and assemble the equipment at the patient's bedside. Insert the closed injectant system tubing into the 500-ml bag of I.V. solution. Connect the 10-ml syringe to the system tubing, and prime the tubing with I.V. solution until it's free from air. Then clamp the tubing. (See *Cardiac output setup*.)
▶ Confirm the patient's identity using two patient identifiers according to your facility's policy. **JC**

Using room-temperature injectant

▶ After clamping the tubing, connect the primed system to the stopcock of

the proximal injectant lumen of the PA catheter.
▶ Next, connect the temperature probe from the CO computer to the closed injectant system's flow-through housing device. Connect the CO computer cable to the thermistor connector on the PA catheter, and verify the blood temperature reading. Finally, turn on the CO computer, and enter the correct computation constant, as provided by the catheter's manufacturer. The constant is determined by the volume and temperature of the injectant as well as the size and type of catheter. **MFR**

AGE FACTOR

For children, you'll need to adjust the computation constant to reflect a smaller volume and a smaller catheter size.

Using iced injectant

▶ After clamping the tubing, place the coiled segment into the Styrofoam container and add crushed ice and water to cover the entire coil. Let the solution cool for 15 to 20 minutes.
▶ After clamping the tubing, connect the primed system to the stopcock of the proximal injectant lumen of the PA catheter.
▶ Next, connect the temperature probe from the CO computer to the

closed injectant system's flow-through housing device. Connect the CO computer cable to the thermistor connector on the PA catheter and verify the blood temperature reading. Finally, turn on the CO computer and enter the correct computation constant, as provided by the catheter's manufacturer. The constant is determined by the volume and temperature of the injectant as well as the size and type of catheter. **MFR**

▶ Inject the solution to flow past the temperature sensor while observing the injectant temperature that registers on the computer. Verify that the injectant temperature is between 43° and 54° F (6.1° and 12.2° C).

The rest of the steps are the same as those for the room-temperature injectant closed delivery system.

▶ Make sure the patient is in a comfortable position. Tell him not to move during the procedure because movement can cause an error in measurement. **CS1**

▶ Explain to the patient that the procedure helps determine how well his heart is pumping and that he'll feel no discomfort.

▶ Verify the presence of a PA waveform on the cardiac monitor.

▶ Unclamp the I.V. tubing and withdraw exactly 10 ml of cooled solution before reclamping the tubing. **CS2**

 AGE FACTOR

With children, use 3 ml or less.

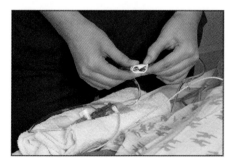

▶ Turn the stopcock at the catheter injectant hub to open a fluid path between the injectant lumen of the PA catheter and syringe.

▶ Press the START button on the cardiac output computer, or wait for the INJECT message to flash.

▶ Inject the solution smoothly within 4 seconds, making sure it doesn't leak at the connectors.

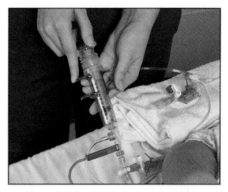

▶ If available, analyze the contour of the thermodilution washout curve on a strip chart recorder for a rapid upstroke and a gradual, smooth return to baseline.

▶ Wait 1 minute between injections, and repeat the procedure until three values are within 10% to 15% of the median value. Compute the average, and record the patient's CO.

▶ Return the stopcock to its original position, and make sure the injectant delivery system tubing is clamped.

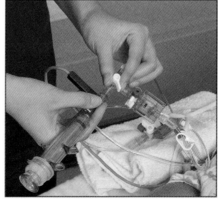

▶ Verify the presence of a PA waveform on the cardiac monitor.

▶ Discontinue CO measurements when the patient is hemodynamically

stable and weaned from his vasoactive and inotropic medications. You can leave the PA catheter inserted for pressure measurements.

▶ Disconnect and discard the injectant delivery system and the I.V. bag. Cover any exposed stopcocks with air-occlusive caps.

▶ Monitor the patient for signs and symptoms of inadequate perfusion, including restlessness, fatigue, changes in level of consciousness, decreased capillary refill time, diminished peripheral pulses, oliguria, and pale, cool skin.

Special considerations

▶ The normal range for CO is 4 to 8 L/minute. The adequacy of a patient's CO is better assessed by calculating his cardiac index (CI), adjusted for his body size.

▶ To calculate the patient's CI, divide his CO by his body surface area (BSA), a function of height and weight. For example, a CO of 4 L/minute might be adequate for a 65″, 120-lb (165-cm, 54-kg) patient (normally a BSA of 1.59 and a CI of 2.5) but would be inadequate for a 74″ 230-lb (188-cm, 104-kg) patient (normally a BSA of 2.26 and a CI of 1.8). Normal CI for an adult ranges from 2.5 to 4.2 L/minute/m^2; for a pregnant woman, 3.5 to 6.5 L/minute/m^2.

AGE FACTOR

Normal CI for infants and children is 3.5 to 4 L/minute/m^2. Normal CI for elderly adults is 2 to 2.5 L/minute/m^2.

▶ Add the fluid volume injected for CO determinations to the patient's total intake. Injectant delivery of 30 ml/hour will contribute 720 ml to the patient's 24-hour intake.

EVIDENCE-BASED RESEARCH

Sequential compression devices and cardiac output

Killu, K., et al. "Effect of lower limb compression devices on thermodilution cardiac output measurement," *Critical Care Medicine* 35(5):1307-11, May 2007.

Level VI
Evidence from a single descriptive or qualitative study

Description
Pulmonary artery catheters and lower limb sequential compression devices (SCDs) are two pieces of equipment that are commonly found in intensive care units (ICUs). Pulmonary artery catheters are frequently used to determine cardiac output using the thermodilution method. This study's objective was to determine if cardiac output measurements obtained using the thermodilution method were altered when they were measured during the inflation phase of SCDs. A total of 43 patients in two ICUs who had a pulmonary artery catheter and bilateral

lower limb SCDs were included in the study. The four cardiac output measurements were taken: with the SCDs off; during the first 2 to 4 seconds of inflation; during the 4 to 8 seconds of inflation; and again with the SCDs off.

Findings
Cardiac output was consistently lower when measured during the SCD inflation cycle. There was a decrease in cardiac output ranging from 7.58% to 49.5%. The mean decrease in cardiac output during the first 2 to 4 seconds of inflation was 24.5% and 20.6% during seconds 4 to 8.

Conclusions
A falsely low cardiac output value will result from taking the measurement using pulmonary artery catheter during the inflation cycle of lower limb SCDs. This study only focused on cardiac output measurements made by thermodilution methods, not using continuous cardiac output measure-

ment pulmonary artery catheters. It isn't known at this point if continuous cardiac output measurements will be affected the same way.

Nursing practice implications
Nurses in the ICU often care for patients who have SCDs and a pulmonary artery catheter for cardiac output measurement. They should be aware of the SCD cycle when obtaining cardiac output measurement using the thermodilution method. The following nursing practice implications are important:
▶ Turn off or pause the SCD compressor while obtaining cardiac output measurements when using the thermodilution method.
▶ Turn the SCD compressor back on after obtaining the cardiac output to help prevent deep vein thrombosis from forming.
▶ Educate staff on stopping SCDs during cardiac output measurement using the thermodilution method.

▶ After CO measurement, make sure the clamp on the injectant bag is secured to prevent inadvertent delivery of the injectant to the patient.

References

Bridges, E.J. "Pulmonary Artery Pressure Monitoring: When, How, and What Else to Use," *AACN Advanced Critical Care* 17(3):286-303, July-September 2006.

Engoren, M., and Barbee, D. "Comparison of Cardiac Output Determination by Bioimpedance, Thermodilution, and the Fick Method," *American Journal of Critical Care* 14(1):40-45, January 2005.

Giuliano, K.K., et al. "Backrest Angle and Cardiac Output Measurement in Critically Ill Patients," *Nursing Research* 52(4):242-8, July-August 2003. **CS1**

Jhanji, S., et al. "Cardiac Output Monitoring: Basic Science and Clinical Applications," *Anaesthesia* 63(2):172-81, February 2008.

Johnson, K.L. "Diagnostic Measures to Evaluate Oxygenation in Critically Ill Adults: Implications and Limitations," *AACN Clinical Issues* 15(4):506-24, October-December 2004.

McCloy, K., et al. "Effects of Injectate Volume on Thermodilution Measurements of Cardiac Output In Patients with Low

Ventriuclar Ejection Fractions," *American Journal of Critical Care* 8(2):86-92, March 1999. **CS2**

Payen, D., and Gayat, E. "Which General Intensive Care Unit Patients can Benefit from Placement of the Pulmonary Artery Catheter?" *Critical Care* 10(Suppl 3):S7, 2006.

Cardiopulmonary resuscitation

Cardiopulmonary resuscitation (CPR) is a basic life support (BLS) procedure that seeks to restore and maintain the patient's respiration and circulation after his heartbeat and breathing have stopped—cardiac arrest. Another BLS procedure is clearing the obstructed airway. (See "Foreign-body airway management," page 214.) BLS procedures should be performed according to the 2005 American Heart Association (AHA) guidelines.

Most adults who experience sudden cardiac arrest develop ventricular fibrillation and require defibrillation; CPR alone doesn't improve their chance of survival. Therefore, you must assess the victim and then contact emergency medical services (EMS) or call a code before starting CPR. Timing is critical because early access to EMS, early CPR, and early defibrillation greatly improve a patient's chance of survival. **AHA**

Equipment

CPR requires no special equipment except a hard surface on which to place the patient.

Implementation **AHA**

See the AHA's *BLS algorithm* on page 76, and follow the step-by-step instructions for CPR for the health care provider as described.

One-person rescue

▶ If you're the sole rescuer, expect to determine unresponsiveness, call for help, open the patient's airway, check for breathing, assess for circulation, and begin compressions.

▶ Assess the victim to determine if he's unconscious. Gently shake his shoulders and shout, "Are you okay?" This helps ensure that you don't start CPR on a person who's conscious. Check whether he has an injury, particularly to the head or neck. If you suspect a head or neck injury, move him as little as possible to reduce the risk of paralysis (as shown at the top of the next column).

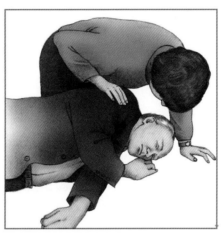

▶ Call out for help. Send someone to contact EMS or call a code, and get the automatic external defibrillator (AED). Place the victim in a supine position on a hard, flat surface. When moving him, roll his head and torso as a unit. Avoid twisting or pulling his neck, shoulders, or hips.

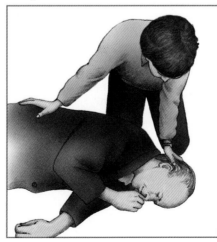

▶ Kneel near his shoulders. This position will give you easy access to his head and chest.

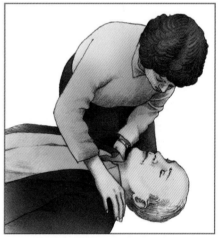

▶ In many cases, the muscles controlling the victim's tongue will be relaxed, causing the tongue to obstruct the airway. If the victim doesn't appear to have a neck injury, use the head-tilt, chin-lift maneuver to open his airway. To accomplish this, first place your hand that's closer to the victim's head on his forehead. Then apply firm pressure. The pressure should be firm enough to tilt the victim's head back. Next, place the fingertips of your other hand under the bony part of his lower jaw near the chin.

BLS algorithm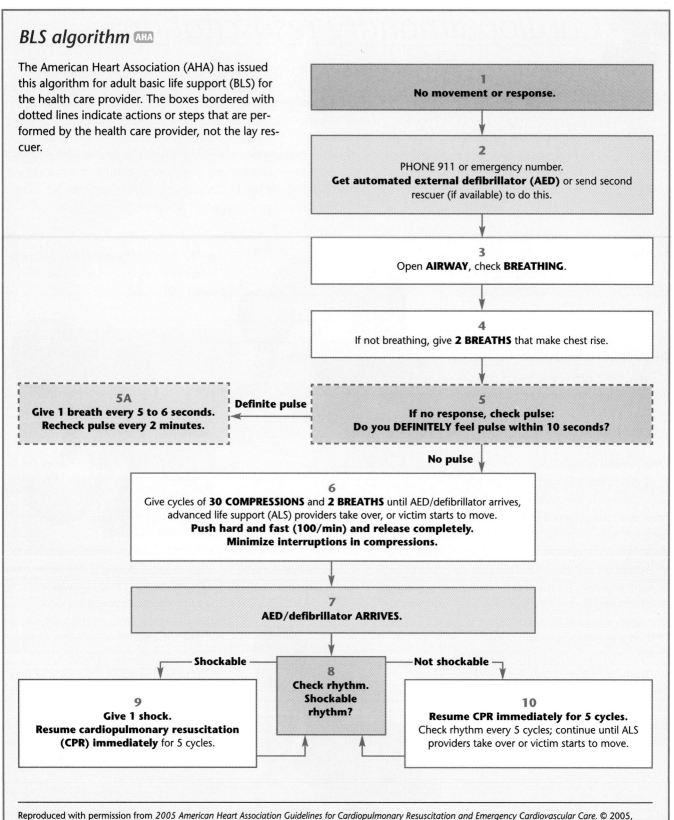

The American Heart Association (AHA) has issued this algorithm for adult basic life support (BLS) for the health care provider. The boxes bordered with dotted lines indicate actions or steps that are performed by the health care provider, not the lay rescuer.

1
No movement or response.

2
PHONE 911 or emergency number.
Get automated external defibrillator (AED) or send second rescuer (if available) to do this.

3
Open **AIRWAY**, check **BREATHING**.

4
If not breathing, give **2 BREATHS** that make chest rise.

5
If no response, check pulse:
Do you DEFINITELY feel pulse within 10 seconds?

— **Definite pulse** →

5A
**Give 1 breath every 5 to 6 seconds.
Recheck pulse every 2 minutes.**

No pulse ↓

6
Give cycles of **30 COMPRESSIONS** and **2 BREATHS** until AED/defibrillator arrives, advanced life support (ALS) providers take over, or victim starts to move.
**Push hard and fast (100/min) and release completely.
Minimize interruptions in compressions.**

7
AED/defibrillator ARRIVES.

8
**Check rhythm.
Shockable rhythm?**

— **Shockable** —

9
**Give 1 shock.
Resume cardiopulmonary resuscitation (CPR) immediately** for 5 cycles.

— **Not shockable** —

10
Resume CPR immediately for 5 cycles.
Check rhythm every 5 cycles; continue until ALS providers take over or victim starts to move.

Now lift the victim's chin. At the same time, keep his mouth partially open.

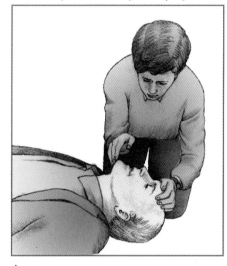

▶ If you suspect a neck injury, use the jaw-thrust maneuver instead of the head-tilt, chin-lift maneuver without head extension. Kneel at the victim's head with your elbows on the ground. Rest your thumbs on his lower jaw near the corners of the mouth, pointing your thumbs toward his feet. Then place your fingertips around the lower jaw. To open the airway, lift the lower jaw with your fingertips.

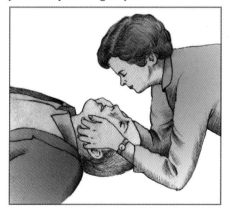

▶ While maintaining the open airway, look, listen, and feel for breathing. Place your ear over the victim's mouth and nose. Now, listen for the sound of air moving, and note whether his chest rises and falls. You may also feel airflow on your cheek. If he starts to breathe, keep the airway open and continue checking his breathing until help arrives.

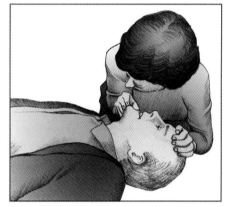

▶ If you don't detect adequate breathing within 10 seconds after you open his airway, begin rescue breathing. Pinch his nostrils shut with the thumb and index finger of the hand you've had on his forehead.

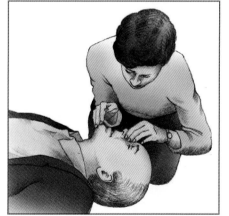

▶ Take a regular (not deep) breath, and place your mouth over the victim's mouth, creating a tight seal. Give 2 breaths, each over 1 second. Each ventilation should have enough volume to produce a visible chest rise.

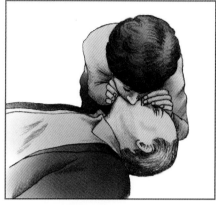

▶ If the first ventilation isn't successful, reposition the victim's head, and try again. If you still aren't successful, he may have a foreign-body airway obstruction. Check for loose dentures. If dentures or other objects are blocking the airway, follow the procedure for clearing an airway obstruction.

▶ Keep one hand on the victim's forehead so his airway remains open. With your other hand, palpate the carotid artery that's closer to you. To do this, place your index and middle fingers in the groove between the trachea and the sternocleidomastoid muscle. Palpate for 10 seconds.

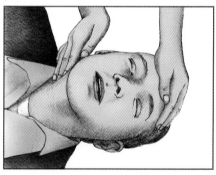

▶ If you detect a pulse, don't begin chest compressions. Instead, perform rescue breathing by giving the victim 10 to 12 ventilations per minute (or one every 5 to 6 seconds). Each breath should be given over 1 second and cause a visible chest rise. After 2 minutes, recheck his pulse but spend only 10 seconds doing so.

▶ If there's no pulse, start giving chest compressions. Make sure the patient is lying on a hard surface. Make sure your knees are apart for a wide base of support. Using the hand closer to his feet, locate the lower margin of the rib cage. Then move your fingertips along the margin to the notch where the ribs meet the sternum.

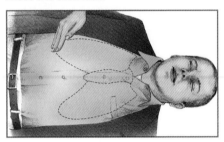

▶ Place your middle finger on the notch and your index finger next to your middle finger. The long axis of the heel of your hand will be aligned with the long axis of the sternum in the center of the chest between the nipples.

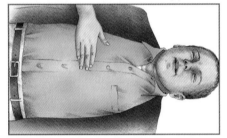

▶ Put the heel of your other hand on the sternum, next to the index finger. The long axis of the heel of your hand will be aligned with the long axis of the sternum.

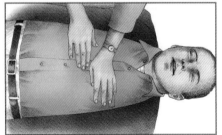

▶ Take the first hand off the notch, and put it on top of the hand on the sternum. Make sure you have one hand directly on top of the other and your fingers aren't on his chest. This posi-

tion will keep the force of the compression on the sternum and reduce the risk of a rib fracture, lung puncture, or liver laceration.

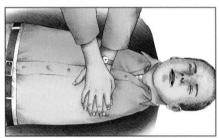

▶ With your elbows locked, arms straight, and your shoulders directly over your hands, you're ready to give chest compressions. Using the weight of your upper body, compress the victim's sternum $1\frac{1}{2}''$ (3.5 to 5 cm), delivering the pressure through the heels of your hands. After each compression, release the pressure and allow the chest to return to its normal position so that the heart can fill with blood. Don't change your hand position during compressions—you might injure the victim.

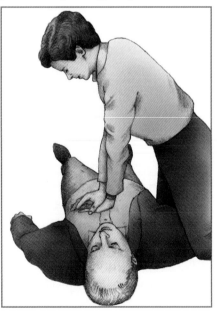

▶ Give 30 chest compressions at a rate of about 100 per minute. Push hard and fast. Open the airway, and give 2 ventilations. Then find the proper hand position again, and deliver 30 more compressions.

▶ Continue chest compressions until EMS arrives or another rescuer arrives with the AED. Health care providers should interrupt chest compressions as infrequently as possible. Interruptions should last for no more than 10 seconds except for special interventions, such as use of the AED or insertion of an airway.

Two-person rescue
If another rescuer arrives while you're giving CPR, follow these steps:

▶ If the EMS team hasn't arrived, tell the second rescuer to repeat the call for help. If he isn't a health care professional, ask him to stand by. Then, after about 2 minutes or 5 cycles of compressions and ventilations, you should switch. The switch should occur in less than 5 seconds.

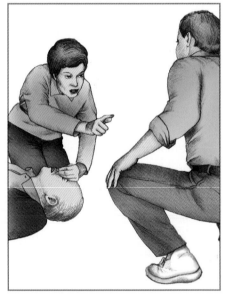

▶ If the rescuer is another health care professional, the two of you can perform two-person CPR. He should start assisting after you've finished 5 cycles of 30 compressions, 2 ventilations, and a pulse check.

▶ The second rescuer should get into place opposite you. While you're checking for a pulse, he should be finding the proper hand placement for delivering chest compressions.

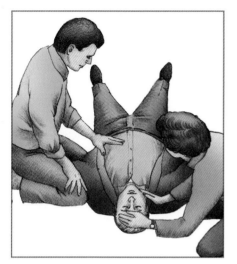

▶ If you don't detect a pulse, say, "No pulse, continue CPR" and give 2 ventilations. Then the second rescuer should begin delivering compressions at a rate of 100 per minute. Compressions and ventilations should be administered at a ratio of 30 compressions to 2 ventilations. The compressor (at this point, the second rescuer) should count out loud so the ventilator can anticipate when to give ventilations. To ensure that the ventilations are effective, watch for a visible chest rise.

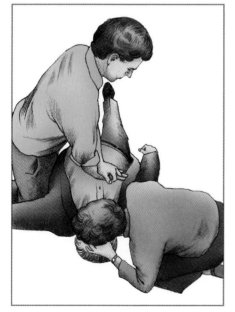

▶ The compressor role should switch after 5 cycles of compressions and ventilations. The switch should occur in less than 5 seconds.

▶ As shown below, both of you should continue giving CPR until an AED or defibrillator arrives, the advanced cardiac life support provider takes over, or the victim starts to move.

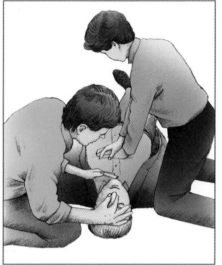

Special considerations

▶ Some health care professionals may hesitate to give mouth-to-mouth rescue breaths. For this reason, the AHA recommends that all health care professionals learn how to use disposable airway equipment. AHA

▶ Improper hand placement during compressions may result in fractured ribs, a lacerated liver, or punctured lungs. Gastric distention, a common complication, results from giving too much air during ventilation.

References

American Association for Respiratory Care. "Clinical Practice Guideline. Resuscitation and Defibrillation in the Health-Care Setting—2004 Revision and Update," *Respiratory Care* 89(9):1085-1099, September 2004.

American Heart Association. "2005 Guidelines for Cardiopulmonary Resuscitation and Emergency Cardiovascular Care: The International Consensus on Science," *Circulation* 112(22 Suppl):IV-1-IV-221, November 2005.

American Heart Association. "Highlights of the 2005 American Heart Association Guidelines for Cardiopulmonary Resuscitation and Emergency Cardiovascular Care," *Currents* 16(4):1-27, Winter 2005-2006.

Craig, K.J., and Hopkins-Pepe, L. "Understanding the New AHA Guidelines, Part I," *Nursing* 36(4):53, April 2006.

Li, Y., et al. "Identifying Potentially Shockable Rhythms without Interrupting Cardiopulmonary Resuscitation," *Critical Care Medicine* 36(1):198-203, January 2008.

Yannopoulos, D., et al. "Clinical and Hemodynamic Comparison of 15:2 and 30:2 Compression-to-ventilation Ratios for Cardiopulmonary Resuscitation," *Critical Care Medicine* 34(5):1444-449, May 2006.

Cast preparation

A cast is a hard mold that encases a body part—usually an extremity—to provide immobilization without discomfort. It can be used to treat injuries (including fractures), correct orthopedic conditions (such as deformities), or promote healing after general or plastic surgery, amputation, or nerve and vascular repair. Casts may be constructed of plaster, fiberglass, or other synthetic materials. Plaster, a commonly used material, is inexpensive, nontoxic, nonflammable, easy to mold, and rarely causes allergic reactions or skin irritation. However, fiberglass is lighter, stronger, and more resilient than plaster. Because fiberglass dries rapidly, it's more difficult to mold, but it can bear body weight immediately, if needed. **ASPN** (See *Types of cylindrical casts*.)

Typically, a practitioner applies a cast, and a nurse prepares the patient and the equipment and assists during the procedure. With special preparation, a nurse may apply or change a standard cast, but an orthopedist must reduce and set the fracture.

Contraindications for casting may include skin diseases, peripheral vascular disease, diabetes mellitus, open or draining wounds, and susceptibility to skin irritations. However, these aren't strict contraindications—the practitioner must weigh the potential risks and benefits for each patient.

Equipment

Tubular stockinette ◆ casting material ◆ plaster rolls ◆ plaster splints (if necessary) ◆ bucket of water ◆ sink equipped with plaster trap ◆ linen-saver pad ◆ sheet wadding ◆ sponge or felt padding (if necessary) ◆ local anesthetic (if necessary) ◆ pillows or bath blankets ◆ optional: rubber gloves, cast stand.

Gather the tubular stockinette, cast material, and plaster splints in the appropriate sizes. Wear rubber gloves, especially if applying a fiberglass cast.

Implementation

▶ Gently squeeze the packaged casting material to make sure the envelopes don't have air leaks.

▶ Follow the manufacturer's directions for water temperature when preparing plaster. Place all equipment within the practitioner's reach. **MFR**

▶ Explain the procedure to allay the patient's fears. If plaster is being used, make sure he understands that heat will build under the cast because of a chemical reaction between the water and plaster. Also begin explaining some aspects of proper cast care to

prepare him for patient teaching and to assess his knowledge level.

▶ Cover the appropriate parts of the patient's bedding and gown with a linen-saver pad.

▶ If the cast is applied to the wrist or arm, remove any rings that may interfere with circulation in the fingers.

▶ Assess the condition of the skin in the affected area, noting redness, contusions, or open wounds. This will make it easier to evaluate complaints the patient may have after the cast is applied.

▶ If the patient has severe contusions or open wounds, prepare him for a local anesthetic if the practitioner will administer one.

▶ Assess the patient's neurovascular status to establish baseline measurements. Palpate distal pulses; assess the color, temperature, and capillary refill of the appropriate fingers or toes; and check his neurologic function, including sensation and motion, in the affected and unaffected extremities.

▶ Help the practitioner position the limb, as ordered. (Commonly, the limb is immobilized in the neutral position.)

▶ Support the limb in the prescribed position while the practitioner applies

the tubular stockinette and sheet wadding. The stockinette should extend beyond the ends of the cast to pad the edges. (If the patient has an open wound or a severe contusion, the practitioner may not use the stockinette.) He then wraps the limb in sheet wadding, starting at the distal end, and applies extra wadding to the distal and proximal ends of the cast area as well as any points of prominence. As he applies the sheet wadding, check for wrinkles.

▶ If needed, help the practitioner place an extra layer of sponge or felt padding over the area where the cast scissors will be used.

▶ Prepare the various cast materials, as ordered.

Preparing a plaster cast

▶ Place a roll of plaster casting on its end in the bucket of water. Be sure to immerse it completely. When air bubbles stop rising from the roll, remove it, gently squeeze out the excess water, and hand the casting material to the practitioner, who will begin applying it to the extremity. As he applies the first roll, prepare a second roll in the same

Types of cylindrical casts

Made of plaster, fiberglass, or synthetic material, casts may be applied almost anywhere on the body—to support a single finger or the entire body. Common casts are shown below.

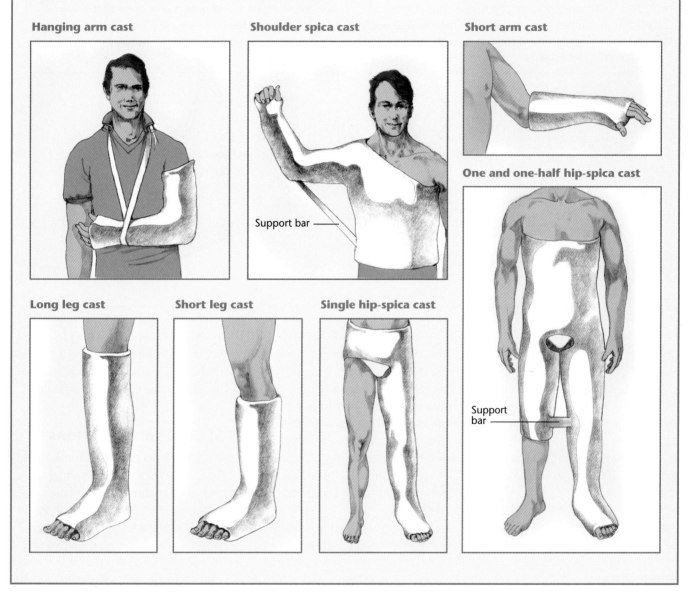

Hanging arm cast

Shoulder spica cast

Support bar

Short arm cast

One and one-half hip-spica cast

Support bar

Long leg cast

Short leg cast

Single hip-spica cast

manner. (Stay at least one roll ahead of the practitioner during the procedure.)

▶ After the practitioner applies each roll, he'll smooth it to remove wrinkles, spread the plaster into the cloth webbing, and empty air pockets. If he's using plaster splints, he'll apply them in the middle layers of the cast. Before wrapping the last roll, he'll pull the ends of the tubular stockinette over the cast edges to create padded ends, prevent cast crumbling, and reduce skin irritation. He'll then use the final roll to keep the ends of the stockinette in place.

Preparing a fiberglass cast

▶ If you're using water-activated fiberglass, immerse the tape rolls in tepid water for 10 to 15 minutes to initiate the chemical reaction that causes the cast to harden. Open one roll at a time. Avoid squeezing out excess water before application.

▶ If you're using light-cured fiberglass, you can unroll the material more slowly. This casting remains soft and malleable until it's exposed to ultraviolet light, which sets it.

How to petal a cast

Rough cast edges can be cushioned by petaling them with adhesive tape or moleskin. To do this, first cut several 4" x 2" (10 x 5 cm) strips. Round off one end of each strip to keep it from curling. Then, making sure the rounded end of the strip is on the outside of the cast, tuck the straight end just inside the cast edge.

Smooth the moleskin with your finger until you're sure it's secured inside and out. Repeat the procedure, overlapping the moleskin pieces until you've gone all the way around the cast edge.

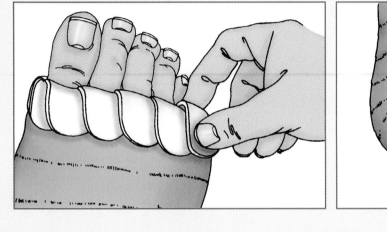 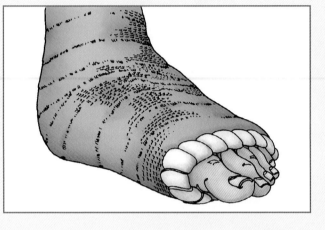

Preparing a cotton and polyester cast

▶ Open the casting materials one roll at a time because cotton and polyester casting must be applied within 3 minutes—before humidity in the air hardens the tape.

▶ Immerse the roll in cold water, and squeeze it four times to ensure uniform wetness.

▶ Remove the dripping material from the bucket. Tell the patient that it will be applied immediately. Forewarn him that the material will feel warm, giving off heat as it sets.

Completing the cast

▶ As necessary, "petal" the cast's edges to reduce roughness and to cushion pressure points. **ASPN** (See *How to petal a cast.*)

▶ Use a cast stand or your palm to support the cast in the therapeutic position until it becomes firm to the touch (usually 6 to 8 minutes).

▶ To check circulation in the casted limb, palpate the distal pulse, and assess the color, temperature, and capillary refill of the fingers or toes. Determine the patient's neurologic status by asking him if he's experiencing paresthesia in the extremity or decreased motion of the extremity's uncovered joints. Assess the unaffected extremity in the same manner and compare findings. **ASPN**

▶ Elevate the limb above heart level with pillows or bath blankets, as ordered, to facilitate venous return and reduce edema. Make sure pressure is evenly distributed under the cast to prevent it from molding incorrectly to the limb. **ASPN**

▶ The practitioner will then order X-rays to ensure proper positioning.

▶ Instruct the patient to notify the practitioner of pain, a foul odor, drainage, or a burning sensation under the cast. (After the cast hardens, the practitioner may cut a window in it to inspect the painful or burning area.)

▶ Pour the water from the plaster bucket into a sink containing a plaster trap. Don't use a regular sink because the plaster will block the plumbing.

Special considerations

▶ A fiberglass cast dries immediately after application. A plaster extremity cast dries in about 24 to 48 hours; a plaster spica or body cast, in 48 to 72 hours. During this drying period, the cast must be properly positioned to prevent a surface depression that could cause pressure areas or dependent edema. The patient neurovascular status must be assessed, drainage monitored, and the condition of the cast checked periodically. **ASPN**

▶ After the cast dries completely, it looks white and shiny and no longer feels damp or soft. Care consists of monitoring for changes in the drainage pattern, preventing skin breakdown near the cast, and averting the complications of immobility.

Removing a plaster cast

Typically, a cast is removed when a fracture heals or requires further manipulation. Less-common indications include cast damage, a pressure ulcer under the cast, excessive drainage or bleeding, and a constrictive cast.

Explain the procedure to the patient. Tell him he'll feel some heat and vibration as the cast is split with the cast saw. If the patient is a child, tell him that the saw is very noisy but won't cut the skin beneath. Warn the patient that when the padding is cut, he'll see discolored skin and signs of poor muscle tone. Reassure him that you'll stay with him. The illustrations below show how a plaster cast is removed.

| The practitioner cuts one side of the cast and then the other. As he does so, closely monitor the patient's anxiety level. | Next, the practitioner opens the cast pieces with a spreader. | Finally, using cast scissors, the practitioner cuts through the cast padding. |

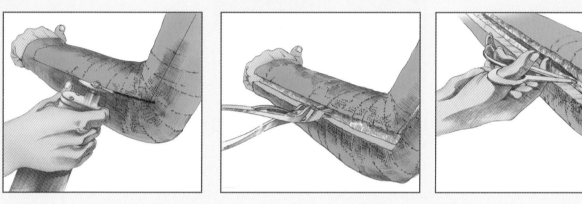

When the cast is removed, provide skin care to remove accumulated dead skin and to begin restoring the extremity's normal appearance.

▶ Patient teaching must begin immediately after the cast is applied and should continue until the patient or a family member can care for the cast.

▶ Never use the bed or a table to support the cast as it sets because incorrect molding can result, causing pressure necrosis of underlying tissue. Also, don't use rubber- or plastic-covered pillows before the cast hardens because they can trap heat under the cast.

▶ If a cast is applied after surgery or traumatic injury, remember that the most accurate way to assess for bleeding is to monitor the patient's vital signs. A visible blood spot on the cast can be misleading: One drop of blood can produce a circle 3" (7.6 cm) in diameter.

▶ Casts may need to be opened to assess the underlying skin and pulses, or to relieve pressure in a specific area. In a windowed cast, a specific area is cut out to allow inspection of the underlying skin or to relieve pressure. A bivalved cast is split medially and laterally, creating anterior and posterior sections. One of the sections may be removed to relieve pressure while the remaining section maintains immobilization.

▶ The practitioner usually removes the cast at the appropriate time, with a nurse assisting. (See *Removing a plaster cast.*) Tell the patient that when the cast is removed, his casted limb will appear thinner and flabbier than the uncasted limb. In addition, his skin will appear yellowish or gray from the accumulated

dead skin and oils from the glands near the skin surface. Reassure him that with exercise and good skin care, his limb will return to normal.

▶ Complications of improper cast application include compartment syndrome, palsy, paresthesia, ischemia, ischemic myositis, pressure necrosis and, eventually, misalignment or nonunion of fractured bones.

References

Smeltzer, S.C., et al. *Brunner & Suddarth's Textbook of Medical-Surgical Nursing,* 11th ed. Philadelphia: Lippincott Williams & Wilkins, 2008.

Smith, G., et al. "Fiberglass Cast Application," *American Journal of Emergency Medicine* 23(3):347-50, May 2005.

Catheter irrigation

To avoid introducing microorganisms into the bladder, the nurse irrigates an indwelling catheter to remove an obstruction, such as a blood clot that develops after bladder, kidney, or prostate surgery. In some cases, the nurse may instill a medication that works directly on the bladder wall. Whenever possible, the catheter should be irrigated through a closed system to decrease the risk of infection. **CDC**

Equipment

Ordered irrigating solution (such as normal saline solution) ◆ sterile basin ◆ two alcohol pads ◆ gloves ◆ linen-saver pad ◆ intake and output sheet ◆ 30- to 60-ml syringe ◆ 18G blunt-end needle (if system is not needleless) ◆ clamp.

Commercially packaged kits containing sterile irrigating solution, a graduated receptacle, and a 50-ml catheter tip syringe may be available.

Implementation

▶ Check the expiration date on the irrigating solution. To prevent vesical spasms during instillation of the solution, warm it to room temperature.
▶ Confirm the patient's identity using two patient identifiers according to your facility's policy. **JC**
▶ Wash your hands, and assemble the equipment at the bedside. Explain the procedure to the patient, and provide privacy. **CDC**
▶ Expose the catheter's aspiration or needleless port and place the linen-saver pad under it to protect the bed linens.
▶ Create a sterile field at the patient's bedside. Using sterile technique, pour the prescribed amount of solution into the basin. **CDC**
▶ Place the tip of the syringe into the solution, and fill the syringe with the appropriate amount of solution (as shown at the top of the next column).

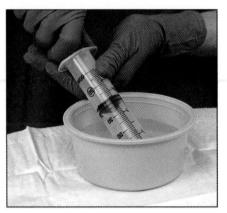

▶ Clean the aspiration or needleless port with an alcohol pad to remove as many bacterial contaminants as possible.

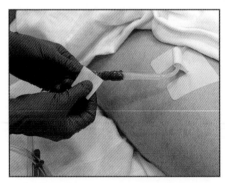

▶ Clamp the catheter tubing below the aspiration port.

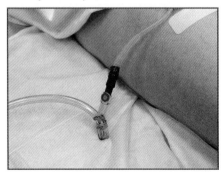

▶ Attach the syringe to the needleless port, or insert the blunt-tip needle in the port if a needleless system isn't in place.
▶ Instill the irrigating solution into the catheter. If necessary, refill the syringe and repeat this step until you've instilled the prescribed amount of irrigating solution.
▶ Remove the syringe and unclamp the drainage tube to allow the irrigant and urine to flow into the drainage bag.
▶ Make sure the catheter tubing is secured to the patient's leg and that the drainage bag is below the level of the bladder.
▶ Dispose of all used supplies properly.

Special considerations

▶ If you encounter resistance during instillation of the irrigating solution, don't try to force the solution into the bladder. Instead, stop the procedure, and notify the practitioner. If an indwelling catheter becomes totally obstructed, obtain an order to remove it and replace it with a new one to prevent bladder distention, acute renal failure, urinary stasis, and subsequent infection.
▶ The practitioner may order a continuous irrigation system. This decreases the risk of infection by eliminating the need to disconnect the catheter and drainage tube repeatedly. (See "Continuous bladder irrigation" page 136.)

▶ Encourage catheterized patients not on restricted fluid intake to increase intake to 3,000 ml per day to help flush the urinary system and reduce sediment formation.

References

Rew, M. "Caring for Catheterized Patients: Urinary Catheter Maintenance," *British Journal of Nursing* 14(2):87-92, January-February 2005.

Taylor, C., et al. *Fundamentals of Nursing: The Art and Science of Nursing Care,* 6th ed. Philadelphia: Lippincott Williams & Wilkins, 2008.

Central venous access device use

A central venous (CV) access device is a sterile catheter that's inserted through a large vein, such as the subclavian or jugular vein, and the tip of the catheter is placed in the superior vena cava. **INS** (See *Central venous pathways*.)

CV access devices allow long-term administration in situations requiring safe, repeated access to the venous system for administration of drugs, fluids and nutrition, and blood products.

Other benefits of central venous (CV) therapy include ease in monitoring CV pressure, drawing blood samples, administering large fluid volumes and irritating substances (such as total parenteral nutrition), and providing long-term venous access. However, CV therapy also increases the risk of complications, such as pneumothorax, sepsis, thrombus formation, and vessel and adjacent organ perforation (all life-threatening conditions). Also, the CV access device may decrease patient mobility, is difficult to insert, and costs more than a peripheral I.V. catheter.

Equipment

For inserting a CV access device: Skin preparation kit, if necessary ◆ sterile gloves and gowns ◆ blanket ◆ linen-saver pad ◆ sterile towel ◆ large sterile drape ◆ masks ◆ alcohol pads ◆ chlorhexidine sponges ◆ normal saline solution ◆ 3-ml syringe with 25G 1″ needle ◆ 1% or 2% injectable lidocaine ◆ dextrose 5% in water ◆ syringes for blood sample collection ◆ suture material ◆ two 14G or 16G CV access devices ◆ I.V. solution with administration set prepared for use ◆ infusion pump, as needed ◆ sterile 4″ × 4″ gauze pads ◆ catheter securement device or sterile tape or sterile surgical strips ◆ sterile scissors ◆ pre-filled syringes with flush solution ◆ transparent semipermeable dressing ◆ sterile marker ◆ sterile labels.

For flushing a catheter: Syringes prefilled with flush solutions ◆ alcohol pad.

For changing an injection cap: Alcohol pad ◆ sterile injection cap ◆ padded clamp.

For obtaining a blood sample: Gloves ◆ alcohol pad ◆ 10-ml syringe filled with flush solution ◆ 2 10-ml syringes with needleless hub (or other size syringe as appropriate) ◆ blood collection tubes ◆ laboratory slip ◆ labels ◆ BIOHAZARD transport bag.

For removing a CV access device: Clean gloves ◆ sterile suture removal set ◆ alcohol pads ◆ sterile gloves ◆ antimicrobial swab ◆ sterile 4″ × 4″ gauze pads ◆ forceps ◆ tape ◆ sterile, plastic adhesive-backed dressing or transparent semipermeable dressing ◆ agar plate, if necessary for culture ◆ antiseptic ointment.

Some facilities have prepared trays containing most of the equipment for catheter insertion. The type of catheter selected depends on the type of therapy to be used.

Implementation

▶ Before inserting a CV access device, confirm the catheter type and size with the practitioner; usually, a 14G or 16G catheter is selected.

▶ Set up the I.V. solution, and prime the administration set using strict sterile technique. Attach the line to the infusion pump, if ordered.

▶ Recheck all connections to make sure they're tight.

▶ Label all medications, medication containers, and other solutions on and off the sterile field. **JC**

▶ As ordered, notify the radiology department that a chest X-ray will be needed. **INS**

▶ Confirm the patient's identity using two patient identifiers according to your facility's policy. **JC**

▶ Wash your hands thoroughly to prevent the spread of microorganisms. **CDC AACN**

Inserting a CV access device

▶ Reinforce the practitioner's explanation of the procedure, and answer the patient's questions. Ensure that the patient has signed a consent form, if necessary, and check his history for hypersensitivity to iodine, latex, or the local anesthetic.

▶ Place the patient in Trendelenburg's position to dilate the veins and reduce the risk of an air embolism.

▶ For subclavian insertion, place a rolled blanket lengthwise between the shoulders to increase venous distention. For jugular insertion, place a rolled blanket under the opposite shoulder to extend the neck, making anatomic landmarks more visible. Place a linen-saver pad under the patient to prevent soiling the bed.

▶ Turn the patient's head away from the site to prevent possible contamination from airborne pathogens and to

Central venous pathways

The illustrations below show several common pathways for central venous (CV) access device insertion. Typically, a CV access device is inserted in the subclavian or internal jugular vein. The access device may terminate in the superior vena cava or, rarely, the right atrium.

Insertion: Subclavian vein
Termination: Superior vena cava

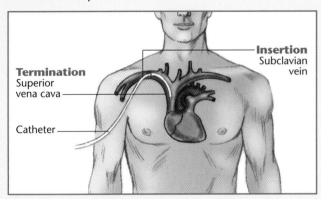

Insertion: Subclavian vein
Termination: Right atrium

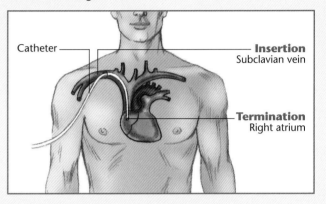

Insertion: Internal jugular vein
Termination: Superior vena cava

Insertion: Through a subcutaneous tunnel to the subclavian vein (Dacron cuff helps hold catheter in place)
Termination: Superior vena cava

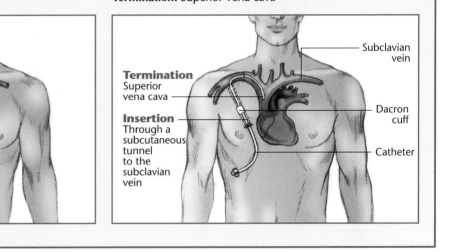

make the site more accessible. Or, if dictated by your facility's policy, place a mask on the patient unless this increases his anxiety or is contraindicated because of his respiratory status.

▶ Prepare the insertion site. You may need to wash the skin with soap and water first. Clip the hair close to the skin rather than shaving. Shaving may cause skin irritation and create multiple small open wounds, increasing the risk of infection. **CDC** **INS**

▶ Establish a sterile field on a table, using a sterile towel or the wrapping from the instrument tray.

▶ Put on a mask and sterile gloves and gown, and clean the area around the insertion site with the chlorhexidine sponge, using a back and forth scrubbing motion. **CDC** **AACN** **INS**

▶ After the practitioner puts on a sterile mask, gown, and gloves and drapes the area with a large sterile drape to create a sterile field, open the packaging of the 3-ml syringe and 25G needle, and give the syringe to him, using sterile technique. **INS** **AACN** **CDC**

▶ Wipe the top of the lidocaine vial with an alcohol pad and invert it. The practitioner then fills the 3-ml syringe and injects the anesthetic into the site.

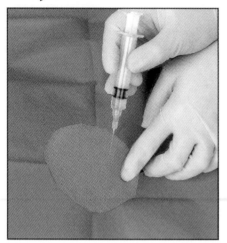

▶ Open the access device package, and give the catheter to the practitioner, using sterile technique. The practitioner then inserts the CV access device.

▶ During this time, prepare the I.V. administration set for immediate attachment to the access device hub. Ask the patient to perform Valsalva's maneuver while the practitioner attaches the I.V. line to the access device hub. This increases intrathoracic pressure, reducing the possibility of an air embolus.

▶ After the practitioner attaches the I.V. line to the access device hub, set the flow rate at a keep-vein-open rate to maintain venous access. (Alternatively, the access device may be capped and flushed with heparin.) The practitioner then sutures the access device in place.

▶ After an X-ray confirms correct access device placement in the superior vena cava, set the flow rate, as ordered. **INS**

▶ Use antimicrobial solution to remove dried blood that could harbor microorganisms. Secure the access device with a catheter securement device, or sterile tape or sterile surgical strips. Apply a transparent semipermeable dressing over the insertion site. **INS** **CDC** Ex-

pect some serosanguineous drainage during the first 24 hours.

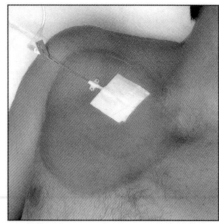

▶ Label the dressing with the time and date of access device insertion and catheter length, if not imprinted on the access device.

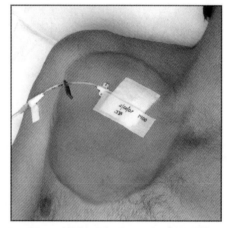

▶ Place the patient in a comfortable position and reassess his status.

Flushing the catheter

▶ To maintain patency, flush the access device routinely according to your facility's policy. **INS** If the system is being maintained as a saline lock and the infusions are intermittent, the flushing procedure will vary according to policy, the medication administration schedule, and the type of access device.

▶ All lumens of a multilumen access device must be flushed regularly. Most facilities use a heparin flush solution available in premixed 10-ml syringes. Recommended concentrations vary

from 10 to 100 units of heparin per milliliter. **INS** Use normal saline solution instead of heparin to maintain patency in three-way valved devices, such as the Groshong type, because research suggests that heparin isn't always needed to keep the line open. **MFR**

▶ The recommended frequency for flushing CV access devices varies from once every 8 hours to once weekly.

▶ The recommended amount of flushing solution also varies. Most facilities recommend using 3 to 5 ml of solution to flush the access device, although some facility policies call for as much as 10 ml of solution. Different access devices require different amounts of solution.

▶ To perform the flushing procedure, start by cleaning the cap or needleless access port with an alcohol pad. Allow the cap to dry. **INS** **CDC**

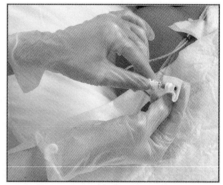

▶ Access the cap, and aspirate 3 to 5 ml of blood to confirm the proper function and patency of the CV access device. **INS**

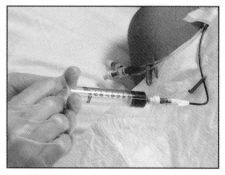

▶ Inject the recommended type and amount of flush solution.

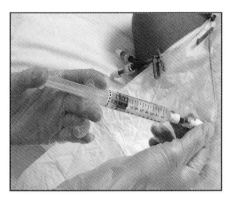 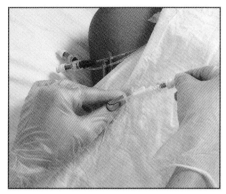

▶ After flushing the access device, maintain positive pressure by keeping your thumb on the plunger of the syringe while withdrawing the syringe. This prevents blood backflow and clotting in the line. If flushing a valved access device, close the clamp before the last of the flush solution leaves the syringe. **INS**

Changing the injection cap
▶ CV access devices used for intermittent infusions have needleless injection caps. These caps must be luer-lock types to prevent inadvertent disconnection and an air embolism. These caps contain a small amount of empty space, so you don't have to pre-flush the cap before connecting it.
▶ The frequency of cap changes varies according to your facility's policy and how often the cap is used; however, if the integrity of the product is compromised, it should be changed immediately. Use strict sterile technique when changing the cap. **INS**
▶ Clean the connection site with an alcohol pad. **INS** **CDC**
▶ Instruct the patient to perform Valsalva's maneuver while you quickly disconnect the old cap and connect the new cap using sterile technique. If he can't perform this maneuver, use a padded clamp to prevent air from entering the catheter (as shown at the top of the next column).

Obtaining a blood sample from a CV access device
▶ Explain the procedure to the patient, and place him in a supine position with the head slightly elevated.
▶ Wash your hands, and put on gloves. **CDC**
▶ Clamp the access device lumen, and clean the injection surface with an alcohol pad. **CDC** **INS**
▶ Attach an empty 10 ml-syringe to the hub, release the clamp, and aspirate the discard volume to clear the access device of dead space and blood diluted by flush solution.
▶ Clamp the access device, and remove the syringe for discard.
▶ Wipe the injection surface with alcohol, and connect the empty syringe or blood collection tube to the access device, release the clamp, and withdraw the blood sample. If using a blood collection tube with a rubber diaphragm, swab the area with alcohol before using.
▶ Clamp the access device, and remove the syringe.
▶ Wipe the injection surface with alcohol, and connect the syringe with normal saline solution.
▶ Open the clamp, and flush with solution. Close the clamp. **INS**
▶ Repeat the flushing procedure with a heparin flush solution per your facility's policy if the patient doesn't have a continuous infusion prescribed.

▶ If you used a syringe instead of a blood collection tube, transfer the blood into the appropriate blood collection tube after wiping it with an alcohol swab.
▶ Label the specimens with the name, room number, and date and time of collection.

Removing a CV access device
▶ If you'll be removing the CV access device, first check the patient's record for the most recent placement (confirmed by an X-ray) to trace its path as it exits the body. Make sure assistance is available if a complication (such as uncontrolled bleeding) occurs during access device removal. (Some blood vessels, such as the subclavian vein, can be difficult to compress.) Before you remove the access device, explain the procedure to the patient. **INS**
▶ Place the patient in a supine position to prevent an air embolism.
▶ Wash your hands, and put on clean gloves and a mask. **CDC** **AACN**
▶ Turn off all infusions, and prepare a sterile field using a sterile drape.
▶ Remove and discard the old dressing, and change to sterile gloves.
▶ Inspect the site for signs of drainage and inflammation. Clean the site with antimicrobial solution.
▶ Clip the sutures and, using forceps, remove the access device in a slow, even motion. Have the patient perform Valsalva's maneuver as it's withdrawn to prevent an air embolism.

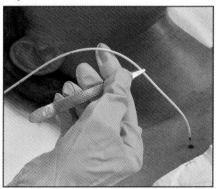

▶ Apply pressure with a sterile gauze pad immediately after removing the access device.

▶ Apply antiseptic ointment to the insertion site to seal it. Cover the site with a gauze pad, and tape a transparent semipermeable dressing over the gauze. Label the dressing with the date and time of the removal and your initials. Keep the site covered until epithelization has occurred. **INS CDC**

▶ Inspect the access device tip, and measure the length of the access device to ensure that the access device has been completely removed. If you suspect that the access device hasn't been completely removed, notify the practitioner immediately, and monitor the patient closely for signs of distress.

If you suspect an infection, swab the access device on a fresh agar plate and send it to the laboratory for culture. **INS**

▶ Dispose of the I.V. tubing and equipment properly.

Special considerations

CLINICAL ALERT

Be alert for such signs of air embolism as sudden onset of pallor, cyanosis, dyspnea, coughing, and tachycardia, progressing to syncope and shock. If any of these signs occur, place the patient on his left side in Trendelenburg's position, and notify the practitioner.

▶ After insertion, also watch for signs of pneumothorax, such as shortness of breath, uneven chest movement, tachycardia, and chest pain. Notify the practitioner immediately if such signs appear.

▶ Change the dressing every 48 hours if a gauze dressing is used and every 7 days if a transparent dressing is used, according to your facility's policy, or whenever it becomes moist or soiled. Change the tubing every 72 hours and solution every 24 hours or according to your facility's policy while the CV access device is in place. Dressing, tubing, and solution changes for a CV access device should be performed using sterile technique. **INS CDC AACN** (See

---

Key steps in changing a central venous dressing

Expect to change your patient's central venous dressing every 48 hours if it's a gauze dressing and at least every 7 days if it's transparent. Many facilities specify dressing changes whenever the dressing becomes soiled, moist, or loose. The following illustrations show the key steps you'll perform.

First, put on clean gloves, and remove the old dressing by pulling it toward the exit site of a long-term access device or toward the insertion site of a short-term access device. This technique helps you avoid pulling out the line. Remove and discard your gloves.

Next, put on sterile gloves, and clean the skin around the site three times using an alcohol pad. Start at the center and move outward, using a circular motion.

Allow the skin to dry, and clean the site with antimicrobial swabs.

After the solution has dried, cover the site with a dressing, such as the transparent semipermeable dressing, as shown below. Write the time and date on the dressing.

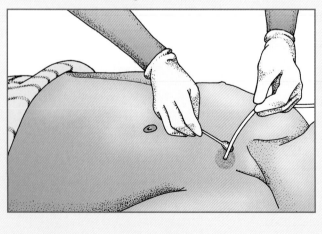
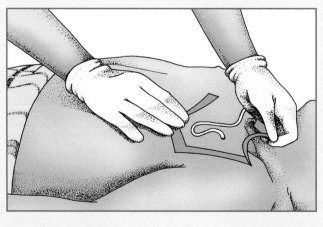

EVIDENCE-BASED RESEARCH

Catheter-associated infections outside the intensive care unit

Marschall, J., et al. "Catheter-associated bloodstream infections in general medical patients outside the intensive care unit: A surveillance study," *Infection Control and Hospital Epidemiology* 28(8):905-9, August 2007.

Level IV
Evidence from a well-designed case-control and cohort studies

Description
Catheter-associated bloodstream infections are frequently associated with patients with central venous access devices, and also patients in the intensive care unit (ICU). This study looked at the incidences of catheter-associated bloodstream infections that occurred in patients with central venous access devices on four regular medical floors at a large teaching hospital. All patients admitted to the four floors over a 13-month period were included in the study. There were a total of 33,174 patient-days, of which 7,337 catheter-days were observed. The ratio of catheter-days to patient-days was 0.22, similar for all four units.

Findings
Forty-two episodes of catheter-associated bloodstream infections were identified during the study period. Incidence was 5.7 infections per 1,000 catheter-days. Fifty-seven percent of the cases were caused by gram-positive bacteria; 17% caused by gram-negative bacteria; 12% by *Candida albicans;* and 12% with a polymicrobial origin. Thirty five of the patients had nontunneled central venous access devices in place.

Conclusion
The medical floors had significantly lower central venous access device use compared to ICUs, but the catheter-associated bloodstream infection rate was similar to that of the ICUs.

Nursing practice implications
Nurses are the ones responsible for central venous access device care and maintenance. The catheter-associated bloodstream infections prevention strategies that are used in ICUs should also be used on general medical floors. The following nursing practice implications are important:
▶ Educate staff on proper care and maintenance of central venous access devices.
▶ Monitor all patients with central venous access devices for signs of infection.
▶ Perform central venous access device care according to your facility's policy or the Centers for Disease Control and Prevention and Infusion Nurses Society guidelines.
▶ Discuss discontinuation of the access device with the practitioner as the patient no longer needs central venous access.
▶ Continue to study and follow catheter-associated bloodstream infection rates in all areas of a facility.

Key steps in changing a central venous dressing.)
▶ Assess the site for signs of infection, such as discharge, inflammation, and tenderness.
▶ To prevent an air embolism, close the access device clamp or have the patient perform Valsalva's maneuver each time the access device hub is open to air. (A Groshong type doesn't require clamping because it has an internal valve.)
▶ If you have trouble aspirating blood, the access device tip may be poorly positioned. Ask the patient to cough, reposition him on his side, raise his arms above his head, or put him in a sitting position.

References

Brungs, S.M., and Render, M.L. "Using Evidence-Based Practice to Reduce Central Line Infections," *Clinical Journal of Oncology Nursing* 10(6):723-25, December 2006.

Centers for Disease Control and Prevention. "Guidelines for the Prevention of Intravascular Catheter-Related Infections," *MMWR* 51(RR-10):1-26, August 2002.

Crawford, A.G., et al. "Cost-Benefit Analysis of Chlorhexidine Gluconate Dressing in the Prevention of Catheter-Related Bloodstream Infections," *Infection Control and Hospital Epidemiology* 25(8):668-74, August 2004.

Hadaway, L. "Keeping Central Line Infection at Bay," *Nursing* 36(4):58-63, April 2006.

Ingram, P., et al. "The Safe Removal of Central Venous Catheters," *Nursing Standards* 20(49):42-46, August 2006.

Lynn-McHale Wiegand, D.J., and Carlson, K.K., eds. *AACN Procedure Manual for Critical Care*, 5th ed. Philadelphia: W.B. Saunders Co., 2005.

Merrer, J., et al. "Complications of Femoral and Subclavian Venous Catheterization in Critically Ill Patients:

A Randomized Controlled Trial," *JAMA* 286(6):700-707, August 2001.

Posa, P.J., et al. "Elimination of Central Line-Associated Bloodstream Infections: Application of the Evidence," *AACN Advanced Critical Care* 17(4):446-54, October-December 2006.

"Standard 35. Injection and Access Caps. Infusion Nursing Standards of Practice," *Journal of Infusion Nursing* 29(1S):S35-36, January-February 2006.

"Standard 37. Site Selection. Infusion Nursing Standards of Practice," *Journal of Infusion Nursing* 29(1S):S37-39, January-February 2006.

"Standard 38. Catheter Selection. Infusion Nursing Standards of Practice," *Journal of Infusion Nursing* 29(1S):S39-40, January-February 2006.

"Standard 39. Hair Removal. Infusion Nursing Standards of Practice," *Journal of Infusion Nursing* 29(1S):S40-41, January-February 2006.

"Standard 40. Local Anesthesia. Infusion Nursing Standards of Practice," *Journal of Infusion Nursing* 29(1S):S41, January-February 2006.

"Standard 41. Access Site Preparation. Infusion Nursing Standards of Practice," *Journal of Infusion Nursing* 29(1S):S41-42, January-February 2006.

"Standard 44. Dressings. Infusion Nursing Standards of Practice," *Journal of Infusion Nursing* 29(1S):S44-45, January-February 2006.

"Standard 49. Catheter Removal. Infusion Nursing Standards of Practice," *Journal of Infusion Nursing* 29(1S):S51-55, January-February 2006.

"Standard 50. Flushing. Infusion Nursing Standards of Practice," *Journal of Infusion Nursing* 29(1S):S55-57, January-February 2006.

"Standard 51. Catheter Site Care. Infusion Nursing Standards of Practice," *Journal of Infusion Nursing* 29(1S):S57-58, January-February 2006.

"Standard 58. Culturing for Suspected Infusion-related Infections. Infusion Nursing Standards of Practice," *Journal of Infusion Nursing* 29(1S):S63-64, January-February 2006.

"Standard 66. Phlebotomy. Infusion Nursing Standards of Practice," *Journal of Infusion Nursing* 29(1S):S71-73, January-February 2006.

Central venous pressure monitoring

For central venous pressure (CVP) monitoring, the practitioner inserts a catheter through a vein and advances it until its tip lies in or near the right atrium. Because no major valves lie at the junction of the vena cava and right atrium, the pressure at end diastole reflects back to the catheter. When connected to a pressure monitoring kit, the catheter measures CVP—an index of right ventricular function.

CVP monitoring helps to assess cardiac function, to evaluate venous return to the heart, and to indirectly gauge how well the heart is pumping. The central venous (CV) line also provides access to a large vessel for rapid, high-volume fluid administration and allows frequent blood withdrawal for laboratory samples.

Normal CVP ranges from 2 to 6 mm Hg (5 to 10 cm H_2O). Any condition that alters venous return, circulating blood volume, or cardiac performance may affect CVP. If circulating volume increases (such as with enhanced venous return to the heart), CVP rises. If circulating volume decreases (such as with reduced venous return), CVP drops.

Equipment

For monitoring CVP: Pressure monitoring kit with disposable pressure transducer ◆ leveling device ◆ bedside pressure module ◆ continuous I.V. flush solution ◆ pressure bag.

For removing a CV catheter: Sterile gloves ◆ suture removal set ◆ sterile gauze pads ◆ antimicrobial ointment ◆ dressing ◆ tape.

Implementation

▶ Confirm the patient's identity using two patient identifiers according to your facility's policy. **JC**
▶ Gather the necessary equipment. Explain the procedure to the patient to reduce his anxiety.
▶ Assist the practitioner as he inserts the CV catheter. (The procedure is similar to that used for pulmonary artery pressure monitoring, except that the catheter is advanced only as far as the superior vena cava.)

Obtaining continuous CVP readings

▶ Make sure the CV access device or the proximal lumen of a pulmonary artery catheter is attached to the system. (If the patient has a CV access device with multiple lumens, one lumen may be dedicated to continuous CVP monitoring and the other lumens used for fluid administration.)
▶ Set up a pressure transducer system. (See "Transducer system setup," page 556.) Connect noncompliant pressure tubing from the CV catheter hub to the transducer. Then connect the flush solution container to a flush device.
▶ To obtain values, position the patient supine with the head of the bed between 0 and 45 degrees. If he can't tolerate this position, use semi-Fowler's position. **CS**

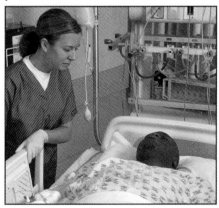

▶ Locate the level of the right atrium by identifying the phlebostatic axis. Zero the transducer, leveling the transducer air-fluid interface stopcock with the right atrium. Read the CVP value from the digital display on the monitor, and note the waveform. Make sure the patient is still when the reading is taken to prevent artifact. Be sure to use this position for all subsequent readings.

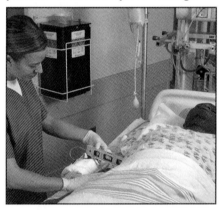

Removing a CV catheter

▶ You may assist the practitioner in removing a CV catheter. (In some states, a nurse is permitted to remove the catheter with a practitioner's order or when acting under advanced collaborative standards of practice.)
▶ If the head of the bed is elevated, to minimize the risk of air embolism during catheter removal, place the patient in Trendelenburg's position if the line was inserted using a superior approach. If he can't tolerate this, position him supine.

Differentiating normal from abnormal CVP waveforms

These illustrations show a normal central venous pressure (CVP) waveform and abnormal CVP waveforms, along with possible causes of abnormal waveforms.

Normal waveforms

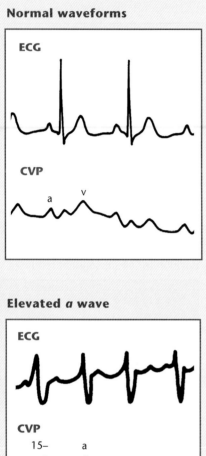

Elevated a wave

Physiologic causes
▶ Increased resistance to ventricular filling
▶ Increased atrial contraction

Associated conditions
▶ Heart failure
▶ Tricuspid stenosis
▶ Pulmonary hypertension

Elevated v wave

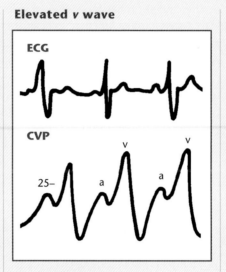

Physiologic causes
▶ Regurgitating flow

Associated conditions
▶ Tricuspid insufficiency
▶ Inadequate closure of the tricuspid valve due to heart failure

Absent a wave

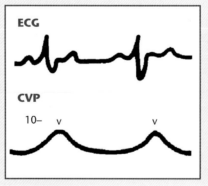

Physiologic causes
▶ Decreased or absent atrial contraction

Associated conditions
▶ Atrial fibrillation
▶ Junctional arrhythmias
▶ Ventricular pacing

Elevated a and v waves

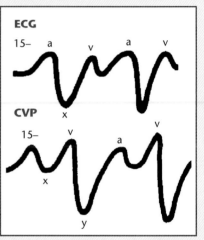

Physiologic causes
▶ Increased resistance to ventricular filling, which causes an elevated a wave
▶ Functional regurgitation, which causes an elevated v wave

Associated conditions
▶ Cardiac tamponade (smaller y descent than x descent)
▶ Constrictive pericardial disease (y descent exceeds x descent)
▶ Heart failure
▶ Hypervolemia
▶ Atrial hypertrophy

▶ Turn the patient's head to the side opposite the catheter insertion site. Remove the dressing, and expose the insertion site. If sutures are in place, remove them carefully.

▶ Turn the I.V. solution off.

▶ Put on sterile gloves. **CDC**

▶ Pull the catheter out in a slow, smooth motion and then apply pressure to the insertion site.

▶ Clean the insertion site, apply antimicrobial ointment, and cover it with a dressing, as ordered. Remove your gloves, and wash your hands. **INS**

▶ Assess the patient for signs of respiratory distress, which may indicate an air embolism.

Special considerations

▶ As ordered, arrange for daily chest X-rays to check catheter placement. **INS AACN**

▶ Care for the insertion site according to your facility's policy. Change a gauze dressing every 48 hours and a transparent dressing every 7 days, whenever the dressing becomes moist, or according to your facility's policy. **INS AACN CDC**

▶ Be sure to wash your hands before performing dressing changes and to use sterile technique and sterile gloves when redressing the site. When removing the old dressing, observe for signs of infection, such as redness, and note any patient complaints of tenderness. Cover the site with a sterile gauze dressing or a clear occlusive dressing.

▶ After the initial CVP reading, reevaluate readings frequently to establish a baseline for the patient. Authorities recommend obtaining readings at 15-, 30-, and 60-minute intervals to establish a baseline. If the patient's CVP fluctuates by more than 2 cm H_2O, suspect a change in his clinical status, and report this finding to the practitioner. (See *Differentiating normal from abnormal CVP waveforms*.)

▶ Change the I.V. solution every 24 hours and the I.V. tubing every 96 hours, according to your facility's policy. Label the I.V. solution, tubing, and dressing with the date, time, and your initials. **INS AACN CDC**

References

Brungs, S.M., and Render, M.L. "Using Evidence-Based Practice to Reduce Central Line Infections," *Clinical Journal of Oncology Nursing* 10(6):723-25, December 2006.

Danks, L.A. "Central Venous Catheters: A Review of Skin Cleansing and Dressings," *British Journal of Nursing* 15(12):650-54, June-July 2006.

Day, M.W. "Tension Pneumothorax from Central Line Placement," *Nursing* 36(11):80, November 2006.

Dobbin, K., et al. "Pulmonary Artery Pressure Measurement in Patients with Elevated Pressures: Effect of Backrest Elevation and Method of Measurement," *American Journal of Critical Care* 1(2):61-9, September 1992. **CS**

Hadaway, L.C. "Keeping Central Line Infection at Bay," *Nursing* 36(4):58-63, April 2006.

Ho, A.M., et al. "Accuracy of Central Venous Pressure Monitoring during Simultaneous Continuous Infusion through the Same Catheter," *Anaesthesia* 60(10):1027-30, October 2005.

Lynn-McHale Wiegand, D.J., and Carlson, K.K., eds. *AACN Procedure Manual for Critical Care,* 5th ed. Philadelphia: W.B. Saunders Co., 2005.

Posa, P., et al. "Elimination of Central Line-Associated Bloodstream Infections: Application of the Evidence," *AACN Advanced Critical Care* 17(4):446-54, October-December 2006.

Weinstein, S. *Plumer's Principles & Practice of Intravenous Therapy,* 8th ed. Philadelphia: Lippincott Williams & Wilkins, 2007.

Cerebrospinal fluid drainage

Cerebrospinal fluid (CSF) drainage aims to reduce CSF pressure to the desired level and then to maintain it at that level. Fluid is withdrawn from the lateral ventricle (ventriculostomy). Ventricular drainage is used to reduce increased intracranial pressure (ICP). External CSF drainage is used most commonly to manage increased ICP and to facilitate spinal or cerebral dural healing after traumatic injury or surgery. In either case, CSF is drained by a catheter or a ventriculostomy tube in a sterile, closed drainage collection system.

Other therapeutic uses include ICP monitoring via the ventriculostomy; direct instillation of medications, contrast media, or air for diagnostic radiology; and aspiration of CSF for laboratory analysis.

To place the ventricular drain, the physician inserts a ventricular catheter through a burr hole in the patient's skull. Usually, this is done in the operating room, with the patient receiving a general anesthetic. (See *CSF drainage*.)

CSF drainage

Closed drainage system

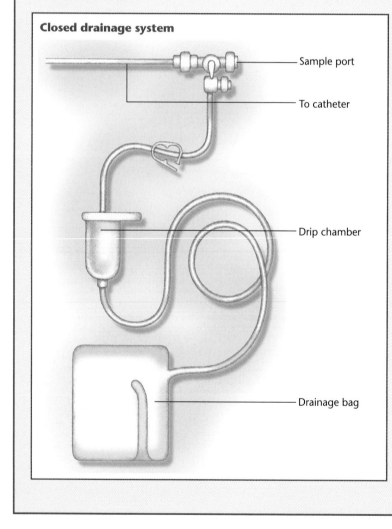

- Sample port
- To catheter
- Drip chamber
- Drainage bag

Cerebrospinal fluid (CSF) drainage aims to control intracranial pressure (ICP) during treatment for traumatic injury or other conditions that cause a rise in ICP.

For a ventricular drain, the physician makes a burr hole in the patient's skull and inserts the catheter into the ventricle. The distal end of the catheter is connected to a closed drainage system.

The ventricular system is usually attached to this drainage system to permit drainage of CSF, if needed.

Equipment

Overbed table ◆ sterile gloves ◆ antiseptic solution ◆ sterile fenestrated drape ◆ 3-ml syringe for local anesthetic ◆ 25G ³/₄″ needle for injecting anesthetic ◆ local anesthetic (usually 1% lidocaine) ◆ sterile gauze ◆ clippers, if needed ◆ #5 French whistle-tip catheter or ventriculostomy tube ◆ external drainage set (includes drainage tubing and sterile collection bag) ◆ suture material ◆ sterile dressing ◆ paper tape ◆ I.V. pole ◆ ventriculostomy tray and twist drill ◆ sterile marker ◆ sterile labels ◆ optional: pain medication.

Implementation

▶ Open all equipment using sterile technique. Check all packaging for breaks in seals and for expiration dates. **CDC**

▶ Label all medications, medication containers, and other solutions on and off the sterile field. **JC**

▶ Confirm the patient's identity using two patient identifiers according to your facility's policy. **JC**

▶ Consent should be obtained by the physician from the patient or a responsible family member and should be documented according to your facility's policy.

▶ Wash your hands thoroughly. **CDC**

▶ Perform a baseline neurologic assessment, including vital signs, to help detect alterations or signs of deterioration.

▶ Administer pain medications or sedation, as ordered.

Inserting a ventricular drain

▶ Place the patient in the supine or side-lying position.

▶ Place the equipment tray on the overbed table, and unwrap the tray.

▶ Adjust the height of the bed so that the physician can perform the procedure comfortably.

▶ Illuminate the area of the catheter insertion site.

▶ The physician will clean the insertion site, administer a local anesthetic, and clip the hair from the area of the insertion site. He'll put on sterile gloves and drape the insertion site. **CDC**

▶ To insert the drain, the physician will request a ventriculostomy tray with a twist drill. After completing the ventriculostomy, he'll connect the drainage system and suture the ventriculostomy in place. Then he'll cover the insertion site with a sterile dressing.

▶ After the physician places the catheter, connect it to the external drainage system tubing. Secure connection points with tape or a connector. Place the collection system, including drip chamber and collection bag, on an I.V. pole.

Monitoring CSF drainage

▶ Maintain a continuous hourly output of CSF by raising or lowering the drainage system drip chamber. To maintain CSF outflow, the drip chamber should be slightly lower than or at the level of the lumbar drain insertion site. Sometimes, you may need to carefully raise or lower the drip chamber to increase or decrease CSF flow. For ventricular drains, ensure that the flow chamber of the ICP monitoring setup remains positioned, as ordered. You should also correlate changes in ICP to the drainage (as shown at the top of the next column).

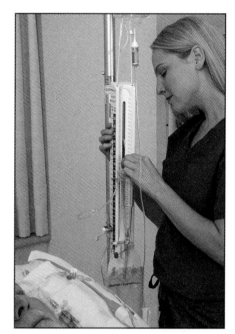

▶ To drain CSF as ordered, put on gloves, and then turn the main stopcock on to drainage. This allows CSF to collect in the graduated flow chamber. Document the time and the amount of CSF obtained. Then turn the stopcock off to drainage. To drain the CSF from this chamber into the drainage bag, release the clamp below the flow chamber. Never empty the drainage bag. Instead, replace it when it's full using sterile technique.

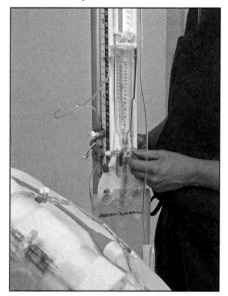

▶ Check the dressing frequently for drainage, which could indicate CSF leakage.

▶ Check the tubing for patency by watching the CSF drops in the drip chamber.

▶ Observe CSF for color, clarity, amount, blood, and sediment. CSF specimens for laboratory analysis should be obtained from the collection port attached to the tubing, not from the collection bag.

▶ Change the collection bag when it's full or every 24 hours, according to your facility's policy.

Special considerations

▶ Maintaining a continual hourly output of CSF is essential to prevent overdrainage or underdrainage. Underdrainage or lack of CSF may reflect kinked tubing, catheter displacement, or a drip chamber placed higher than the catheter insertion site. Overdrainage can occur if the drip chamber is placed too far below the catheter insertion site.

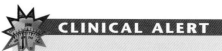

CLINICAL ALERT

If drainage accumulates too rapidly, clamp the system, notify the physician immediately, and perform a complete neurologic assessment because this constitutes a potential neurosurgical emergency.

▶ Raising or lowering the head of the bed can affect the CSF flow rate. When changing the patient's position, reposition the drip chamber.

▶ Patients may experience a chronic headache during continuous CSF drainage. Assess for signs of hemorrhage, which may include headache. Reassure the patient that this isn't unusual; administer analgesics, as appropriate.

▶ For ventricular drains, make sure ICP waveforms are being monitored continuously.

▶ Follow strict sterile technique when connecting tubing, flushing, or taking samples from the drainage system and during dressing changes. **CDC**

References

American Association of Neuroscience Nurses. *Core Curriculum for Neuroscience Nursing,* 4th ed. Philadelphia: W.B. Saunders Co., 2004.

Bota, D.P., et al. "Ventriculostomy-Related Infections in Critically Ill Patients: A 6-Year Experience," *Journal of Neurosurgery* 103(3):468-72, September 2005.

Hickey, J.V. *The Clinical Practice of Neurological and Neurosurgical Nursing,* 5th ed. Philadelphia: Lippincott Williams & Wilkins, 2003.

Lo, C.H., et al. "External Ventricular Infections are Independent of Drain Durations: An Argument against Elective Revision," *Journal of Neurosurgery* 106(3):378-83, March 2007.

Lynn-McHale Weigand, D.J., and Carlson, K.K., eds. *AACN Procedure Manual for Critical Care,* 5th ed. Philadelphia: W.B. Saunders Co., 2005.

March, K. "Intracranial Pressure Monitoring: Why Monitor?" *AACN Clinical Issues* 16(4):456-75, October-December 2005.

Chemotherapeutic drug administration

Administration of chemotherapeutic drugs requires skills in addition to those used when giving other drugs. For example, some drugs require special equipment or must be given through an unusual route; others become unstable after a period of time; and still others must be protected from light. Finally, the drug dosage must be exact to avoid possibly fatal complications. For these reasons, only specially trained nurses and physicians should give chemotherapeutic drugs.

Chemotherapeutic drugs may be administered through several routes. The administration route depends on the drug's pharmacodynamics and the tumor's characteristics. Although the I.V. route (using peripheral or central veins) is used most commonly, these drugs may also be given orally, subcutaneously, or I.M. Alternative approaches, such as intraperitoneal chemotherapy and the Ommaya reservoir, may also be used. (See *Alternative approaches to chemotherapy*.)

Alternative approaches to chemotherapy

Administering chemotherapeutic drugs into the peritoneal cavity—intraperitoneal chemotherapy—has several benefits for patients with malignant ascites or ovarian cancer that has spread to the peritoneum. This method passes drugs directly to the tumor area in the peritoneal cavity, exposing malignant cells to high concentrations of chemotherapy—up to 1,000 times the amount that can be safely given systemically. What's more, the semipermeable peritoneal membrane permits prolonged exposure of malignant cells to the drug.

An Ommaya reservoir, also known as a *subcutaneous cerebrospinal fluid (CSF) reservoir,* allows delivery of long-term drug therapy to the CSF via the brain's ventricles. The reservoir spares the patient repeated lumbar punctures to administer chemotherapeutic drugs. It's most commonly used for treating central nervous system (CNS) leukemia, malignant CNS disease, and meningeal carcinomatosis. Besides providing convenient, comparatively painless access to the CSF, the Ommaya reservoir permits consistent and predictable drug distribution throughout the subarachnoid space and CNS.

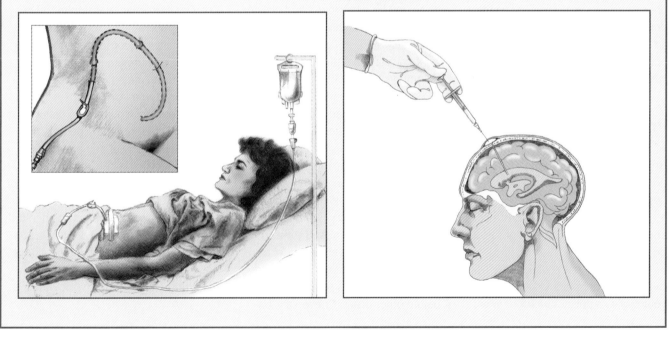

Classifying chemotherapeutic drugs

If the practitioner has ordered the intermittent administration of a vesicant drug, you can give it either by instilling the drug into the side port of an infusing I.V. line or by direct I.V. push through an intermittent infusion device. If the vesicant drug is to be infused continuously, you should administer it only through a central venous line or an implanted port. **INS** On the other hand, nonvesicant agents (including irritants) may be given by direct I.V. push through an intermittent infusion device, through the side port of an infusing I.V. line, or as a continuous infusion.

Irritants

Irritants can cause a local venous response with or without a skin reaction. Chemotherapeutic irritants include:
▶ carboplatin (Paraplatin)
▶ carmustine (BiCNU)
▶ dacarbazine (DTIC-Dome)
▶ etoposide (VePesid)
▶ ifosfamide (IFEX)
▶ irinotecan (Camptosar)
▶ streptozocin (Zanosar)
▶ topotecan (Hycamtin).

Vesicants

Vesicants cause a reaction so severe that blisters form and tissue is damaged or destroyed. Chemotherapeutic vesicants include:
▶ dactinomycin (Cosmegen)
▶ daunorubicin (Cerubidine)
▶ doxorubicin (Adriamycin)
▶ idarubicin (Idamycin)
▶ mechlorethamine (Mustargen)
▶ mitomycin (Mutamycin)
▶ mitoxantrone (Novantrone)
▶ vinblastine (Velban)
▶ vincristine (Oncovin)
▶ vinorelbine (Navelbine).

Nonvesicants

Nonvesicants don't cause irritation or damage. Chemotherapeutic nonvesicants include:
▶ asparaginase (Elspar)
▶ bleomycin (Blenoxane)
▶ cyclophosphamide (Cytoxan)
▶ cytarabine (Cytosar-U)
▶ floxuridine (FUDR)
▶ fluorouracil (Efudex).

Equipment

Prescribed drug ◆ gloves ◆ aluminum foil or a brown paper bag (if the drug is photosensitive) ◆ normal saline solution ◆ syringes and needleless adapters ◆ infusion pump ◆ impervious containers labeled CAUTION: BIO-HAZARD.

Implementation

▶ Verify the drug, dosage, and administration route by checking the medication record against the practitioner's order. **JC INS ONS**
▶ Make sure you know the immediate and delayed adverse effects of the ordered drug. **INS**
▶ Confirm the patient's identity using two patient identifiers according to your facility's policy. **INS JC**

▶ Assess the patient's physical condition, and review his medical history.
▶ Make sure you understand what chemotherapeutic agent needs to be given and by what route, and provide the necessary teaching and support to the patient and his family. **INS**
▶ If your facility utilizes a bar code scanning system, be sure to scan your ID badge, the patient's ID bracelet, and the medication's bar code. **JC ISMP**
▶ Determine the best site to administer the drug. When selecting the site, consider drug compatibilities, frequency of administration, and vesicant potential of the drug. (See *Classifying chemotherapeutic drugs*.) Check your facility's policy before administering a vesicant. Because vein integrity decreases with time, some facilities require that vesicants be administered before other drugs. Conversely, be-

cause vesicants increase vein fragility, some facilities require that vesicants be given after other drugs. **INS**
▶ Evaluate the patient's condition, paying particular attention to the results of recent laboratory studies, specifically the complete blood count, blood urea nitrogen level, platelet count, urine creatinine level, and liver function studies. **ONS INS**
▶ Determine whether the patient has received chemotherapy before, and note the severity of any previous adverse effects.
▶ Check the patient's drug history for medications that might interact with chemotherapy. As a rule, you shouldn't mix chemotherapeutic drugs with other medications. If you have questions or concerns about giving the chemotherapeutic drug, talk with the

practitioner or pharmacist before you give it.

▶ Next, double-check the patient's chart for the complete chemotherapy protocol order, including the patient's name, drug's name and dosage, and route, rate, and frequency of administration. Be aware that some facilities require two nurses to verify the dosage order of high-alert medications and to check the drug and amount being administered. **INS**

▶ Check to see whether the practitioner has ordered an antiemetic, fluids, a diuretic, or electrolyte supplements to be given before, during, or after chemotherapy administration.

▶ Evaluate the patient's and his family's understanding of chemotherapy, and make sure the patient or a responsible family member has signed the consent form.

▶ Next, put on gloves. Keep them on through all stages of handling the drug. **OSHA ONS INS**

▶ Before administering the drug, perform a new venipuncture proximal to the old site. Avoid giving chemotherapeutic drugs through an existing I.V. line. To identify an administration site, examine the patient's veins, starting with his hand and proceeding to his forearm.

▶ When an appropriate line is in place, infuse 10 to 20 ml of normal saline solution to test vein patency. Never test vein patency with a chemotherapeutic drug. Next, administer the drug as appropriate and according to your facility's policy.

▶ During I.V. administration, closely monitor the patient for signs of a hypersensitivity reaction or extravasation. Check for adequate blood return after 5 ml of the drug has been infused or according to your facility's guidelines. **ONS**

▶ After infusion of the medication, infuse 20 ml of normal saline solution.

Do this between administrations of different chemotherapeutic drugs and before discontinuing the I.V. line.

▶ Dispose of used needles and syringes carefully. To prevent aerosol dispersion of chemotherapeutic drugs, don't clip needles. Place them intact in an impervious container for incineration. Dispose of I.V. bags, bottles, gloves, and tubing in a properly labeled and covered trash container. **CDC OSHA ONS**

▶ Wash your hands thoroughly with soap and warm water after giving chemotherapeutic drugs, even though you have worn gloves. **CDC ONS**

Special considerations

▶ Observe the I.V. site frequently for signs of extravasation and an allergic reaction (swelling, redness, urticaria). If you suspect extravasation, stop the infusion immediately. Leave the I.V. catheter in place, and notify the practitioner. A conservative method for treating extravasation involves aspirating any residual drug from the tubing and I.V. catheter, instilling an I.V. antidote, and then removing the I.V. catheter. Afterward, you may apply heat or cold to the site and elevate the affected limb. **ONS INS**

▶ During infusion, some drugs need protection from direct sunlight to avoid possible drug breakdown. If this is the case, cover the vial with a brown paper bag or aluminum foil.

▶ When giving vesicants, avoid sites where damage to underlying tendons or nerves may occur (veins in the antecubital fossa, near the wrist, or in the dorsal surface of the hand). **INS**

▶ Observe the patient at regular intervals and after treatment for adverse reactions. Monitor his vital signs throughout the infusion to assess changes during chemotherapy administration.

▶ Maintain a list of the types and amounts of drugs the patient has received. This is especially important if he has received drugs that have a cumulative effect and that can be toxic to such organs as the heart and kidneys.

▶ Common adverse effects of chemotherapy are nausea and vomiting, ranging from mild to debilitating. Another major complication is bone marrow suppression, leading to neutropenia and thrombocytopenia. Other adverse effects include intestinal irritation, stomatitis, pulmonary fibrosis, cardiotoxicity, nephrotoxicity, neurotoxicity, hearing loss, anemia, alopecia, urticaria, radiation recall (if drugs are given with or soon after radiation therapy), anorexia, esophagitis, diarrhea, and constipation.

References

Brown, K., et al. *Chemotherapy and Biotherapy Guidelines and Recommendations for Practice.* Pittsburgh: Oncology Nursing Society, 2001.

Sauerland, C., et al. "Vesicant Extravasation Part I. Mechanisms, Pathogens, and Nursing Care to Reduce Risk," *Oncology Nurse Forum* 33(6):1134-141, November 2006.

"Standard 37. Site Selection. Infusion Nursing Standards of Practice," *Journal of Infusion Nursing* 29(1S):S37-39, January-February 2006.

"Standard 54. Infiltration. Infusion Nursing Standards of Practice," *Journal of Infusion Nursing* 29(1S):S59-60, January-February 2006.

"Standard 55. Extravasation. Infusion Nursing Standards of Practice," *Journal of Infusion Nursing* 29(1S):S61-62, January-February 2006.

"Standard 69. Antineoplastic and Biologic Therapy. Infusion Nursing Standards of Practice," *Journal of Infusion Nursing* 29(1S):S69-71, January-February 2006.

Tipton, J.M., et al. "Putting Evidence into Practice: Evidence-Based Interventions to Prevent, Manage, and Treat Chemotherapy-Induced Nausea and Vomiting," *Clinical Journal of Oncology Nursing* 11(1):69-78, February 2007.

U.S. Department of Labor. Occupational Safety & Health Administration. "Controlling Occupational Exposure to Harmful Drugs," *In:* TED 1-0.15A, Section VI, Chapter 2. *OSHA Technical Manual.* Washington, D.C.: OSHA, January 1999. Available: *www.osha.gov/dts/osta_vi/otm_vi_2.htm.*

Wickham, R., et al. "Vesicant Extravasation Part II: Evidence-Based Management and Continuing Controversies," *Oncology Nursing Forum* 33(6):1143-150, November 2006.

Wilson, L. "Oncology Safety: Safe Environment/Safe Practice for Patients and Providers," *ONS News* 21(8 Suppl):29-30, 2006.

Wyatt, A., et al. "Cutaneous Reactions to Chemotherapy and Their Management," *American Journal of Clinical Dermatology* 7(1):45-63, 2006.

Chest physiotherapy

Chest physiotherapy includes postural drainage, chest percussion and vibration, and coughing and deep-breathing exercises. Together, these techniques mobilize and eliminate secretions, reexpand lung tissue, and promote efficient use of respiratory muscles. Of critical importance to the bedridden patient, chest physiotherapy helps prevent or treat atelectasis and may also help prevent pneumonia—two respiratory complications that can seriously impede recovery.

Postural drainage performed in conjunction with percussion and vibration encourages peripheral pulmonary secretions to empty (by gravity) into the major bronchi or trachea and is accomplished by sequential repositioning of the patient. Usually, secretions drain best with the patient positioned so that the bronchi are perpendicular to the floor. Lower and middle lobe bronchi usually empty best with the patient in the head-down position; upper lobe bronchi, in the head-up position. (See *Positioning a patient for postural drainage*, pages 104 and 105.)

Percussing the chest with cupped hands mechanically dislodges thick, tenacious secretions from the bronchial walls. Vibration can be used with percussion or as an alternative to it in a patient who's frail, in pain, or recovering from thoracic surgery or trauma.

Candidates for chest physiotherapy include patients who expectorate large amounts of sputum, such as those with bronchiectasis and cystic fibrosis. In critical care patients, including those on mechanical ventilation, postural drainage therapy (PDT) should be performed every 4 to 6 hours, as indicated. PDT frequency should be determined by assessing response to therapy. Acute care patient orders should be reevaluated, based on patient response to therapy, at least every 72 hours or with a change in patient status. **AARC**

Contraindications may include active pulmonary bleeding with hemoptysis and the immediate posthemorrhage stage, fractured ribs or an unstable chest wall, lung contusions, pulmonary tuberculosis, untreated pneumothorax, acute asthma or bronchospasm, lung abscess or tumor, bony metastasis, head injury, and recent myocardial infarction.

Equipment

Stethoscope ◆ pillows ◆ tilt or postural drainage table (if available) or adjustable hospital bed ◆ emesis basin ◆ facial tissues ◆ suction equipment ◆ equipment for oral care ◆ trash bag ◆ optional: sterile specimen container, mechanical ventilator, supplemental oxygen.

Implementation

▶ Gather the equipment at the patient's bedside. Set up suction equipment, and test its function.
▶ Confirm the patient's identity using two patient identifiers according to your facility's policy. **JC**

▶ Explain the procedure to the patient, provide privacy, and wash your hands.
▶ Auscultate the patient's lungs to determine baseline respiratory status.
▶ Position the patient as ordered. In generalized disease, drainage usually begins with the lower lobes, continues with the middle lobes, and ends with the upper lobes. In localized disease, drainage begins with the affected lobes and then proceeds to the other lobes to avoid spreading the disease to uninvolved areas.
▶ Instruct the patient to remain in each position for 3 to 15 minutes. During this time, perform percussion and vibration as ordered. (See *Performing percussion and vibration,* page 106.)

▶ After postural drainage, percussion, or vibration, instruct the patient to cough to remove loosened secretions. First, tell him to inhale deeply through his nose and then exhale in three short huffs. Then have him inhale deeply again and cough through a slightly open mouth. Three consecutive coughs are highly effective. An effective cough sounds deep, low, and hollow; an ineffective one, high-pitched. Have the patient perform exercises for about 1 minute and then rest for 2 minutes. Gradually progress to a 10-minute exercise period four times daily. **CS**
▶ Provide oral hygiene because secretions may have a foul taste or a stale odor.
▶ Auscultate the patient's lungs to evaluate the effectiveness of therapy.

(Text continues on page 106.)

Positioning a patient for postural drainage

The following illustrations show the various postural drainage positions and the areas of the lungs affected by each.

Lower lobes:
Posterior basal segments
Elevate the foot of the bed 30 degrees. Have the patient lie prone with his head lowered. Position pillows under his chest and abdomen. Percuss his lower ribs on both sides of his spine.

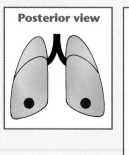

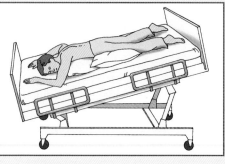

Lower lobes:
Lateral basal segments
Elevate the foot of the bed 30 degrees. Instruct the patient to lie on his abdomen with his head lowered and his upper leg flexed over a pillow for support. Then have him rotate a quarter turn upward. Percuss his lower ribs on the uppermost portion of his lateral chest wall.

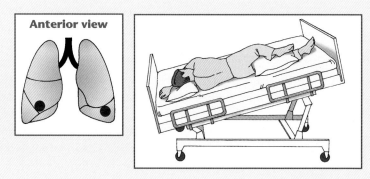

Lower lobes:
Anterior basal segments
Elevate the foot of the bed 30 degrees. Instruct the patient to lie on his side with his head lowered. Then place pillows as shown. Percuss with a slightly cupped hand over his lower ribs just beneath the axilla. If an acutely ill patient has trouble breathing in this position, adjust the bed to an angle he can tolerate. Then begin percussion.

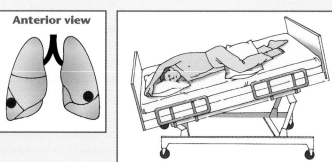

Lower lobes:
Superior segments
With the bed flat, have the patient lie on his abdomen. Place two pillows under his hips. Percuss on both sides of his spine at the lower tip of his scapulae.

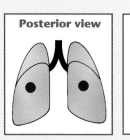

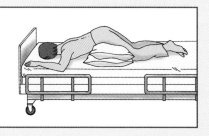

Right middle lobe:
Medial and lateral segments
Elevate the foot of the bed 15 degrees. Have the patient lie on his left side with his head down and his knees flexed. Then have him rotate a quarter turn backward. Place a pillow beneath him. Percuss with your hand moderately cupped over the right nipple. For a woman, cup your hand so that its heel is under the armpit and your fingers extend forward beneath the breast.

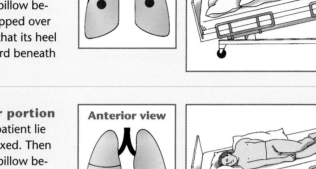

Left upper lobe:
Superior and inferior segments, lingular portion
Elevate the foot of the bed 15 degrees. Have the patient lie on his right side with his head down and knees flexed. Then have him rotate a quarter turn backward. Place a pillow behind him, from shoulders to hips. Percuss with your hand moderately cupped over his left nipple. For a woman, cup your hand so that its heel is beneath the armpit and your fingers extend forward beneath the breast.

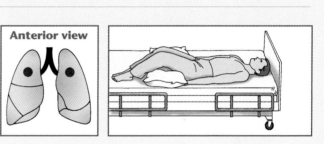

Upper lobes:
Anterior segments
Make sure the bed is flat. Have the patient lie on his back with a pillow folded under his knees. Then have him rotate slightly away from the side being drained. Percuss between his clavicle and nipple.

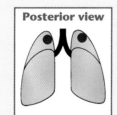
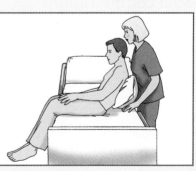

Upper lobes:
Apical segments
Keep the bed flat. Have the patient lean back at a 30-degree angle against you and a pillow. Percuss with a cupped hand between his clavicles and the top of each scapula.

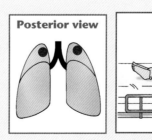
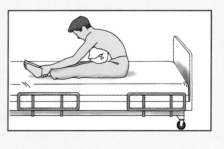

Upper lobes:
Posterior segments
Keep the bed flat. Have the patient lean over a pillow at a 30-degree angle. Percuss and clap his upper back on each side.

Performing percussion and vibration

To perform percussion, instruct the patient to breathe slowly and deeply, using the diaphragm, to promote relaxation. Hold your hands in a cupped shape, with fingers flexed and thumbs pressed tightly against your index fingers. Percuss each segment for 1 to 2 minutes by alternating your hands against the patient in a rhythmic manner. Listen for a hollow sound on percussion to verify correct performance of the technique.

To perform vibration, ask the patient to inhale deeply and then exhale slowly through pursed lips. During exhalation, firmly press your fingers and palms against the chest wall. Tense the muscles of your arms and shoulders in an isometric contraction to send fine vibrations through the chest wall. Vibrate during five exhalations over each chest segment.

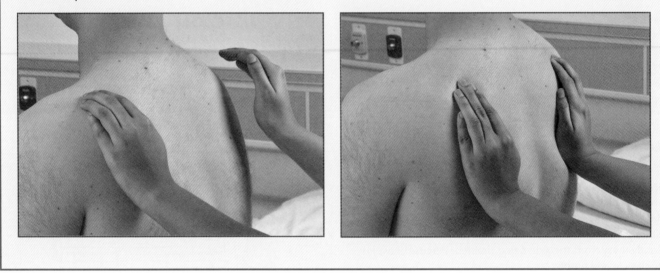

Special considerations

▶ For optimal effectiveness and safety, modify chest physiotherapy according to the patient's condition. Also, suction the patient who has an ineffective cough reflex. If the patient tires quickly during therapy, shorten the sessions because fatigue leads to shallow respirations and increased hypoxia.

▶ Maintain adequate hydration in the patient receiving chest physiotherapy to prevent mucus dehydration and promote easier mobilization. Avoid performing postural drainage immediately before or within 1 1/2 hours after meals to avoid nausea, vomiting, and aspiration of food or vomitus.

▶ Because chest percussion can induce bronchospasm, any adjunct treatment (for example, intermittent positive-pressure breathing, aerosol, or neb-

ulizer therapy) should precede chest physiotherapy.

▶ Refrain from percussing over the spine, liver, kidneys, or spleen to avoid injury. Also avoid performing percussion on bare skin or the female patient's breasts. Percuss over soft clothing (but not over buttons, snaps, or zippers), or place a thin towel over the chest wall. Remember to remove jewelry that might scratch or bruise the patient.

▶ Explain coughing and deep-breathing exercises preoperatively so that the patient can practice them when he's pain-free and better able to concentrate. Postoperatively, splint the patient's incision using your hands or, if possible, teach the patient to splint it himself to minimize pain during coughing.

▶ Try to schedule the last session just before bedtime to help maximize the patient's oxygenation while he's sleeping.

References

McCarven, B., et al. "Vibration and Its Effects on the Respiratory System," *Australian Journal of Physiotherapy* 52(1):39-43, 2006.

McCool, F.D., et al. "Non-Pharmacological Airway Clearance Therapies: AACP Evidence-Based Clinical Practice Guidelines," *Chest* 129(1 Suppl):2505-595, January 2006. **CS**

Pruitt, B., et al. "Clearing Away Pulmonary Secretions," *Nursing* 35(7):36-41, July 2005.

Taylor, C., et al. *Fundamentals of Nursing: The Art and Science of Nursing Care,* 5th ed. Philadelphia: Lippincott Williams & Wilkins, 2008.

Chest tube insertion

The pleural space normally contains a thin layer of lubricating fluid that allows the viscera and parietal pleura to move without friction during respiration. An excess of air (pneumothorax), fluid (hemothorax or pleural effusion), or both in this space alters intrapleural pressure and causes partial or complete lung collapse.

Chest tube insertion allows drainage of air or fluid from the pleural space. Usually performed by a physician with a nurse assisting, this procedure requires sterile technique. The insertion site varies depending on the patient's condition and the physician's judgment. For pneumothorax, the second to third intercostal spaces are the usual sites because air rises to the top of the intrapleural space. For hemothorax or pleural effusion, the fourth to sixth intercostal spaces are common sites because fluid settles to the lower levels of the intrapleural space. For removal of air and fluid, a chest tube is inserted into a high and low site.

After insertion, one or more chest tubes are connected to a thoracic drainage system that removes air, fluid, or both from the pleural space and prevents backflow into that space, thus promoting lung reexpansion. (See "Thoracic drainage," page 524.)

Equipment

Two pairs of sterile gloves ◆ sterile drape ◆ vial of 1% lidocaine ◆ antiseptic solution ◆ 10-ml syringe ◆ alcohol pad ◆ 22G 1″ needle ◆ 25G ³/₈″ needle ◆ sterile scalpel (usually with #11 blade) ◆ two rubber-tipped clamps for each chest tube inserted ◆ sterile 4″ × 4″ gauze pads ◆ two sterile 4″ × 4″ drain dressings ◆ 3″ or 4″ sturdy, elastic tape ◆ 1″ adhesive tape for connections ◆ chest tube of appropriate size (#16 to #20 French catheter for air or serous fluid; #28 to #40 French catheter for blood, pus, or thick fluid), with or without a trocar ◆ sterile Kelly clamp ◆ suture material (usually 2-0 silk with cutting needle) ◆ thoracic drainage system with tubing ◆ sterile Y-connector (for two chest tubes on the same side) ◆ petroleum gauze ◆ sterile water.

Prepackaged sterile chest tube trays are commercially available and usually contain most of the equipment needed.

Implementation

▶ Check the expiration date on the sterile packages, and inspect for tears. Then assemble all equipment in the patient's room, and set up the thoracic drainage system. **CDC**

▶ Label all medications, medication containers, and other solutions on and off the sterile field. **JC**

▶ Place the thoracic drainage system next to the patient's bed below his chest level to facilitate drainage. **CS**

▶ Confirm the patient's identity using two patient identifiers according to your facility's policy. **JC**

▶ In a nonemergency, make sure the patient has signed the appropriate consent form.

▶ Explain the procedure to the patient, provide privacy, and wash your hands.

▶ Record baseline vital signs and respiratory assessment. Place oxygen on the patient as needed.

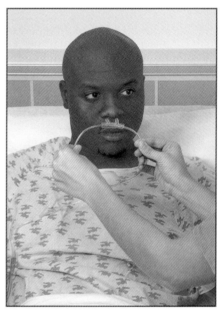

▶ Position the patient appropriately. If he has a pneumothorax, place him in high Fowler's, semi-Fowler's, or the supine position. If the patient has a hemothorax, have him lean over the overbed table or straddle a chair with his arms dangling over the back. For either pneumothorax or hemothorax, the patient may lie on his unaffected side with his arms extended over his head.

▶ When you've positioned the patient properly, place the chest tube tray on the overbed table. Open it using sterile technique.

▶ The physician puts on sterile gloves and prepares the insertion site by cleaning the area with antiseptic solution.

▶ Wipe the rubber stopper of the lidocaine vial with an alcohol pad. Then invert the bottle, and hold it for the physician to withdraw the anesthetic.

▶ After the physician anesthetizes the site, he makes a small incision and inserts the chest tube. Next, he either immediately connects the chest tube to the thoracic drainage system or momentarily clamps the tube close to the patient's chest until he can connect it to the drainage system. He may then secure the tube to the skin with a suture.

▶ As the physician is inserting the chest tube, reassure the patient and assist the physician, as necessary.

▶ Immediately after the drainage system is connected, instruct the patient to take a deep breath, hold it momentarily, and slowly exhale to assist drainage of the pleural space and lung reexpansion.

▶ Open the packages containing the petroleum gauze, 4″ × 4″ drain dressings, and gauze pads, and put on sterile gloves. Then place the petroleum gauze and two 4″ × 4″ drain dressings around the insertion site, one from the top and the other from the bottom. Place several 4″ × 4″ gauze pads on top of the drain dressings. Tape the dressings, covering them completely to form an occlusive dressing.

▶ Securely tape the chest tube to the patient's chest distal to the insertion site to help prevent accidental tube dislodgment.

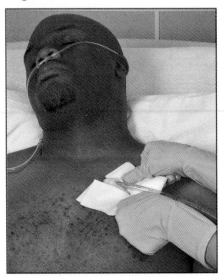

▶ Securely tape the junction of the chest tube and the drainage tube to prevent their separation.

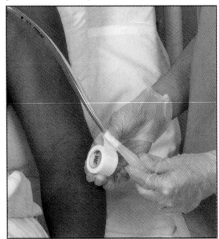

▶ Check the status of the drainage tubing. Be sure the tubing remains at the level of the patient and no dependent loops are present.

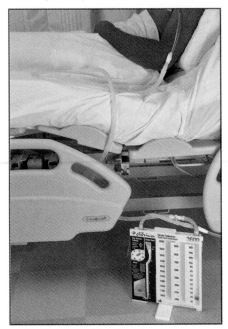

▶ A portable chest X-ray is then done to check tube position.

▶ Take the patient's vital signs every 15 minutes for 1 hour and then as his condition indicates. Auscultate his lungs at least every 4 hours following the procedure to assess air exchange in the affected lung. Diminished or absent breath sounds indicate that the lung hasn't reexpanded.

▶ Monitor and record the drainage in the drainage collection chamber. (See "Thoracic drainage," page 524.)

Special considerations

▶ Remember that routine changing of the chest tube isn't recommended because of the risk of tension pneumothorax.

▶ During patient transport, keep the thoracic drainage system below chest level. Don't clamp the chest tube or tip the drainage system during transport. **CS**

▶ If the chest tube comes out, cover the site immediately with 4″ × 4″ gauze pads, and tape them in place. Stay with the patient, and monitor his vital signs every 10 minutes. Observe him for signs of tension pneumothorax (hypotension, distended jugular veins, absent or decreased breath sounds, tracheal shift, hypoxemia, weak and rapid pulse, dyspnea, tachypnea, diaphoresis, and chest pain). Have another staff member notify the physician, and gather the equipment needed to reinsert the tube.

▶ Place the rubber-tipped clamps at the bedside. If the commercial system cracks or a tube disconnects, clamp the chest tube momentarily as close to the insertion site as possible. Because no air or liquid can escape from the pleural space while the tube is clamped, observe the patient closely for signs of tension pneumothorax while the clamp is in place. Instead of clamping the tube, you can submerge the distal end of the tube in a container of normal saline solution to create a temporary water seal while you replace the drainage system. Check your facility's policy for the proper procedure.

References

Allibone, L. "Principles for Inserting and Managing Chest Drains," *Nursing Times* 101(42):45-49, October 2005.

Carroll, P. "Keeping Up with Mobile Chest Drains," *RN* 68(10):26-31, October 2005.

Coughlin, A.M., and Parchinsky, C. "Go with the Flow of Chest Tube Therapy," *Nursing* 36(3):36-41, March 2006.

Lynn-McHale Wiegand, D.J., and Carlson, K.K., eds. *AACN Procedure Manual for Critical Care,* 5th ed. Philadelphia: W.B. Saunders Co., 2006.

Roman, M., and Mercado, D. "Review of Chest Tube Use," *Medsurg Nursing* 15(1):41-43, February 2006.

Schmelz, J.O., et al. "Effects of Position of Chest Drainage Tube on Volume Drained and Pressure," *American Journal of Critical Care* 8(5):319-23, September 1999 **CS**

Closed-wound drain management

Typically inserted during surgery in anticipation of substantial postoperative drainage, a closed-wound drain promotes healing and prevents swelling by suctioning the exudate that accumulates at the wound site. By removing this fluid, the closed-wound drain helps reduce the risk of infection and skin breakdown as well as the number of dressing changes to be used. The drain is usually emptied every 4 to 8 hours. Hemovac and Jackson-Pratt closed drainage systems are used most commonly. (See *Types of closed drainage systems*.)

A closed-wound drain consists of perforated tubing connected to a portable vacuum unit. The distal end of the tubing lies within the wound and usually leaves the body from a site other than the primary suture line to preserve the integrity of the surgical wound. The tubing exit site is treated as an additional surgical wound; the drain is usually sutured to the skin.

Equipment

Graduated cylinder ◆ sterile laboratory container, if needed ◆ alcohol pads ◆ gloves ◆ gown ◆ face shield ◆ sterile gauze pads ◆ antiseptic cleaning agent ◆ antiseptic swabs ◆ optional: label.

Implementation

▶ Check the practitioner's order, and assess the patient's condition.
▶ Explain the procedure to the patient, provide privacy, and wash your hands.
▶ Unclip the vacuum unit from the patient's bed or gown.
▶ Using sterile technique, release the vacuum by removing the spout plug on the collection chamber. The container expands completely as it draws in air.
▶ Empty the unit's contents into a graduated cylinder, and note the amount and appearance of the drainage. If diagnostic tests will be performed on the fluid specimen, pour the drainage directly into a sterile laboratory container, note the amount and appearance, and send it to the laboratory (as shown at the top of the next column).

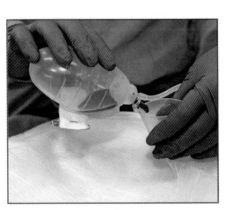

▶ Maintaining sterile technique, use an alcohol pad to clean the unit's spout and plug.
▶ To reestablish the vacuum that creates the drain's suction power, fully compress the vacuum unit. With one hand holding the unit compressed to maintain the vacuum, replace the spout plug with your other hand.

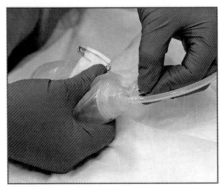

▶ Check the patency of the equipment. Make sure the tubing is free from twists, kinks, and leaks because the drainage system must be airtight to work properly. The vacuum unit should remain compressed when you release manual pressure; rapid reinflation indicates an air leak. If this occurs, recompress the unit, and make sure the spout plug is secure.
▶ Secure the vacuum unit to the patient's gown. Fasten it below wound level to promote drainage. To prevent possible dislodgment, don't apply tension on drainage tubing when fastening the unit.
▶ Remove and discard your gloves, and wash your hands thoroughly.
▶ Observe the sutures that secure the drain to the patient's skin; look for signs of pulling or tearing and for swelling or infection of surrounding skin. Gently clean the sutures with sterile gauze pads soaked in an antiseptic cleaning agent or with an antiseptic swab.
▶ Properly dispose of drainage and solutions, and clean or dispose of soiled equipment and supplies according to your facility's policy.

Types of closed drainage systems

There are two common types of closed drainage systems. The Jackson-Pratt drain collects exudate in a bulblike device that's typically used with breast and abdominal surgery.

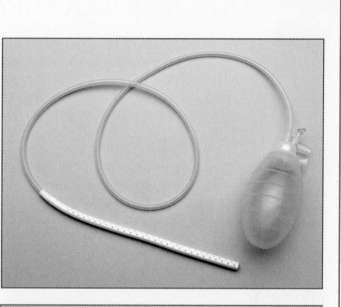

The Hemovac drain is used when blood drainage is expected after surgery, such as with abdominal and orthopedic surgeries.

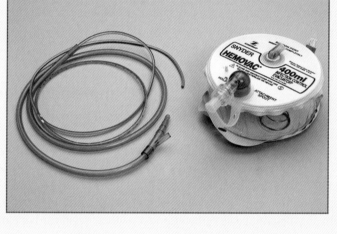

Special considerations

▶ Empty the drain, and measure its contents once during each shift if drainage has accumulated; more often if drainage is excessive. Removing excess drainage maintains maximum suction and avoids straining the drain's suture line.

▶ If the patient has more than one closed drain, number the drains so you can record drainage from each site.

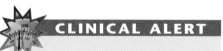

CLINICAL ALERT

Be careful not to mistake chest tubes with water seal drainage devices for closed-wound drains because the care of these devices differs from closed-wound drainage systems, and the vacuum of a chest tube should never be released.

References

Jeter, K. "Closed Suction Wound Drainage System," *Journal of Wound, Ostomy, and Continence Nursing* 31(2):51, March-April 2004.

Patel, V.P., et al. "Factors Associated with Prolonged Wound Drainage after Primary Total Hip and Knee Arthroplasty," *Journal of Bone and Joint Surgery* 89(1):33-38, January 2007.

Code management

The goals of any code are to restore the patient's spontaneous heartbeat and respirations and to prevent hypoxic damage to the brain and other vital organs. Fulfilling these goals requires a team approach. Ideally, the team should consist of health care workers trained in advanced cardiac life support (ACLS), although nurses trained in basic life support (BLS) may also be a part of the team. BLS and ACLS procedures and protocols should be performed according to the 2005 American Heart Association (AHA) guidelines.

Because ventricular fibrillation commonly precedes sudden cardiac arrest, initial resuscitative efforts focus on rapid recognition of arrhythmias and, when indicated, defibrillation. If monitoring equipment isn't available, you should simply perform BLS measures. Of course, the scope of your responsibilities in any situation depends on your facility's policies and procedures and your state's nurse practice act.

A code may be called for patients with absent pulse, apnea, ventricular fibrillation, ventricular tachycardia, or asystole. Some facilities allow family members to be present during a code; check your facility's policy regarding this issue.

Equipment

Oral, nasal, and endotracheal (ET) airways ◆ one-way valve masks ◆ oxygen source ◆ oxygen flowmeter ◆ intubation supplies, including end-tidal carbon dioxide detector or esophageal detector ◆ handheld resuscitation bag ◆ suction supplies ◆ nasogastric (NG) tube ◆ goggles, masks, and gloves ◆ cardiac arrest board ◆ peripheral I.V. supplies, including 14G and 18G peripheral I.V. catheters ◆ central I.V. supplies, including an 18G thin-wall catheter, a 6-cm needle catheter, and a 16G 15- to 20-cm catheter ◆ I.V. administration sets (including macrodrip and microdrip) ◆ I.V. fluids, including dextrose 5% in water (D_5W), normal saline solution, and lactated Ringer's solution ◆ electrocardiogram (ECG) monitor and leads ◆ cardioverter-defibrillator ◆ conductive medium ◆ cardiac drugs, including adenosine, epinephrine, lidocaine, procainamide, vasopressin, amiodarone, atropine, isoproterenol, dopamine, calcium chloride, and dobutamine.

Because effective emergency care depends on reliable and accessible equipment, the equipment as well as the personnel must be ready for a code at any time. (See *Organizing your crash cart.*) You should also be familiar with the cardiac drugs you may have to administer.

Implementation

▶ If you're the first to arrive at the site of a code, call for help, and instruct another person to retrieve the emergency equipment. Then, assess the patient's level of consciousness (LOC), assess airway, breathing, and circulation, and then begin cardiopulmonary resuscitation (CPR). Use a pocket mask, if available, to ventilate the patient. **AHA**

▶ When the emergency equipment arrives, have the second BLS provider place the cardiac arrest board under the patient and assist with two-rescuer CPR. Meanwhile, have the nurse assigned to the patient relate the patient's medical history and describe the events leading to cardiac arrest.

▶ A third person, either a nurse certified in BLS or a respiratory therapist, will then attach the handheld resuscitation bag to the oxygen source and begin to ventilate the patient with 100% oxygen.

▶ When the ACLS-trained nurse arrives, she'll expose the patient's chest and apply defibrillator pads. She'll then apply the paddles to the patient's chest to obtain a "quick look" at the patient's cardiac rhythm. If the patient is in ventricular fibrillation, ACLS protocol calls for defibrillation as soon as possible with 360 joules. Then, resume CPR immediately. A rhythm check isn't done at this time. After 5 cycles of CPR, and if a rhythm is detected, perform a pulse check. (See *ACLS pulseless arrest algorithm,* pages 114 and 115.) The ACLS-trained nurse will act as code leader until the practitioner arrives. **AHA**

▶ If not already in place, apply ECG electrodes and attach the patient to the defibrillator's cardiac monitor. Avoid placing electrodes on bony prominences or hairy areas. Also avoid the areas where the defibrillator pads will be placed and where chest compressions will be given. **MFR**

▶ After 5 cycles of CPR, the patient's rhythm will be checked and, if necessary, another shock will be given at the same dose; you'll then continue CPR while the defibrillator is charging. After another 5 cycles of CPR, the patient's rhythm will be checked, and another

Organizing your crash cart

When responding to a code, you can't waste time searching the drawers of your crash cart for the equipment you need. One way to make sure you know the precise location of everything is to follow the ABCD plan to maintain an organized crash cart. Label the crash cart drawers with the letters A, B, C, and D, and fill them as described below.

A: Airway control drawer

The airway control drawer should contain all the equipment necessary for maintaining a patient's airway, including:
▶ oral, nasal, and endotracheal (ET) airways
▶ an intubation tray containing a laryngoscope and blades
▶ an extra laryngoscope
▶ lidocaine ointment
▶ tape or ET tube securement device
▶ a 10-ml syringe to inflate the ET balloon
▶ extra batteries and lightbulbs
▶ suction devices.

B: Breathing drawer

The breathing drawer should contain all of the equipment needed to support the patient's ventilation and oxygenation. Maintain gastric compression with nasogastric tubes. Support oxygenation with:
▶ nasal cannulas
▶ face masks
▶ Venturi masks.

C: Circulation drawer

In the circulation drawer, place anything needed to start a central or peripheral I.V. line, such as:
▶ catheters
▶ tubing
▶ start kits
▶ pump tubing
▶ 250-ml or 500-ml bags of I.V. solutions (dextrose 5% in water and normal saline solution).

D: Drug drawer

The drug drawer should contain all medications needed for advanced cardiac life support.

---

shock will be given at the same dose, if necessary. **AHA**

▶ As CPR continues, you or an ACLS-trained nurse will then start two peripheral I.V. lines with large-bore I.V. catheters. Be sure to use only a large vein, such as the antecubital vein, to allow for rapid fluid administration and to prevent drug extravasation.

▶ As soon as the I.V. catheter is in place, begin an infusion of normal saline solution to help prevent circulatory collapse. Although D_5W continues to be acceptable, the latest ACLS guidelines encourage the use of normal saline solution because D_5W can produce hyperglycemic effects during a cardiac arrest. **AHA**

▶ While one nurse starts the I.V. lines, the other nurse sets up portable or wall suction equipment and suctions the patient's oral secretions, as necessary, to maintain an open airway.

▶ The ACLS-trained nurse will then prepare and administer emergency cardiac drugs, as needed. Keep in mind that drugs administered through a central line reach the myocardium more quickly than those administered through a peripheral line.

▶ The ACLS pulseless arrest algorithm shows the timing of drug administration and shock administration. Drug doses should be given immediately after a rhythm check. **AHA**

▶ If the patient doesn't have an accessible I.V. catheter, you may administer such medications as epinephrine, lidocaine, vasopressin, and atropine through an ET tube. To do so, dilute the drugs in 10 ml of normal saline solution or sterile water and then instill them into the patient's ET tube. Afterward, ventilate the patient manually to improve absorption by distributing the drug throughout the bronchial tree. **AHA**

▶ The ACLS-trained nurse will also prepare for, and assist with, ET intubation or other advanced airway. Compression interruption should be minimized during advanced airway placement.

▶ Suction the patient, as needed. After the patient has been intubated, the practitioner should use clinical assessment and confirmation devices to check ET tube placement. Assessment includes visualizing chest expansion and auscultating for equal breath sounds and breath sounds over the epigastrium. Devices used to check tube placement include exhaled carbon dioxide detectors and esophageal detectors. When the tube is correctly positioned, tape it securely. To serve as a reference, mark the point on the tube level with the patient's lips. **AHA**

▶ Meanwhile, other members of the code team should keep a written record of the events. Other duties in-

(Text continues on page 116.)

ACLS pulseless arrest algorithm AHA

This American Heart Association algorithm outlines the steps an advanced cardiac life support (ACLS)-certified nurse should take to treat rhythms that produce cardiac arrest, such as ventricular fibrillation (VF), rapid ventricular tachycardia (VT), pulseless electrical activity (PEA), and asystole. If you aren't ACLS-certified, this algorithm will help you know what to expect in such an emergency.

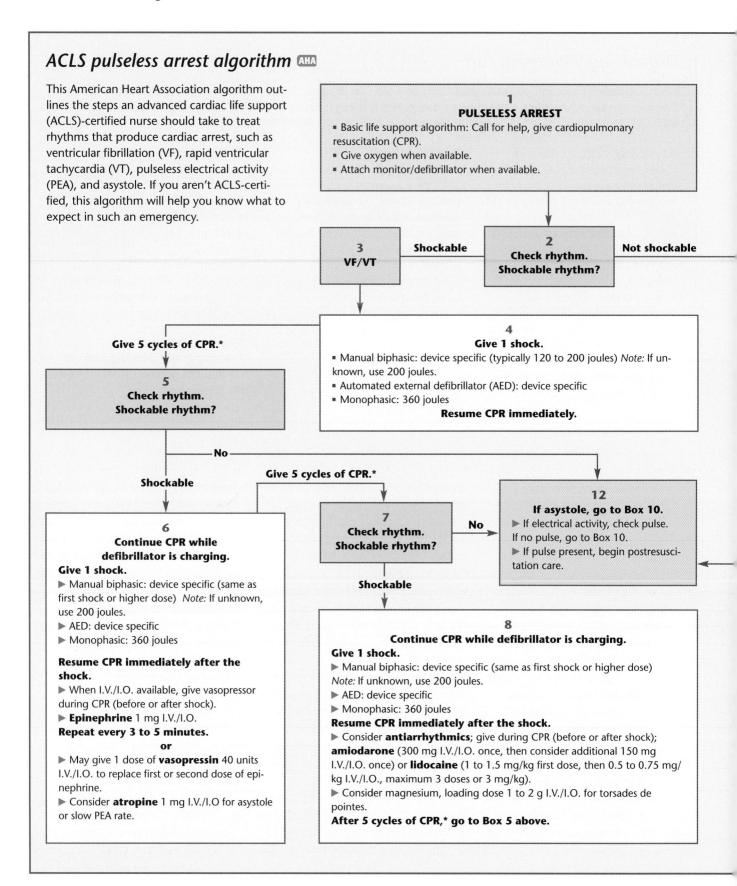

1
PULSELESS ARREST
- Basic life support algorithm: Call for help, give cardiopulmonary resuscitation (CPR).
- Give oxygen when available.
- Attach monitor/defibrillator when available.

2
Check rhythm.
Shockable rhythm?

3
VF/VT

Shockable

Not shockable

Give 5 cycles of CPR.*

4
Give 1 shock.
- Manual biphasic: device specific (typically 120 to 200 joules) *Note:* If unknown, use 200 joules.
- Automated external defibrillator (AED): device specific
- Monophasic: 360 joules
Resume CPR immediately.

5
Check rhythm.
Shockable rhythm?

No

Shockable

Give 5 cycles of CPR.*

6
Continue CPR while defibrillator is charging.
Give 1 shock.
▶ Manual biphasic: device specific (same as first shock or higher dose) *Note:* If unknown, use 200 joules.
▶ AED: device specific
▶ Monophasic: 360 joules

Resume CPR immediately after the shock.
▶ When I.V./I.O. available, give vasopressor during CPR (before or after shock).
▶ **Epinephrine** 1 mg I.V./I.O.
Repeat every 3 to 5 minutes.
or
▶ May give 1 dose of **vasopressin** 40 units I.V./I.O. to replace first or second dose of epinephrine.
▶ Consider **atropine** 1 mg I.V./I.O for asystole or slow PEA rate.

7
Check rhythm.
Shockable rhythm?

No

Shockable

12
If asystole, go to Box 10.
▶ If electrical activity, check pulse. If no pulse, go to Box 10.
▶ If pulse present, begin postresuscitation care.

8
Continue CPR while defibrillator is charging.
Give 1 shock.
▶ Manual biphasic: device specific (same as first shock or higher dose) *Note:* If unknown, use 200 joules.
▶ AED: device specific
▶ Monophasic: 360 joules
Resume CPR immediately after the shock.
▶ Consider **antiarrhythmics**; give during CPR (before or after shock); **amiodarone** (300 mg I.V./I.O. once, then consider additional 150 mg I.V./I.O. once) or **lidocaine** (1 to 1.5 mg/kg first dose, then 0.5 to 0.75 mg/kg I.V./I.O., maximum 3 doses or 3 mg/kg).
▶ Consider magnesium, loading dose 1 to 2 g I.V./I.O. for torsades de pointes.
After 5 cycles of CPR,* go to Box 5 above.

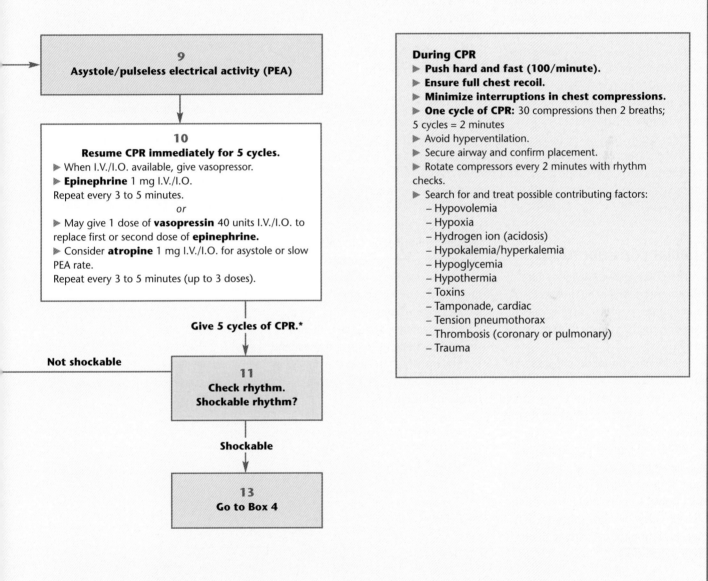

9
Asystole/pulseless electrical activity (PEA)

10
Resume CPR immediately for 5 cycles.
▶ When I.V./I.O. available, give vasopressor.
▶ **Epinephrine** 1 mg I.V./I.O.
Repeat every 3 to 5 minutes.
or
▶ May give 1 dose of **vasopressin** 40 units I.V./I.O. to replace first or second dose of **epinephrine.**
▶ Consider **atropine** 1 mg I.V./I.O. for asystole or slow PEA rate.
Repeat every 3 to 5 minutes (up to 3 doses).

*Give 5 cycles of CPR.**

Not shockable

11
Check rhythm.
Shockable rhythm?

Shockable

13
Go to Box 4

During CPR
▶ **Push hard and fast (100/minute).**
▶ **Ensure full chest recoil.**
▶ **Minimize interruptions in chest compressions.**
▶ **One cycle of CPR:** 30 compressions then 2 breaths; 5 cycles = 2 minutes
▶ Avoid hyperventilation.
▶ Secure airway and confirm placement.
▶ Rotate compressors every 2 minutes with rhythm checks.
▶ Search for and treat possible contributing factors:
 – Hypovolemia
 – Hypoxia
 – Hydrogen ion (acidosis)
 – Hypokalemia/hyperkalemia
 – Hypoglycemia
 – Hypothermia
 – Toxins
 – Tamponade, cardiac
 – Tension pneumothorax
 – Thrombosis (coronary or pulmonary)
 – Trauma

*After an advanced airway is placed, rescuers no longer deliver "cycles" of CPR. Give continuous chest compressions without pauses for breaths. Give 8 to 10 breaths/minute. Check rhythm every 2 minutes.

Reproduced with permission from *2005 American Heart Association Guidelines for Cardiopulmonary Resuscitation and Emergency Cardiovascular Care.* © 2005, American Heart Association.

clude prompting participants about when to perform certain activities (such as when to check a pulse or take vital signs), overseeing the effectiveness of CPR, and keeping track of the time between therapies. Each team member should know what each participant's role is to prevent duplicating effort. Finally, someone from the team should make sure the primary nurse's other patients are reassigned to another nurse.

▶ If the family is present during the code, have someone, such as a clergy member or social worker, remain with them. Be sure to keep the family regularly informed of the patient's status.

▶ If the family isn't at the facility, contact them as soon as possible. Encourage them not to drive to the facility, but offer to call someone who can give them a ride.

Special considerations

▶ The 2005 AHA guidelines stress that compressions shouldn't be interrupted unless a shock is being delivered or a rhythm check is being performed.

▶ Health care providers shouldn't attempt to check for a pulse after a shock is delivered, but the pulse check should occur after 5 cycles of CPR, if a rhythm is detected. **AHA**

▶ When the patient's condition has stabilized, assess his LOC, breath sounds, heart sounds, peripheral perfusion, bowel sounds, and urine output. Measure his vital signs every 15 minutes, and monitor his cardiac rhythm continuously. **AHA**

▶ Make sure the patient receives an adequate supply of oxygen, whether through a mask or ventilator. **AHA**

▶ Check the infusion rates of all I.V. fluids, and use infusion pumps to deliver vasoactive drugs. To evaluate the effectiveness of fluid therapy, insert an indwelling catheter if the patient doesn't already have one. Also insert an NG tube to relieve or prevent gastric distention.

▶ If appropriate, reassure the patient and explain what's happening. Allow the patient's family to visit as soon as possible. If the patient dies, notify the family, and allow them to see the patient as soon as possible.

▶ To make sure your code team performs optimally, schedule a time to review the code.

▶ Even when performed correctly, CPR can cause fractured ribs, liver laceration, lung puncture, and gastric distention. Defibrillation can cause electric shock, and emergency intubation can result in esophageal or tracheal laceration, subcutaneous emphysema, or accidental right mainstem bronchus intubation. (Decreased or absent breath sounds on the left side of the chest and normal breath sounds on the right may signal accidental right mainstem bronchus intubation.)

References

American Heart Association. "2005 Guidelines for Cardiopulmonary Resuscitation and Emergency Cardiovascular Care: The International Consensus on Science," *Circulation* 112(22 Suppl):IV-1-IV-221, November 2005.

American Heart Association. "Highlights of the 2005 American Heart Association Guidelines for Cardiopulmonary Resuscitation and Emergency Cardiovascular Care," *Currents* 16(4):1-27, Winter 2005-2006.

Emergency Nurses Association. "Family Presence at the Bedside during Invasive Procedures or Resuscitation. Position Statement." Available: *www.ena.org/about/position/PDFs/4E6C256B26994E319F66C65748BFBDBF.pdf*.

Halm, M.A. "Family Presence during Resuscitation: A Critical Review of the Literature," *American Journal of Critical Care* 14(6):494-511, November 2005.

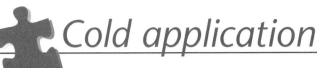

Cold application

The application of cold constricts blood vessels; inhibits local circulation, suppuration, and tissue metabolism; relieves vascular congestion; slows bacterial activity in infections; reduces body temperature; and may act as a temporary anesthetic during brief, painful procedures. Because treatment with cold also relieves inflammation, reduces edema, and slows bleeding, it may provide effective initial treatment after eye injuries, strains, sprains, bruises, muscle spasms, and burns. Cold doesn't reduce existing edema, however, because it inhibits reabsorption of excess fluid.

Cold may be applied in dry or moist forms, but ice shouldn't be placed directly on a patient's skin because it may further damage tissue. Moist application is more penetrating than dry because moisture facilitates conduction. Devices for applying cold include an ice bag or collar, aquathermia pad (which can produce cold or heat), and chemical cold packs and ice packs. Devices for applying moist cold include cold compresses for small body areas and cold packs for large areas.

Apply cold treatments cautiously on patients with impaired circulation, on children, and on elderly or arthritic patients because of the risk of ischemic tissue damage.

Equipment

Patient thermometer ◆ towel ◆ adhesive tape or roller gauze ◆ gloves, if necessary.

For an ice bag or collar: Tap water ◆ ice chips ◆ absorbent, protective cloth covering.

For an aquathermia pad: Distilled water ◆ temperature-adjustment key ◆ absorbent, protective cloth covering.

For a chemical cold pack: Single-use packs are available for applying dry cold. These lightweight plastic packs contain a chemical that turns cold when activated. Reusable, sealed cold packs, filled with an alcohol-based solution, are also available. These packs may be stored frozen until use and, after exterior disinfection, may be refrozen and used again. Other chemical packs are activated by striking, squeezing, or kneading them.

For a cold compress or pack: Basin of ice chips ◆ container of tap water ◆ bath thermometer ◆ compress material (4″ × 4″ gauze pads or washcloths) or pack material (towels or flannel) ◆ linen-saver pad ◆ waterproof covering.

Implementation

▶ Confirm the patient's identity using two patient identifiers according to your facility's policy. **JC**
▶ Check the practitioner's order, and assess the patient's condition.
▶ Explain the procedure to the patient, provide privacy, and make sure the room is warm and free from drafts. Wash your hands thoroughly.
▶ Record the patient's temperature, pulse, and respirations to serve as a baseline.
▶ Expose only the treatment site to avoid chilling the patient.

Applying an ice bag or collar, an aquathermia pad, or a chemical cold pack

▶ For an ice bag or collar, select a device of the correct size, fill it with cold tap water, and check for leaks. Empty the device, and fill it about halfway with crushed ice. Squeeze the device to expel air that might reduce conduction. Fasten the cap, and wipe moisture from the outside of the device (as shown at the top of the next column).

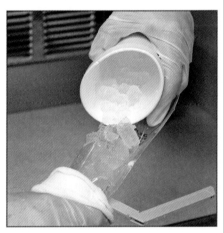

▶ Wrap the bag or collar in a cloth covering, and secure the cover with tape or roller gauze. The protective cover prevents tissue trauma and absorbs condensation.

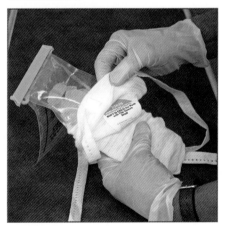

▶ For an aquathermia pad, check the cord for frayed or damaged insulation. Then fill the control unit two-thirds full with distilled water. Don't use tap water because it leaves mineral deposits in the unit. Check for leaks, and then tilt the unit several times to clear the pad's tubing of air. Tighten the cap. After ensuring that the hoses between the control unit and pad are free from tangles, place the unit on the bedside table slightly above the patient so that gravity can assist water flow. If the central supply department hasn't preset the temperature, use the temperature-adjustment key to adjust the control unit setting to the lowest temperature. Cover the pad with an absorbent, protective cloth, and secure the cover with tape or roller gauze. Plug in the unit, and turn it on. Allow the pad to cool for 2 minutes before placing it on the patient. **MFR**

▶ For a chemical cold pack, select a pack of the appropriate size, and follow the manufacturer's directions (strike, squeeze, or knead) to activate the cold-producing chemicals. Make certain that the container hasn't been broken during activation. Wrap the pack in a cloth cover, and secure the cover with tape or roller gauze.

▶ Place the covered cold device on the treatment site, and begin timing the application.

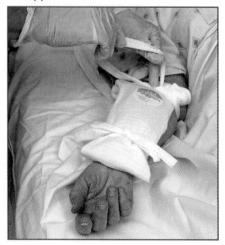

▶ Observe the site frequently for signs of tissue intolerance, such as blanching, mottling, cyanosis, maceration, and blisters. Also be alert for shivering and complaints of burning or numbness. If these signs or symptoms develop, discontinue treatment, and notify the practitioner.

▶ Refill or replace the cold device, as necessary, to maintain the correct temperature. Change the protective cover if it becomes wet.

▶ Remove the device after the prescribed treatment period (usually 30 minutes as reflex vasodilation begins to occur after that time).

Applying a cold compress or pack

▶ For a cold compress or pack, cool a container of tap water by placing it in a basin of ice or by adding ice to the water. Using a bath thermometer for guidance, adjust the water temperature to 59° F (15° C) or as ordered. Immerse the compress or pack material in the water.

▶ Place a linen-saver pad under the site.

▶ Remove the compress or pack from the water, and wring it out to prevent dripping. Apply it to the treatment site, and begin timing the application.

▶ Cover the compress or pack with a waterproof covering to provide insulation and to keep the surrounding area dry. Secure the covering with tape or roller gauze to prevent it from slipping.

▶ Check the application site frequently for signs of tissue intolerance, and note complaints of burning or numbness. If these symptoms develop, discontinue treatment, and notify the practitioner.

▶ Change the compress or pack, as needed, to maintain the correct temperature. Remove it after the prescribed treatment period (usually 20 minutes).

Concluding all cold applications

▶ Dry the patient's skin and redress the treatment site according to the practitioner's orders. Then position the patient comfortably and take his temperature, pulse, and respirations for comparison with baseline.

▶ Dispose of liquids and soiled materials properly. If the cold treatment will be repeated, clean and store the equipment in the patient's room, out of his reach; otherwise, return it to storage.

Special considerations

▶ Apply cold immediately after an injury to minimize edema. Although colder temperatures can be tolerated for a longer time when the treatment site is small, don't continue any application for longer than 1 hour to avoid reflex vasodilation. The application of temperatures below 59° F (15° C) also causes local reflex vasodilation.

▶ Use sterile technique when applying cold to an open wound or to a lesion that may open during treatment. Also maintain sterile technique during eye treatment, with separate sterile equipment for each eye to prevent cross-contamination.

▶ Avoid securing cooling devices with pins because an accidental puncture could allow extremely cold fluids to leak out and burn the patient's skin.

▶ If the patient is unconscious, anesthetized, neurologically impaired, irrational, or otherwise insensitive to cold, stay with him throughout the treatment, and check the application site frequently for complications.

References

Craven, R.F., and Hirnle, C.J. *Fundamentals of Nursing: Human Health and Function,* 6th ed. Philadelphia: Lippincott Williams & Wilkins, 2009.

Kanlayanaphotoporn, R., et al. "Comparison of Skin Surface Temperature during the Application of Various Cryotherapy Modalities," *Archives of Physical Medicine and Rehabilitation* 86(7):1411-415, July 2005.

Laureanofilho, J.R., et al. "The Influence of Cryotherapy on Reduction of Swelling, Pain, and Trimus after Third Molar Extraction: A Preliminary Study," *Journal of the American Dental Association* 136(6):774-78, June 2005.

Ownby, K.K. "Effects of Ice Massage on Neuropathic Pain in Persons with AIDS," *The Journal of the Association of Nurses and AIDS Care* 17(5):15-22, September-October 2006.

Taylor, C., et al. *Fundamentals of Nursing: The Art and Science of Nursing Care,* 6th ed. Philadelphia: Lippincott Williams & Wilkins, 2008.

Colostomy and ileostomy care

A patient with an ascending or transverse colostomy or an ileostomy must wear an external pouch to collect emerging fecal matter, which will be watery or pasty. Besides collecting waste matter, the pouch helps to control odor and protect the stoma and peristomal skin. Most disposable pouching systems can be used for 2 to 7 days; some models last longer.

All pouching systems need to be changed immediately if a leak develops, and every pouch must be emptied when it's one-third to one-half full. The patient with an ileostomy may need to empty his pouch four or five times daily.

The best time to change the pouching system is when the bowel is least active, usually between 2 and 4 hours after meals. After a few months, most patients can predict the best changing time.

The selection of a pouching system should take into consideration which system provides the best adhesive seal and skin protection for the patient. The type of pouch selected also depends on the stoma's location and structure, availability of supplies, wear time, consistency of effluent, personal preference, and finances.

Equipment

Pouching system ◆ stoma measuring guide ◆ stoma paste (if drainage is watery to pasty or stoma secretes excess mucus) ◆ scissors ◆ clippers ◆ washcloth and towel ◆ closure clamp ◆ toilet or bedpan ◆ water or pouch cleaning solution ◆ gloves ◆ facial tissues ◆ optional: paper tape, mild nonmoisturizing soap, liquid skin sealant, pouch deodorant.

Pouching systems may be drainable or closed-bottomed, disposable or reusable, adhesive-backed, and one-piece or two-piece. (See *Comparing ostomy pouching systems*.)

Implementation

▶ Provide privacy and emotional support.

Fitting the pouch and skin barrier

▶ For a pouch with an attached skin barrier, measure the stoma with the stoma measuring guide. Select the opening size that matches the stoma.

▶ For an adhesive-backed pouch with a separate skin barrier, measure the stoma with the measuring guide, and select the opening that matches the stoma. Trace the selected size opening onto the paper back of the skin barrier's adhesive side. Cut out the opening. (If the pouch has precut openings, which can be handy for a round stoma, select an opening that is $1/8''$ larger than the stoma. If the pouch comes without an opening, cut the hole $1/8''$ wider than the measured tracing.) The cut-to-fit system works best for an irregularly shaped stoma. **WOCN**

▶ For a two-piece pouching system with flanges, see *Applying a skin barrier and pouch*, page 122.

▶ Avoid fitting the pouch too tightly because the stoma has no pain receptors. A constrictive opening could injure the stoma or skin tissue without the patient feeling discomfort. Also avoid cutting the opening too big because this may expose the skin to fecal matter and moisture. **WOCN**

▶ The patient with a descending or sigmoid colostomy who has formed stools and whose ostomy doesn't secrete much mucus may choose to wear only a pouch. In this case, make sure the pouch opening closely matches the stoma size.

▶ From 6 weeks to 1 year after surgery, the stoma will shrink to its permanent size. At that point, pattern-making preparations will be unnecessary unless the patient gains weight, has additional surgery, or injures the stoma.

Applying or changing the pouch

▶ Collect all equipment.

▶ Wash your hands, and provide privacy.

▶ Explain the procedure to the patient. As you perform each step, explain what you're doing and why because the patient will eventually perform the procedure himself.

▶ Put on gloves. **CDC**

▶ Remove and discard the old pouch.

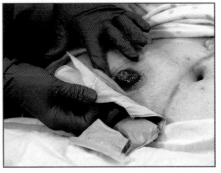

▶ Wipe the stoma and peristomal skin gently with a facial tissue (as shown at the top of the next column).

Comparing ostomy pouching systems

Manufactured in many shapes and sizes, ostomy pouches are fashioned for comfort, safety, and easy application. For example, a disposable closed-end pouch may meet the needs of a patient who irrigates, who wants added security, or who wants to discard the pouch after each bowel movement. Another patient may prefer a reusable, drainable pouch. Some commonly available pouches are described below.

Disposable pouches

The patient who must empty his pouch often (because of diarrhea or a new colostomy or ileostomy) may prefer a one-piece, drainable, disposable pouch with a closure clamp attached to a skin barrier (below left).

These transparent or opaque, odor-proof plastic pouches come with attached adhesive or karaya seals. Some pouches have microporous adhesive. The bottom opening allows for easy draining. This pouch may be used permanently or temporarily, until stoma size stabilizes.

Also disposable and made of transparent or opaque odor-proof plastic, a one-piece disposable closed-end pouch (below right) may come in a kit with adhesive seal, skin barrier, or carbon filter for gas release. A patient with a regular bowel elimination pattern may choose this style for additional security and confidence.

A two-piece disposable drainable pouch with separate skin barrier permits frequent changes and also minimizes skin breakdown. Also made of transparent or opaque odor-proof plastic, this style usually snaps to the skin barrier with a flange mechanism.

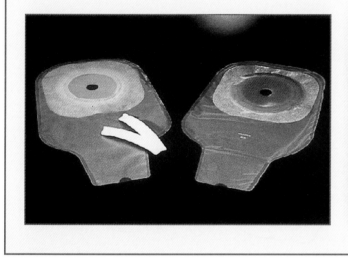

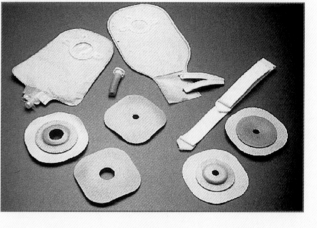

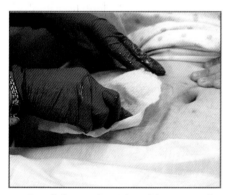

► Carefully wash with mild soap and water, and dry the peristomal skin by patting gently. Allow the skin to dry thoroughly. Inspect the peristomal skin and stoma. If necessary, clip surrounding hair (in a direction away from the stoma) to promote a better seal and avoid skin irritation from hair pulling against the adhesive. **WOCN**

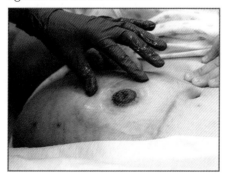

► If applying a separate skin barrier, peel the paper backing off the prepared skin barrier, center the barrier over the stoma, and press gently to ensure adhesion.

► You may want to outline the stoma on the back of the skin barrier (depending on the product) with a thin ring of stoma paste to provide extra skin protection. (Skip this step if the patient has a sigmoid or descending colostomy, formed stools, and little mucus.) **MFR**

► Remove the paper backing from the adhesive side of the pouching system,

Applying a skin barrier and pouch

Fitting a skin barrier and ostomy pouch properly can be done in a few steps. Shown here is a two-piece pouching system with flanges, which is commonly used.

Measure the stoma using a measuring guide.

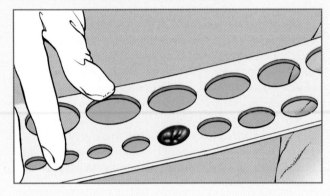

Trace the appropriate circle carefully on the back of the skin barrier.

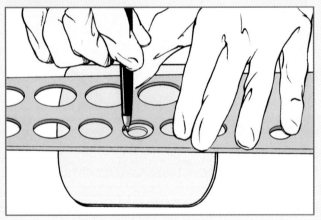

Cut the circular opening in the skin barrier. Bevel the edges to keep them from irritating the patient.

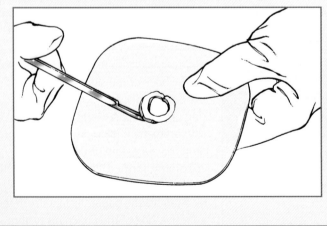

Remove the backing from the skin barrier, and moisten it or apply barrier paste, as needed, along the edge of the circular opening.

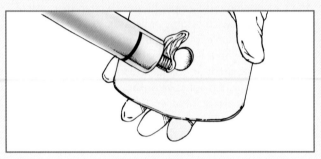

Center the skin barrier over the stoma, adhesive side down, and gently press it to the skin.

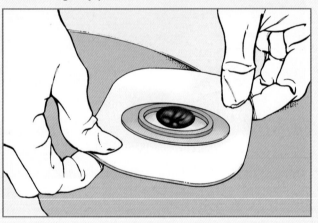

Gently press the pouch opening onto the ring until it snaps into place.

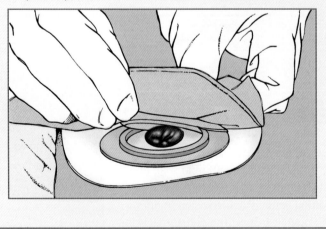

and center the pouch opening over the stoma. Press gently to secure.

▶ For a pouching system with flanges, align the lip of the pouch flange with the bottom edge of the skin barrier flange. Gently press around the circumference of the pouch flange, beginning at the bottom, until the pouch securely adheres to the barrier flange. (The pouch will click into its secured position.) Holding the barrier against the skin, gently pull on the pouch to confirm the seal between flanges.

▶ Encourage the patient to stay quietly in position for about 5 minutes to improve adherence. The patient's body warmth also helps to improve adherence and soften a rigid skin barrier. **MFR**

▶ Leave a bit of air in the pouch to allow drainage to fall to the bottom.

▶ Apply the closure clamp, if necessary.

▶ If desired, apply paper tape in a picture-frame fashion to the pouch edges for additional security.

Emptying the pouch

▶ Put on gloves. **CDC**

▶ Tilt the bottom of the pouch upward and remove the closure clamp.

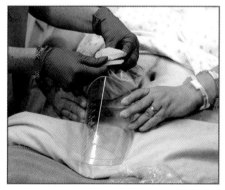

▶ Turn up a cuff on the lower end of the pouch, and allow it to drain into the toilet or graduated container (as shown at the top of the next column).

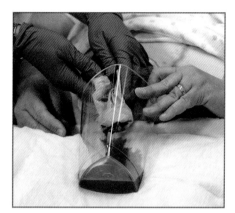

▶ Wipe the bottom of the pouch, and reapply the closure clamp.

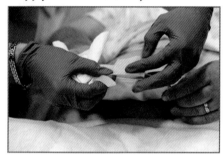

▶ If desired, the bottom portion of the pouch can be rinsed with cool tap water. Don't aim water up near the top of the pouch because this may loosen the seal on the skin.

▶ A two-piece flanged system can also be emptied by unsnapping the pouch. Let the drainage flow into the toilet.

▶ Release flatus through the gas release valve if the pouch has one. Otherwise, release flatus by tilting the pouch bottom upward, releasing the clamp, and expelling the flatus. To release flatus from a flanged system, loosen the seal between the flanges. (Some pouches have gas release valves.)

▶ Never make a pinhole in a pouch to release gas because doing so will destroy the odor-proof seal. **MFR**

▶ Remove and discard your gloves.

Special considerations

▶ After performing and explaining the procedure to the patient, encourage the patient's increasing involvement in self-care.

▶ Use adhesive solvents and removers only after patch-testing the patient's skin because some products may irritate the skin or produce hypersensitivity reactions. Consider using a liquid skin sealant, if available, to give skin tissue additional protection from drainage and adhesive irritants.

▶ Remove the pouching system if the patient reports burning or itching beneath it or purulent drainage around the stoma. Notify the practitioner of skin irritation, breakdown, rash, or unusual appearance of the stoma or peristomal area.

▶ Use commercial pouch deodorants, if desired. However, most pouches are odor-free, and odor should only be evident when you empty the pouch or if it leaks. Before discharge, suggest that the patient avoid odor-causing foods, such as fish, eggs, onions, and garlic.

▶ If the patient wears a reusable pouching system, suggest that he obtain two or more systems so that he can wear one while the other dries after cleaning with soap and water or a commercially prepared cleaning solution.

References

Colwell, J.C., and Fichera, A. "Care of the Obese Patient with an Ostomy," *Journal of Wound, Ostomy, and Continence Nursing* 32(6):378-83, November-December 2005.

Pontierei-Lewis, V. "Basics of Ostomy Care," *Medsurg Nursing* 15(4):199-202, August 2006.

Taylor, C., et al. *Fundamentals of Nursing: The Art and Science of Nursing Care,* 6th ed. Philadelphia: Lippincott Williams & Wilkins, 2008.

Turnbull, G.B. "Using Education to Increase Self-Care for the Person with an Ostomy," *Ostomy/Wound Management* 52(9):16, 18, September 2006.

Colostomy irrigation

Irrigation of a colostomy can serve two purposes: It allows a patient with a descending or sigmoid colostomy to regulate bowel function, and it cleans the large bowel before and after tests, surgery, or other procedures.

Colostomy irrigation may begin as soon as bowel function resumes after surgery. However, most clinicians recommend waiting until bowel movements are more predictable. Initially, the nurse or the patient irrigates the colostomy at the same time every day, recording the amount of output and any spillage between irrigations. Between 4 and 6 weeks may pass before colostomy irrigation establishes a predictable elimination pattern.

Equipment

Colostomy irrigation set (contains an irrigation drain or sleeve, water-soluble lubricant, drainage pouch clamp, and irrigation bag with clamp, tubing, and cone tip) ◆ 1 L (1 qt) of tap water irrigant warmed to about 105° F (40.6° C) ◆ normal saline solution (for cleansing enemas) ◆ I.V. pole or wall hook ◆ washcloth and towel ◆ water ◆ ostomy pouching system ◆ linen-saver pad ◆ gown, goggles, and gloves ◆ optional: bedpan or chair, mild nonmoisturizing soap, rubber band or clip, small dressing or bandage, stoma cap.

Implementation

▶ Set up the irrigation bag with tubing and cone tip. If irrigation will take place with the patient in bed, place the bedpan beside the bed, and elevate the head of the bed 45 to 90 degrees, if allowed. If irrigation will take place in the bathroom, have the patient sit on the toilet or on a chair facing the toilet, whichever he finds more comfortable.

▶ Fill the irrigation bag with warmed tap water (or normal saline solution, if the irrigation is for bowel cleansing). Hang the bag on the I.V. pole or wall hook. The bottom of the bag should be at the patient's shoulder level to prevent the fluid from entering the bowel too quickly. Most irrigation sets also have a clamp that regulates the flow rate.

▶ Prime the tubing with irrigant to prevent air from entering the colon and possibly causing cramps and gas pains.

▶ Confirm the patient's identity using two patient identifiers according to your facility's policy. **JC**

▶ Explain every step of the procedure to the patient because he'll probably be irrigating the colostomy himself.

▶ Provide privacy, and wash your hands.

▶ If the patient is in bed, place a linen-saver pad under him to protect the sheets from soiling.

▶ Put on gloves and personal protective equipment. **JC**

▶ Remove the ostomy pouch if the patient uses one.

▶ Place the irrigation sleeve over the stoma. If the patient has a two-piece pouching system with flanges, snap off the pouch and save it. Snap on the irrigation sleeve.

▶ Place the open-ended bottom of the irrigation sleeve in the bedpan or toilet to promote drainage by gravity. If necessary, cut the sleeve so that it meets the water level inside the bedpan or toilet. Effluent may splash from a short sleeve or may not drain from a long sleeve.

▶ Lubricate your gloved small finger with water-soluble lubricant and insert the finger into the stoma. If you're teaching the patient, have him do this to determine the bowel angle at which to insert the cone safely. Expect the stoma to tighten when the finger enters the bowel and then to relax in a few seconds.

▶ Lubricate the cone with water-soluble lubricant to prevent it from irritating the mucosa.

▶ Insert the cone into the top opening of the irrigation sleeve and then into the stoma. Angle the cone to match the bowel angle. Insert it gently but snugly.

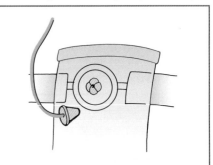

▶ Unclamp the irrigation tubing, and allow the water to flow slowly. If you don't have a clamp to control the irrigant's flow rate, pinch the tubing to control the flow. The water should enter the colon over 5 to 10 minutes. (If the patient reports cramping, slow or stop the flow, keep the cone in place, and have the patient take a few deep breaths until the cramping stops.) Cramping during irrigation may result from a bowel that is ready to empty, water that is too cold, a rapid flow rate, or air in the tubing.

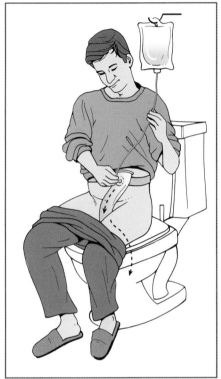

▶ Have the patient remain stationary for 15 or 20 minutes so that the initial effluent can drain.

▶ If the patient is ambulatory, he can stay in the bathroom until all effluent empties, or he can clamp the bottom of the drainage sleeve with a rubber band or clip and return to bed. Explain that ambulation and activity stimulate elimination. Suggest that the nonambulatory patient lean forward or massage his abdomen to stimulate elimination.

▶ Wait about 45 minutes for the bowel to finish eliminating the irrigant and effluent. Then remove the irrigation sleeve.

▶ If the irrigation was intended to clean the bowel, repeat the procedure with warmed normal saline solution until the return solution appears clear.

▶ Using a washcloth, mild soap, and water, gently clean the area around the stoma. Rinse and dry the area thoroughly with a clean towel.

▶ Inspect the skin and stoma for changes in appearance. Usually dark pink to red, stoma color may change with the patient's status. Notify the practitioner of marked stoma color changes because a pale hue may result from anemia, and substantial darkening suggests a change in blood flow to the stoma.

▶ Apply a clean pouch. If the patient has a regular bowel elimination pattern, he may prefer a small dressing, bandage, or commercial stoma cap.

▶ Discard a disposable irrigation sleeve. Rinse a reusable irrigation sleeve, and hang it to dry along with the irrigation bag, tubing, and cone.

Special considerations

▶ Irrigating a colostomy to establish a regular bowel elimination pattern doesn't work for all patients. If the bowel continues to move between irrigations, try decreasing the volume of irrigant. Increasing the irrigant won't help because it serves only to stimulate peristalsis. Keep a record of results. Also consider irrigating every other day.

▶ Irrigation may help to regulate bowel function in patients with a descending or sigmoid colostomy because this is the bowel's stool storage area. However, a patient with an ascending or transverse colostomy won't benefit from irrigation. Also, a patient with a descending or sigmoid colostomy who's missing part of the ascending or transverse colon may not be able to irrigate successfully because his ostomy may function like an ascending or transverse colostomy.

▶ If diarrhea develops, discontinue irrigations until stools form again. Keep in mind that irrigation alone won't achieve regularity for the patient. He must also observe a complementary diet and exercise regimen.

▶ If the patient has a strictured stoma that prohibits cone insertion, remove the cone from the irrigation tubing, and replace it with a soft silicone catheter. Angle the catheter gently 2″ to 4″ (5 to 10 cm) into the bowel to instill the irrigant. Don't force the catheter into the stoma, and don't insert it farther than the recommended length because you may perforate the bowel.

References

Craven, R.F., and Hirnle, C.J. *Fundamentals of Nursing: Human Health and Function,* 6th ed. Philadelphia: Lippincott Williams & Wilkins, 2009.

Karadag, A., et al. "Colostomy Irrigation: Results of 25 Cases with Particular Reference to Quality of Life," *Journal of Clinical Nursing* 14(4):479-85, April 2005.

Pullen, R.L., Jr. "Teaching Your Patient to Irrigate a Colostomy," *Nursing* 36(4):22, April 2006.

Taylor, C., et al. *Fundamentals of Nursing: The Art and Science of Nursing Care,* 6th ed. Philadelphia: Lippincott Williams & Wilkins, 2008.

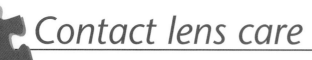

Contact lens care

Illness or emergency treatment may require that you insert or remove and store a patient's contact lenses. Proper handling and lens-care techniques help prevent eye injury and infection as well as lens loss or damage. **AOA** Appropriate lens-handling techniques depend in large part on what type of lenses the patient wears.

All contact lenses float on the corneal tear layer. Rigid lenses typically have a smaller diameter than the cornea; soft lens diameter typically exceeds that of the cornea. Because they're larger and more pliable, soft lenses tend to mold themselves more closely to the eye for a more stable fit than rigid lenses.

Keep in mind that handling contact lenses improperly can provide a direct source of contamination to the eye. **AOA**

Equipment

Lens storage case or two small medicine cups and adhesive tape ◆ gloves ◆ patient's equipment for contact lens care, if available ◆ sterile normal saline solution or soaking solution ◆ flashlight, if needed ◆ optional: suction cup.

Implementation

▶ If a commercial lens storage case isn't available, place enough sterile normal saline solution into two small medicine cups to submerge a lens in each one. To avoid confusing the left and right lenses, which may have different prescriptions, mark one cup "L" and the other cup "R," and place the corresponding lens in each cup.

▶ Tell the patient what you're about to do, wash your hands, and put on gloves to help prevent ocular infection.

Inserting rigid lenses

▶ Wet one lens with solution, and gently rub it between your thumb and index finger, or place it on your palm and rub it with your opposite index finger. Rinse well with the solution, leaving a small amount in the lens.

▶ Place the lens, convex side down, on the tip of the index finger of your dominant hand.

▶ Instruct the patient to gaze upward slightly. Separate the eyelids with your other thumb and index finger, and place the lens directly and gently on the cornea. You need not press it to the eye; the tear film will attract it naturally at the first touch. Using the same procedure, insert the opposite lens.

Inserting soft lenses

▶ To see if the lens is inside out, bend it between your thumb and index finger or fill it with saline or soaking solution. If the lens tends to roll inward or the edge points slightly inward, it's oriented correctly. If the edge points outward or the lens tends to collapse over your fingertip, it's probably inside out and should be reversed.

▶ Wet the lens with fresh normal saline solution, and rub it gently between your thumb and index finger, or place it on your palm and rub it with your opposite index finger. Rinse well.

▶ Place the lens, convex side down, on the tip of the index finger of your dominant hand.

▶ Instruct the patient to gaze upward slightly. Separate the eyelids with your other thumb and index finger, and place the lens on the sclera, just below the cornea. Then, slide the lens gently upward with your finger until it centers

on the cornea. Using the same procedure, insert the opposite lens.

Removing rigid lenses

▶ Before removing a lens, position the patient supine to prevent the lens from popping out onto the floor, risking loss or damage.

▶ Place one thumb against the patient's upper eyelid and the other thumb against the lower eyelid. Move the lids toward each other while gently pressing inward against the eye to trap the lens edge and break the suction. Extract the lens from the patient's eyelashes.

▶ Depending on the lens type and thickness, it may pop out when the suction breaks. You may want to try to break the suction with one hand while cupping the other hand below the patient's eye to catch the lens as it falls.

▶ Sometimes the lens will pop out on its own if you ask the patient to blink after stretching the corner of the eyelids toward the temporal bone, thus tightening the lid edges against the globe of the eye (as shown at the top of the next column).

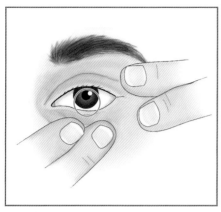

▶ After removal, place the lens in the proper well of the storage case (L or R) with enough of the appropriate storage solution to cover it. Alternatively, place the lens in a labeled medicine cup with solution, and secure adhesive tape over the top of the cup to prevent loss of the lens.

▶ Remove and care for the opposite lens using the same technique.

Removing soft lenses

▶ Place the patient in the supine position. Using your nondominant hand, raise the patient's upper eyelid and hold it against the orbital rim.

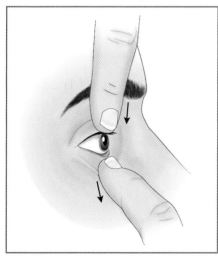

▶ Lightly place the forefinger of your other hand on the lens, and move it down onto the sclera below the cornea. Then pinch the lens between your forefinger and thumb; it should pop off (as shown at the top of the next column).

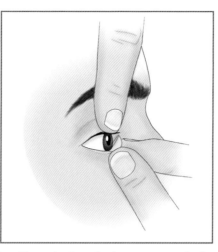

▶ Place the lens in the proper well of the storage case with enough of the appropriate storage solution to cover it. Alternatively, place the lens in a labeled medicine cup with solution, and secure adhesive tape over the top of the cup to prevent loss of the lens.

▶ Remove and care for the other lens using the same technique.

Cleaning lenses

▶ Because lens-cleaning steps vary with lens type and with each manufacturer's and practitioner's instructions, ask the patient to guide you step-by-step through his normal cleaning routine. **MFR**

▶ If the patient can't tell you how to clean his lenses properly, remember that all lens types require two steps: cleaning and disinfection.

▶ Cleaning involves rubbing the lens with a surfactant solution designed to remove most surface deposits. For most patients, especially those who wear soft lenses, the cleaning step may also include use of an enzyme agent to remove protein deposits against which surfactant cleaners are typically ineffective. Enzyme cleaning involves soaking lenses overnight in a solution in which you've dissolved special enzyme tablets. **AOA**

▶ Disinfection, which doesn't require rubbing, may be accomplished through chemical means or by heat. This step aims to rid the lens of infectious organisms.

▶ If you must clean a patient's lenses, use only his own solutions. This minimizes the risk of allergic reactions to substances included in other solution brands. Never touch the nozzle of a solution bottle to the lens, your fingers, or anything else to avoid contaminating the solution in the bottle. **AOA**

Special considerations

▶ If the patient's eyes appear dry or if you have trouble moving the lens on the eye, instill several drops of sterile normal saline solution, and wait a few minutes before trying again to remove the lens to prevent corneal damage. If you still can't remove the lens easily, notify the practitioner. Avoid instilling eye medication while the patient is wearing lenses. The lenses could trap the medication, possibly causing eye irritation or lens damage.

▶ Don't allow soft lenses, which are 40 % to 60 % water, to dry out. If they do, soak them in sterile normal saline solution, and they may return to their natural shape.

▶ If an unconscious patient is admitted to the emergency department, check for contact lenses by opening each eyelid and searching with a small flashlight. If you detect lenses, remove them immediately because tears can't circulate freely beneath the lenses with the eyelids closed, possibly leading to corneal oxygen depletion or infection.

▶ Advise contact lens wearers to carry appropriate identification to speed lens removal and ensure proper care in an emergency.

▶ If a patient can't provide adequate care for his lenses during hospitalization, encourage him to send them home with a family member. If you aren't sure how to care for the lenses in the interim, store them in sterile normal saline solution until the family member can take them home.

References

Alfonso, E.C., et al. "Fungal Keratitis Associated with Non-Therapeutic Soft Contact Lenses," *American Journal of Ophthalmology* 142(1):154-55, July 2006.

Cohen, E.J. "Fusarium Keratitis Associated with Soft Contact Lens Wear," *Archives of Ophthalmology* 125(8):1183-184, August 2006.

Collins, M.J., et al. "The Biomechanics of Rigid Contact Lens Removal," *Contact Lens & Anterior Eye* 28(3):121-25, September 2005.

Foulks, G.N. "Prolonging Contact Lens Wear and Making Contact Lens Wear Safer," *American Journal of Ophthalmology* 141(2):369-73, February 2006.

Niyadurupola, N., and Illingworth, C.D. "Acanthamoeba Keratitis Associated with Misuse of Daily Disposable Contact Lenses," *Contact Lens & Anterior Eye* 29(5):269-71, December 2006.

Continent ileostomy care

An alternative to a conventional ileostomy, a continent, or pouch, ileostomy (also called a Koch ileostomy or an ileal pouch) features an internal reservoir fashioned from the terminal ileum (see *Understanding pouch construction*). This procedure may be used for patients who require proctocolectomy for chronic ulcerative colitis or multiple polyposis. Other patients may have a traditional ileostomy converted to a continent ileostomy. This procedure is contraindicated in patients with Crohn's disease or gross obesity. Patients who need emergency surgery and those who can't care for the pouch are also unlikely to have this procedure.

Equipment

For postoperative care: Bedside drainage bag ◆ normal saline solution ◆ 50-ml catheter-tipped syringe ◆ gloves ◆ water ◆ washcloth and towel ◆ skin sealant ◆ precut drain dressing ◆ 4″ × 4″ × 1″ foam ◆ Montgomery straps ◆ optional: catheter securement device.

For draining the pouch: Gloves ◆ drainage catheter ◆ water-soluble lubricant ◆ normal saline solution or water ◆ 50-ml catheter-tipped syringe ◆ dressing supplies (drain dressing, foam, Montgomery straps).

Implementation

Postoperative care

▶ When the patient returns to his room, attach the drainage catheter emerging from the ileostomy to a bedside drainage bag.

▶ Irrigate the catheter with 30 ml of normal saline solution, as ordered and

Understanding pouch construction

Depending on the patient and related factors during intestinal surgery, the surgeon may construct a pouch to collect fecal matter internally. To make such a pouch, the surgeon loops about 12″ (30.5 cm) of ileum and sutures the inner sides together.

He opens the loop with a U-shaped cut and seams the inside to create a smooth lining. Then he fashions a nipple or valve between what is becoming the pouch and what will be the stoma. He folds the open ileum over, sews the pouch closed, and fixes the pouch to the abdominal wall.

Because the pouch holds fecal matter in reserve, the patient benefits from not having to change and empty ostomy equipment. Instead, he empties and irrigates the pouch, as needed, by inserting a catheter though the stoma and into the pouch.

Initially after surgery, the nurse performs this procedure until the patient can do it himself.

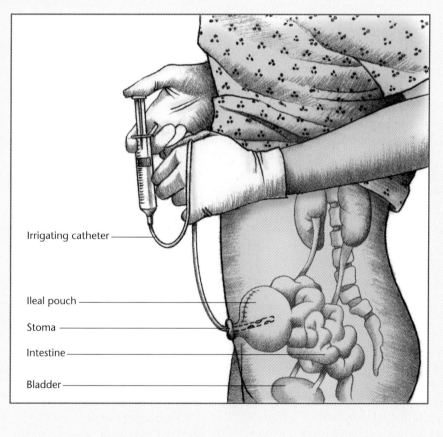

Irrigating catheter

Ileal pouch

Stoma

Intestine

Bladder

needed, to prevent catheter obstruction and allow fluid return by gravity. During the early postoperative period, keep the pouch empty; drainage will be serosanguineous.

▶ Monitor fluid intake and output.

▶ Check the catheter frequently after the patient begins eating solid food to ensure that neither mucus nor undigested food particles block it.

▶ If the patient complains of abdominal cramps, distention, and nausea—symptoms of bowel obstruction—the catheter may be clogged. Gently irrigate with 20 to 30 ml of water or normal saline solution until the catheter drains freely. Then move the catheter slightly or rotate it gently to help clear the obstruction. Finally, try milking the catheter. If these measures fail, notify the practitioner.

▶ Check the stoma frequently for color, edema, and bleeding. Normally pink to red, a stoma that turns dark red or blue-red may have a compromised blood supply.

▶ To care for the stoma and peristomal skin, put on gloves. Remove the dressing, gently clean the peristomal area with water, and pat it dry. Use a skin sealant around the stoma to prevent skin irritation. **WOCN**

▶ One way to apply a stoma dressing is to slip a precut drain dressing around the catheter to cover the stoma. Cut a hole slightly larger than the lumen of the catheter in the center of a 4″ × 4″ × 1″ piece of foam. Disconnect the catheter from the drainage bag, and insert the distal end of the catheter through the hole in the foam. Slide the foam pad onto the dressing. Secure the foam in place with Montgomery straps. Secure the catheter by wrapping the strap ties around it or by using a commercial catheter securing device. Then reconnect the catheter to the drainage bag. (The drainage catheter will be removed by the surgeon when he determines that the suture line has healed.) **WOCN**

▶ Assess the peristomal skin for irritation from moisture.

▶ To reduce discomfort from gas pains, encourage the patient to ambulate. Also recommend that he avoid swallowing air (to minimize gas pains) by chewing food well, limiting conversation while eating, and not drinking from a straw.

Draining the pouch

▶ Provide privacy, explain the procedure to the patient, and wash your hands.

▶ Put on gloves. **CDC**

▶ Have the patient with a pouch conversion sit on the toilet to help him feel more at ease during the procedure.

▶ Remove the stoma dressing.

▶ Encourage the patient to relax his abdominal muscles to allow the catheter to slide easily into the pouch.

▶ Lubricate the tip of the drainage catheter tip with the water-soluble lubricant, and insert it into the stoma. Gently push the catheter downward. (The direction of insertion may vary depending on the patient.)

▶ When the catheter reaches the nipple valve of the internal pouch or reservoir (after about 2″ or 2½″ [5 or 6.5 cm]), you'll feel resistance. Instruct the patient to take a deep breath as you exert gentle pressure on the catheter to insert it through the valve. If this fails, have the patient lie supine and rest for a few minutes. Then, with the patient still supine, try to insert the catheter again.

▶ Gently advance the catheter to the suture marking made by the surgeon.

▶ Let the pouch drain completely. This usually takes 5 to 10 minutes. With thick drainage or a clogged catheter, the process may take 30 minutes.

▶ If the tube clogs, irrigate with 30 ml of water or normal saline using the 50-ml catheter-tip syringe. Also, rotate and milk the tube. If these steps fail, remove, rinse, and reinsert the catheter.

▶ Remove the catheter after completing drainage.

▶ Measure output, subtracting the amount of irrigant used.

▶ Rinse the catheter thoroughly with warm water.

▶ Clean the peristomal area, and apply a fresh stoma dressing.

Special considerations

▶ Never aspirate fluid from the catheter because the resulting negative pressure may damage inflamed tissue.

▶ The first few times you intubate the pouch, the patient may be tense, making insertion difficult. Encourage relaxation. To shorten drainage time, have the patient cough, press gently on his abdomen over the pouch, or suddenly tighten his abdominal muscles and then relax them.

▶ Keep an accurate record of intake and output to ensure fluid and electrolyte balance. The average daily output should be 1,000 ml. Report inadequate or excessive output (more than 1,400 ml daily).

▶ A leg drainage bag may be attached to the patient's thigh during ambulation.

References

Burch, J. "The Pre- and Postoperative Nursing Care for Patients with a Stoma," *British Journal of Nursing* 14(6):310-18, March 2005.

Herlufson, P., et al. "Study of Peristomal Skin Disorders in Patients with Permanent Stomas," *British Journal of Nursing* 15(16):854-62, September 2006.

Taylor, C., et al. *Fundamentals of Nursing: The Art and Science of Nursing Care,* 6th ed. Philadelphia: Lippincott Williams & Wilkins, 2008.

Continuous ambulatory peritoneal dialysis

Continuous ambulatory peritoneal dialysis (CAPD) is used most commonly for patients with end-stage renal disease. CAPD can be a welcome alternative to hemodialysis because it gives the patient more independence and requires less travel for treatments. It also provides more stable fluid and electrolyte levels than conventional hemodialysis. (See *How peritoneal dialysis works,* page 132.)

CAPD requires insertion of a permanent peritoneal catheter (such as a Tenckhoff catheter) to circulate dialysate in the peritoneal cavity constantly. (See *Comparing peritoneal dialysis catheters,* page 133.) Inserted under local anesthetic, the catheter is sutured in place and its distal portion tunneled subcutaneously to the skin surface. There, it serves as a port for the dialysate, which flows in and out of the peritoneal cavity by gravity.

Patients or family members can usually learn to perform CAPD after only 2 weeks of training. In addition, because the patient can resume normal daily activities between solution changes, CAPD helps promote independence and a return to a near-normal lifestyle. It also less expensive than hemodialysis.

Conditions that may prohibit CAPD include recent abdominal surgery, abdominal adhesions, an infected abdominal wall, diaphragmatic tears, ileus, and respiratory insufficiency.

Equipment

To infuse dialysate: Prescribed amount of dialysate (usually in 2-L bags) ◆ heating pad or commercial warmer ◆ three face masks ◆ 42″ (106.7-cm) connective tubing with drain clamp ◆ six to eight packages of sterile 4″ × 4″ gauze pads ◆ medication, if ordered ◆ antiseptic pads ◆ hypoallergenic tape ◆ plastic snap-top container ◆ antiseptic solution ◆ sterile basin ◆ container of alcohol ◆ sterile gloves ◆ belt or fabric pouch ◆ two sterile waterproof paper drapes (one fenestrated) ◆ optional: syringes, labeled specimen container.

To discontinue dialysis temporarily: Three sterile waterproof paper barriers (two fenestrated) ◆ 4″ × 4″ gauze pads (for cleaning and dressing the catheter) ◆ two face masks ◆ sterile basin ◆ hypoallergenic tape ◆ antiseptic solution ◆ sterile gloves ◆ sterile rubber catheter cap.

All equipment for infusing the dialysate and discontinuing the procedure must be sterile. Commercially prepared sterile CAPD kits are available.

Implementation

▶ Check the concentration of the dialysate against the practitioner's order. Also check the expiration date and appearance of the solution—it should be clear, not cloudy.

▶ Warm the solution to body temperature with a heating pad or a commercial warmer if one is available. Don't warm the solution in a microwave oven because the temperature is unpredictable. To minimize the risk of contaminating the bag's port, leave the dialysate container's wrapper in place. This also keeps the bag dry, which makes examining it for leakage easier after you remove the wrapper.

▶ Wash your hands, and put on a surgical mask. Remove the dialysate container from the warming setup, and remove its protective wrapper. Squeeze the bag firmly to check for leaks. **CDC**

▶ If ordered, use a syringe to add any prescribed medication to the dialysate, using sterile technique to avoid contamination. (The ideal approach is to add medication under a laminar flow hood.) Disinfect multiple-dose vials in a 5-minute antiseptic soak. Insert the connective tubing into the dialysate container. Open the drain clamp to prime the tube. Then close the clamp.

▶ Place an antiseptic pad on the dialysate container's port. Cover the port with a dry gauze pad, and secure the pad with tape. Remove and discard the surgical mask. Tear the tape so it will be ready to secure the new dressing. Commercial devices with antiseptic pads are available for covering the dialysate container and tubing connection.

▶ Confirm the patient's identity using two patient identifiers according to your facility's policy. **JC**

▶ Weigh the patient to establish a baseline level. Weigh him at the same time every day to help monitor fluid balance. **ANNA**

How peritoneal dialysis works

Peritoneal dialysis works through a combination of diffusion and osmosis.

Diffusion

In diffusion, particles move through a semipermeable membrane from an area of high-solute concentration to an area of low-solute concentration.

In peritoneal dialysis, the water-based dialysate being infused contains glucose, sodium chloride, calcium, magnesium, acetate or lactate, and no waste products. Therefore, the waste products and excess electrolytes in the blood cross through the semipermeable peritoneal membrane into the dialysate. Removing the waste-filled dialysate and replacing it with fresh solution keeps the waste concentration low and encourages further diffusion.

Osmosis

In osmosis, fluids move through a semipermeable membrane from an area of low-solute concentration to an area of high-solute concentration.

In peritoneal dialysis, dextrose is added to the dialysate to give it a higher solute concentration than the blood, creating a high osmotic gradient. Water migrates from the blood through the membrane at the beginning of each infusion, when the osmotic gradient is highest.

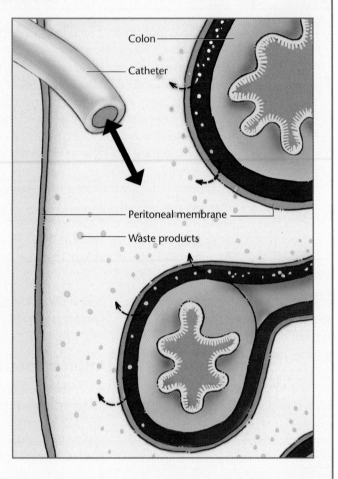

Colon

Catheter

Peritoneal membrane

Waste products

Infusing dialysate

▶ Assemble all equipment at the patient's bedside, and explain the procedure to him. Prepare the sterile field by placing a waterproof, sterile paper drape on a dry surface near the patient. Take care to maintain the drape's sterility.

▶ Fill the snap-top container with antiseptic solution, and place it on the sterile field. Place the basin on the sterile field. Then place four pairs of sterile gauze pads in the sterile basin, and saturate them with the antiseptic solution. Drop the remaining gauze pads on the

sterile field. Loosen the cap on the alcohol container, and place it next to the sterile field.

▶ Put on a clean surgical mask, and provide one for the patient. **CDC**

▶ Carefully remove the dressing covering the peritoneal catheter and discard it. Be careful not to touch the catheter or skin. Check skin integrity at the catheter site, and look for signs of infection such as purulent drainage. If drainage is present, obtain a swab specimen, put it in a labeled specimen container, and notify the practitioner.

▶ Put on the sterile gloves, and palpate the insertion site and subcutaneous tunnel route for tenderness or pain. If these symptoms occur, notify the practitioner. **ANNA**

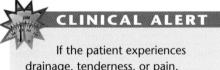

CLINICAL ALERT

If the patient experiences drainage, tenderness, or pain, don't proceed with the infusion without specific orders.

▶ Wrap one gauze pad saturated with antiseptic solution around the distal

Comparing peritoneal dialysis catheters

The first step in any type of peritoneal dialysis is insertion of a catheter to allow instillation of dialyzing solution. The surgeon may insert one of the three catheters described here.

Tenckhoff catheter

To implant a Tenckhoff catheter, the surgeon inserts the first 6¾" (17 cm) of the catheter into the patient's abdomen. The next 2¾" (7-cm) segment, which may have a Dacron cuff at one or both ends, is imbedded subcutaneously. Within a few days after insertion, the patient's tissues grow around the cuffs, forming a tight barrier against bacterial infiltration. The remaining 3⅞" (10 cm) of the catheter extends outside of the abdomen and is equipped with a metal adapter at the tip that connects to dialyzer tubing.

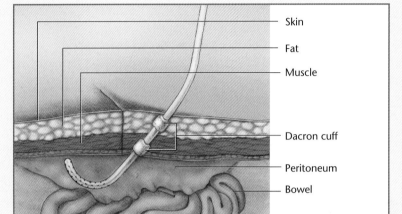

Skin
Fat
Muscle
Dacron cuff
Peritoneum
Bowel

Flanged-collar catheter

To insert this kind of catheter, the surgeon positions its flanged collar just below the dermis so that the device extends through the abdominal wall. He keeps the distal end of the cuff from extending into the peritoneum, where it could cause adhesions.

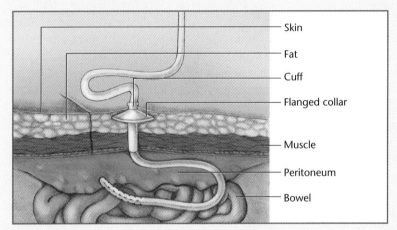

Skin
Fat
Cuff
Flanged collar
Muscle
Peritoneum
Bowel

Column-disk peritoneal catheter

To insert a column-disk peritoneal catheter (CDPC), the surgeon rolls up the flexible disk section of the implant, inserts it into the peritoneal cavity, and retracts it against the abdominal wall. The implant's first cuff rests just outside the peritoneal membrane, and its second cuff rests just underneath the skin.

Because the CDPC doesn't float freely in the peritoneal cavity, it keeps inflowing dialyzing solution from being directed at the sensitive organs, which increases patient comfort during dialysis.

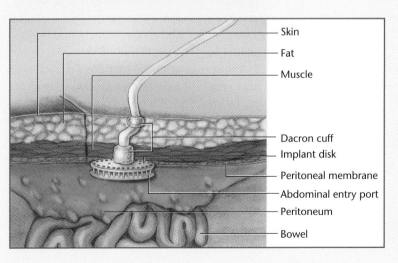

Skin
Fat
Muscle
Dacron cuff
Implant disk
Peritoneal membrane
Abdominal entry port
Peritoneum
Bowel

end of the catheter, and leave it in place for 5 minutes. Clean the catheter and insertion site with the rest of the gauze pads, moving in concentric circles away from the insertion site. Use straight strokes to clean the catheter, beginning at the insertion site and moving outward. Use a clean area of the pad for each stroke. Loosen the catheter cap one notch, and clean the exposed area. Place each used pad at the base of the catheter to help support it. After using the third pair of pads, place the fenestrated paper drape around the base of the catheter. Continue cleaning the catheter for another minute with one of the remaining pads soaked with antiseptic solution.

▶ Remove the antiseptic pad on the catheter cap, remove the cap, and use the remaining antiseptic pad to clean the end of the catheter hub. Attach the connective tubing from the dialysate container to the catheter. Be sure to secure the luer-lock connector tightly.

▶ Open the drain clamp on the dialysate container to allow solution to enter the peritoneal cavity by gravity over a period of 5 to 10 minutes. Leave a small amount of fluid in the bag to make folding it easier. Close the drain clamp.

▶ Fold the bag, and secure it with a belt, or tuck it in the patient's clothing or a small fabric pouch.

▶ After the prescribed dwell time (usually 4 to 6 hours), unfold the bag, open the clamp, and allow peritoneal fluid to drain back into the bag by gravity.

▶ When drainage is complete, attach a new bag of dialysate, and repeat the infusion.

▶ Discard used supplies appropriately.

Discontinuing dialysis temporarily

▶ Wash your hands, put on a surgical mask, and provide one for the patient. Explain the procedure to him. **CDC**

▶ Using sterile gloves, remove and discard the dressing over the peritoneal catheter.

▶ Set up a sterile field next to the patient by covering a clean, dry surface with a waterproof drape. Be sure to maintain the drape's sterility. Place all equipment on the sterile field, and place the 4″ × 4″ gauze pads in the basin. Saturate them with the antiseptic solution. Open the 4″ × 4″ gauze pads to be used as the dressing, and drop them onto the sterile field. Tear pieces of tape, as needed.

▶ Tape the dialysate tubing to the side rail of the bed to keep the catheter and tubing off the patient's abdomen.

▶ Change to another pair of sterile gloves. Then place one of the fenestrated drapes around the base of the catheter.

▶ Use a pair of antiseptic pads to clean about 6″ (15 cm) of the dialysis tubing. Clean for 1 minute, moving in one direction only, away from the catheter. Then clean the catheter, moving from the insertion site to the junction of the catheter and dialysis tubing. Place used pads at the base of the catheter to prop it up. Use two more pairs of pads to clean the junction for a total of 3 minutes.

▶ Place the second fenestrated paper drape over the first at the base of the catheter. With the fourth pair of pads, clean the junction of the catheter and 6″ of the dialysate tubing for another minute.

▶ Disconnect the dialysate tubing from the catheter. Pick up the catheter cap, and fasten it to the catheter, making sure it fits securely over both notches of the hard plastic catheter tip.

▶ Clean the insertion site and a 2″ (5-cm) radius around it with antiseptic pads, working from the insertion site outward. Let the skin air-dry before applying the dressing.

▶ Remove the tape, and discard used supplies appropriately.

Special considerations

▶ Absolute contraindications for CAPD include:

— documented loss of peritoneal function or extensive abdominal adhesions that limit dialysate flow

— physical or mental incapacity to perform peritoneal dialysis and no assistance available at home

— mechanical defects that prevent effective dialysis, which can't be corrected, or increase the risk of infection (such as surgically irreparable hernia, omphalocele, gastroschisis, diaphragmatic hernia, and bladder extrophy).

▶ Relative contraindications for CAPD include:

— fresh intra-abdominal foreign bodies (for example, 4-month wait after abdominal vascular prostheses, recent ventricular-peritoneal shunt)

— peritoneal leaks or infection, or infection of the abdominal wall or skin

— body size limitations—either a patient who's too small to tolerate adequate dialysate or a patient who's too large to be effectively dialyzed

— inability to tolerate the necessary volumes of dialysate for peritoneal dialysis to be successful

— inflammatory or ischemic bowel disease or recurrent episodes of diverticulitis

— morbid obesity in short individuals or patients suffering from severe malnutrition.

▶ If inflow and outflow are slow or absent, check the tubing for kinks. You can also try raising the solution or repositioning the patient to increase the inflow rate. Repositioning the patient or applying manual pressure to the lateral aspects of the patient's abdomen may also help increase drainage.

▶ Peritonitis is the most frequent complication of CAPD. Although treatable, it can permanently scar the peritoneal membrane, decreasing its permeability and reducing the efficiency of dialysis.

▶ Excessive fluid loss may result from a concentrated (4.25%) dialysate solution, improper or inaccurate monitoring of inflow and outflow, or inadequate oral fluid intake. Excessive fluid retention may result from improper or inaccurate monitoring of inflow and outflow, or excessive salt or oral fluid intake.

References

American Nephrology Nurses Association. *ANNA Standards of Clinical Practice for Nephrology Nursing,* 4th edition. Pitman, N.J.: 2005.

Finkelstein, F.O., et al. "The Role of Chronic Peritoneal Dialysis in the Management of the Patient with Chronic Kidney Disease," *Contributions to Nephrology* 150:235-39, 2006.

National Kidney Foundation. "Clinical Practice Guidelines for Peritoneal Dialysis Adequacy Update 2000," *American Journal of Kidney Diseases* 37(1 Suppl):S65-S136, January 2001.

National Kidney and Urologic Diseases Information Clearinghouse. "Peritoneal Dialysis Dose and Adequacy," *NIH Publications* No. 04-4587, May 2004. Available at *http://kidney.niddk.nih.gov/Kudiseases/pubs/peritonealdose/.*

Selby, N.M., et al. "Automated Peritoneal Dialysis Has Significant Effects on Systemic Hemodynamics," *Peritoneal Dialysis International* 26(3):306-308, May-June 2006.

Continuous bladder irrigation

Continuous bladder irrigation can help prevent urinary tract obstruction by flushing out small blood clots that form after prostate or bladder surgery. It may also be used to treat an irritated, inflamed, or infected bladder lining.

This procedure requires placement of a triple-lumen catheter: One lumen controls balloon inflation, one allows irrigant inflow, and one allows irrigant outflow. The continuous flow of irrigating solution through the bladder also creates a mild tamponade that may help prevent venous hemorrhage. (See *Setup for continuous bladder irrigation*.) Although the patient typically receives the catheter while he's in the operating room after prostate or bladder surgery, he may have it inserted at the bedside if he isn't a surgical patient.

Equipment

Sterile irrigating solution ◆ sterile tubing for use with bladder irrigating system ◆ alcohol or antiseptic pad ◆ drainage bag and tubing ◆ I.V. pole.

Implementation

▶ Confirm the patient's identity using two patient identifiers according to your facility's policy. **JC**
▶ Wash your hands. Assemble all equipment at the patient's bedside. Explain the procedure, and provide privacy.
▶ Insert the spike of the tubing into the container of irrigating solution.

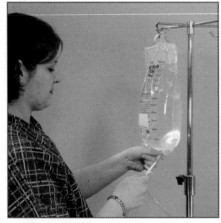

▶ Squeeze the drip chamber on the spike of the tubing.
▶ Open the flow clamp, and flush the tubing to remove air, which could cause

bladder distention. Then close the clamp.

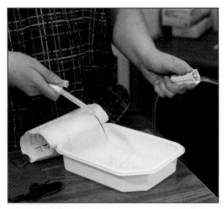

▶ To begin, hang the bag of irrigating solution on the I.V. pole.
▶ Clean the opening to the inflow lumen of the catheter with the alcohol or antiseptic pad. **CDC**
▶ Insert the distal end of the tubing securely into the inflow lumen (third port) of the catheter.

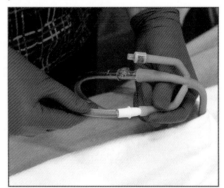

▶ Make sure the catheter's outflow lumen is securely attached to the drainage bag tubing.
▶ Open the flow clamp under the container of irrigating solution, and set the drip rate, as ordered.

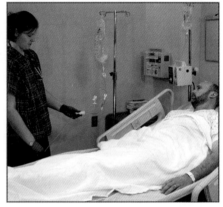

▶ To prevent air from entering the system, don't let the primary container empty completely before replacing it.
▶ Empty the drainage bag about every 4 hours, or as often as needed. Use sterile technique to avoid the risk of contamination.
▶ Monitor the patient's vital signs at least every 4 hours during irrigation; increase the frequency if the patient becomes unstable.
▶ Monitor urine output at least hourly for the first 4 hours. Check for bladder distention or abdominal pain.

Setup for continuous bladder irrigation

In continuous bladder irrigation, a triple-lumen catheter allows irrigating solution to flow into the bladder through one lumen and flow out through another, as shown in the inset. The third lumen is used to inflate the balloon that holds the catheter in place.

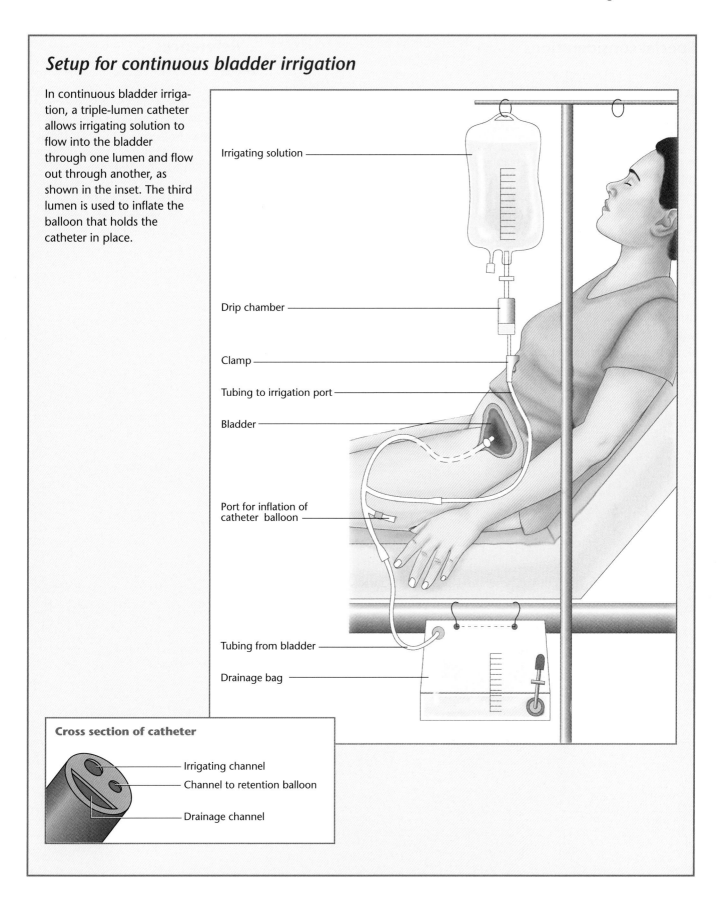

Irrigating solution

Drip chamber

Clamp

Tubing to irrigation port

Bladder

Port for inflation of catheter balloon

Tubing from bladder

Drainage bag

Cross section of catheter

Irrigating channel

Channel to retention balloon

Drainage channel

Special considerations

▶ Check the inflow and outflow lines periodically for kinks to make sure the solution is running freely. If the solution flows rapidly, check the lines frequently.

▶ As an alternative to flow clamp administration, an administration pump may be used, requiring the pump tubing to be primed. Set the flow rate as ordered by the practitioner. The volume infused is used to help calculate the urine output.

▶ Measure the outflow volume accurately. It should equal or, allowing for urine production, slightly exceed inflow volume. If inflow volume exceeds outflow volume postoperatively, suspect bladder rupture at the suture lines or renal damage, and notify the practitioner immediately.

▶ Also assess outflow for changes in appearance and for blood clots, especially if irrigation is being performed postoperatively to control bleeding. If drainage is bright red, irrigating solution should usually be infused rapidly with the clamp wide open until drainage clears. Notify the practitioner at once if you suspect hemorrhage. If drainage is clear, the solution is usually given at a rate of 40 to 60 drops/minute. The practitioner typically specifies the rate for antibiotic solutions.

▶ Encourage oral fluid intake of 2 to 3 qt (2 to 3 L)/day unless contraindicated by another medical condition.

References

Cutts, B. "Developing and Implementing a New Bladder Irrigation Chart," *Nursing Standard* 20(8):48-52, November 2005.

Defoor, W., et al. "Safety of Gentamicin Bladder Irrigations in Complex Urological Cases," *Journal of Urology* 175(5):1861-864, May 2006.

Smeltzer, S.C., et al. *Brunner & Suddarth's Textbook of Medical-Surgical Nursing,* 11th ed. Philadelphia: Lippincott Williams & Wilkins, 2008.

Continuous passive motion device

A continuous passive motion (CPM) device is frequently used after joint surgery—particularly after total knee arthroplasty. The device increases range of motion in the joint as the flexion and extension settings are adjusted during therapy. In addition, the negative effects of immobility are minimized due to increased circulation from the passive movement of the limb. There's also stimulation of healing within the articular cartilage and reduction in adhesions and swelling.

The practitioner determines the amount of flexion and extension of the joint and the cycle rate (the number of revolutions per minute) as well as the length of time it's to be used.

Although the CPM device is usually used on the knee, it may be appropriate for other joints as well.

Equipment

CPM device ◆ single-patient-use soft-goods kit ◆ tape measure ◆ goniometer ◆ nonsterile gloves, if indicated.

Implementation

▶ Check the practitioner's order for the CPM settings, frequency, and duration.
▶ Gather the appropriate equipment.
▶ Apply the soft-goods padding to the CPM device. **MFR**
▶ Confirm the patient's identity using two patient identifiers according to your facility's policy. **JC**
▶ Explain the procedure to the patient to reduce anxiety and encourage compliance.
▶ Assess the patient's pain level, and administer the prescribed analgesic, if needed. Allow time for the full effect of the analgesic to occur before starting the machine.
▶ Wash your hands and put on gloves, if indicated, to prevent possible contact with blood or body fluids. **CDC**
▶ Provide privacy. Place the bed at a comfortable working height.
▶ Determine the distance between the gluteal crease and the popliteal space using the measuring tape.
▶ Also measure the length of the lower leg from the knee to $^{1}/_{4}''$ (0.6 cm) beyond the bottom of the foot.

▶ Adjust the thigh length and foot plate position on the CPM machine based on your measurements. **MFR**
▶ Position the patient in the middle of the bed.
▶ Support the affected extremity, elevating it to allow placement of the padded CPM device on the bed. Gently lower the leg onto the device.

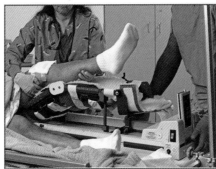

▶ Make sure the knee is resting at the hinged joint of the CPM machine and that the leg is slightly abducted.
▶ Adjust the footplate to maintain a neutral position for the patient's foot. Assess the patient's position to make sure the leg isn't internally or externally rotated to prevent injury.

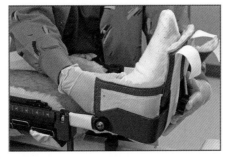

▶ Secure the restraining straps under the CPM device and around the leg to hold the leg in position. Check that two fingers fit between the strap and the leg to prevent injury from excessive pressure from the strap.

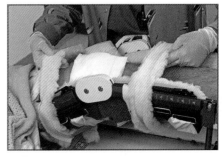

▶ Turn the unit on at the main power switch, and set the controls to the level prescribed by the practitioner.
▶ Instruct the patient in the use of the STOP/GO button.
▶ Set the device to ON, and start the therapy by pressing the GO button. Monitor the patient and the device through the first few cycles. Verify the angle of flexion when the device reaches its greatest height by measuring with a goniometer to ensure the device is set to the prescribed parameters.

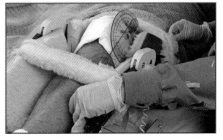

▶ Return the bed to the lowest position for patient safety. Make sure the call bell and other necessary items are within reach.

▶ Check the patient's level of comfort frequently, and perform skin and neurovascular assessments at least every 8 hours or according to your facility's policy.

▶ Remove gloves and wash your hands.

Special considerations

▶ The use of the CPM device is in addition to physical therapy during the rehabilitation process.

▶ Encourage the patient to use the CPM machine, as prescribed, to promote healing and function of the joint. Effective and timely pain control is important to ensuring the patient's cooperation.

▶ Show the patient how to use the device and patient controls. Make the patient aware of setting changes and goals of CPM therapy.

▶ Teach the patient signs and symptoms of neurovascular impairment to report, such as numbness or tingling, sudden pain, or coolness of the affected limb.

References

Altizer, L. "Patient Education for Total Hip or Knee Replacement," *Orthopaedic Nursing* 23(4):283-88, July-August 2004.

Denis, M., et al. "Effectiveness of Continuous Passive Motion and Conventional Physical Therapy after Total Knee Arthroplasty: A Randomized Clinical Trial," *Physical Therapy* 86(2):174-85, February 2006.

Milne, S., et al. "Continuous Passive Motion following Total Knee Arthroplasty," *Cochrane Database of Systematic Reviews* (2):CD004260, 2003.

Taylor, C., et al. *Fundamentals of Nursing: The Art and Science of Nursing Care,* 6th ed. Philadelphia: Lippincott Williams & Wilkins, 2008.

Continuous positive airway pressure

Continuous positive airway pressure (CPAP) is used to provide low flow pressure into the airways to help hold the airway open, mobilize secretions, and treat atelectasis—all of which eases the work of breathing. Nonintubated patients receive CPAP through a high flow generating system, and its use may eliminate the need for intubation. CPAP is also commonly used to treat chronic obstructive sleep apnea because it prevents the palate and tongue from collapsing and obstructing the airways. Many patients are started on CPAP in the hospital and then continue CPAP use at home. CPAP has traditionally been administered through a face mask, but newer, more comfortable methods include the face pillow and nasal mask.

It may also be administered to an intubated patient through a ventilator setting.

CPAP is contraindicated in patients with chronic obstructive lung disease, bullous lung disease, low cardiac output, or tension pneumothorax due to the increase in thoracic pressure.

Equipment

Nasal mask, nasal pillows, or face mask properly sized ◆ permanent marker ◆ CPAP machine ◆ oxygen delivery tubing ◆ washcloth ◆ water ◆ optional: oxygen source, oxygen tubing, pulse oximetry.

Implementation

▶ Set up the CPAP machine according to manufacturer's instructions. Position the CPAP machine so the tubing easily reaches the patient, and plug in the machine. Don't plug the CPAP machine into an outlet with another plug in it, and don't use an extension cord to reach the outlet. **MFR**
▶ Check the practitioner's order.
▶ Connect the oxygen delivery tubing to the air outlet valve on the CPAP unit, if ordered.
▶ Confirm the patient's identity using two patient identifiers according to your facility's policy. **JC**
▶ Explain the procedure to the patient to decrease anxiety and increase compliance.
▶ Wash your hands.
▶ Have the patient wash his face with the washcloth and water to remove facial oils and help achieve a better fit.

▶ Check the face mask, nasal mask, or nasal pillow to make sure the cushion isn't hard or broken. If it is, replace it.

Nasal mask
▶ Place the nasal mask so the longer straps are located at the top of the mask.

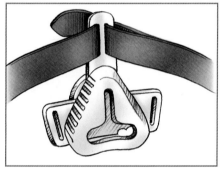

▶ Make sure that the Velcro is facing away from you, and thread the four tabs through the slots on the sides and top of the mask.

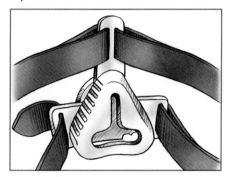

▶ Pull the straps through the slots and fasten them using the Velcro.
▶ Place the mask over the patient's nose, and position the headgear over his head.
▶ Gradually tighten all the straps on the mask until a seal is obtained. The mask doesn't have to be tight to fit correctly—it just has to have a seal.

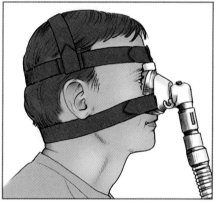

▶ Use the permanent marker to mark the straps with the final position to eliminate having to fit the mask each time the patient wears it.

Nasal pillow
▶ Insert the nasal pillows into the shell, making sure they fit correctly and that there's no air leaking around them (shown at the top left of the next page).

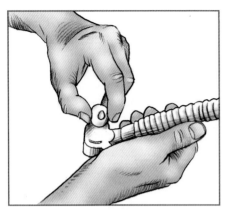

▶ Place the headgear around the patient's head, and use the Velcro straps to achieve the proper fit. When the straps are in the correct place, remove the headgear without undoing the straps.

▶ Attach the nasal pillow to the headgear by wrapping the Velcro around the tubing, leaving room for rotation.

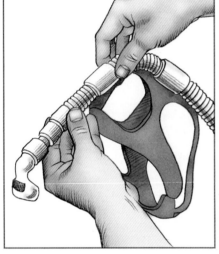

▶ Place the completely assembled headgear back on the patient, and position the nasal pillows comfortably.

▶ Attach the shell strap across the shell, and adjust the tension of the strap until there's a seal in both nostrils (as shown at the top of the next column).

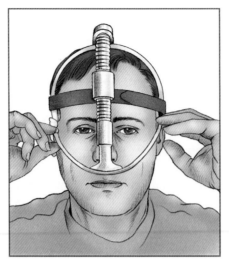

▶ Be careful not to block the exhalation port on the back side of the shell.

Face mask

▶ Hold the mask against the patient's face, and position the headgear over his head.

▶ Using the Velcro straps, adjust the straps as with the nasal mask until there are no leaks present.

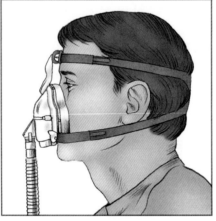

▶ Connect the flexible tubing to the mask, and turn on the airflow.

Administering CPAP

▶ After the administration device is correctly fitted on the patient, turn on the pressure generator.

▶ Turn on the CPAP unit before turning on the oxygen flow to the ordered level.

▶ If ordered, monitor the patient's pulse oximetry during treatment.

▶ When the treatment is over, in the morning or on discontinuation of the order, turn off the pressure generator, and remove the headgear and appliance from the patient.

▶ Clean the equipment according to your facility's policy, and store it properly.

Special considerations

▶ If the mask isn't properly fitted, the patient may complain of dry or sore eyes. If this is the case, remove the mask and headgear and readjust them to minimize leaks.

▶ The patient may need to use a humidifier with the CPAP unit if he complains of a runny nose or dryness or burning in his nose and throat. Discuss this with the practitioner, and obtain an order for humidification.

▶ Always make sure there's air coming out of the unit when the power is turned on.

▶ Because CPAP via a mask can cause nausea and vomiting, it shouldn't be used in a patient who's unresponsive or at risk for aspiration.

References

American Association for Respiratory Care. "AARC Clinical Practice Guideline: Pulse Oximetry," *Respiratory Care* 36(12):1406-409, December 1991.

American Association for Respiratory Care. "AARC Clinical Practice Guideline: Use of Positive Airway Pressure Adjuncts to Bronchial Hygiene Therapy," *Respiratory Care* 28(5):516-21, May 1993.

Collop, N. "The Effect of Obstructive Sleep Apnea on Chronic Medical Disorders," *Cleveland Clinic Journal of Medicine* 74(1):72-78, January 2007.

Davidhizar, R.E., and Hart, A.N. "Living with a CPAP Machine," *Journal of Practical Nursing* 55(3):20-22, Fall 2005.

Dikerson, S.S., and Kennedy, M.C. "CPAP Devices: Encouraging Patients with Sleep Apnea," *Rehabilitation Nurse* 31(3):114-22, May-June 2006.

Kaneko, Y. "Cardiovascular Effects of Continuous Positive Airway Pressure in Patients with Heart Failure and Obstructive Sleep Apnea," *New England Journal of Medicine* 348(13):1233-241, March 2003.

Mador, M.J., et al. "Effect of Heated Humidification on Compliance and Quality of Life in Patients with Sleep Apnea Using Nasal Continuous Positive Airway Pressure," *Chest* 126(4):2151-158, October 2005.

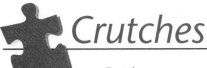

Crutches

Crutches remove weight from one or both legs, enabling the patient to support himself with his hands and arms. Typically prescribed for a patient with lower-extremity injury or weakness, crutches require balance, stamina, and upper-body strength for successful use. Crutch selection and walking gait depend on the patient's condition.

Equipment

Crutches with axillary pads, handgrips, and rubber suction tips ◆ optional: walking belt.

Three types of crutches are commonly used. Standard aluminum or wooden crutches are used by the patient with a sprain, strain, or cast. Aluminum forearm crutches are used by the paraplegic or other patient using the swing-through gait. They have a collar that fits around the forearm and a horizontal handgrip that provides support. Platform crutches are used by the arthritic patient who has an upper-extremity deficit that prevents weight bearing through the wrist. They provide padded surfaces for the upper extremities.

Implementation

▶ After choosing the appropriate crutches, adjust their height with the patient standing or, if necessary, recumbent. (See *Fitting a patient for a crutch*.)

▶ Consult with the patient's practitioner and physical therapist to coordinate rehabilitation orders and teaching.

Fitting a patient for a crutch

To measure for an axilla crutch, position the crutch so that it extends from a point 4" to 6" (10 to 15 cm) to the side and 4" to 6" in front of the patient's feet to 1½" to 2" (4 to 5 cm) below the axillae (about the width of two fingers). Then adjust the handgrips so that the patient's elbows are flexed at a 30-degree angle when he's standing with the crutches in the resting position and the wrists at a 15-degree angle.

To fit a forearm crutch, have the patient flex his elbow so the crease in his wrist is at his hip. Then measure his forearm from 3" (7.6 cm) below the elbow, and add the distance between his wrist and the floor.

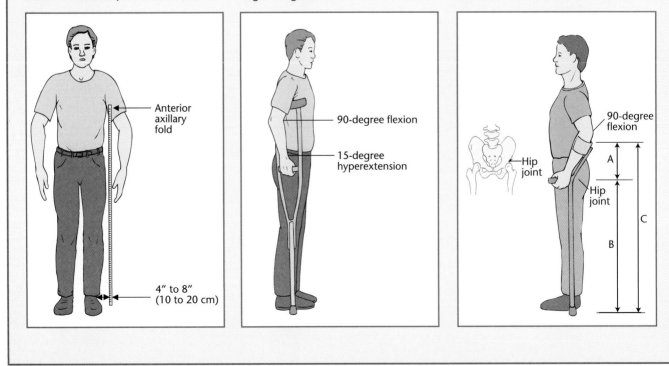

Crutch gaits

Guide for using the 4-point, 3-point, 2-point, swing-to, and swing-through gaits. Start at the bottom and move forward.
Note: Shaded areas indicate weight bearing.

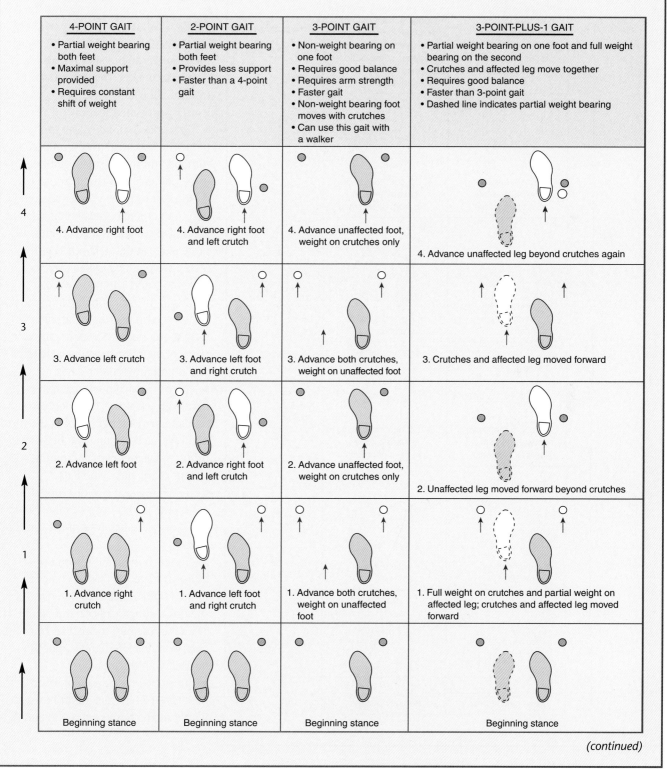

4-POINT GAIT	2-POINT GAIT	3-POINT GAIT	3-POINT-PLUS-1 GAIT
• Partial weight bearing both feet • Maximal support provided • Requires constant shift of weight	• Partial weight bearing both feet • Provides less support • Faster than a 4-point gait	• Non-weight bearing on one foot • Requires good balance • Requires arm strength • Faster gait • Non-weight bearing foot moves with crutches • Can use this gait with a walker	• Partial weight bearing on one foot and full weight bearing on the second • Crutches and affected leg move together • Requires good balance • Faster than 3-point gait • Dashed line indicates partial weight bearing
4. Advance right foot	4. Advance right foot and left crutch	4. Advance unaffected foot, weight on crutches only	4. Advance unaffected leg beyond crutches again
3. Advance left crutch	3. Advance left foot and right crutch	3. Advance both crutches, weight on unaffected foot	3. Crutches and affected leg moved forward
2. Advance left foot	2. Advance right foot and left crutch	2. Advance unaffected foot, weight on crutches only	2. Unaffected leg moved forward beyond crutches
1. Advance right crutch	1. Advance left foot and right crutch	1. Advance both crutches, weight on unaffected foot	1. Full weight on crutches and partial weight on affected leg; crutches and affected leg moved forward
Beginning stance	Beginning stance	Beginning stance	Beginning stance

(continued)

Crutch gaits *(continued)*

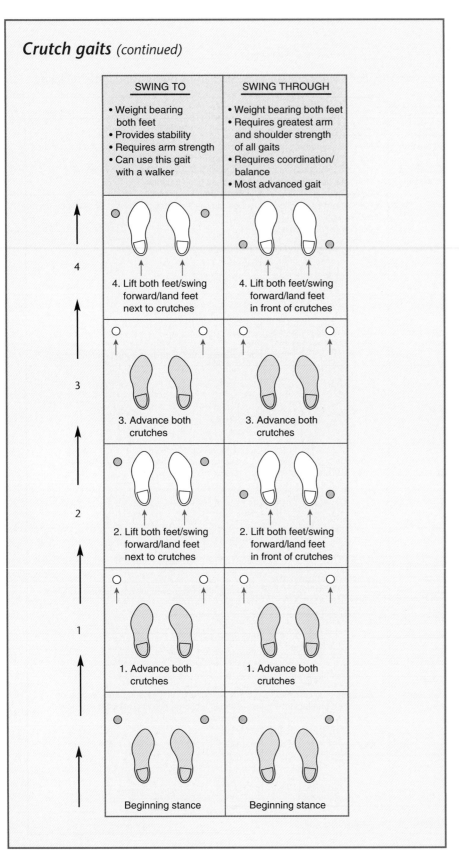

	SWING TO	SWING THROUGH
	• Weight bearing both feet • Provides stability • Requires arm strength • Can use this gait with a walker	• Weight bearing both feet • Requires greatest arm and shoulder strength of all gaits • Requires coordination/balance • Most advanced gait
4	4. Lift both feet/swing forward/land feet next to crutches	4. Lift both feet/swing forward/land feet in front of crutches
3	3. Advance both crutches	3. Advance both crutches
2	2. Lift both feet/swing forward/land feet next to crutches	2. Lift both feet/swing forward/land feet in front of crutches
1	1. Advance both crutches	1. Advance both crutches
	Beginning stance	Beginning stance

▶ Describe the gait you'll teach and the reason for your choice. Then demonstrate the gait, as necessary. Have the patient give a return demonstration.

▶ Place a walking belt around the patient's waist, if necessary, to help prevent falls. Tell the patient to position the crutches and to shift his weight from side to side. Then place him in front of a full-length mirror to facilitate learning and coordination.

▶ Teach the four-point gait to the patient who can bear weight on both legs. Although this is the safest gait because three points are always in contact with the floor, it requires greater coordination than others because of its constant shifting of weight. If the patient gains proficiency at this gait, teach him the faster two-point gait. (See *Crutch gaits,* pages 145 and 146.)

▶ Teach the three-point gait to the patient who can bear only partial or no weight on one leg. Stress the importance of taking steps of equal length and duration with no pauses.

▶ Teach the two-point gait to the patient with weak legs but good coordination and arm strength. This is the most natural crutch-walking gait because it mimics walking, with alternating swings of the arms and legs.

▶ Teach the swing-to or swing-through gaits—the fastest ones—to the patient with complete paralysis of the hips and legs.

▶ To teach the patient who uses crutches to get up from a chair, tell him to hold both crutches in one hand, with the tips resting firmly on the floor. Then instruct him to push up from the chair with his free hand, supporting himself with the crutches.

▶ To sit down, the patient reverses the process: Tell him to support himself with the crutches in one hand and to lower himself with the other.

▶ To teach the patient to ascend stairs using the three-point gait, tell him to lead with the uninvolved leg and to follow with both the crutches and the involved leg. To descend stairs, he should lead with the crutches and the involved leg and follow with the good leg. He may find it helpful to remember "The good goes up; the bad goes down."

Special considerations

▶ Encourage arm- and shoulder-strengthening exercises to prepare the patient for crutch walking. If possible, consult with physical therapy to teach the patient two techniques—one fast and one slow—so he can alternate between them to prevent excessive muscle fatigue and can adjust more easily to various walking conditions.

References

Clark, B.C., et al. "Leg Muscle Activity during Walking with Assistive Devices at Varying Levels of Weight Bearing," *Archives of Physical Medicine and Rehabilitation* 85(9):1555-60, September 2004.

Craven, R.F., and Hirnle, C.J. *Fundamentals of Nursing: Human Health and Function,* 6th ed. Philadelphia: Lippincott Williams & Wilkins, 2009.

Dabke, H.V., et al. "How Accurate is Partial Weight Bearing?" *Clinical Orthopaedics and Related Research* (421):282-86, April 2004.

Youdas, J.W., et al. "Partial Weight-Bearing Gait using Conventional Assistive Devices," *Archives of Physical Medicine and Rehabilitation* 86(3):394-98, March 2005.

D

Defibrillation

The 2005 American Heart Association guidelines identify defibrillation as the standard treatment for ventricular fibrillation (VF), with subsequent cardiopulmonary resuscitation (CPR). CPR prolongs VF and delays the time that defibrillation can occur. And, because CPR alone isn't likely to correct VF, early defibrillation is critical. **AHA** Defibrillation involves using electrode paddles to direct an electric current through the patient's heart. The current causes the myocardium to depolarize which, in turn, encourages the sinoatrial node to resume control of the heart's electrical activity. Successful defibrillation depends on the appropriate selection of energy to generate sufficient flow through the heart to achieve defibrillation while minimizing injury to the heart. (See *Using a defibrillator*.)

Equipment

Defibrillator with electrocardiogram (ECG) monitor and recorder ◆ oxygen therapy equipment ◆ handheld resuscitation bag ◆ airway equipment ◆ emergency pacing equipment ◆ emergency cardiac medications ◆ blood pressure monitoring equipment.

Implementation

▶ Make sure that the defibrillation pads are attached to the defibrillator. If the pads aren't pregelled, be sure to have conductive gel or paste on hand to place on the patient before placing the pads or paddles. **MFR**

▶ Assess the patient to determine if he lacks a pulse. Call for help and perform CPR until the defibrillator and other emergency equipment arrive. **AHA**

▶ If the defibrillator has "quick-look" capability, place the paddles on the patient's chest to quickly view his cardiac rhythm. Otherwise, connect the monitoring leads of the defibrillator to the patient, and assess his cardiac rhythm.

▶ Expose the patient's chest, and apply the defibrillator pads at the paddle placement positions. For anterolateral placement, place one paddle to the right of the upper sternum, just below the right clavicle, and the other over the fifth or sixth intercostal space at the left anterior axillary line. For anteroposterior placement, place the anterior pad directly over the heart at the precordium, to the left of the lower sternal border. Place the posterior pad under the patient's body beneath the heart and immediately below the scapulae (but not under the vertebral column).

✴ CLINICAL ALERT

Never place the defibrillator pads directly over an implanted pacemaker. This may damage the pacemaker.

▶ Turn on the defibrillator and, if performing external defibrillation, set the energy level for 360 joules for an adult patient when using a monophasic defibrillator. Use clinically appropriate energy levels for biphasic defibrillators (usually 120 to 200 joules). **AHA**

▶ Charge the pads by pressing the charge buttons, which are located either on the machine or on the pads themselves.

▶ Press the paddles firmly against the patient's chest, using 25 lb (11.3 kg) of pressure. **CS**

▶ Reassess the patient's cardiac rhythm.

▶ If the patient remains in VF or pulseless ventricular tachycardia, instruct all personnel to stand clear of the patient and the bed. Visually verify that all personnel are clear of the patient and the bed before discharging the current.

Using a defibrillator

Because ventricular fibrillation (VF) can be fatal if not corrected, the success of defibrillation depends largely on early recognition and quick treatment of this arrhythmia. In addition to treating VF, defibrillation may also be used to treat pulseless ventricular tachycardia. **AHA**

To treat your patient as quickly as possible, you should familiarize yourself with the defibrillator available at your facility. The photo shown here depicts a standard defibrillator.

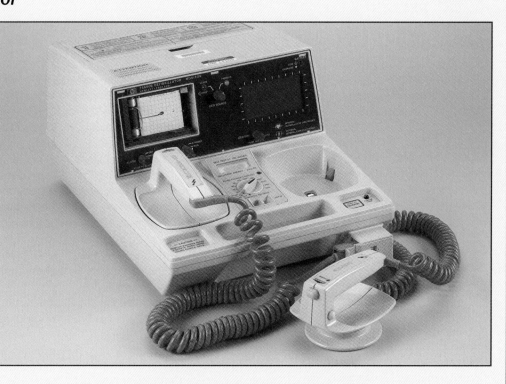

▶ Discharge the current by pressing both paddle charge buttons simultaneously.

▶ Resume CPR immediately for five cycles. **AHA**

▶ Reassess the patient's cardiac rhythm.

▶ If necessary, prepare to defibrillate a second time. Instruct someone to reset the energy level on the defibrillator to 360 joules or the biphasic energy equivalent and continue CPR while the defibrillator is charging. Announce that you're preparing to defibrillate, and follow the procedure described above. **AHA**

▶ Resume CPR immediately for five cycles. Begin administering appropriate medications, such as epinephrine or vasopressin. **AHA**

▶ Reassess the patient. If defibrillation is again necessary, instruct someone to

reset the energy level to 360 joules or the biphasic energy equivalent. Then follow the same procedure as before.

▶ Resume CPR immediately for five cycles. Continue to administer medications, adding antiarrhythmics or magnesium, as appropriate. **AHA**

▶ If defibrillation restores a normal rhythm, check the patient's central and peripheral pulses and obtain a blood pressure reading, heart rate, and respiratory rate. Assess the patient's level of consciousness, cardiac rhythm, breath sounds, skin color, and urine output. Obtain baseline arterial blood gas levels and a 12-lead ECG. Provide supplemental oxygen, ventilation, and medications, as needed. Check the patient's chest for electrical burns and treat them, as ordered, with corticosteroid or lanolin-based creams. Also prepare the defibrillator for immediate reuse.

Special considerations

▶ Defibrillators vary from one manufacturer to the next, so familiarize yourself with your facility's equipment. Defibrillator operation should be checked at least once per shift and after each use. **MFR**

▶ Defibrillation can be affected by several factors, including paddle size and placement, the condition of the patient's myocardium, the duration of the arrhythmia, chest resistance, and the number of countershocks. **CS**

▶ Remove transdermal medications from the chest (and back if using anterior-posterior placement) because the medication may interfere with the conduction of the current or produce a chest burn.

EVIDENCE-BASED RESEARCH

Delayed defibrillation

Chan, P.S., et al. "Delayed time to defibrillation after in-hospital cardiac arrest," *New England Journal of Medicine* 358(1):9-17, January 2008.

Level V
Evidence from systematic reviews of descriptive and qualitative studies

Description
Expert guidelines advise defibrillation within 2 minutes after an in-hospital cardiac arrest caused by ventricular arrhythmia. There have been very few studies done on delayed defibrillation and survival. This study looked at 6,789 patients who suffered cardiac arrest due to ventricular fibrillation or pulseless ventricular tachycardia at 369 hospitals in the National Registry of Cardiopulmonary Resuscitation. The definition of delayed defibrillation that was used was a length of time greater than 2 minutes from known onset of arrest until defibrillation.

Findings
The average time to defibrillation was one minute. Delayed time to defibrillation occurred in 30% of patients. Several characteristics identified with delayed defibrillation included black race; noncardiac admitting diagnosis; cardiac arrest at a hospital with fewer than 250 beds; unmonitored hospital unit; and arrest occurring between 5 p.m. and 8 a.m. or on a weekend.

Patients who had delayed defibrillation had a significantly lower survival percentage. Only 22.2% of patients with delayed defibrillation survived to discharge, compared with 39.3% of patients without delayed defibrillation.

Conclusion
Delayed defibrillation, although common, is associated with lower rates of survival after in-hospital cardiac arrest.

Nursing practice implications
Nurses are often the ones to find a patient in cardiac arrest, and they are also usually the first responders to an in-hospital cardiac arrest. Rapid defibrillation of the patient with a ventricular arrhythmia should be the nurse's priority in these situations. The following practice implications are important:
► Know where the defibrillator and crash cart are located on the unit.
► Perform quality assurance checks on the defibrillator at least every day, or according to your facility's policy, to make sure it is in working order.
► Prepare the defibrillator for use again immediately after it has been used.
► Educate the staff on the importance of rapid defibrillation.
► Conduct reviews on all patients who experienced a cardiac arrest and determine the time to defibrillation, as well as determine reasons for delayed defibrillation.

References

American Heart Association. "2005 Guidelines for Cardiopulmonary Resuscitation and Emergency Cardiovascular Care: The International Consensus on Science," *Circulation* 112(22 Suppl):IV-1-IV-221, November 2005.

American Heart Association. "Highlights of the 2005 American Heart Association Guidelines for CPR and ECG," *Currents* 16(4):1-27, Winter 2005-2006.

Kerber, R.E., et al. "Transthoracic resistance in human defibrillation. Influence of body weight, chest size, serial shocks, paddle size and paddle contact pressure," *Circulation* 63(3):676-82, March 1981. **CS**

Koster, R.W., et al. "Definition of Successful Defibrillation," *Critical Care Medicine* 34(12 Suppl):5423-426, December 2006.

Kudenchuk, P.J., et al. "Transthoracic Incremental Monophasic versus Biphasic Defibrillation by Emergency Responders (TIMBER): A Randomized Comparison of Monophasic with Biphasic Waveform Ascending Energy Defibrillation for the Resuscitation of Out-of-Hospital Cardiac Arrest Due to Ventricular Fibrillation," *Circulation* 114(19):2010-2018, November 2006.

Lynn-McHale Wiegand, D.J., and Carlson, K.K., eds. *AACN Procedure Manual for Critical Care*, 5th ed. Philadelphia: W.B. Saunders Co., 2005.

Direct heat application

Heat applied directly to the patient's body raises tissue temperature and enhances the inflammatory process by causing vasodilation and increasing local circulation. This promotes leukocytosis, suppuration, drainage, and healing. Heat also increases tissue metabolism, reduces pain caused by muscle spasm, and decreases congestion in deep visceral organs.

Direct heat may be dry or moist. Dry heat can be delivered at a higher temperature and for a longer time. Devices for applying dry heat include the hot-water bottle, electric heating pad, aquathermia pad, and chemical hot pack.

Moist heat softens crusts and exudates, penetrates deeper than dry heat, doesn't dry the skin, produces less perspiration, and usually is more comfortable for the patient. Devices for applying moist heat include warm compresses for small body areas and warm packs for large areas.

Direct heat treatment can't be used on patients at risk for hemorrhage. It's also contraindicated if the patient has a sprained limb in the acute stage (because vasodilation would increase pain and swelling) or if he has a condition associated with acute inflammation such as appendicitis. Direct heat should be applied cautiously to pediatric and elderly patients and to patients with impaired renal, cardiac, or respiratory function; arteriosclerosis or atherosclerosis; or impaired sensation. It should be applied with extreme caution to heat-sensitive areas, such as with areas of scar tissue and stomas.

Equipment

Patient thermometer ◆ towel ◆ adhesive tape or roller gauze ◆ absorbent, protective cloth covering ◆ gloves, if the patient has an open lesion.

For a hot-water bottle: Hot tap water ◆ pitcher ◆ bath (utility) thermometer ◆ absorbent, protective cloth covering.

For an electric heating pad: Absorbent, protective cloth covering.

For an aquathermia pad: Distilled water ◆ temperature-adjustment key ◆ absorbent, protective cloth covering.

For a chemical hot pack (disposable): Absorbent, protective cloth covering.

For a warm compress or pack (sterile or nonsterile): Basin of hot tap water or container of sterile water, normal saline or other solution, as ordered ◆ hot-water bottle, aquathermia pad, or chemical hot pack ◆ linen-saver pad ◆ bath thermometer ◆ optional: forceps.

The following items may be sterile or nonsterile, as needed: compress material (flannel, 4″ × 4″ gauze pads) or pack material (absorbent towels, large absorbent pads) ◆ cotton-tipped applicators ◆ forceps ◆ bowl or basin ◆ bath (utility) thermometer ◆ waterproof covering ◆ towel ◆ dressing.

Implementation

▶ Before beginning the procedure, you must prepare the equipment.

▶ If you're using a hot water bottle, fill the bottle with hot tap water to detect leaks and warm the bottle; then empty it. Run hot tap water into a pitcher, and measure the water temperature with the bath thermometer. Adjust the temperature, as ordered, usually to 115° to 125° F (46.1° to 51.7° C) for adults.

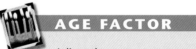

AGE FACTOR

Adjust the water temperature to 105° to 115° F (40.6° to 46.1° C) for children younger than age 2 or elderly patients.

▶ Next, pour hot water into the bottle, filling it one-half to two-thirds full. Partially filling the bottle keeps it lightweight and flexible to mold to the treatment area. Squeeze the bottle until the water reaches the neck to expel any air that would make the bottle inflexible and reduce heat conduction. Fasten the top and cover the bag with an absorbent cloth. Secure the cover with tape or roller gauze.

▶ For an electric heating pad, check the cord for frayed or damaged insulation. Then plug in the pad and adjust the control switch to the desired setting. Wrap the pad in a protective cloth covering, and secure the cover with tape or roller gauze.

▶ For an aquathermia pad: Check the cord for safety, as above, and fill the control unit two-thirds full with distilled water. Don't use tap water because it leaves mineral deposits in the unit. Check for leaks, and then tilt the unit in several directions to clear the pad's tubing of air. Tighten the cap, and then loosen it a quarter turn to allow heat expansion within the unit. After making sure the hoses between the control unit and the pad are free from tangles, place the unit on the bedside table, slightly above the patient so that gravity can assist water flow. If the central supply department hasn't preset the temperature, use the temperature-adjustment key provided to set the temperature on the control unit. The usual temperature is 105° F (40.6° C). Then place the pad in a protective cloth covering, and secure the cover with tape or roller gauze. Plug in the unit, turn it on, and allow the pad to warm for 2 minutes.

▶ If you're using a chemical heat pack, select a pack of the correct size. Then follow the manufacturer's directions (strike, squeeze, or knead) to activate the heat-producing chemicals. Place the pack in a protective cloth covering, and secure the cover with tape or roller gauze.

▶ For a warm sterile compress: Warm the container of sterile water or solution by setting it in a sink or basin of hot water. Measure its temperature with a sterile bath thermometer. If a sterile thermometer is unavailable, pour some heated sterile solution into a clean container, check the temperature with a regular bath thermometer, and then discard the tested solution. Adjust the temperature by adding hot or cold water to the sink or basin until the solution reaches 131° F (55° C) for adults.

AGE FACTOR

Adjust the water temperature to 105° F for children or elderly patients or for an eye compress.

▶ Pour the heated solution into a sterile bowl or basin. Then, using sterile technique, soak the compress or pack in the heated solution. If necessary, prepare a hot-water bottle, aquathermia pad, or chemical hot pack to keep the compress or pack warm.

▶ For a nonsterile warm compress or pack: Fill a bowl or basin with hot tap water or other solution, and measure the temperature of the fluid with a bath thermometer. Adjust the temperature, as ordered, usually to 131° F (55° C) for adults.

AGE FACTOR

Adjust the water temperature to 105° F for children or elderly patients or for an eye compress.

Then soak the compress or pack in the hot liquid. If necessary, prepare a hot-water bottle, aquathermia pad, or chemical hot pack to keep the compress or pack warm.

▶ Check the practitioner's order.

▶ Assess the patient's condition.

▶ Confirm the patient's identity using two patient identifiers according to your facility's policy. **JC**

▶ Explain the procedure to the patient, and tell him not to lean or lie directly on the heating device because this reduces air space and increases the risk of burns. Warn him against adjusting the temperature of the heating device or adding hot water to a hot-water bottle. Advise him to report pain immediately and to remove the device, if necessary.

▶ Provide privacy and make sure the room is warm and free from drafts. Wash your hands.

▶ Take the patient's temperature, pulse, and respiration to serve as a baseline. If heat treatment is being applied to raise the patient's body temperature, monitor his temperature, pulse, and respirations throughout the application.

▶ Expose only the treatment area because vasodilation will make the patient feel chilly.

Applying a hot-water bottle, an electric heating pad, an aquathermia pad, or a chemical hot pack

▶ Before applying the heating device, press it against your inner forearm to test its temperature and heat distribution. If it heats unevenly, obtain a new device.

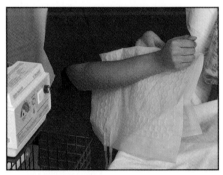

▶ Apply the device to the treatment area and, if necessary, secure it with tape or roller gauze. Begin timing the application.

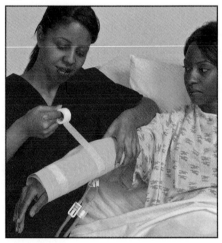

▶ Assess the patient's skin condition frequently, and remove the device if you observe increased swelling or excessive redness, blistering, maceration, or pallor or if the patient reports discomfort. Refill the hot-water bottle, as necessary, to maintain the correct temperature.

▶ Remove the device after 20 to 30 minutes or as ordered.

▶ Dry the patient's skin with a towel and re-dress the site, if necessary. Take the patient's temperature, pulse, and respiration for comparison with the baseline. Position him comfortably in bed.

▶ If the treatment is to be repeated, store the equipment in the patient's room, out of his reach; otherwise, return it to its proper place.

Applying a warm compress or pack

▶ Place a linen-saver pad under the site.

▶ Remove the warm compress or pack from the bowl or basin. (Use sterile forceps throughout the procedure, if necessary.)

▶ Wring excess solution from the compress or pack (using sterile forceps, if needed). Excess moisture increases the risk of burns.

▶ Apply the compress gently to the affected site (using forceps, if warranted). After a few seconds, lift the compress (with forceps, if needed) and check the skin for excessive redness, maceration, or blistering. When you're sure the compress isn't causing a burn, mold it firmly to the skin to keep air out, which reduces the temperature and effectiveness of the compress. Work quickly so the compress retains its heat.

▶ Apply a waterproof covering (sterile, if necessary) to the compress. Secure it with tape or roller gauze to prevent it from slipping.

▶ Place a hot-water bottle, aquathermia pad, or chemical hot pack over the compress and waterproof covering to maintain the correct temperature. Begin timing the application.

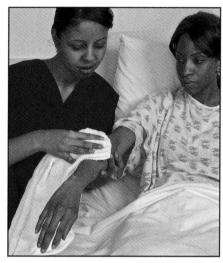

▶ Check the patient's skin every 5 minutes for tissue tolerance. Remove the device if the skin shows excessive redness, maceration, or blistering or if the patient experiences pain or discomfort. Change the compress, as needed, to maintain the correct temperature.

▶ After 15 to 20 minutes or as ordered, remove the compress. (Use forceps, if warranted.) Discard the compress into a waterproof trash bag.

▶ Dry the patient's skin with a towel (sterile, if necessary). Note the condition of the skin and redress the area, if necessary. Take the patient's temperature, pulse, and respiration for comparison with the baseline. Then make sure the patient is comfortable.

Special considerations

▶ If the patient is unconscious, anesthetized, irrational, neurologically impaired, or insensitive to heat, stay with him throughout the treatment.

▶ When direct heat is ordered to decrease congestion within internal organs, the application must cover a large enough area to increase blood volume at the skin's surface. For relief of pelvic organ congestion, for example, apply heat over the patient's lower abdomen,

hips, and thighs. To achieve local relief, you may concentrate heat only over the specified area.

▶ As an alternative method of applying sterile moist compresses, use a bedside sterilizer to sterilize the compresses. Saturate the compress with tap water or another solution and wring it dry. Then place it in the bedside sterilizer at 275° F (135° C) for 15 minutes. Remove the compress with sterile forceps or sterile gloves, and wring out the excess solution. Then place the compress in a sterile bowl, and measure its temperature with a sterile thermometer.

▶ Be sure to follow the manufacturer's instructions for heating compresses, and avoid over-heating.

References

Cosqray, N.A., et al. "Effect of Heat Modalities on Hamstring Length: A Comparison of Pneumatherm, Moist Heat Pack, and a Control," *Journal of Orthopedic Sports and Physical Therapy* 34(7):377-84, July 2004.

Craven, R.F., and Hirnle, C.J. *Fundamentals of Nursing: Human Health and Function,* 6th ed. Philadelphia: Lippincott Williams & Wilkins, 2009.

Mayer, J.M., et al. "Treating Acute Low Back Pain with Continuous Low-level Heat Wrap Therapy and/or Exercises: A Randomized Controlled Trial," *The Spine Journal* 5(4):395-403, July-August 2005.

Taylor, C., et al. *Fundamentals of Nursing: The Art and Science of Nursing Care,* 6th ed. Philadelphia: Lippincott Williams & Wilkins, 2008.

E

Ear irrigation

Irrigating the ear involves washing the external auditory canal with a stream of solution to clean the canal of discharges, to soften and remove impacted cerumen, or to dislodge a foreign body. Irrigation may also be used to relieve localized inflammation and discomfort. The procedure must be performed carefully to avoid causing patient discomfort or vertigo and to avoid increasing the risk of otitis externa. Because irrigation may contaminate the middle ear if the tympanic membrane is ruptured, an otoscopic examination always precedes ear irrigation.

This procedure is contraindicated when a foreign body (such as a pea) obstructs the auditory canal. The foreign body may swell when it comes in contact with an irrigant or other solution, causing intense pain and complicating removal of the object. Ear irrigation is also contraindicated if the patient has a cold, a fever, an ear infection, or an injured or ruptured tympanic membrane. The presence of a hearing aid battery in the ear also prohibits irrigation because battery acid could leak, and irrigation would spread caustic material throughout the canal.

Equipment

Ear irrigation syringe ◆ gloves ◆ otoscope with aural speculum ◆ prescribed irrigant ◆ large basin ◆ linen-saver pad and bath towel ◆ emesis basin ◆ cotton balls or cotton-tipped applicators ◆ 4″ × 4″ gauze pad ◆ optional: adjustable light.

Implementation

▶ Put the container of irrigant into the large basin filled with hot water to warm the solution to body temperature. Avoid extreme temperature changes because they can affect inner ear fluids, causing nausea and dizziness. Test the temperature of the solution by sprinkling a few drops on your inner wrist.

▶ Confirm the patient's identity using two patient identifiers according to your facility's policy. **JC**

▶ Explain the procedure to the patient, provide privacy, and wash your hands and put on gloves.

▶ If you haven't already done so, use the otoscope to inspect the auditory canal that will be irrigated.

▶ Help the patient to a sitting position. Tilt his head forward and slightly toward the affected side. This will help prevent the solution from running down his neck. If he can't sit, have him lie on his back and tilt his head slightly forward and toward the affected ear.

▶ If the patient is sitting, place the linen-saver pad (covered with the bath towel) on his shoulder and upper arm, under the affected ear. If he's lying down, cover his pillow and the area under the affected ear.

▶ Have the patient hold the emesis basin close to his head under the affected ear.

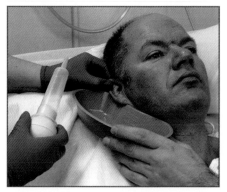

▶ Clean the auricle and meatus of the auditory canal with a cotton ball or cotton-tipped applicator moistened with normal saline solution or the prescribed irrigating solution.

▶ Draw the irrigant into the syringe and expel any air.

▶ Straighten the auditory canal, then insert the syringe tip and start the flow. (See *How to irrigate the ear canal*.)

▶ During irrigation, observe the patient for signs of pain or dizziness. If he reports either, stop the procedure, recheck the temperature of the irrigant, inspect the patient's ear with the otoscope, and resume irrigation, as indicated.

▶ When the syringe is empty, remove it and inspect the return flow. Then refill the syringe and continue the irrigation until the return flow is clear. Never use more than 500 ml of irrigant during this procedure.

▶ Remove the syringe and inspect the ear canal for cleanliness with the otoscope.

▶ Dry the patient's auricle and neck.

▶ Remove the bath towel and place a 4″ × 4″ gauze pad under his ear to promote drainage of residual debris and solution.

Special considerations

▶ Avoid dropping or squirting irrigant on the tympanic membrane because this may startle the patient and cause discomfort.

▶ If the practitioner directs you to place a cotton pledget in the ear canal to retain some of the solution, pack the cotton loosely. Instruct the patient not to remove it.

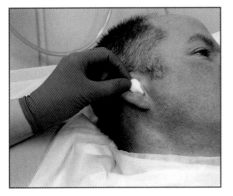

How to irrigate the ear canal

Follow these guidelines for irrigating the ear canal.

▶ Gently pull the auricle up and back to straighten the ear canal (as shown at right). (For a child, pull the ear down and back.)

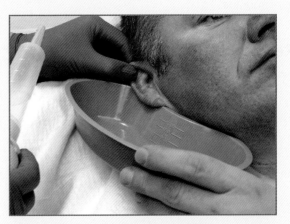

▶ Have the patient hold an emesis basin beneath the ear to catch returning irrigant. Position the tip of the irrigating syringe at the meatus of the auditory canal (as shown at right). Don't block the meatus because you'll impede backflow and raise pressure in the canal.

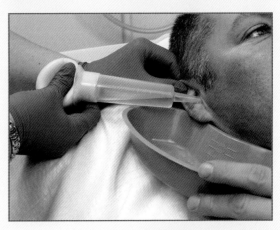

▶ Tilt the patient's head toward you, and point the syringe tip upward and toward the posterior ear canal (as shown at right). This angle prevents damage to the tympanic membrane and guards against pushing debris farther into the canal.

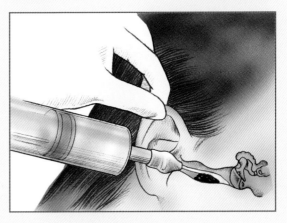

▶ Direct a steady stream of irrigant against the upper wall of the ear canal, and inspect return fluid for cloudiness, cerumen, blood, or foreign matter.

▶ Possible complications of ear irrigation include vertigo, nausea, otitis externa, and otitis media. Forceful instillation of irrigant can rupture the tympanic membrane.

References

Heim, S.W., and Maughan, K.L. "Foreign Bodies in the Ear, Nose, and Throat," *American Family Physician* 76(8):1185-189, October 2007.

Keegan, D.A., and Bannister, S.L. "A Novel Method for the Removal of Ear Cerumen," *Canadian Medical Association Journal* 173(12):1496-497, December 2005.

Taylor, C., et al. *Fundamentals of Nursing: The Art and Science of Nursing Care,* 6th ed. Philadelphia: Lippincott Williams & Wilkins, 2008.

Eardrop instillation

Eardrops may be instilled to treat infection and inflammation, soften cerumen for later removal, produce local anesthesia, or facilitate removal of an insect trapped in the ear by immobilizing and smothering it.

Instillation of eardrops is usually contraindicated if the patient has a perforated eardrum, but it may be permitted with certain medications and adherence to sterile technique. Other conditions may also prohibit instillation of certain medications into the ear. For example, instillation of drops containing hydrocortisone is contraindicated if the patient has herpes, another viral infection, or a fungal infection.

Equipment

Prescribed eardrops ◆ patient's medication record and chart ◆ light source ◆ facial tissue or cotton-tipped applicator ◆ optional: cotton ball, bowl of warm water.

Implementation

▶ Warm the medication to body temperature in the bowl of warm water or carry it in your pocket for 30 minutes before administration. If necessary, test the temperature of the medication by placing a drop on your wrist. (If the medication is too hot, it may burn the patient's eardrum.)

▶ Verify the order on the patient's medication record by checking it against the practitioner's order. **JC** **ISMP**

▶ Wash your hands. **CDC**

▶ Confirm the patient's identity using two patient identifiers according to your facility's policy. **JC**

▶ If your facility utilizes a bar code scanning system, be sure to scan your ID badge, the patient's ID bracelet, and the medication's bar code. **JC** **ISMP**

▶ Provide privacy, if possible. Explain the procedure to the patient.

▶ Have the patient lie on the side opposite the affected ear.

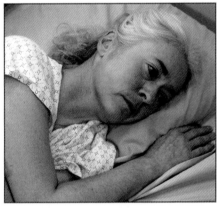

▶ Straighten the patient's ear canal. For an adult, pull the auricle of the ear up and back. (See *Positioning the patient for eardrop instillation,* page 158.)

▶ Using a light source, examine the ear canal for drainage. If you find any, clean the canal with a tissue or cotton-tipped applicator because drainage can reduce the medication's effectiveness.

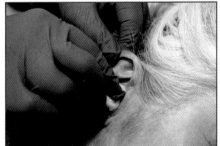

▶ Compare the label on the eardrops with the order on the patient's medication record. Check the label again while drawing the medication into the dropper. Check the label for the final time

before returning the eardrops to the shelf or drawer. **ISMP**

▶ To avoid damaging the ear canal with the dropper, gently support the hand holding the dropper against the patient's head. Straighten the patient's ear canal once again, and instill the ordered number of drops. To avoid patient discomfort, aim the dropper so that the drops fall against the sides of the ear canal, not on the eardrum. Hold the ear canal in position until you see the medication disappear down the canal. Then release the ear.

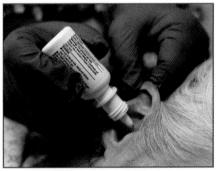

▶ Instruct the patient to remain in the side-lying position for 5 to 10 minutes to let the medication run down into the ear canal.

▶ If ordered, tuck the cotton ball loosely into the opening of the ear canal to prevent the medication from leaking out. However, be careful not to insert it too deeply into the canal be-

Positioning the patient for eardrop instillation

Before instilling eardrops, have the patient lie on his side. Then straighten the patient's ear canal to help the medication reach the eardrum. For an adult, gently pull the auricle *up and back;* for an infant or a young child, gently pull the auricle *down and back.*

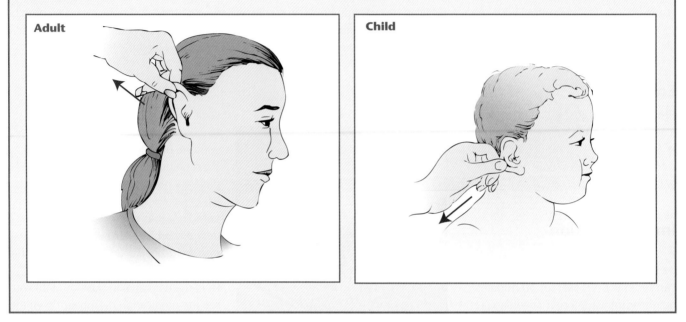

Adult

Child

cause this would prevent drainage of secretions and increase pressure on the eardrum.

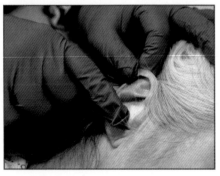

▶ Clean and dry the outer ear.
▶ If ordered, repeat the procedure in the other ear after 5 to 10 minutes.
▶ Assist the patient into a comfortable position.
▶ Wash your hands.

Special considerations

▶ Remember that some conditions make the normally tender ear canal even more sensitive; therefore, be especially gentle when performing this procedure.
▶ To prevent injury to the eardrum, never insert a cotton-tipped applicator into the ear canal past the point where you can see the tip. After applying eardrops to soften the cerumen, irrigate the ear, as ordered, to facilitate its removal.
▶ If the patient has vertigo, keep the side rails of the bed up and help the patient during the procedure, as needed. Also, move slowly and unhurriedly to avoid exacerbating the vertigo.
▶ Teach the patient to instill the eardrops correctly so that treatment can continue at home, if necessary. Review the procedure and let the patient try it while you observe.

References

The Joint Commission. *Comprehensive Accreditation Manual for Hospitals: The Official Handbook.* Standard MM.1.10. Oakbrook Terrace, Ill. : The Joint Commission, 2007.

The Joint Commission. *Comprehensive Accreditation Manual for Hospitals: The Official Handbook.* Standard MM.3.10. Oakbrook Terrace, Ill. : The Joint Commission, 2007.

The Joint Commission. *Comprehensive Accreditation Manual for Hospitals: The Official Handbook.* Standard MM.4.10. Oakbrook Terrace, Ill. : The Joint Commission, 2007.

The Joint Commission. *Comprehensive Accreditation Manual for Hospitals: The Official Handbook.* Standard MM.4.20. Oakbrook Terrace, Ill. : The Joint Commission, 2007.

The Joint Commission. *Comprehensive Accreditation Manual for Hospitals: The Official Handbook.* Standard MM.4.30.

Oakbrook Terrace, Ill. : The Joint Commission, 2007.

The Joint Commission. *Comprehensive Accreditation Manual for Hospitals: The Official Handbook.* Standard MM.5.10. Oakbrook Terrace, Ill. : The Joint Commission, 2007.

The Joint Commission. *Comprehensive Accreditation Manual for Hospitals: The Official Handbook.* Standard MM.6.10. Oakbrook Terrace, Ill. : The Joint Commission, 2007.

The Joint Commission. *Comprehensive Accreditation Manual for Hospitals: The Official Handbook.* Standard MM.6.20. Oakbrook Terrace, Ill. : The Joint Commission, 2007.

Taylor, C., et al. *Fundamentals of Nursing: The Art and Science of Nursing Care,* 6th ed. Philadelphia: Lippincott Williams & Wilkins, 2008.

Elastic bandage application

Elastic bandages exert gentle, even pressure on a body part. By supporting blood vessels, these rolled bandages promote venous return and prevent pooling of blood in the legs. They're typically used in place of antiembolism stockings to prevent thrombophlebitis and pulmonary embolism in postoperative or bedridden patients who can't stimulate venous return by muscle activity.

Elastic bandages also minimize joint swelling after trauma to the musculoskeletal system. Used with a splint, they immobilize a fracture during healing. They can also provide hemostatic pressure and anchor dressings over a fresh wound or after surgical procedures such as vein stripping.

Equipment

Elastic bandage of appropriate width ◆ tape, pins, or self-closures ◆ gauze pads or absorbent cotton.

Bandages usually come in 2″ to 6″ widths and 4′ and 6′ (1.2- and 1.8-m) lengths. The 3″ width is adaptable to most applications. Most elastic bandages come with self-closures.

Implementation

▶ Select a bandage that wraps the affected body part completely but isn't excessively long. In most cases, use a narrower bandage for wrapping the foot, lower leg, hand, or arm, and a wider bandage for the thigh or trunk. The bandage should be clean and rolled before application.
▶ Confirm the patient's identity using two patient identifiers according to your facility's policy. **JC**
▶ Check the practitioner's order.
▶ Examine the area to be wrapped for lesions or skin breakdown. If these conditions are present, consult the practitioner before applying the elastic bandage.
▶ Explain the procedure to the patient, provide privacy, and wash your hands thoroughly. Position him comfortably, with the body part to be bandaged in normal functioning position to promote circulation and prevent deformity and discomfort.

▶ Avoid applying a bandage to a dependent extremity. If you're wrapping an extremity, elevate it for 15 to 30 minutes before application to facilitate venous return.
▶ Apply the bandage so that two skin surfaces don't remain in contact when wrapped. Place gauze or absorbent cotton, as needed, between skin surfaces, such as between toes and fingers and under breasts and arms, to prevent skin irritation.
▶ Hold the bandage with the roll facing upward in one hand and the free end of the bandage in the other hand. Hold the bandage roll close to the part being bandaged to ensure even tension and pressure.

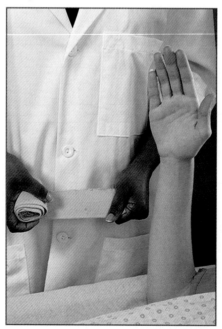

▶ Unroll the bandage as you wrap the body part in a spiral or spiral-reverse method. Never unroll the entire bandage before wrapping because this could produce uneven pressure, which interferes with blood circulation and cell perfusion.
▶ Overlap each layer of bandage by one-half to two-thirds the width of the strip. (See *Bandaging techniques*.)
▶ Wrap firmly but not too tightly. As you wrap, ask the patient to tell you if the bandage feels comfortable. If he complains of tingling, itching, numbness, or pain, loosen the bandage.
▶ Begin wrapping an extremity at the most distal part and work proximally to promote venous return.
▶ When wrapping an extremity, anchor the bandage initially by circling the body part twice. To prevent the bandage from slipping out of place on the foot, wrap it in a figure eight around the foot, the ankle, and then the foot again before continuing. The same technique works on any joint, such as the knee, wrist, or elbow. Include the heel when wrapping the foot, but never wrap the toes (or fingers) unless absolutely necessary because the distal extremities are used to detect impaired circulation.
▶ When you're finished wrapping, secure the end of the bandage with the self-closures, or use tape or pins, being careful not to scratch or pinch the patient.

Bandaging techniques

Circular
Each turn encircles the previous one, covering it completely. Use this technique to anchor a bandage.

Spiral
Each turn partially overlaps the previous one. Use this technique to wrap a long, straight body part or one of increasing circumference.

Spiral-reverse
Anchor the bandage and then reverse direction halfway through each spiral turn. Use this technique to accommodate the increasing circumference of a body part.

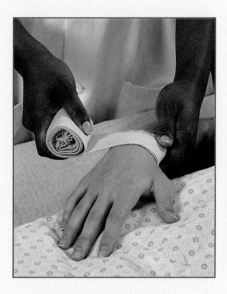

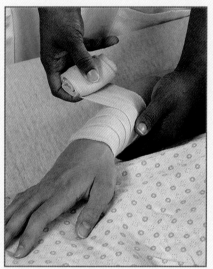

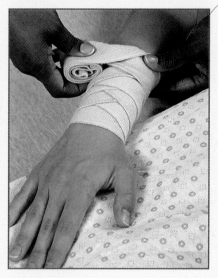

Figure eight
Anchor below the joint, and then use alternating ascending and descending turns to form a figure-eight. Use this technique around joints.

Recurrent
This technique includes a combination of recurrent and circular turns. Hold the bandage as you make each recurrent turn and then use the circular turns as a final anchor. Use this technique for a stump, a hand, or the scalp.

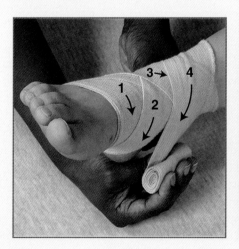

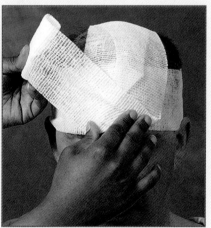

EVIDENCE-BASED RESEARCH

Compression bandages and orthostatic hypotension

Podoleanu, C., et al. "Lower limb and abdominal compression bandages prevent progressive orthostatic hypotension in elderly persons: a randomized single-blind controlled study," *Journal of the American College of Cardiology* 48(7):1425-32, October 2006.

Level II

Evidence obtained from at least one well-designed randomized controlled trial

Description

Orthostatic hypotension is a drop in blood pressure that occurs when changing position, usually to a more upright position. Orthostatic hypotension often occurs in elderly patients, and is a common cause of falls. This study looked at whether compression bandages placed on the lower legs and abdomen helped prevent orthostatic hypotension and its symptoms. 21 patients with an average age of 70 years were subjected to two tilt-test procedures. One occurred with elastic bandages on the legs and abdomen,

and the other without. The leg bandage was applied for 10 minutes, and then the abdominal bandage was applied for another 10 minutes. The patient's symptoms were evaluated on the seven-item Specific Symptom Score (SSS) questionnaire before and after 1 month of therapy.

Findings

Patients with the sham elastic bandages had more of a decrease in their blood pressure after tilting than patients with active bandages. About 90% of patients with active bandages were asymptomatic after tilting, compared with only 53% of the patients with sham elastic bandages. The overall SSS score before therapy was 35.2, and decreased to 22.5 after 1 month of therapy with active bandages.

Conclusions

Lower limb compression bandage avoids decreased orthostatic systolic blood pressure and reduces symptoms in elderly patients with progressive orthostatic hypotension.

Nursing practice implications: Nurses often care for elderly patients who are affected by orthostatic hypotension to some degree. By using elastic bandages on the patient's legs and abdomen, the nurses could help lessen the effect of orthostatic hypotension on the patient. The following nursing practice implications are important:

▶ Assess patients for orthostatic hypotension.

▶ Assist all patients with orthostatic hypotension in standing to help prevent falls.

▶ Teach patients with orthostatic hypotension how to gradually change their position.

▶ Conduct fall risk assessments, including the presence of orthostatic hypotension, on all patients.

▶ Discuss elastic bandage use with the practitioner and, if appropriate, teach the patient how to apply the elastic bandages.

▶ Check distal circulation after the bandage is in place because the elastic may tighten as you wrap.

▶ Elevate a wrapped extremity for 15 to 30 minutes to facilitate venous return.

Special considerations

▶ Check distal circulation once or twice every 8 hours. Lift the distal end of the bandage, and assess the skin underneath for color, temperature, and integrity.

▶ Remove the bandage every 8 hours or whenever it's loose and wrinkled. Roll it up as you unwrap to ready it for reuse. Observe the area and provide skin care before rewrapping the bandage.

▶ Change the bandage at least once daily. Bathe the skin, dry it thoroughly, and observe for irritation and breakdown before applying a fresh bandage.

▶ Avoid leaving gaps in bandage layers or exposed skin surfaces because this may result in uneven pressure on the body part.

▶ Observe the patient for an allergic reaction because some patients can't tolerate the sizing in a new bandage. Laundering it reduces this risk.

▶ Launder the bandage daily or whenever it becomes limp; laundering restores its elasticity. Always keep two bandages handy so one can be applied while the other bandage is being laundered.

▶ When using an elastic bandage after a surgical procedure on an extremity (such as vein stripping) or with a splint to immobilize a fracture, remove it only as ordered rather than every 8 hours.

References

Coull, A., et al. "Class 3C Compression Bandaging for Venous Ulcers: Comparison of Spiral and Figure-Eight Techniques," *Journal of Advanced Nursing* 54(3):274-83, May 2006.

Fletcher, J. "The Importance of Correctly Choosing a Bandage and Bandaging Technique," *Nursing Times* 100(32):52-53, August 2004.

Lynn, P. *Taylor's Clinical Nursing Skills,* 2nd ed. Philadelphia: Lippincott Williams & Wilkins, 2008.

Electrocardiography

One of the most valuable and frequently used diagnostic tools, electrocardiography displays the heart's electrical activity as waveforms. Impulses moving through the heart's conduction system create electric currents that can be monitored on the body's surface. Electrodes attached to the skin can detect these electric currents and transmit them to an instrument that produces a record (the electrocardiogram [ECG]) of cardiac activity.

Electrocardiography can be used to identify myocardial ischemia and infarction, rhythm and conduction disturbances, chamber enlargement, electrolyte imbalances, and the effects of drugs on the heart.

The standard 12-lead ECG uses a series of electrodes placed on the extremities and the chest wall to assess the heart from 12 different views (leads). The 12 leads consist of three standard bipolar limb leads (designated I, II, III), three unipolar augmented leads (aV_R, aV_L, aV_F), and six unipolar precordial leads (V_1 to V_6). The limb leads and augmented leads show the heart from the frontal plane. The precordial leads show the heart from the horizontal plane. All electrodes are attached to the patient at once, and the machine prints a simultaneous view of all leads. (See *Understanding ECG leads*.)

The ECG device measures and averages the differences between the electrical potential of the electrode sites for each lead and graphs them over time. This creates the standard ECG complex, called PQRST. The P wave represents atrial depolarization; the QRS complex, ventricular depolarization; and the T wave, ventricular repolarization. (See *Reviewing ECG waveforms and components,* page 166.)

Equipment

ECG machine ◆ recording paper ◆ disposable pregelled electrodes ◆ 4″ × 4″ gauze pads ◆ optional: clippers, marking pen.

Implementation

▶ Confirm the patient's identity using two patient identifiers according to your facility's policy. **JC**

▶ Place the ECG machine close to the patient's bed, and plug the power cord into the wall outlet. If the patient is already connected to a cardiac monitor, remove the electrodes to accommodate the precordial leads and minimize electrical interference on the ECG tracing. Keep the patient away from objects that might cause electrical interference, such as equipment, fixtures, and power cords. **MFR**

▶ As you set up the machine to record a 12-lead ECG, explain the procedure to the patient.

▶ Have the patient lie in a supine position in the center of the bed with his arms at his sides. You may raise the head of the bed to promote his comfort. Expose his arms and legs, and drape him appropriately. His arms and legs should be relaxed to minimize muscle trembling, which can cause electrical interference.

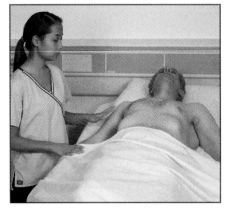

▶ If the bed is too narrow, place the patient's hands under his buttocks to prevent muscle tension. Also use this technique if the patient is shivering or trembling. Make sure his feet aren't touching the bed board.

▶ Select flat, fleshy areas to place the electrodes. Avoid muscular and bony areas. If the patient has an amputated limb, choose a site on the stump.

▶ If an area is excessively hairy, clip it. Clean excess oil or other substances from the skin to enhance electrode contact.

▶ Peel off the contact paper of the disposable electrodes, and apply them directly to the prepared site. To guarantee the best connection to the leadwire, position disposable electrodes on the legs with the lead connection pointing superiorly.

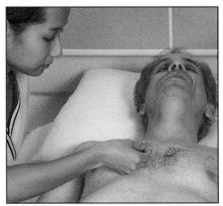

Understanding ECG leads

Each of the leads on a 12-lead electrocardiogram (ECG) views the heart from a different angle. These illustrations show the direction of electrical activity (depolarization) monitored by each lead and the 12 views of the heart.

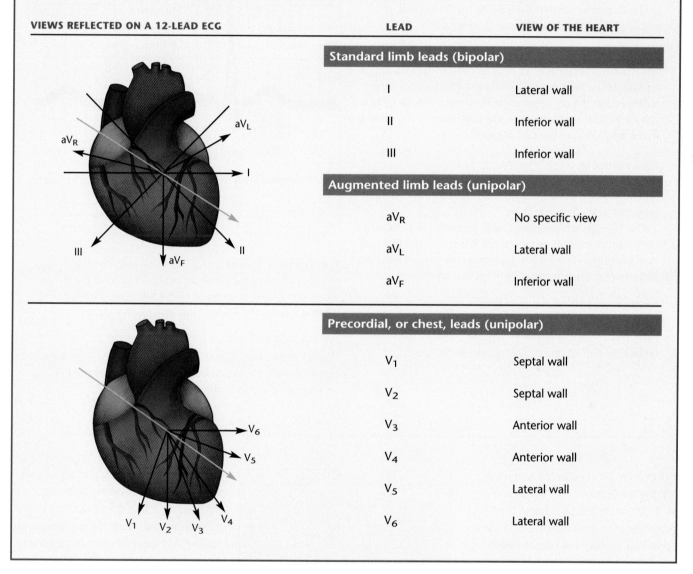

VIEWS REFLECTED ON A 12-LEAD ECG

LEAD	VIEW OF THE HEART
Standard limb leads (bipolar)	
I	Lateral wall
II	Inferior wall
III	Inferior wall
Augmented limb leads (unipolar)	
aV_R	No specific view
aV_L	Lateral wall
aV_F	Inferior wall
Precordial, or chest, leads (unipolar)	
V_1	Septal wall
V_2	Septal wall
V_3	Anterior wall
V_4	Anterior wall
V_5	Lateral wall
V_6	Lateral wall

▶ Connect the limb leadwires to the electrodes. Make sure the metal parts of the electrodes are clean and bright. Dirty or corroded electrodes prevent a good electrical connection.

▶ Expose the patient's chest. Put a disposable electrode at each electrode position. (See *Positioning chest electrodes,* page 167.)

If your patient is a woman, be sure to place the chest electrodes below the breast tissue. In a large-breasted woman, you may need to displace the breast tissue laterally.

▶ Check to see that the paper speed selector is set to the standard 25 mm/second and that the machine is set to full voltage. The machine will record a normal standardization

mark—a square that's the height of two large squares or 10 small squares on the recording paper. Then, if necessary, enter the appropriate patient identification data.

▶ If any part of the waveform extends beyond the paper when you record the ECG, adjust the normal standardization to half-standardization. Note this adjustment on the ECG strip because this

Reviewing ECG waveforms and components

An electrocardiogram (ECG) waveform has three basic components: the P wave, QRS complex, and T wave. These elements can be further divided into the PR interval, J point, ST segment, U wave, and QT interval.

P wave and PR interval
The P wave represents atrial depolarization. The PR interval represents the time it takes an impulse to travel from the atria through the atrioventricular nodes and bundle of His. The PR interval measures from the beginning of the P wave to the beginning of the QRS complex.

QRS complex
The QRS complex represents ventricular depolarization (the time it takes for the impulse to travel through the bundle branches to the Purkinje fibers).

   The Q wave, when present, appears as the first negative deflection in the QRS complex; the R wave, as the first positive deflection. The S wave appears as the second negative deflection or the first negative deflection after the R wave.

J point and ST segment
Marking the end of the QRS complex, the J point also indicates the beginning of the ST segment. The ST segment represents part of ventricular repolarization.

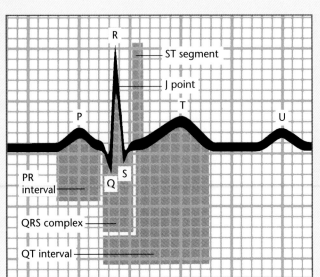

T wave and U wave
Usually following the same deflection pattern as the P wave, the T wave represents ventricular repolarization. The U wave follows the T wave, but isn't always seen.

QT interval
The QT interval represents ventricular depolarization and repolarization. It extends from the beginning of the QRS complex to the end of the T wave.

---

will need to be considered when interpreting the results.

▶ Now you're ready to begin the recording. Ask the patient to relax and breathe normally. Tell him to lie still and not to talk when you record his ECG. Then press the AUTO button. Observe the tracing quality. The machine will record all 12 leads automatically, recording three consecutive leads simultaneously. Some machines have a display screen so you can preview waveforms before the machine records them on paper (as shown in the next column).

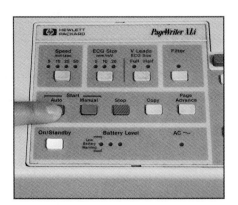

▶ When the machine finishes recording the 12-lead ECG, remove the electrodes and clean the patient's skin. After disconnecting the leadwires from the electrodes, dispose of or clean the electrodes, as indicated.

▶ If serial ECGs are expected, consider marking the electrode positions on the patient's skin. Consistent lead placement enhances the comparison of serial ECGs and eliminates inaccuracy due to lead placement. **CS**

Special considerations

▶ Small areas of hair on the patient's chest or extremities may be clipped, but this usually isn't necessary.

▶ If the patient's skin is exceptionally oily, scaly, or diaphoretic, rub the electrode site with a dry 4″ × 4″ gauze or alcohol pad before applying the elec-

Positioning chest electrodes

To ensure accurate test results, position chest electrodes as follows:

V_1: Fourth intercostal space at right sternal border
V_2: Fourth intercostal space at left sternal border
V_3: Halfway between V_2 and V_4
V_4: Fifth intercostal space at midclavicular line
V_5: Fifth intercostal space at anterior axillary line (halfway between V_4 and V_6)
V_6: Fifth intercostal space at midaxillary line, level with V_4

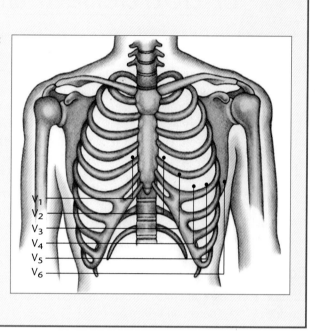

trode to help reduce interference in the tracing.

▶ During the procedure, ask the patient to breathe normally. If his respirations distort the recording, ask him to hold his breath briefly to reduce baseline wander in the tracing.

▶ If the patient has a pacemaker, you can perform an ECG with or without a magnet, according to the practitioner's order. Be sure to note the presence of a pacemaker and the use of the magnet on the strip.

References

American College of Cardiology and American Heart Association. "ACC/AHA Clinical Competence Statement on Electrocardiography and Ambulatory Electrocardiography," *Circulation* 104(25):3169-178, December 2001.

Davies, A. "Recognizing and Reducing Interference on 12-lead Electrocardiograms," *British Journal of Nursing* 16(13):800-804, July 2007.

Jowett, N.I., et al. "Modified Electrode Placement Must be Recorded when Performing 12-lead Electrocardiograms," *Postgraduate Medical Journal* 81(952):122-5, February 2005. **CS**

Lynn-McHale Wiegand, D.J., and Carlson, K.K., eds. *AACN Procedure Manual for Critical Care,* 5th ed. Philadelphia: W.B. Saunders Co., 2005.

Noordzij, P.G., et al. "Prognostic Value of Routine Preoperative Electrocardiography in Patients Undergoing Noncardiac Surgery," *American Journal of Cardiology* 97(7):1103-106, April 2006.

Endotracheal drug administration

When an I.V. line isn't readily available, drugs can be administered into the respiratory system through an endotracheal (ET) tube. This route allows uninterrupted resuscitation efforts and avoids such complications as coronary artery laceration, cardiac tamponade, and pneumothorax, which can occur when emergency drugs are administered intracardially.

Drugs given endotracheally usually have a longer duration of action than drugs given I.V. because they're absorbed in the alveoli. However, many of the drugs achieve a lower blood level when administered via the ET tube than I.V. For these reasons, repeat doses and continuous infusions must be adjusted to prevent adverse effects. Drugs most commonly given by this route include atropine, epinephrine, lidocaine, naloxone, and vasopressin. **AHA**

Endotracheal drugs are usually administered in an emergency by a physician, an emergency medical technician, or a critical care nurse. Although guidelines may vary depending on state, county, or city regulations, the basic administration method is the same. (See *Administering endotracheal drugs*.)

Equipment

ET tube ◆ gloves ◆ end-tidal carbon dioxide ($ETCO_2$) detection device or esophageal detection device ◆ handheld resuscitation bag ◆ prescribed drug ◆ syringe or adapter ◆ sterile water or normal saline solution.

Administering endotracheal drugs

In an emergency, some drugs may be given through an endotracheal (ET) tube if I.V. access isn't available. They may be given using the syringe method or the adapter method.

Before injecting any drug, check for proper placement of the ET tube, using an end-tidal carbon dioxide detector or an esophageal detection device. Make sure that the patient is supine and that her head is level with or slightly higher than her trunk.

Syringe method
Remove the needle before injecting medication into the ET tube. Insert the tip of the syringe into the ET tube, and inject the drug deep into the tube (as shown below).

Adapter method
An adapter for endotracheal drug administration provides a more closed system of drug delivery than the syringe method. A special adapter placed on the end of the ET tube (as shown below) allows needle insertion and drug delivery through the closed stopcock.

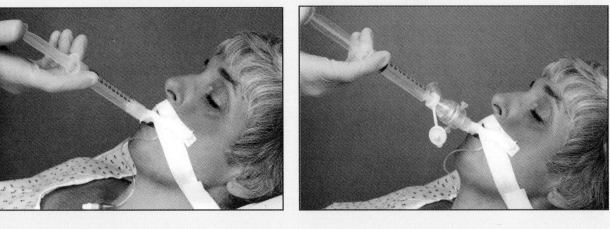

Implementation

▶ Verify the order on the patient's medication record by checking it against the practitioner's order. In an emergency, verify the practitioner's verbal order. **JC**

▶ Draw the drug up into a syringe. Dilute it in 10 ml of sterile water or normal saline solution. Dilution increases drug volume and contact with lung tissue. **AHA** **CS**

▶ Wash your hands and put on gloves. **CDC**

▶ Move the patient into the supine position, and make sure his head is level with or slightly higher than his trunk.

▶ Check ET tube placement by using an ETCO$_2$ or esophageal detection device. Ventilate the patient three to five times with the resuscitation bag. Then remove the bag. **AHA**

▶ Remove the needle from the syringe, and insert the tip of the syringe into the ET tube. Inject the drug deep into the tube.

▶ After injecting the drug, reattach the resuscitation bag, and ventilate the patient briskly. This propels the drug into the lungs, oxygenates the patient, and clears the tube.

▶ Discard the syringe in an appropriate sharps container.

▶ Remove and discard your gloves.

Special considerations

▶ Be aware that the drug's onset of action may be quicker than it would be by I.V. administration. If the patient doesn't respond quickly, the practitioner may order a repeat dose.

References

American Heart Association. "2005 Guidelines for Cardiopulmonary Resuscitation and Emergency Cardiovascular Care: Advanced Cardiac Life Support," *Circulation* 112(24 Suppl):IV-58, December 2005.

Hahnel, J.H., et al. "Plasma Lidocaine Levels and PaO$_2$ with Endobronchial Administration: Dilution with Normal Saline or Distilled Water?" *Annals of Emergency Medicine* 19(11):1314-7, November 1990. **CS**

Kockare, M., et al. "Comparison between Direct Humidification and Nebulization of the Respiratory Tract at Mechanical Ventilation: Distribution of Saline Solution Studied by Gamma Camera," *Journal of Clinical Nursing* 15(3):301-307, March 2006.

Endotracheal intubation

Endotracheal (ET) intubation involves the oral or nasal insertion of a flexible tube through the larynx into the trachea for the purposes of controlling the airway and mechanically ventilating the patient. Performed by a physician, anesthetist, respiratory therapist, or other practitioner educated in the procedure, ET intubation usually occurs in emergencies, such as cardiopulmonary arrest, or in diseases such as epiglottiditis. However, intubation may also occur under more controlled circumstances such as just before surgery. If a health care worker isn't authorized to perform ET intubation, alternative measures, such as a laryngeal mask airway or an esophageal-tracheal Combitube, may be used.

Advantages of the procedure are that it establishes and maintains a patent airway, protects against aspiration by sealing off the trachea from the digestive tract, permits removal of tracheobronchial secretions in patients who can't cough effectively, and provides a route for mechanical ventilation. Disadvantages are that it bypasses normal respiratory defenses against infection, reduces cough effectiveness, and prevents verbal communication.

Oral ET intubation is contraindicated in patients with severe airway trauma or obstruction that won't permit safe passage of an ET tube. It may also be contraindicated in cervical spine injury because the need for complete immobilization makes ET intubation difficult.

Equipment

Two ET tubes (one spare) in appropriate size ◆ 10-ml syringe ◆ stethoscope ◆ gloves ◆ lighted laryngoscope with a handle and blades of various sizes, curved and straight ◆ sedative ◆ local anesthetic spray ◆ mucosal vasoconstricting agent (for nasal intubation) ◆ overbed or other table ◆ water-soluble lubricant ◆ adhesive or other strong tape or commercial tube holder ◆ compound benzoin tincture ◆ goggles ◆ oral airway or bite block (for oral intubation) ◆ suction equipment ◆ handheld resuscitation bag with sterile swivel adapter ◆ humidified oxygen source ◆ end tidal carbon dioxide (ETCO$_2$) detector ◆ optional: prepackaged intubation tray, stylet.

Implementation

▶ Select an ET tube of the appropriate size—typically, 2.5 to 5.5 mm, uncuffed, for children and 6 to 10 mm, cuffed, for adults. The typical size of an oral tube is 7 to 8 mm for women and 8 to 9 mm for men. Select a slightly smaller tube for nasal intubation.

▶ Check the light in the laryngoscope by snapping the appropriate-sized blade into place; if the bulb doesn't light, replace the batteries or the laryngoscope (whichever is quicker).

▶ Using sterile technique, open the package containing the ET tube and, if desired, open the other supplies on an overbed table.

▶ To ease insertion, you may lubricate the first 1″ (2.5 cm) of the distal end of the ET tube with the water-soluble lubricant, using sterile technique. Use only water-soluble lubricant because it can be absorbed by mucous membranes.

▶ Attach the syringe to the port on the tube's exterior pilot cuff. Slowly inflate the cuff, observing for uniform inflation. Then use the syringe to deflate the cuff. **MFR**

▶ A stylet may be used on oral intubations to stiffen the tube. The entire stylet may be lubricated. Insert the stylet into the tube so that its distal tip lies about ½″ (1.3 cm) inside the distal end of the tube. Make sure the stylet doesn't protrude from the tube to avoid vocal cord trauma.

▶ Prepare the humidified oxygen source and the suction equipment for immediate use.

▶ If the patient is in bed, remove the headboard to provide easier access.

▶ Administer sedatives, as ordered, to induce amnesia or analgesia and help calm and relax the conscious patient. Remove dentures and bridgework, if present.

▶ Hyperventilate with 100% oxygen using a handheld resuscitation bag; continue until the tube is inserted to prevent hypoxia.

▶ Place the patient supine in the sniffing position so that his mouth, pharynx, and trachea are extended. For a blind intubation, place the patient's head and neck in a neutral position (as shown at the top of the next column).

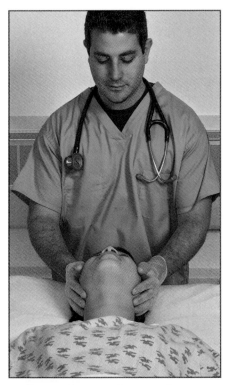

▶ Put on gloves and personal protective equipment. **CDC**

▶ For oral intubation, a local anesthetic (such as lidocaine) may be sprayed deep into the posterior pharynx to diminish the gag reflex and reduce patient discomfort. For nasal intubation, spray a local anesthetic and a mucosal vasoconstrictor into the nasal passages to anesthetize the nasal turbinates and reduce the risk of bleeding.

▶ If necessary, suction the patient's pharynx just before tube insertion to improve visualization of the patient's pharynx and vocal cords.

▶ Time each intubation attempt, limiting attempts to less than 30 seconds to prevent hypoxia. Hyperventilate the patient between attempts, if necessary.

Intubation with direct visualization

▶ Stand at the head of the patient's bed. Using your right hand, hold the patient's mouth open by crossing your index finger over your thumb, placing your thumb on the patient's upper teeth and your index finger on his lower teeth. This technique provides greater leverage.

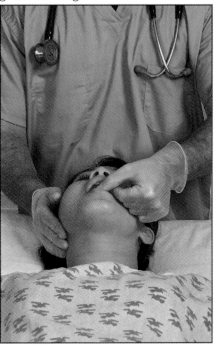

▶ Grasp the laryngoscope handle in your left hand, and gently slide the blade into the right side of the patient's mouth. Center the blade, and push the patient's tongue to the left. Hold the patient's lower lip away from his teeth.

▶ Advance the blade to expose the epiglottis.

▶ Lift the laryngoscope handle upward and away from your body at a 45-degree angle to reveal the vocal cords. Avoid pivoting the laryngoscope against the patient's teeth to avoid damaging them.

▶ If desired, have an assistant apply pressure to the cricoid ring to occlude the esophagus and minimize gastric regurgitation.

▶ Insert the ET tube into the right side of the patient's mouth.

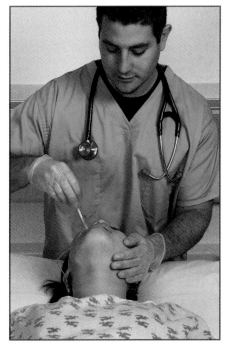

▶ Guide the tube into the vertical openings of the larynx between the vocal cords, being careful not to mistake the horizontal opening of the esophagus for the larynx. If the vocal cords are closed because of a spasm, wait a few seconds for them to relax; then gently guide the tube past them to avoid traumatic injury.

▶ Advance the tube until the cuff disappears beyond the vocal cords. Avoid advancing the tube farther to avoid occluding a major bronchus and precipitating lung collapse.

▶ Holding the ET tube in place, quickly remove the stylet, if present.

Blind nasotracheal intubation

▶ Pass the ET tube along the floor of the nasal cavity. If necessary, use gentle force to pass the tube through the nasopharynx and into the pharynx.

▶ Listen and feel for air movement through the tube as it's advanced to ensure that the tube is properly placed in the airway.

▶ Slip the tube between the vocal cords when the patient inhales because the vocal cords separate on inhalation.

▶ When the tube is past the vocal cords, breath sounds should become louder. If at any time during tube advancement breath sounds disappear, withdraw the tube until they reappear.

After intubation

▶ Remove the laryngoscope. If the patient was intubated orally, insert an oral airway or a bite block to prevent the patient from obstructing airflow or puncturing the tube with his teeth.

▶ Inflate the tube's cuff with 5 to 10 cc of air until you feel resistance. When the patient is mechanically ventilated, you'll use the minimal-leak technique or the minimal occlusive volume technique to establish correct inflation of the cuff. (For instructions, see "Tracheal cuff–pressure measurement," page 527.)

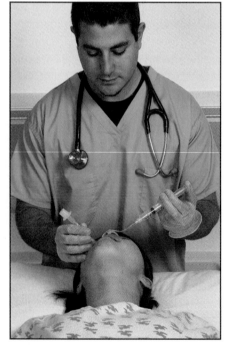

▶ Confirm ET tube placement by listening for bilateral breath sounds, observing chest expansion, and using such techniques as capnography or capnometry. **AHA**

▶ The 2005 American Heart Association guidelines recommend confirming ET tube placement using techniques other than physical examination, such as esophageal detector devices, qualitative ETCO₂ indicators, and capnographic and capnometric devices. Be aware that devices that rely on exhaled carbon dioxide may not be accurate in patients in cardiac arrest because of reduced lung perfusion and in patients with large amounts of dead space in the lungs as in a large pulmonary embolus. Other methods that complement nonphysical examination techniques include observing for bilateral chest expansion, auscultating for bilateral breath sounds or an absence of abdominal sounds, feeling for warm exhalations, and observing for condensation in the ET tube. **AHA CS1**

▶ If you don't hear breath sounds, auscultate over the stomach while ventilating with the resuscitation bag. Stomach distention, belching, or a gurgling sound indicates esophageal intubation. Immediately deflate the cuff and remove the tube. After reoxygenating the patient to prevent hypoxia, repeat insertion using a sterile tube to prevent contamination of the trachea.

▶ Auscultate bilaterally to exclude the possibility of endobronchial intubation. If you fail to hear breath sounds on both sides of the chest, you may have inserted the tube into one of the mainstem bronchi; such insertion occludes the other bronchus and lung and results in atelectasis on the obstructed side. Or, the tube may be resting on the carina, resulting in dry secretions that obstruct both bronchi. (The patient's

coughing and fighting the ventilator will alert you to the problem.) To correct these situations, deflate the cuff, withdraw the tube 1 to 2 mm, auscultate for bilateral breath sounds, and reinflate the cuff.

▶ When you've confirmed correct tube placement, administer oxygen or initiate mechanical ventilation, and suction, if indicated.

▶ To secure tube position, apply compound benzoin tincture to each cheek and let it dry. Tape the tube firmly with adhesive or other strong tape or use a commercial tube holder. (See *Methods to secure an ET tube.*)

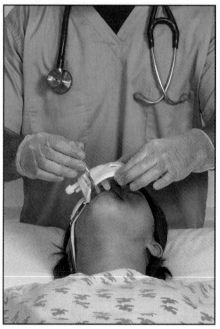

▶ Clearly note the centimeter marking on the tube where it exits the patient's mouth or nose. By periodically monitoring this mark, you can detect tube displacement. **AHA**

► Make sure a chest X-ray is taken to verify ET tube position. **AHA**

► Place a swivel adapter between the tube and the humidified oxygen source to allow for intermittent suctioning and to reduce tube tension (as shown at right).

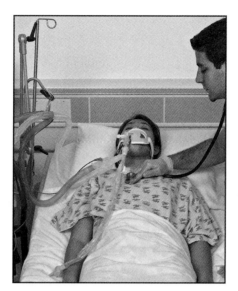

► Place the patient on his side with his head in a comfortable position to avoid tube kinking and airway obstruction.

► Provide frequent oral care to the orally intubated patient, and position the ET tube to prevent formation of pressure ulcers and avoid excessive pressure on the sides of the mouth. Provide frequent nasal and oral care to the nasally intubated patient to prevent formation of pressure ulcers and drying of oral mucous membranes. **AACN** **CDC**

► Suction secretions through the ET tube as the patient's condition indicates to clear secretions and prevent mucus plugs from obstructing the tube.

(Text continues on page 176.)

Methods to secure an ET tube

An endotracheal (ET) tube should be secured with a tracheal tube holder for either the adult or infant patient, as recommended by the American Heart Association and the American Pediatric Association. Alternatively, the tube may be taped in place to prevent dislodgment.

Before securing an ET tube, make sure the patient's face is clean, dry, and free from beard stubble. If possible, suction his mouth and dry the tube just before taping. Check the reference mark on the tube to ensure correct placement. After securing the ET tube, always check for bilateral breath sounds to ensure that it hasn't been displaced by manipulation.

To secure the ET tube, use one of the following methods.

Method 1

ET tube holders are available that help secure a tracheal tube in place. Made of hard plastic or of softer materials, the tube holder is a convenient way to secure an ET tube. The strap is placed around the patient's neck and secured around the tube with Velcro fasteners.

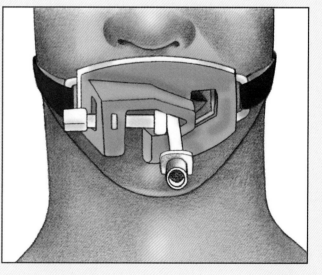

(continued)

Methods to secure an ET tube *(continued)*

Method 2

Cut two 2″ (5.1-cm) strips and two 15″ (38.1-cm) strips of 1″ cloth adhesive tape. Then cut a 13″ (33-cm) slit in one end of each 15″ strip (as shown below). (Some facilities require the tape to encircle the patient's head; check your facility's policy and procedure manual.)

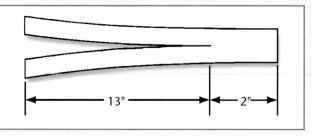

Apply compound benzoin tincture to the patient's cheeks. Place the 2″ strips on his cheeks, creating a new surface on which to anchor the tape securing the tube. If the patient's skin is excoriated or at risk, you can use a transparent semi-permeable dressing to protect the skin.

Apply the benzoin tincture to the tape on the patient's face and to the part of the tube where you'll be applying the tape. On the side of the mouth where the tube will be anchored, place the unslit end of the long tape on top of the tape on the patient's cheek.

Wrap the top half of the tape around the tube twice, pulling the tape tightly around the tube. Then, directing the tape over the patient's upper lip, place the end of the tape on his other cheek. Cut off excess tape. Use the lower half of the tape to secure an oral airway, if necessary (as shown below).

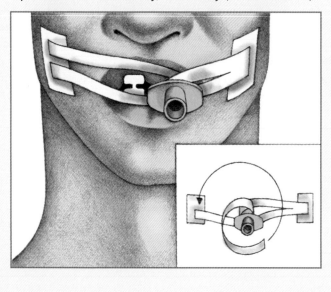

Or, twist the lower half of the tape around the tube twice, and attach it to the original cheek (as shown below). Taping in opposite directions places equal traction on the tube.

If you've taped in an oral airway or are concerned about the tube's stability, apply the other 15″ strip of tape in the same manner, starting on the other side of the patient's face (as shown below). If the tape around the tube is too bulky, use only the upper part of the tape and cut off the lower part. If the patient has copious oral secretions, seal the tape by cutting a 1″ (2.5 cm) piece of paper tape, coating it with benzoin tincture, and placing the paper tape over the adhesive tape.

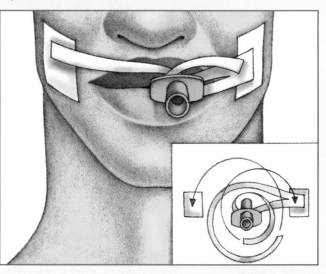

Method 3

Cut one piece of 1" cloth adhesive tape long enough to wrap around the patient's head and overlap in front. Then cut an 8" (20.3-cm) piece of tape and center it on the longer piece, sticky sides together. Next, cut a 5" (12.7-cm) slit in each end of the longer tape (as shown below).

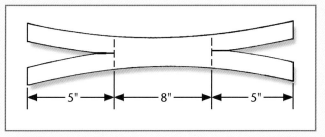

Apply benzoin tincture to the patient's cheeks, under his nose, and under his lower lip. Don't spray benzoin directly on his face because the vapors can be irritating if inhaled and can also harm the eyes.

Place the top half of one end of the tape under the patient's nose, and wrap the lower half around the ET tube. Place the lower half of the other end of the tape along his lower lip, and wrap the top half around the tube (as shown below).

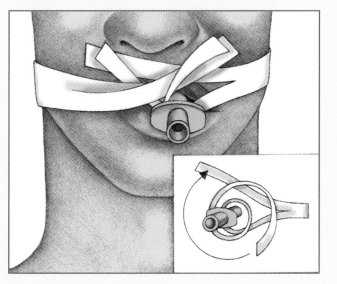

Method 4

Cut a tracheostomy tie in two pieces, one a few inches longer than the other, and cut two 6" (15.2-cm) pieces of 1" cloth adhesive tape. Then cut a 2" (5.1 cm) slit in one end of both pieces of tape. Fold back the other end of the tape ½" (1.3 cm) so that the sticky sides are together, and cut a small hole in it (as shown below).

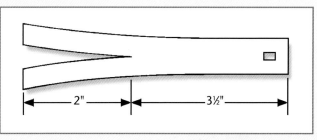

Apply benzoin tincture to the part of the ET tube that will be taped. Wrap the split ends of each piece of tape around the tube, one piece on each side. Overlap the tape to secure it.

Apply the free ends of the tape to both sides of the patient's face. Then insert tracheostomy ties through the holes in the tape and knot the ties (as shown below).

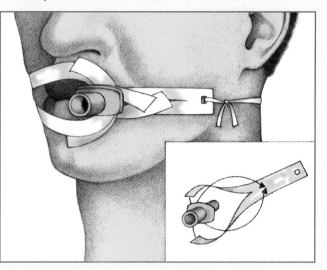

Bring the longer tie behind the patient's neck. Knotting the ties on the side prevents the patient from lying on the knot and developing a pressure ulcer.

Special considerations

▶ Always record the volume of air needed to inflate the cuff. A gradual increase in this volume indicates tracheal dilation or erosion. A sudden increase in volume indicates rupture of the cuff and requires immediate reintubation if the patient is being ventilated or if he requires continuous cuff inflation to maintain a high concentration of delivered oxygen. When the cuff has been inflated, measure its pressure at least every 8 hours to avoid overinflation. Normal cuff pressure is about 18 mm Hg. **CS2**

References

American Heart Association. "2005 AHA Guidelines for Cardiopulmonary Resuscitation and Emergency Cardiovascular Care: International Consensus on Science," *Circulation* 112(22 Suppl):IV-1-IV-211, November 2005.

Lynn-McHale Wiegand, D.J., and Carlson, K.K., eds. *AACN Procedure Manual for Critical Care,* 5th ed. Philadelphia: W.B. Saunders Co., 2005.

Takeda, T., et al. "The Assessment of Three Methods to Verify Tracheal Tube Placement in the Emergency Setting," *Resuscitation* 56(2):153-7, February 2003. **CS1**

Vyas, D., et al. "Measurement of Tracheal Tube Cuff Pressure in Critical Care," *Anaesthesia* 57(3):275-7, March 2002. **CS2**

Weitzel, N., et al. "Blind Nasotracheal Intubation for Patients with Penetrating Neck Trauma," *Journal of Trauma* 56(5):1097-101, May 2004.

Werner, S.L., et al. "Pilot Study to Evaluate the Accuracy of Ultrasonography in Confirming Endotracheal Tube Placement," *Annals of Emergency Medicine* 49(1):75-80, January 2007.

Endotracheal tube care

The intubated patient requires meticulous care to ensure airway patency and prevent complications until he can maintain independent ventilation. Care includes frequent assessment of airway status, maintenance of proper cuff pressure to prevent tissue ischemia and necrosis, repositioning of the endotracheal (ET) tube to avoid traumatic manipulation, and constant monitoring for complications.

Equipment

For repositioning the tube: 10-ml syringe ◆ compound benzoin tincture ◆ stethoscope ◆ adhesive or hypoallergenic tape or commercial tube holder ◆ suction equipment ◆ sedative or 2% lidocaine ◆ gloves ◆ handheld resuscitation bag with mask (in case of accidental extubation).

For removing the tube: 10-ml syringe ◆ suction equipment ◆ supplemental oxygen source with mask ◆ cool-mist large-volume nebulizer ◆ handheld resuscitation bag with mask ◆ gloves ◆ equipment for reintubation.

Implementation

▶ Confirm the patient's identity using two patient identifiers according to your facility's policy. **JC**

▶ Explain the procedure to the patient even if he doesn't appear to be alert.

▶ Provide privacy, wash your hands thoroughly, and put on gloves. **CDC**

▶ Before starting any procedure involving the ET tube, make sure supplemental oxygen and a handheld resuscitation bag are available at the bedside.

Repositioning the ET tube

▶ Get help from a respiratory therapist or another nurse to prevent accidental extubation during the procedure if the patient coughs.

▶ Hyperoxygenate the patient, and then suction the patient's trachea through the ET tube to remove secretions. Then suction the patient's pharynx to remove secretions that may have accumulated above the tube cuff. This helps to prevent aspiration of secretions during cuff deflation. **AARC** **AACN** **CS1**

▶ To prevent traumatic manipulation of the tube, instruct the assisting nurse to hold it as you carefully untape the tube or unfasten the commercial tube holder. When freeing the tube, locate a landmark, such as a number on the tube, or measure the distance from the patient's mouth to the top of the tube so that you have a reference point when moving the tube. **AHA**

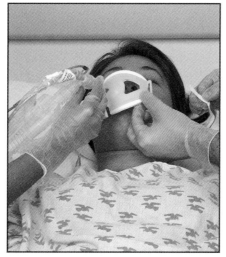

▶ Deflate the cuff by attaching a 10-ml syringe to the pilot balloon port and aspirating air until you meet resistance and the pilot balloon deflates. Deflate the cuff before moving the tube because the cuff forms a seal within the trachea and movement of an inflated cuff can damage the tracheal wall and vocal cords. **AARC**

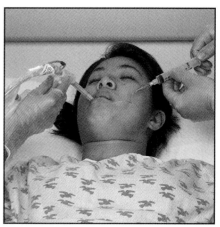

▶ Reposition the tube as necessary, noting new landmarks or measuring the length. Then immediately reinflate the cuff. To do this, instruct the patient to inhale, and slowly inflate the cuff using a 10-ml syringe attached to the pilot balloon port. As you do this, use your stethoscope to auscultate the patient's neck to determine the presence of an air leak (as shown below).

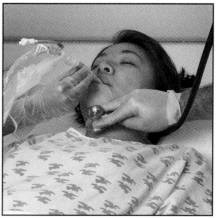

When air leakage ceases, stop cuff inflation and, while still auscultating the patient's neck, aspirate a small amount of air until you detect a slight leak. If

the patient is being mechanically ventilated, aspirate to create a minimal air
leak during the inspiratory phase of
respiration because the positive pressure of the ventilator during inspiration
will create a larger leak around the cuff.
Note the number of cubic centimeters
of air required to achieve a minimal air
leak. **AARC**

▶ Measure cuff pressure, and compare the reading with previous pressure
readings to prevent overinflation. Then
use compound benzoin tincture and
tape to secure the tube in place, or re-
fasten the commercial tube holder. **CS2**

▶ Make sure the patient is comfortable and the airway is patent. Properly
clean or dispose of equipment. **CDC**

▶ When the cuff is inflated, measure
its pressure at least every 8 hours to
avoid overinflation. (See "Tracheal cuff–
pressure measurement," page 527.) **CS2**

▶ Auscultate the lungs to ensure bilateral breath sounds.

Removing the ET tube

▶ When you're authorized to remove
the tube, obtain another nurse's assistance to prevent traumatic manipulation of the tube when it's untaped or
unfastened.

▶ Elevate the head of the patient's
bed to approximately 90 degrees.

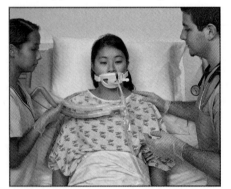

▶ Suction the patient's oropharynx
and nasopharynx. **AACN** **CDC** **AARC**

▶ Using a handheld resuscitation bag
or the mechanical ventilator, give the
patient several deep breaths through
the ET tube to hyperinflate his lungs

and increase his oxygen reserve. **AARC**
AACN **CS1**

▶ Attach a 10-ml syringe to the pilot
balloon port, and aspirate air until you
meet resistance and the pilot balloon
deflates. If you fail to detect an air leak
around the deflated cuff, notify the
practitioner immediately and don't
proceed with extubation. Absence of
an air leak may indicate marked tracheal edema, which can result in total
airway obstruction if the ET tube is removed. **AARC**

▶ If you detect the proper air leak, untape or unfasten the ET tube while the
assisting nurse stabilizes the tube.

▶ Insert a sterile suction catheter
through the ET tube. Then apply suction and ask the patient to take a deep
breath and to open his mouth fully and
pretend to cry out.

▶ Simultaneously remove the ET tube
and the suction catheter in one
smooth, outward and downward motion, following the natural curve of the
patient's mouth. Suctioning during extubation removes secretions retained at
the end of the tube and prevents aspiration.

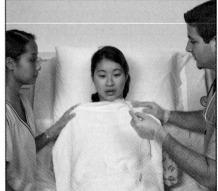

▶ Give the patient supplemental oxygen.

▶ Encourage the patient to cough and
deep-breathe. Remind him that a sore
throat and hoarseness are to be expected and will gradually subside.

▶ Make sure the patient is comfortable and the airway is patent. Clean or
dispose of equipment. **CDC**

▶ After extubation, auscultate the patient's lungs frequently and watch for
signs of respiratory distress. Be especially alert for stridor or other evidence
of upper airway obstruction. If ordered,
draw an arterial sample for blood gas
analysis. **AARC**

Special considerations

▶ When repositioning an ET tube, be
especially careful in patients with highly sensitive airways. Sedation or direct
instillation of 2% lidocaine to numb the
airway may be indicated in such patients. Because the lidocaine is absorbed systemically, you must have a
practitioner's order to use it.

▶ After extubation of a patient who
has been intubated for an extended period, keep reintubation supplies readily
available for at least 12 hours or until
you're sure he can tolerate extubation.

▶ Never extubate a patient unless
someone skilled at intubation is readily
available.

▶ If you inadvertently cut the pilot balloon on the cuff, immediately call the
person responsible for intubation in
your facility, who will remove the damaged ET tube and replace it with one
that's intact. Don't remove the tube because a tube with an air leak is better
than no airway.

References

Akca, O. "Endotracheal Tube Cuff Leak:
Can Optimum Management of Cuff
Pressure Prevent Pneumonia?" *Critical
Care Medicine* 35(6):1624-626, June
2007.

American Heart Association. "2005 AHA
Guidelines for Cardiopulmonary Resus-
citation and Emergency Cardiovascular
Care: International Consensus on Sci-
ence," *Circulation* 112(22 Suppl):IV-1-
IV-211, November 2005.

EVIDENCE-BASED RESEARCH

Decreasing ventilator-associated pneumonia

Koeman, M., et al. "Oral decontamination with chlorhexidine reduces the incidence of ventilator-associated pneumonia," *American Journal of Respiratory and Critical Care Medicine* 173(12):1348-355, June 2006.

Level II

Evidence obtained from at least one well-designed randomized controlled trial

Description

Of all infections acquired as a result of health care, ventilator-associated pneumonia (VAP) is the most frequently occurring one that causes increased sickness and death. One of the major causes of VAP is poor oral care. It has been thought that using oral decontamination with antibiotics may help decrease the incidence of VAP, but that practice isn't recommended because of the increase of antibiotic-resistant organisms. This study compared oral decontamination with chlorhexidine or chlorhexidine/colistin and if it would decrease the incidence of VAP and also

oral and endotracheal colonization. Included in the study were 385 patients who required mechanical ventilation for longer than 48 hours; they were divided into three groups: chlorhexidine, chlorhexidine/colistin, or placebo. The trial medication was applied to the buccal cavity every 6 hours. Oropharyngeal swabs were obtained daily and analyzed for the number of gram-positive and gram-negative bacteria.

Findings

Of the 385 patients, 130 received the placed, 127 chlorhexidine, and 128 chlorhexidine/colistin. The baseline characteristics of all the patients were equivalent. Both groups who received the treatment medication had a decreased daily risk of VAP compared with the group who received the placebo. Chlorhexidine/colistin provided the most significant reduction in both gram-positive and gram-negative bacteria, where chlorhexidine mostly reduced gram-positive bacteria. Chlorhexidine/colistin also decreased endo-

tracheal colonization to a greater extent than chlorhexidine alone.

Conclusions

Use of either chlorhexidine or chlorhexidine/colistin as an oral decontaminate would help decrease the patient's risk of developing VAP.

Nursing practice implications: Nurses must provide frequent oral care to ventilated patients. Both the American Association of Critical Care Nurses and the Centers for Disease Control and Prevention state that frequent and thorough oral care helps decrease the risk of VAP. The following nursing practice implications are important:

▶ Provide frequent oral care to all patients who are mechanically ventilated.
▶ Suction the patient's mouth frequently to help decrease the number of bacteria present.
▶ Suction the patient before deflating the endotracheal tube cuff.
▶ Monitor the patient's secretions for signs and symptoms of an infection.
▶ Administer antibiotics as ordered.

Birkett, K.M., et al. "Reporting Unplanned Extubation," *Intensive and Critical Care Nursing* 21(2):65-75, April 2005.

Centers for Disease Control and Prevention. "Guidelines for Preventing Healthcare–Associated Pneumonia, 2003: Recommendations of CDC and the Healthcare Infection Control Practices Advisory Committee," *MMWR* 53(RR-3):1-40, March 2004.

Chao, D.C., and Scheinhorn, D.J. "Determining the Best Threshold of Rapid Shallow Breathing Index in a Therapist-Implemented Patient-Specific Weaning Protocol," *Respiratory Care* 52(2):159-65, February 2007.

Chluay, M. "Arterial Blood Gas Changes with a Hyperinflation and Hyperoxygenation Suctioning Intervention in Critically Ill Patients," *Heart & Lung* 17(6 Pt 1):654-61, November 1988. **CS1**

"Evidence-Based Guidelines for Weaning and Discontinuing Ventilatory Support: A Collective Task Force Facilitated by the American College of Chest Physicians, the American Association for Respiratory Care, and the American College of Critical Care Medicine," *Respiratory Care* 47(1):69-90, January 2002.

Frutos-Vivar, F., et al. "Risk Factors for Extubation Failure in Patients Following a

Successful Spontaneous Breathing Trial," *Chest* 130(6):1664-671, December 2006.

Lynn-McHale Wiegand, D.J., and Carlson, K.K., eds. *AACN Procedure Manual for Critical Care,* 5th ed. Philadelphia: W.B. Saunders Co., 2005.

Vollman, K. "Oral Hygiene in the Intubated Patient," *Critical Care Nurse* 26(4):54, August 2006.

Vyas, D., et al. "Measurement of Tracheal Tube Cuff Pressure in Critical Care," *Anaesthesia* 57(3):275-7, March 2002. **CS2**

End-tidal carbon dioxide monitoring

Monitoring of end-tidal carbon dioxide ($ETCO_2$) determines the carbon dioxide (CO_2) concentration in exhaled gas. In this technique, a photodetector measures the amount of infrared light absorbed by airway gas during inspiration and expiration. (Light absorption increases along with the CO_2 concentration.) A monitor converts these data to a CO_2 value and a corresponding waveform, or capnogram, if capnography is used. (See *How $ETCO_2$ monitoring works.*)

$ETCO_2$ monitoring provides information about the patient's pulmonary, cardiac, and metabolic status, which aids patient management and helps to prevent clinical compromise. This technique has become standard during anesthesia administration and mechanical ventilation.

$ETCO_2$ monitoring may be used to help wean a patient with a stable acid-base balance from mechanical ventilation. It also reduces the need for frequent arterial blood gas (ABG) measurements, especially when combined with pulse oximetry. Other uses for $ETCO_2$ monitoring include assessing resuscitation efforts and identifying the return of spontaneous circulation. **CS** Because no CO_2 is exhaled when breathing stops, this technique also detects apnea. $ETCO_2$ monitoring can also be used during endotracheal (ET) tube placement to avert neurologic injury (and even death) by confirming correct ET tube placement and detecting accidental esophageal intubation. **AARC** **AHA**

Ongoing $ETCO_2$ monitoring throughout intubation may also prove valuable because an ET tube may become dislodged during manipulation or patient movement or transport. **AHA**

Equipment

Mainstream or sidestream CO_2 monitor ◆ CO_2 sensor ◆ airway adapter, as recommended by the manufacturer ◆ gloves ◆ $ETCO_2$ sensor.

Implementation

▶ Confirm the patient's identity using two patient identifiers according to your facility's policy. **JC**
▶ If the patient requires ET intubation, an $ETCO_2$ detector or monitor is usually applied immediately after the tube is inserted. If he doesn't require intubation or is already intubated and alert, explain the purpose and the expected duration of monitoring.
▶ Wash your hands. **CDC**
▶ After turning on the monitor and calibrating it (if necessary), position the airway adapter and sensor as the manufacturer directs. For an intubated patient, position the adapter directly on the ET tube. For a nonintubated patient, place the adapter at or near the patient's airway. (An oxygen-delivery cannula may have a sample port through which gas can be aspirated for monitoring.) **MFR**
▶ Turn on all alarms and adjust alarm settings as appropriate for your patient. Make sure the alarm volume is loud enough to hear. **JC**

Special considerations

▶ Wear gloves when handling the airway adapter to prevent cross-contamination. Make sure the adapter is changed with every breathing circuit and ET tube change. **CDC**
▶ Place the adapter on the ET tube to avoid contaminating exhaled gases with fresh gas flow from the ventilator. If you're using a heat and moisture exchanger, you may be able to position the airway adapter between the exchanger and breathing circuit.
▶ If your patient's $ETCO_2$ values differ from his partial pressure of arterial carbon dioxide ($PaCO_2$) level, assess him for factors that can influence $ETCO_2$. Such factors include decreased CO_2 production, increased CO_2 removal caused by hyperventilation, and diminished pulmonary perfusion.
▶ After the patient is started on $ETCO_2$ monitoring, obtain a sample for ABG analysis to determine baseline values. Note the difference between $ETCO_2$ and $PaCO_2$ values (a-$ADCO_2$). Typically, $ETCO_2$ levels are 1 to 6 mm Hg less than $PaCO_2$ levels. As long as a-$ADCO_2$ is normal, you can estimate the $PaCO_2$ level from the $ETCO_2$ level. Monitor a-$ADCO_2$ levels throughout therapy to determine the effectiveness of treatment and detect potential problems. If a-$ADCO_2$ increases, the patient may have reduced pulmonary perfusion.
▶ Remember that $ETCO_2$ monitoring doesn't replace ABG measurements because it doesn't assess oxygenation or blood pH. Supplementing $ETCO_2$ monitoring with pulse oximetry may provide more complete information.
▶ If the CO_2 waveform is available, assess it for height, frequency, rhythm, baseline, and shape to help evaluate

How ETCO$_2$ monitoring works

The optical portion of an end-tidal carbon dioxide (ETCO$_2$) monitor contains an infrared light source, a sample chamber, a special carbon dioxide (CO$_2$) filter, and a photodetector. The infrared light passes through the sample chamber and is absorbed in varying amounts, depending on the amount of CO$_2$ the patient has just exhaled. The photodetector measures CO$_2$ content and relays this information to the microprocessor in the monitor, which displays the CO$_2$ value and waveform.

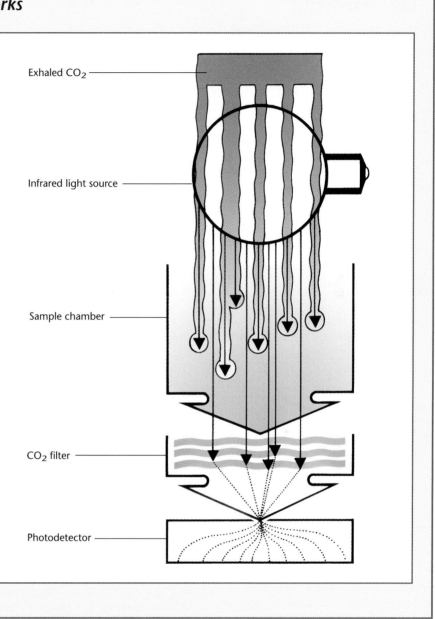

Exhaled CO$_2$

Infrared light source

Sample chamber

CO$_2$ filter

Photodetector

gas exchange. Make sure you know how to recognize a normal waveform and can identify abnormal waveforms and their possible causes. If a printer is available, record and document abnormal waveforms in the patient's medical record. (See *CO$_2$ waveform,* page 182.)

▶ In a nonintubated patient, ETCO$_2$ values may be used to establish trends. Be aware that in a nonintubated pa-

tient, exhaled gas is more likely to mix with ambient air, and exhaled CO$_2$ may be diluted by fresh gas flow from the nasal cannula.

▶ ETCO$_2$ monitoring is usually discontinued when the patient has been weaned effectively from mechanical ventilation or when he's no longer at risk for respiratory compromise. Carefully assess your patient's tolerance for weaning.

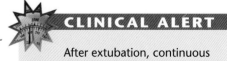

CLINICAL ALERT

After extubation, continuous ETCO$_2$ monitoring may detect the need for reintubation.

CO₂ waveform

The carbon dioxide (CO_2) waveform, or capnogram, produced in end-tidal carbon dioxide ($ETCO_2$) monitoring reflects the course of CO_2 elimination during exhalation. A normal capnogram (shown below) consists of several segments that reflect the various stages of exhalation and inhalation.

Normally, any gas eliminated from the airway during early exhalation is dead-space gas, which hasn't undergone exchange at the alveolocapillary membrane. Measurements taken during this period contain no CO_2. As exhalation continues, CO_2 concentration rises sharply and rapidly. The sensor now detects gas that has undergone exchange, producing measurable quantities of CO_2.

The final stages of alveolar emptying occur during late exhalation. During the alveolar plateau phase, CO_2 concentration rises more gradually because alveolar emptying is more constant.

The point at which the $ETCO_2$ value is derived is at the end of exhalation, when CO_2 concentration peaks. Unless an alveolar plateau is present, this value doesn't accurately estimate alveolar CO_2. During inhalation, the CO_2 concentration declines sharply to zero.

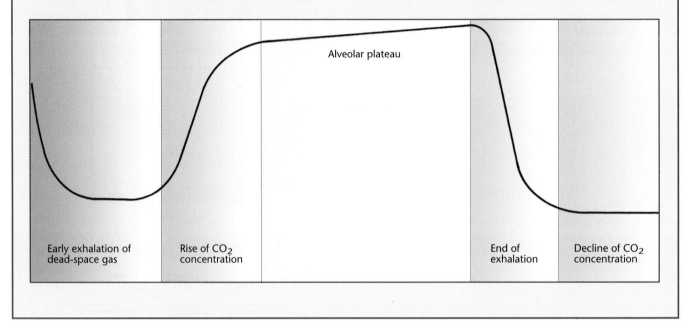

Alveolar plateau

Early exhalation of dead-space gas

Rise of CO_2 concentration

End of exhalation

Decline of CO_2 concentration

▶ Disposable $ETCO_2$ detectors are available. When using a disposable $ETCO_2$ detector, always check its color under fluorescent or natural light because the dome looks pink under incandescent light.

▶ Be aware that the effects of manual resuscitation or ingestion of alcohol or carbonated beverages can alter the detector's findings. Color changes detected after fewer than six ventilations can be misleading. **AHA**

References

Ahrens, T., et al. "End-Tidal Carbon Dioxide Measurements as a Prognostic Indicator of Outcome of Cardiac Arrest," *American Journal of Critical Care* 10(6):391-98, November 2001. **CS**

American Association for Respiratory Care. "AARC Clinical Practice Guidelines: Capnography/Capnometry during Mechanical Ventilation," *Respiratory Care* 48(5):1321-324, May 2003.

Bair, A.E., et al. "Intubation Confirmation Techniques Associated with Unrecognized Non-tracheal Intubations by Prehospital Procedures," *Journal of Emergency Medicine* 28(4):403-407, May 2005.

Lynn-McHale Wiegand, D.J., and Carlson, K.K., eds. *AACN Procedure Manual for Critical Care,* 5th ed. Philadelphia: W.B. Saunders Co., 2006.

Zwerneman, K. "End-tidal Carbon Dioxide Monitoring: A VITAL Sign Worth Watching," *Critical Care Nursing Clinics of North America* 18(2):217-25, June 2006.

Enema administration

Enema administration involves instilling a solution into the rectum and colon. In a retention enema, the patient holds the solution within the rectum or colon for 30 minutes to 1 hour. In a cleansing enema, the patient expels the solution almost completely within 15 minutes. Both types of enema stimulate peristalsis by mechanically distending the colon and stimulating rectal wall nerves.

Enemas are used to clean the lower bowel in preparation for diagnostic or surgical procedures, to relieve distention and promote expulsion of flatus, to lubricate the rectum and colon, and to soften hardened stool for removal. They're contraindicated, however, after recent colon or rectal surgery or myocardial infarction and in a patient with an acute abdominal condition of unknown origin such as suspected appendicitis. Enemas should be administered cautiously to a patient with an arrhythmia.

Equipment

Prescribed solution ◆ bath (utility) thermometer ◆ enema administration bag with attached rectal tube and clamp ◆ I.V. pole ◆ gloves ◆ linen-saver pads ◆ bath blanket ◆ two bedpans with covers, or bedside commode ◆ water-soluble lubricant ◆ toilet tissue ◆ stethoscope ◆ plastic bag for equipment ◆ water ◆ gown ◆ washcloth ◆ soap and water ◆ if observing enteric precautions: plastic trash bags, labels ◆ optional (for patients who can't retain the solution): plastic rectal tube guard, indwelling urinary catheter or rectal catheter with 30-ml balloon and syringe.

Prepackaged disposable enema sets are available, as are small-volume enema solutions in both irrigating and retention types and in pediatric sizes.

Implementation

▶ Prepare the prescribed type and amount of solution, as indicated. The standard volume of an irrigating enema is 750 to 1,000 ml for an adult.

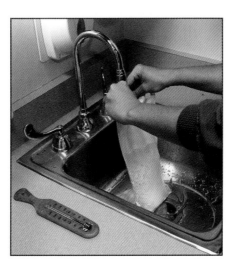

AGE FACTOR

Standard irrigating enema volumes for pediatric patients are 500 to 750 ml for a school-age child, 250 to 500 ml for a toddler or preschooler, and 250 ml or less for an infant.

▶ Warm the solution to reduce patient discomfort. Administer an adult's enema at 105° to 110° F (40.6° to 43.3° C).

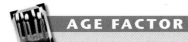

AGE FACTOR

Administer a child's enema at 100° F (37.8° C) to avoid burning rectal tissues.

▶ Clamp the tubing and fill the solution bag with the prescribed solution. Unclamp the tubing, flush the solution through the tubing, and then reclamp it. Hang the solution container on the I.V. pole and take all supplies to the patient's room. If you're using an indwelling urinary catheter or rectal catheter, fill the syringe with 30 ml of water.
▶ Confirm the patient's identity using two patient identifiers according to your facility's policy. **JC**
▶ Check the practitioner's order and assess the patient's condition. **JC**
▶ Assess the patient, paying special attention to his abdomen. Be sure to auscultate for bowel sounds; a cleansing enema will increase peristalsis.
▶ Provide privacy and explain the procedure.
▶ Ask the patient if he's had previous difficulty retaining an enema to determine whether you need to use a rectal tube guard or a catheter.
▶ Wash your hands. **CDC**
▶ Assist the patient, as necessary, in putting on a hospital gown.
▶ Assist the patient into the left-lateral Sims' position. This will facilitate the solution's flow by gravity into the descending colon. If contraindicated or if the patient reports discomfort, reposition him on his back or right side.
▶ Put on gloves. **CDC**

▶ Place linen-saver pads under the patient's buttocks to prevent soiling the linens. Replace the top bed linens with a bath blanket.

▶ Have a bedpan or commode nearby for the patient to use. If the patient may use the bathroom, make sure it will be available when the patient needs it. Have toilet tissue within the patient's reach.

▶ Lubricate the distal tip of the rectal catheter with water-soluble lubricant to facilitate rectal insertion and reduce irritation.

▶ Separate the patient's buttocks and touch the anal sphincter with the rectal tube to stimulate contraction. Then, as the sphincter relaxes, tell the patient to breathe deeply through his mouth as you gently advance the tube.

▶ Advance the tube 2″ to 4″ (5 to 10 cm), aiming it toward the umbilicus. Avoid forcing the tube to prevent rectal wall trauma. If it doesn't advance easily, allow a little solution to flow in to relax the inner sphincter enough to allow passage.

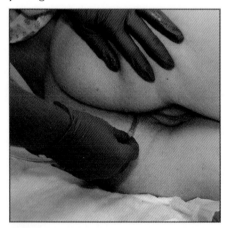

 AGE FACTOR

For a child, insert the tube only 2″ to 3″ (5 to 7.5 cm); for an infant, insert it only 1″ to 1½″ (2.5 to 4 cm).

▶ If the patient feels pain or if the tube meets continued resistance, notify the practitioner. This may signal an unknown stricture or abscess. If the patient has poor sphincter control, use a plastic rectal tube guard.

▶ You can also use an indwelling urinary catheter or a rectal catheter as a rectal tube if your facility's policy permits. Insert the lubricated catheter as you would a rectal tube. Then gently inflate the catheter's balloon with 20 to 30 ml of water. Gently pull the catheter back against the patient's internal anal sphincter to seal off the rectum. If leakage still occurs with the balloon in place, add more water to the balloon in small amounts. When using either catheter, avoid inflating the balloon above 45 ml because overinflation can compromise blood flow to the rectal tissues and may cause necrosis from pressure on the rectal mucosa.

▶ If you're using a rectal tube, hold it in place throughout the procedure because bowel contractions and the pressure of the tube against the anal sphincter can promote tube displacement.

▶ Hold the solution container slightly above bed level, and release the tubing clamp. Then raise the container gradually to start the flow—usually at a rate of 75 to 100 ml/minute for a cleansing enema, but at the slowest possible rate for a retention enema to avoid stimulating peristalsis and to promote retention. Adjust the flow rate of an irrigating enema by raising or lowering the solution container according to the patient's retention ability and comfort. However, be sure not to raise it higher than 18″ (45.7 cm) for an adult, 12″ (30.5 cm) for a child, and 6″ to 8″ (15.2 to 20.3 cm) for an infant because excessive pressure can force colon bacteria into the small intestine or rupture the colon.

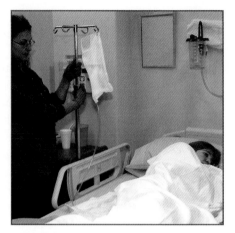

▶ Assess the patient's tolerance frequently during instillation. If he complains of discomfort, cramps, or the need to defecate, stop the flow by pinching or clamping the tubing. Then hold the patient's buttocks together, or firmly press toilet tissue against the anus. Instruct him to gently massage his abdomen and to breathe slowly and deeply through his mouth to help relax his abdominal muscles and promote retention. Resume administration at a slower flow rate after a few minutes when the discomfort passes, but interrupt the flow any time the patient complains of discomfort.

▶ If the flow slows or stops, the catheter tip may be clogged with feces or pressed against the rectal wall. Gently turn the catheter slightly to free it without stimulating defecation. If the catheter tip remains clogged, withdraw the catheter, flush it with solution, and reinsert it.

▶ After administering most of the prescribed amount of solution, clamp the tubing. Stop the flow before the container empties completely to avoid introducing air into the bowel (as shown at the top of the next column).

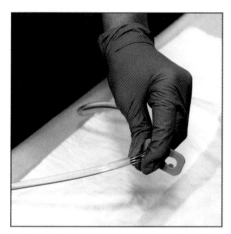

▶ For a flush enema, stop the flow by lowering the solution container below bed level and allowing gravity to siphon the enema from the colon. Continue to raise and lower the container until gas bubbles cease or the patient feels more comfortable and abdominal distention subsides. Don't allow the solution container to empty completely before lowering it because this may introduce air into the bowel.

▶ For a cleansing enema, instruct the patient to retain the solution for 15 minutes, if possible.

▶ For a retention enema, instruct the patient to avoid defecation for the prescribed time. If you're using an indwelling catheter, leave the catheter in place to promote retention.

▶ If the patient is apprehensive, position him on the bedpan and allow him to hold toilet tissue or a rolled washcloth against his anus. Place the call signal within his reach. If he will be using the bathroom or the commode, instruct him to call for help before attempting to get out of bed because the procedure may make the patient—particularly an elderly patient—feel weak or faint. Also instruct him to call you if he feels weak at any time.

▶ When the solution has remained in the colon for the recommended time or for as long as the patient can tolerate it, assist the patient onto a bedpan or to the commode or bathroom as required.

▶ If an indwelling catheter is in place, deflate the balloon and remove the catheter if applicable.

▶ Provide privacy while the patient expels the solution. Instruct the patient not to flush the toilet.

▶ While the patient uses the bathroom, remove and discard any soiled linen and linen-saver pads.

▶ Assist the patient with cleaning, if necessary, and help him to bed. Make sure he feels clean and comfortable and can easily reach the call signal. Place a clean linen-saver pad under him to absorb rectal drainage, and tell him that he may need to expel additional stool or flatus later. Encourage him to rest because the procedure may be tiring.

▶ Cover the bedpan or commode and take it to the utility room for observation, or observe the contents of the toilet, as applicable. Carefully note fecal color, consistency, amount (minimal, moderate, or generous), and foreign matter, such as blood, rectal tissue, worms, pus, mucus, or other unusual matter.

▶ Send specimens to the laboratory, if ordered.

▶ Rinse the bedpan or commode with cold water, and then wash it in hot soapy water. Return it to the patient's bedside.

▶ Properly dispose of the enema equipment. If additional enemas are scheduled, store clean, reusable equipment in a closed plastic bag in the patient's bathroom. Discard your gloves and wash your hands.

▶ Ventilate the room or use an air freshener, if necessary.

Special considerations

▶ Schedule a retention enema before meals because a full stomach may stimulate peristalsis and make retention difficult. Follow an oil-retention enema with a soap and water enema 1 hour later to help expel the softened feces completely.

▶ For the patient who can't tolerate a flat position (for example, a patient with shortness of breath), administer the enema with the head of the bed in the lowest position he can safely and comfortably maintain. For a bedridden patient who needs to expel the enema into a bedpan, raise the head of the bed to approximate a sitting or squatting position. Don't give an enema to a patient who's in a sitting position, unless absolutely necessary, because the solution won't flow high enough into the colon and will only distend the rectum and trigger rapid expulsion.

▶ If the patient has hemorrhoids, instruct him to bear down gently during tube insertion. This causes the anus to open and facilitates insertion.

▶ If the patient fails to expel the solution within 1 hour because of diminished neuromuscular response, you may need to remove the enema solution. First, review your facility's policy because you may need a practitioner's order. Inform the practitioner when a patient can't expel an enema spontaneously because of possible bowel perforation or electrolyte imbalance. To siphon the enema solution from the patient's rectum, assist him to a side-lying position on the bed. Place a bedpan on a bedside chair so that it rests below mattress level. Disconnect the tubing from the solution container, place the distal end in the bedpan, and reinsert the rectal end into the patient's anus. If gravity fails to drain the solution into the bedpan, instill 30 to 50 ml of warm water (105° F [40.6° C] for an adult; 100° F [37.8° C] for a child or infant) through the tube. Then quickly direct the distal end of the tube into the bedpan. In both cases, measure the return to make sure all of the solution has drained.

▶ In patients with fluid and electrolyte disturbances, measure the amount of expelled solution to assess for retention of enema fluid.

▶ Double-bag all enema equipment, and label it as isolation equipment if the patient is on enteric precautions.

▶ If the practitioner orders enemas until returns are clear, give no more than three to avoid excessive irritation of the rectal mucosa. Notify the practitioner if the returned fluid isn't clear after three administrations.

▶ To administer a commercially prepared, small-volume enema, first remove the cap from the rectal tube. Insert the rectal tube into the rectum and squeeze the bottle to deposit the contents in the rectum. Remove the rectal tube, replace the used enema unit in its original container, and discard it.

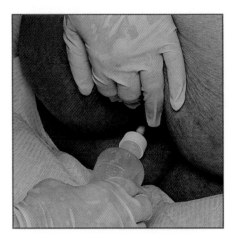

▶ Enemas may produce dizziness or faintness; excessive irritation of the colonic mucosa, resulting from repeated administration or from sensitivity to the enema's ingredients; hyponatremia or hypokalemia from repeated administration of hypotonic solutions; and cardiac arrhythmias, resulting from vasovagal reflex stimulation after insertion of the rectal catheter.

References

Fihn, J.G. "Pain and Cramping with Enema Administration," *Gastroenterology Nursing* 28(3):262, May-June 2005.

Higgins, D. "How to Administer an Enema," *Nursing Times* 102(20):24-25, May 2006.

Schmelzer, M., et al. "Safety and Effectiveness of Large-Volume Enema Solutions," *Applied Nursing Research* 17(4):265-74, November 2004.

Taylor, C., et al. *Fundamentals of Nursing: The Art and Science of Nursing Care,* 6th ed. Philadelphia: Lippincott Williams & Wilkins, 2008.

Epidural analgesics

In this procedure, the practitioner injects or infuses medication into the epidural space, which lies just outside the subarachnoid space where cerebrospinal fluid (CSF) flows. The drug diffuses slowly into the subarachnoid space of the spinal canal and then into the CSF, which carries it directly into the spinal area, bypassing the blood-brain barrier. In some cases, the medication is injected directly into the subarachnoid space.

Epidural analgesia helps manage acute and chronic pain, including moderate to severe postoperative pain. It's especially useful in patients with cancer or degenerative joint disease. Opioids, such as preservative-free morphine and fentanyl, are administered as a bolus dose or by continuous infusion, either alone or in combination with a local anesthetic. **ASA** **ASPN** Infusion through an epidural catheter is preferable because it allows a smaller drug dose to be given continuously.

The epidural catheter eliminates the risks of multiple I.M. injections, minimizes adverse cerebral and systemic effects, and eliminates the analgesic peaks and valleys that usually occur with intermittent I.M. injections. (See *Placement of a permanent epidural catheter,* page 188.)

Epidural analgesia is contraindicated in patients who have local or systemic infection, neurologic disease, coagulopathy, spinal arthritis or a spinal deformity, hypotension, marked hypertension, or in those with an allergy to the prescribed medication and who are undergoing anticoagulant therapy.

Equipment

Volume infusion device and epidural infusion tubing (depending on your facility's policy) ◆ patient's medication record and chart ◆ prescribed epidural solutions ◆ transparent dressing ◆ epidural tray ◆ labels for epidural infusion line ◆ silk tape ◆ optional: monitoring equipment for blood pressure and pulse, apnea monitor, pulse oximeter.

Have on hand the following drugs and equipment for emergency use: naloxone, 0.4 mg I.V.; ephedrine, 50 mg I.V. ◆ oxygen ◆ intubation set ◆ handheld resuscitation bag.

Implementation

▶ Prepare the infusion device according to the manufacturer's instructions and your facility's policy. Obtain an epidural tray.
▶ Make sure that the pharmacy has been notified ahead of time regarding the medication order because epidural solutions require special preparation. Check the medication concentration

and infusion rate against the practitioner's order.
▶ Label all medications and solutions on and off the sterile field. **JC**
▶ Confirm the patient's identity using two patient identifiers according to your facility's policy. **JC**
▶ Explain the procedure and its potential complications to the patient. Tell him that he'll feel some pain as the catheter is inserted. Answer any questions he has. Make sure that a consent form has been properly signed and witnessed.
▶ Position the patient on his side in the knee-chest position, or have him sit on the edge of the bed and lean over a bedside table.
▶ After the catheter is in place, prime the infusion device, confirm the appropriate medication and infusion rate, and then adjust the device for the correct rate.
▶ Help the anesthesiologist connect the infusion tubing to the epidural catheter. Then connect the tubing to the infusion pump.

▶ Bridge-tape all connection sites, and apply an EPIDURAL INFUSION label to the catheter, infusion tubing, and infusion pump to prevent accidental infusion of other drugs. Then start the infusion.
▶ Tell the patient to immediately report any pain. Instruct him to use a pain scale from 0 to 10, with 0 denoting no pain and 10 denoting the worst pain imaginable. A response of 3 or less typically indicates tolerable pain. If the patient reports a higher pain score, the infusion rate may need to be increased. Call the practitioner or change the rate within prescribed limits.
▶ If ordered, place the patient on an apnea monitor for the first 24 hours after beginning the infusion.
▶ Change the dressing over the catheter's exit site every 24 to 48 hours, as needed, or as specified by your facility's policy. The dressing is usually transparent to allow inspection of drainage and commonly appears moist or slightly blood-tinged. Don't use alcohol to clean the insertion site. Use only chlorhexidine or povidone-

Placement of a permanent epidural catheter

An epidural catheter is implanted beneath the patient's skin and inserted near the spinal cord at the L1 interspace. For temporary analgesic therapy (less than 1 week), the catheter may exit directly over the spine and be taped up the patient's back to the shoulder. For prolonged therapy, the catheter may be tunneled subcutaneously to an exit site on the patient's side or abdomen or over his shoulder.

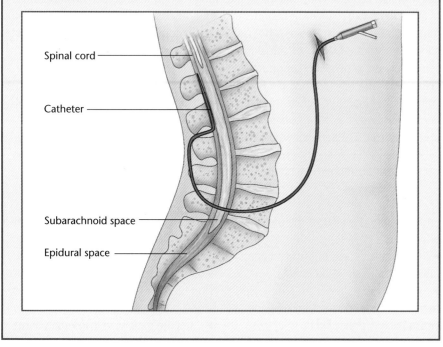

Spinal cord

Catheter

Subarachnoid space

Epidural space

iodine; alcohol may migrate into the catheter space and cause nerve destruction. **ASPMN**

▶ The epidural generally isn't sutured in place, and it's important that you don't manipulate the catheter during a dressing change.

▶ Change the infusion tubing every 48 hours or as specified by your facility's policy.

▶ Change the epidural solution every 24 hours.

Special considerations

▶ Assess the patient's respiratory rate, blood pressure, and oxygen saturation every 2 hours for 8 hours and then every 4 hours for 8 hours during the first 24 hours after starting the infusion. Then assess the patient once per shift, depending on his condition or unless ordered otherwise. Your facility may require more frequent assessments. Notify the practitioner if the patient's respiratory rate is less than 10 breaths/minute or if his systolic blood pressure is less than 90 mm Hg.

▶ Assess the patient's sedation level, mental status, and pain-relief status every hour initially and then every 2 to 4 hours until adequate pain control is achieved. Notify the practitioner if the patient appears drowsy; experiences nausea and vomiting, refractory itching, or an inability to void, which are adverse effects of certain opioid analgesics; or complains of unrelieved pain.

A change in sedation level (the patient becoming somnolent) is an early indicator of the respiratory depressant effects of the opioid.

▶ Assess the patient's lower-extremity motor strength every 2 to 4 hours. If sensorimotor loss (numbness and leg weakness) occurs, large motor nerve fibers have been affected and the dose may need to be decreased. Notify the practitioner because he may need to titrate the dosage to identify the dose that provides adequate pain control without causing excessive numbness and weakness.

▶ Keep in mind that drugs given epidurally diffuse slowly and may cause adverse effects, including excessive sedation, up to 12 hours after the infusion has been discontinued.

▶ The patient should always have a peripheral I.V. line (either continuous infusion or heparin lock) open to allow immediate administration of emergency drugs.

▶ Typically, the anesthesiologist orders analgesics and removes the catheter. However, your facility's policy may allow a specially trained nurse to remove the catheter.

▶ If you feel resistance when removing the catheter, stop and call the practitioner for further orders.

▶ Be sure to save the catheter. The practitioner will want to examine the catheter tip to rule out damage during removal.

▶ Catheter migration occurs when the epidural catheter migrates out of the epidural space toward the skin. If this occurs, the patient will have decreased pain relief and leaking at the catheter site. Notify the practitioner because the infusion needs to be stopped and the catheter removed. Contact the practitioner for further pain management orders.

References

American Society of Anesthesiologists Task Force on Acute Pain Management. "Practice Guidelines for Acute Pain Management in the Perioperative Setting: An Updated Report by the American Society of Anesthesiologists Task Force on Acute Pain Management," *Anesthesiology* 100(6):1573-581, June 2004.

Anim-Somuah, M., et al. "Epidural versus Non-epidural or No Analgesia in Labour," *Cochrane Database of Systemic Reviews* (4):CD000331, 2005.

Coyne, P.J., et al. "Effectively Starting and Titrating Intrathecal Analgesic Therapy in Patients with Refractory Cancer Pain," *Clinical Journal of Oncology Nursing* 9(5):581-83, October 2005.

DePetri, L., et al. "The Use of Intrathecal Morphine for Postoperative Pain Relief after Liver Resection: A Comparison with Epidural Analgesia," *Anesthesia and Analgesia* 102(4):1157-163, April 2006.

Mordechai, M.M., and Brull, S.J. "Spinal Anesthesia," *Current Opinion in Anaesthesiology* 18(5):527-33, October 2005.

Ng, K., et al. "Spinal versus Epidural Anaesthesia for Caesarean Section," *Cochrane Database of Systematic Reviews* (2):CD003765, 2004.

Rathmell, J.P., et al. "The Role of Intrathecal Drugs in the Treatment of Acute Pain," *Anesthesia and Analgesia* 101(Suppl 5):S30-43, November 2005.

Viscusi, E.R. "Emerging Techniques in the Management of Acute Pain: Epidural Analgesia," *Anesthesia and Analgesia* 101(Suppl 5):S23-29, November 2005.

Esophageal airway insertion and removal

Esophageal airways, such as the esophageal gastric tube airway (EGTA) and the esophageal obturator airway (EOA), are used temporarily (for up to 2 hours) to maintain ventilation in comatose patients during cardiac or respiratory arrest. These devices avoid tongue obstruction, prevent air from entering the stomach, and keep stomach contents from entering the trachea. They can be inserted only after a patent airway is established.

Although health care providers must have special training to insert an EGTA or EOA, insertion of these airways is much simpler than endotracheal intubation. One reason is that these devices don't require visualization of the trachea or hyperextension of the neck. This makes them useful for treating patients with suspected spinal cord injuries.

Because conscious and semiconscious patients will reject an esophageal airway, these airways shouldn't be used unless the patient is unconscious and not breathing. They're also contraindicated if facial trauma prevents a snug mask fit or if the patient has an absent or weak gag reflex, has recently ingested toxic chemicals, has esophageal disease, or has taken an overdose of opioids that can be reversed by naloxone.

AGE FACTOR

Because pediatric sizes aren't currently available, esophageal airways shouldn't be used in patients younger than age 16.

Equipment

Esophageal tube ◆ face mask ◆ #16 or #18 French nasogastric (NG) tube (for EGTA) ◆ syringe ◆ intermittent gastric suction equipment ◆ oral suction equipment ◆ goggles and gloves ◆ optional: handheld resuscitation bag, water-soluble lubricant.

Implementation

▶ Assess the patient's condition to determine if he's an appropriate candidate for an esophageal airway.
▶ Gather the equipment. (See *Types of esophageal airways.*)
▶ Fill the face mask with air to check for leaks. Inflate the esophageal tube's cuff with 35 cc of air to check for leaks,

and then deflate the cuff. Connect the esophageal tube to the face mask (the lower opening on an EGTA), and listen for the tube to click to determine proper placement. **MFR**
▶ Put on gloves and personal protective equipment. **CDC**
▶ Lubricate the first 1″ (2.5 cm) of the tube's distal tip with a water-soluble lubricant. With an EGTA, also lubricate the first 1″ of the NG tube's distal tip.
▶ If the patient's condition permits, place him in the supine position with his neck in a neutral or semiflexed position. Remove his dentures, if applicable.
▶ Insert your thumb deeply into the patient's mouth behind the base of his tongue. Place your index and middle fingers of the same hand under the patient's chin, and lift his jaw straight up.
▶ With your other hand, grasp the esophageal tube just below the mask in the same way you would grasp a pencil. This promotes gentle maneuvering of the tube and reduces the risk of pharyngeal trauma.

▶ Still elevating the patient's jaw with one hand, insert the tip of the esophageal tube into the patient's mouth. Gently guide the airway over the tongue into the pharynx and then into the esophagus, following the natural pharyngeal curve. No force is required for proper insertion; the tube should easily seat itself. If you encounter resistance, withdraw the tube slightly and readvance it. When the tube is fully advanced, the mask should fit snugly over the patient's mouth and nose. When this is accomplished, the cuff will lie below the level of the carina. If the cuff is above the carina, it may, when inflated, compress the posterior membranous portion of the trachea and cause tracheal obstruction.
▶ Because the tube may enter the trachea, deliver positive-pressure ventilation before inflating the cuff. Watch for the chest to rise to confirm that the tube is in the esophagus.
▶ When the tube is properly in place in the esophagus, draw 35 cc of air into the syringe, connect the syringe to the tube's cuff-inflation valve, and inflate

Types of esophageal airways

The two most commonly used types of esophageal airways are the esophageal gastric tube airway and the esophageal obturator airway. Both are described below.

Gastric tube airway

A gastric tube airway consists of an inflatable mask and an esophageal tube, as shown at right. The transparent face mask has two ports: a lower one for insertion of an esophageal tube and an upper one for ventilation, which can be maintained with a handheld resuscitation bag. The inside of the mask is soft and pliable; it molds to the patient's face and makes a tight seal, preventing air loss.

The proximal end of the esophageal tube has a one-way, nonrefluxing valve that blocks the esophagus. This valve prevents air from entering the stomach, thus reducing the risk of abdominal distention and aspiration. The distal end of the tube has an inflatable cuff that rests in the esophagus just below the tracheal bifurcation, preventing pressure on the noncartilaginous tracheal wall.

During ventilation, air is directed into the upper port in the mask and, with the esophagus blocked, enters the trachea and lungs.

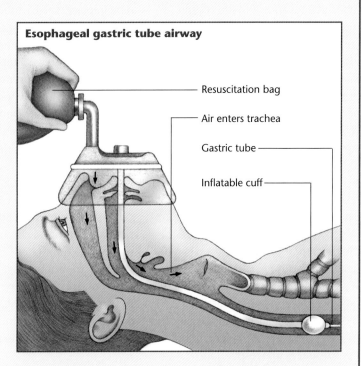

Esophageal gastric tube airway

Resuscitation bag

Air enters trachea

Gastric tube

Inflatable cuff

Obturator airway

An obturator airway consists of an adjustable, inflatable transparent face mask with a single port, attached by a snap lock to a blind esophageal tube. When properly inflated, the transparent mask prevents air from escaping through the nose and mouth, as shown at right.

The esophageal tube has 16 holes at its proximal end through which air or oxygen introduced into the port of the mask is transferred to the trachea. The tube's distal end is closed and circled by an inflatable cuff. When the cuff is inflated, it occludes the esophagus, preventing air from entering the stomach and acting as a barrier against vomitus and involuntary aspiration.

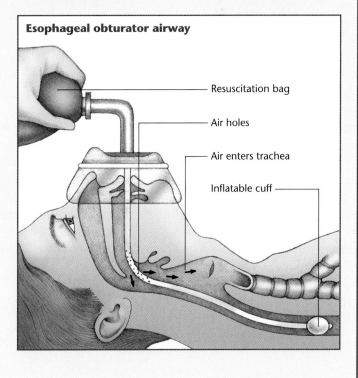

Esophageal obturator airway

Resuscitation bag

Air holes

Air enters trachea

Inflatable cuff

the cuff. Avoid overinflation because this can cause esophageal trauma.

▶ If you've inserted an EGTA, insert the NG tube through the lower port on the face mask and into the esophageal tube, and advance it to the second marking so it reaches 6″ (15.2 cm) beyond the distal end of the esophageal tube. Suction stomach contents using intermittent gastric suction to decompress the stomach. This is particularly necessary after mouth-to-mouth resuscitation, which introduces air into the stomach. Leave the tube in place during resuscitation.

▶ For both airways, attach a handheld resuscitation bag, or attach a mechanical ventilator to the face mask port (upper port) on the EGTA. Up to 100% of the fraction of inspired oxygen can be delivered this way.

▶ Monitor the patient to ensure adequate ventilation. Watch for chest movement, and suction the patient if mucus blocks the EOA tube perforations or interrupts respiration.

Removing an esophageal airway

▶ Assess the patient's condition to determine if airway removal is appropriate. The airway may be removed if respirations are spontaneous and number 16 to 20 breaths/minute. If 2 hours have elapsed since airway insertion and respirations aren't spontaneous and at the normal rate, the patient must be switched to an artificial airway that can be used for long-term ventilation such as an endotracheal (ET) tube.

▶ Detach the mask from the esophageal tube.

▶ If the patient is conscious, place him on his left side, if possible, to avoid aspiration during removal of the esoph-

ageal tube. If he's unconscious and requires an ET tube, insert it or assist with its insertion and inflate the cuff of the ET tube before removing the esophageal tube. With the esophageal tube in place, the ET tube can be guided easily into the trachea, and stomach contents are less likely to be aspirated when the esophageal tube is removed.

▶ Deflate the cuff on the esophageal tube by removing air from the inflation valve with a syringe. Don't try to remove the tube with the cuff inflated because it may perforate the esophagus.

▶ Turn the patient's head to the side, if possible, to avoid aspiration.

▶ Remove the EGTA or EOA in one swift, smooth motion, following the natural pharyngeal curve to avoid esophageal trauma.

▶ Perform oropharyngeal suctioning to remove residual secretions.

▶ Assist the practitioner, as required, in monitoring and maintaining adequate ventilation for the patient.

Special considerations

▶ To ease insertion, you may prefer to direct the airway along the right side of the patient's mouth because the esophagus is located to the right of and behind the trachea. Or you may advance the tube tip upward toward the hard palate, and then invert the tip and glide it along the tongue surface and into the pharynx. This keeps the tube centered, avoids snagging it on the sides of the throat, and eases insertion in the patient with clenched jaws.

▶ Watch the unconscious patient as he regains consciousness. Explain the procedure to him, if possible, to reduce his apprehension. Observe also for retching; if it occurs, remove the airway immediately because the accumulation of vomitus blocked by the airway cuff may perforate the esophagus.

▶ A mechanical ventilator attached to an ET tube or a tracheostomy tube maintains more exact tidal volume than a mechanical ventilator attached to an esophageal airway.

References

Abo, B.N., et al. "Does the Type of Out-of-Hospital Airway Interfere with Other Cardiopulmonary Resuscitation Tasks?" *Resuscitation* 72(2):234-39, February 2007.

American Heart Association. "2005 American Heart Association Guidelines for Cardiopulmonary Resuscitation and Emergency Cardiovascular Care," *Circulation* 112(Suppl IV):VI-19-VI-34, December 2005.

Lynn-McHale Wiegand, D.J., and Carlson, K.K., eds. *AACN Procedure Manual for Critical Care,* 5th ed. Philadelphia: W.B. Saunders Co., 2006.

Smalley, A. "The Esophageal-Tracheal Double-Lumen Airway: Rescue for the Difficult Airway," *AANA Journal* 75(2):129-34, April 2007.

Esophageal tube insertion and removal

Used to control hemorrhage from esophageal or gastric varices, an esophageal tube is inserted nasally or orally and advanced into the esophagus or stomach. The physician usually inserts and removes the tube; however, in an emergency, a nurse may remove it.

When the tube is in place, a gastric balloon secured at the end of the tube can be inflated and drawn tightly against the cardia of the stomach. The inflated balloon secures the tube and exerts pressure on the cardia. The pressure, in turn, controls bleeding varices.

Most tubes also contain an esophageal balloon to control esophageal bleeding. (See *Types of esophageal tubes*, page 194.) Usually, gastric or esophageal balloons are deflated after 24 hours. If the balloon remains inflated longer than 24 hours, pressure necrosis may develop and cause further hemorrhage or perforation.

Equipment

Esophageal tube ◆ nasogastric (NG) tube (if using a Sengstaken-Blakemore tube) ◆ two suction sources ◆ basin of ice ◆ irrigation set ◆ 2 L of normal saline solution ◆ two 60-ml syringes ◆ water-soluble lubricant ◆ $1/2''$ or $1''$ adhesive tape ◆ stethoscope ◆ foam nose guard ◆ four rubber-shod clamps (two clamps and two plastic plugs for a Minnesota tube) ◆ anesthetic spray (as ordered) ◆ traction equipment (football helmet or a basic frame with traction rope, pulleys, and a 1-lb [0.5-kg] weight) ◆ mercury aneroid manometer ◆ Y-connector tube (for Sengstaken-Blakemore or Linton tube) ◆ cup of water with straw ◆ scissors ◆ gloves ◆ gown ◆ waterproof marking pen ◆ goggles ◆ sphygmomanometer.

Implementation

▶ Keep the traction helmet at the bedside or attach traction equipment to the bed so that either is readily available after tube insertion. Place the suction machines nearby and plug them in. Open the irrigation set and fill the container with normal saline solution.

▶ Test the balloons on the esophageal tube for air leaks by inflating them and submerging them in the basin of water. If no bubbles appear in the water, the balloons are intact. Remove them from the water and deflate them. Clamp the tube lumens so that the balloons stay deflated during insertion. **MFR**

▶ To prepare the Minnesota tube, connect the mercury manometer to the gastric pressure monitoring port. Note the pressure when the balloon fills with 100, 200, 300, 400, and 500 cc of air. **MFR**

▶ Check the aspiration lumens for patency, and make sure they're labeled according to their purpose. If they aren't identified, label them carefully with the marking pen.

▶ Chill the tube in a basin of ice. This will stiffen it and facilitate insertion.

▶ Confirm the patient's identity using two patient identifiers according to your facility's policy. **JC**

▶ Explain the procedure and its purpose to the patient, and provide privacy.

▶ Wash your hands, and put on gloves, a gown, and goggles to protect yourself from splashing blood. **CDC**

▶ Assist the patient into semi-Fowler's position, and turn him slightly toward his left side. This position promotes stomach emptying and helps prevent aspiration.

▶ Explain that the physician will inspect the patient's nostrils (for patency).

▶ To determine the length of tubing needed, hold the balloon at the patient's xiphoid process and then extend the tube to the patient's ear and forward to his nose. Using a waterproof pen, mark this point on the tubing.

▶ Inform the patient that the physician will spray his throat and nostril with an anesthetic to minimize discomfort and gagging during intubation.

▶ After lubricating the tip of the tube with water-soluble lubricant, the physician will pass the tube through the more patent nostril. As he does, he'll direct the patient to tilt his chin toward his chest and to swallow when he senses the tip of the tube in the back of his throat. Swallowing helps to advance the tube into the esophagus and prevents intubation of the trachea. (If the physician introduces the tube orally, he'll direct the patient to swallow immediately.) As the patient swallows, the physician quickly advances the tube at least 10 cm beyond the previously marked point on the tube. **MFR**

Types of esophageal tubes

When working with patients who have an esophageal tube, remember the advantages of the most common types.

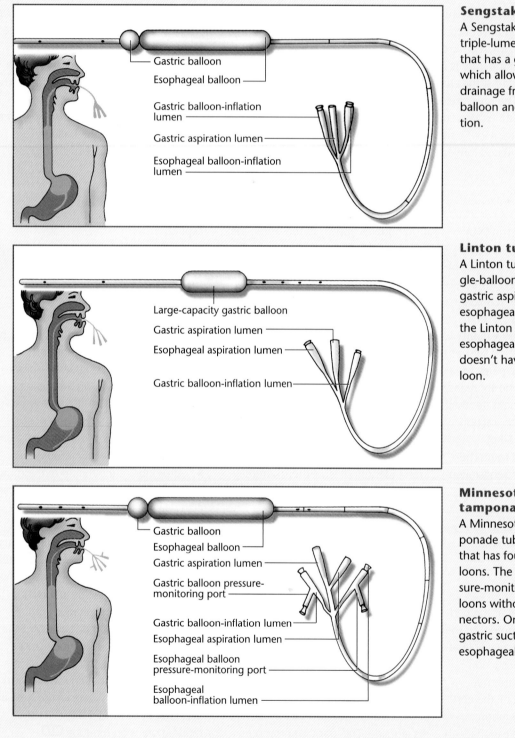

Gastric balloon
Esophageal balloon

Gastric balloon-inflation lumen
Gastric aspiration lumen
Esophageal balloon-inflation lumen

Large-capacity gastric balloon
Gastric aspiration lumen
Esophageal aspiration lumen
Gastric balloon-inflation lumen

Gastric balloon
Esophageal balloon
Gastric aspiration lumen
Gastric balloon pressure-monitoring port
Gastric balloon-inflation lumen
Esophageal aspiration lumen
Esophageal balloon pressure-monitoring port
Esophageal balloon-inflation lumen

Sengstaken-Blakemore tube
A Sengstaken-Blakemore tube is a triple-lumen, double-balloon tube that has a gastric aspiration port, which allows you to obtain drainage from below the gastric balloon and also to instill medication.

Linton tube
A Linton tube is a triple-lumen, single-balloon tube that has a port for gastric aspiration and one for esophageal aspiration. Additionally, the Linton tube reduces the risk of esophageal necrosis because it doesn't have an esophageal balloon.

Minnesota esophagogastric tamponade tube
A Minnesota esophagogastric tamponade tube is an esophageal tube that has four lumens and two balloons. The device provides pressure-monitoring ports for both balloons without the need for Y-connectors. One port is used for gastric suction, the other for esophageal suction.

Securing an esophageal tube

To reduce the risk of the gastric balloon's slipping down or away from the cardia of the stomach, secure an esophageal tube to a football helmet. Tape the tube to the face guard, as shown, and fasten the chinstrap.

To remove the tube quickly, unfasten the chinstrap and pull the helmet slightly forward. Cut the tape and the gastric balloon and esophageal balloon lumens. Be sure to hold on to the tube near the patient's nostril.

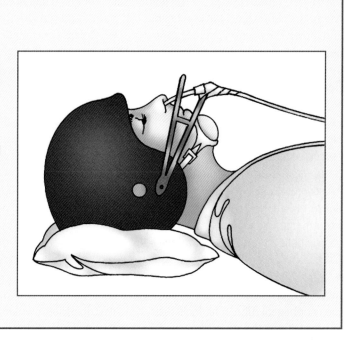

▶ To confirm tube placement, the physician will aspirate stomach contents through the gastric port. After partially inflating the gastric balloon with 50 to 100 cc of air, he'll order an X-ray of the abdomen to confirm correct placement of the balloon. Before fully inflating the balloon, he'll use the 60-ml syringe to irrigate the stomach with normal saline solution and empty the stomach as completely as possible. This helps the patient avoid regurgitating gastric contents when the balloon inflates. **CS**

▶ After confirming tube placement, the physician will fully inflate the gastric balloon (250 to 500 cc of air for a Sengstaken-Blakemore tube, 700 to 800 cc of air for a Linton tube) and clamp the tube. If he's using a Minnesota tube, he'll connect the pressure-monitoring port for the gastric balloon lumen to the mercury manometer and then inflate the balloon in 100-cc increments until it fills with up to 500 cc of air. Then he'll clamp the ports. For the Sengstaken-Blakemore or Minnesota tube, the physician will gently pull on the tube until he feels resistance, which indicates that the gastric balloon is inflated and exerting pressure on the cardia of the stomach. When he senses that the balloon is engaged, he'll place the foam nose guard around the area where the tube emerges from the nostril. **MFR**

▶ Be ready to tape the nose guard in place around the tube. This helps to minimize pressure on the nostril from the traction and decreases the risk of necrosis.

▶ With the nose guard secured, traction can be applied to the tube with a traction rope and a 1-lb weight, or the tube can be pulled gently and taped tightly to the face guard of a football helmet. (See *Securing an esophageal tube*.)

▶ With pulley-and-weight traction, lower the head of the bed to about 25 degrees to produce countertraction.

▶ Lavage the stomach through the gastric aspiration lumen with normal saline solution (iced or tepid) until the return fluid is clear. The resulting vasoconstriction stops the hemorrhage; the lavage empties the stomach. Any blood detected later in the gastric aspirate indicates that bleeding remains uncontrolled.

▶ Attach one of the suction sources to the gastric aspiration lumen. This empties the stomach, helps prevent nausea and possible vomiting, and allows continuous observation of the gastric contents for blood.

▶ If the physician inserted a Sengstaken-Blakemore or a Minnesota tube, he'll inflate the esophageal balloon as he inflates the gastric balloon to compress the esophageal varices and control bleeding.

▶ Set up esophageal suction to prevent accumulation of secretions that may cause vomiting and pulmonary aspiration. This is important because swallowed secretions can't pass into the stomach if the patient has an inflated esophageal balloon in place. If the patient has a Linton or Minnesota tube, attach the suction source to the esophageal aspiration port. If the patient has a Sengstaken-Blakemore tube, advance an NG tube through the other nostril into the esophagus to the point where the esophageal balloon begins, and attach the suction source, as ordered.

Removing the tube

▶ The physician will deflate the esophageal balloon by aspirating the air with a syringe. (He may order the esophageal balloon to be deflated at 5-mm Hg increments every 30 minutes for several hours.) Then, if bleeding doesn't recur, he'll remove the traction from the gastric tube and deflate the gastric balloon (also by aspiration). **MFR**

▶ After disconnecting all suction tubes, the physician will gently remove the esophageal tube. If he feels resistance, he'll aspirate the balloons again. (To remove a Minnesota tube, he'll grasp it near the patient's nostril and cut across all four lumens approximately 3″ [7.5 cm] below that point. This ensures deflation of all balloons.)

▶ After the tube has been removed, assist the patient with mouth care.

Special considerations

▶ If the patient appears cyanotic or if other signs of airway obstruction develop during tube placement, remove the tube immediately because it may have entered the trachea instead of the esophagus. After intubation, keep scissors taped to the head of the bed. If respiratory distress occurs, cut across all lumens while holding the tube at the nares, and remove the tube quickly.

▶ Unless contraindicated, the patient can sip water through a straw during intubation to facilitate tube advancement.

▶ Keep in mind that the intraesophageal balloon pressure varies with respirations and esophageal contractions. Baseline pressure is the important pressure.

▶ The balloon on the Linton tube should stay inflated no longer than 24 hours because necrosis of the cardia may result. Usually, the physician removes the tube only after a trial period (lasting at least 12 hours) with the esophageal balloon deflated or with the gastric balloon tension released from the cardia to check for rebleeding. In some facilities, the physician may deflate the esophageal balloon for 5 to 10 minutes every hour to temporarily relieve pressure on the esophageal mucosa.

▶ Erosion and perforation of the esophagus and gastric mucosa may result from the tension placed on these areas by the balloons during traction. Esophageal rupture may result if the gastric balloon accidentally inflates in the esophagus.

References

Greenwald, B. "The Minnesota Tube: Its Use and Care in Bleeding Esophageal and Gastric Varices," *Gastroenterology Nursing* 27(5):212-17, September-October 2004.

Greenwald, B. "Two Devices That Facilitate the Use of the Minnesota Tube," *Gastroenterology Nursing* 27(6):268-70, November-December 2004.

Lynn-McHale Wiegand, D.J., and Carlson, K.K., eds. *AACN Procedure Manual for Critical Care,* 5th ed. Philadelphia: W.B. Saunders Co., 2005.

Metheny, N., et al. "Effectiveness of pH Measurements in Predicting Feeding Tube Placement: An Update," *Nursing Research* 42(6):324-31, November-December, 1993. **CS**

Zaman, A. "Current Management of Esophageal Varices," *Current Treatment Options in Gastroenterology* 6(6):499-507, December 2003.

Esophageal tube care

Although the physician inserts an esophageal tube, the nurse cares for the patient during and after intubation. Typically, the patient is in the intensive care unit for close observation and constant care. Sedatives may be contraindicated, especially for a patient with portal systemic encephalopathy.

Most important, the patient who has an esophageal tube in place to control variceal bleeding (typically from portal hypertension) must be observed closely for esophageal rupture because varices weaken the esophagus. Additionally, possible traumatic injury from intubation or esophageal balloon inflation increases the risk of rupture. Emergency surgery is usually performed if a rupture occurs, but the operation has a low success rate.

Equipment

Manometer ◆ two 2-L bottles of normal saline solution ◆ irrigation set ◆ water-soluble lubricant ◆ several cotton-tipped applicators ◆ mouth care equipment ◆ nasopharyngeal suction apparatus ◆ several #12 French suction catheters ◆ intake and output record sheets ◆ gloves ◆ goggles ◆ sedatives ◆ traction weights or football helmet ◆ scissors.

Implementation

▶ Confirm the patient's identity using two patient identifiers according to your facility's policy. **JC**
▶ To ease the patient's anxiety, explain the care that you'll give.
▶ Provide privacy. Wash your hands and put on gloves and goggles. **CDC**
▶ Monitor the patient's vital signs every 5 minutes to 1 hour, as ordered. A change in vital signs may signal complications or recurrent bleeding.
▶ If the patient has a Sengstaken-Blakemore or Minnesota tube, check the pressure gauge on the manometer every hour to detect leaks in the esophageal balloon and to verify the set pressure.
▶ Maintain drainage and suction on gastric and esophageal aspiration ports, as ordered. This is important because fluid accumulating in the stomach may cause the patient to regurgitate the

Sengstaken-Blakemore tube

The following illustration shows a Sengstaken-Blakemore tube in a patient. When caring for a patient with an esophageal tube, be careful not to displace the tube, which may cause bleeding.

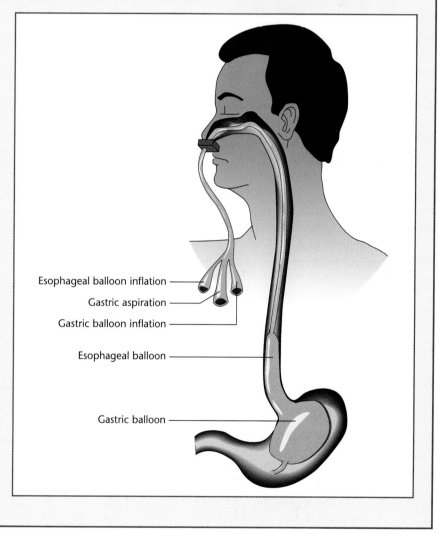

Esophageal balloon inflation

Gastric aspiration

Gastric balloon inflation

Esophageal balloon

Gastric balloon

tube, and fluid accumulating in the esophagus may lead to vomiting and aspiration.

▶ Irrigate the gastric aspiration port, as ordered, using the irrigation set and normal saline solution. Frequent irrigation keeps the tube from clogging. Obstruction in the tube can lead to regurgitation of the tube and vomiting. **MFR**

▶ To prevent pressure ulcers, clean the patient's nostrils, and apply water-soluble lubricant frequently. Use warm water to loosen crusted nasal secretions before applying the lubricant with cotton-tipped applicators. Make sure the tube isn't pressing against the nostril.

▶ Provide mouth care often to rid the patient's mouth of foul-tasting matter and to relieve dryness from mouth breathing.

▶ Use #12 French catheters to provide gentle oral suctioning, if necessary, to help remove secretions.

▶ Offer emotional support. Keep the patient as quiet as possible, and administer sedatives, if ordered and indicated.

▶ Make sure the traction weights hang from the foot of the bed at all times. Never rest them on the bed. Instruct housekeepers and other coworkers not to move the weights because reduced traction may change the position of the tube.

▶ Elevate the head of the bed about 25 degrees to ensure countertraction for the weights.

▶ Keep the patient on complete bed rest because exertion, such as coughing or straining, increases intra-abdominal pressure, which may trigger further bleeding.

▶ Keep the patient in semi-Fowler's position to reduce blood flow into the portal system and to prevent reflux into the esophagus.

▶ Monitor intake and output, as ordered.

Special considerations

▶ Observe the patient carefully for esophageal rupture indicated by signs and symptoms of shock, increased respiratory difficulties, and increased bleeding. Tape scissors to the head of the bed so you can cut the tube quickly to deflate the balloons if asphyxia develops. When performing this emergency intervention, hold the tube firmly close to the nostril before cutting.

▶ If using traction, be sure to release the tension before deflating any balloons. If weights and pulleys supply traction, remove the weights. If a football helmet supplies traction, untape the esophageal tube from the face guard before deflating the balloons. Deflating the balloon under tension triggers a rapid release of the entire tube from the nose, which may injure mucous membranes, initiate recurrent bleeding, and obstruct the airway.

▶ If the physician orders an X-ray study to check the tube's position or to view the chest, lift the patient in the direction of the pulley, and then place the X-ray film behind his back. Never roll him from side to side because pressure exerted on the tube in this way may shift the tube's position. Similarly, lift the patient to make the bed or to assist him with the bedpan.

References

Greenwald, B. "The Minnesota Tube: Its Use and Care in Bleeding Esophageal and Gastric Varices," *Gastroenterology Nursing* 27(5):212-17, September-October 2004.

Lynn-McHale Wiegand, D.J., and Carlson, K.K., eds. *AACN Procedure Manual for Critical Care,* 5th ed. Philadelphia: W.B. Saunders Co., 2005.

Vogel, S.B., et al. "Esophageal Perforation in Adults: Aggressive/Conservative Treatment Lowers Morbidity and Mortality," *Annals of Surgery* 241(6):1016-1021, June 2005.

Eye irrigation

Used mainly to flush secretions, chemicals, and foreign objects from the eye, eye irrigation also provides a way to administer medications for corneal and conjunctival disorders. In an emergency, however, tap water may serve as an irrigant. **CS**

The amount of solution needed to irrigate an eye depends on the contaminant. Secretions require a moderate volume, whereas major chemical burns require a copious amount. Usually, an I.V. bag of normal saline solution (with I.V. tubing attached) supplies enough solution for continuous irrigation of a chemical burn.

Equipment

Gloves ◆ towels ◆ eyelid retractor ◆ 60-ml sterile syringe ◆ sterile basin ◆ emesis basin ◆ optional: proparacaine topical anesthetic.

For moderate-volume irrigation: Prescribed sterile ophthalmic irrigant ◆ sterile cotton-tipped applicators.

For copious irrigation: One or more 1-L bags of normal saline solution ◆ standard I.V. infusion set without needle ◆ I.V. pole.

Implementation

▶ Read the label on the sterile ophthalmic irrigant. Double-check its sterility, strength, and expiration date.
▶ Make sure the solution is warmed to body temperature.
▶ For moderate-volume irrigation, pour the sterile irrigant into the sterile basin. Fill the syringe with 30 to 60 ml of irrigant. If you're using a commercially prepared bottle of sterile irrigant, remove the cap from the irrigant container and place the container within easy reach. Be sure to keep the tip of the container sterile.
▶ For copious irrigation, use sterile technique to set up the I.V. tubing and the bag of normal saline solution. Hang the container on an I.V. pole and adjust the drip regulator valve to ensure an adequate—but not forceful—flow.

▶ Confirm the patient's identity using two patient identifiers according to your facility's policy. **JC**
▶ Wash your hands, put on gloves, and explain the procedure to the patient. **CDC**
▶ Assist the patient into the supine position. Turn his head slightly toward the affected side to prevent solution from flowing over his nose and into the other eye.

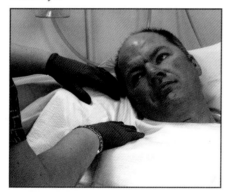

▶ Place a towel under the patient's head and let him hold the emesis basin against his affected side.

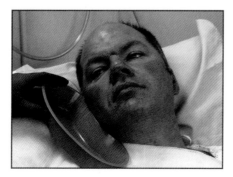

▶ Using the thumb and index finger of your nondominant hand, separate the patient's eyelids.
▶ If ordered, instill proparacaine eyedrops once as a comfort measure.
▶ To irrigate the conjunctival cul-de-sac, continue holding the eyelids apart with your thumb and index finger.

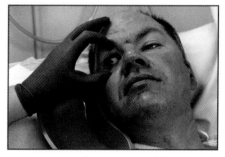

▶ To irrigate the upper eyelid, use an eyelid retractor. The retractor prevents the eyelid from closing involuntarily when solution touches the cornea and conjunctiva.

For moderate irrigation

▶ Holding the syringe about 1″ (2.5 cm) from the eye, direct a constant gentle stream at the inner canthus so that the solution flows across the cornea to the outer canthus.

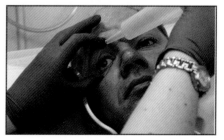

▶ Evert the lower eyelid and then the upper lid to inspect for retained foreign particles.

▶ Remove any foreign particles by gently touching the conjunctiva with sterile, wet cotton-tipped applicators. Don't touch the cornea.

▶ Resume irrigating the eye until it's clean of all visible foreign particles.

For copious irrigation

▶ Hold the control valve on the I.V. tubing about 1″ above the eye, and direct a constant, gentle stream of normal saline solution at the inner canthus. Ask the patient to rotate his eye periodically while you continue the irrigation. This action may dislodge foreign particles.

▶ Evert the lower eyelid and then the upper eyelid to inspect for retained foreign particles.

Concluding the procedure

▶ After eye irrigation, gently dry the eyelid with cotton balls or facial tissues, wiping from the inner to the outer canthus. Use a new cotton ball or tissue for each wipe.

▶ Remove and discard your gloves and wash your hands.

Special considerations

▶ When irrigating both eyes, have the patient tilt his head toward the side being irrigated to avoid cross-contamination.

▶ For chemical burns, irrigate each eye for at least 15 minutes with normal saline solution to dilute and wash the harsh chemical.

References

Ikeda, N., et al. "Alkali Burns of the Eye: Effect of Immediate Copious Irrigation with Tap Water on Their Severity," *Ophthalmologica* 220(4):225-8, September 2006. CS

Taylor, C., et al. *Fundamentals of Nursing: The Art and Science of Nursing Care,* 6th ed. Philadelphia: Lippincott Williams & Wilkins, 2008.

Eye medications

Eye medications—drops, ointments, and disks—serve diagnostic and therapeutic purposes. During an eye examination, eyedrops can be used to anesthetize the eye, dilate the pupil to facilitate examination, and stain the cornea to identify corneal abrasions, scars, and other anomalies. Eye medications can also be used to lubricate the eye, treat certain eye conditions (such as glaucoma and infections), protect the vision of neonates, and lubricate the eye socket for insertion of a prosthetic eye.

Equipment

Prescribed eye medication ◆ patient's medication record and chart ◆ gloves ◆ warm water or normal saline solution ◆ sterile gauze pads ◆ facial tissues ◆ optional: ocular dressing.

Implementation

▶ Make sure the medication is labeled for ophthalmic use. Then check the expiration date. Remember to date the container the first time you use the medication. After it's opened, an eye medication may be used for a maximum of 2 weeks to avoid contamination.

▶ Inspect ocular solutions for cloudiness, discoloration, and precipitation, but remember that some eye medications are suspensions and normally appear cloudy. Don't use any solution that appears abnormal. If the tip of an eye ointment tube has crusted, turn the tip on a sterile gauze pad to remove the crust.

▶ Verify the order on the patient's medication record by checking it against the practitioner's order on his chart. **JC**

▶ Wash your hands.

▶ Check the medication label against the patient's medication record. **ISMP**

CLINICAL ALERT

Make sure you know which eye to treat because different medications or doses may be ordered for each eye.

▶ Confirm the patient's identity using two patient identifiers according to your facility's policy. **JC**

▶ If your facility utilizes a bar code scanning system, be sure to scan your ID badge, the patient's ID bracelet, and the medication's bar code. **JC** **ISMP**

▶ Explain the procedure to the patient, and provide privacy. Put on gloves.

▶ If the patient is wearing an eye dressing, gently remove it. Take care not to contaminate your hands.

▶ Remove discharge by cleaning around the eye with sterile gauze pads moistened with warm water or normal saline solution. With the patient's eye closed, clean from the inner to the outer canthus, using a fresh sterile gauze pad for each stroke.

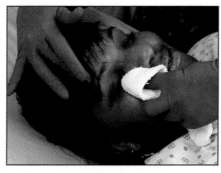

▶ To remove crusted secretions around the eye, moisten a gauze pad with warm water or normal saline solution. Ask the patient to close the eye, and then place the gauze pad over it for 1 or 2 minutes. Remove the pad, and then reapply moist sterile gauze pads, as necessary, until the secretions are soft enough to be removed without traumatizing the mucosa.

▶ Have the patient sit or lie in the supine position. Instruct her to tilt her head back and toward the side of the affected eye so that excess medication can flow away from the tear duct, minimizing systemic absorption through the nasal mucosa.

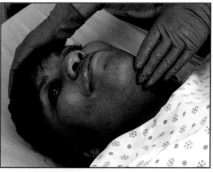

Instilling eyedrops

▶ Remove the dropper cap from the medication container, if necessary, and draw the medication into it. Be careful to avoid contaminating the dropper tip or bottle top.

▶ Before instilling the eyedrops, instruct the patient to look up and away.

▶ You can steady the hand holding the dropper by resting it against the patient's forehead. Then, with your other hand, gently pull down the lower lid of the affected eye and instill the drops in

How to insert and remove an eye medication disk

Small and flexible, an oval eye medication disk consists of three layers: two soft outer layers and a middle layer that contains the medication. Floating between the eyelids and the sclera, the disk stays in the eye while the patient sleeps and even during swimming and athletic activities. The disk frees the patient from having to remember to instill his eyedrops. When the disk is in place, ocular fluid moistens it, releasing the medication. Eye moisture or contact lenses don't adversely affect the disk. The disk can release medication for up to 1 week before needing replacement. Pilocarpine, for example, can be administered this way to treat glaucoma.

Contraindications include conjunctivitis, keratitis, retinal detachment, and any condition in which constriction of the pupil should be avoided.

To insert an eye medication disk

Arrange to insert the disk before the patient goes to bed. This minimizes the blurring that usually occurs immediately after disk insertion.

▶ Wash your hands and put on gloves.

▶ Press your fingertip against the oval disk so that it lies lengthwise across your fingertip. Lift the disk out of its packet.

▶ Gently pull the patient's lower eyelid away from the eye and place the disk in the conjunctival sac. It should lie horizontally, not vertically. The disk will adhere to the eye naturally.

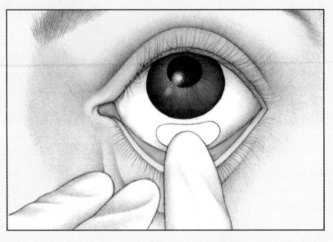

---

the conjunctival sac. Try to avoid placing the drops directly on the eyeball to prevent the patient from experiencing discomfort. If you're instilling more than one drop agent, you should wait 5 or more minutes between agents.

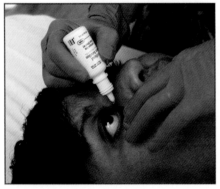

Applying eye ointment

▶ Squeeze a small ribbon of medication on the edge of the conjunctival sac from the inner to the outer canthus. Cut off the ribbon by turning the tube.

You can steady the hand holding the medication tube by bracing it against the patient's forehead or cheek. If you're applying more than one ribbon of medication, wait 10 minutes before applying the second medication.

Using a medication disk

▶ A medication disk can release medication in the eye for up to 1 week before needing to be replaced. (See *How to insert and remove an eye medication disk*.)

After instilling eyedrops or eye ointment

▶ Instruct the patient to close her eyes gently, without squeezing the lids shut. If you instilled drops, tell the patient to blink. If you applied ointment, tell the patient to roll her eyes behind closed lids to help distribute the medication over the surface of the eyeball.

▶ Use a clean tissue to remove excess solution or ointment leaking from the eye. Remember to use a fresh tissue for each eye to prevent cross-contamination.

▶ Apply a new eye dressing, if necessary. (See "Hot and cold eye compresses," page 241.)

▶ Return the medication to the storage area. Make sure you store it according to the label's instructions.

▶ Wash your hands.

Special considerations

▶ When administering an eye medication that may be absorbed systemically (such as atropine), gently press your thumb on the inner canthus for 1 to 2 minutes after instilling drops while the patient closes her eyes. This helps

▶ Pull the lower eyelid out, up, and over the disk. Tell the patient to blink several times. If the disk is still visible, pull the lower lid out and over the disk again. Caution him against rubbing his eye or moving the disk across the cornea.

▶ If the disk falls out, wash your hands, rinse the disk in cool water, and reinsert it. If the disk appears bent, replace it.

▶ If both of the patient's eyes are being treated with medication disks, replace both disks at the same time.

▶ If the disk repeatedly slips out of position, reinsert it under the upper eyelid. To do this, gently lift and evert the upper eyelid, and insert the disk in the conjunctival sac. Then gently pull the lid back into position, and tell the patient to blink several times.

▶ If the patient will continue therapy with an eye medication disk after discharge, teach him how to insert and remove it himself. To check his mastery of these skills, have him demonstrate insertion and removal for you.

To remove an eye medication disk

▶ You can remove an eye medication disk with one or two fingers. To use one finger, put on gloves and evert the lower eyelid to expose the disk. Then use the forefinger of your other hand to slide the disk onto the lid and out of the patient's eye. To use two fingers, evert the lower lid with one hand to expose the disk. Then pinch the disk with the thumb and forefinger of your other hand and remove it from the eye.

▶ If the disk is located in the upper eyelid, apply long circular strokes to the patient's closed eyelid with your finger until you can see the disk in the corner of the patient's eye. When the disk is visible, you can place your finger directly on the disk and move it to the lower sclera. Then remove it as you would a disk located in the lower eyelid.

---

prevent medication from flowing into the tear duct.

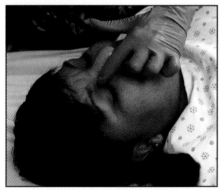

▶ To maintain the drug container's sterility, never touch the tip of the bottle or dropper to the patient's eyeball, lids, or lashes. Discard any solution remaining in the dropper before returning the dropper to the bottle. If the dropper or bottle tip has become contaminated, discard it and obtain another sterile dropper. To prevent cross-contamination, never use a container of eye medication for more than one patient.

▶ Teach the patient to instill eye medications so that treatment can continue at home, if necessary. Review the procedure and ask for a return demonstration.

▶ If ointment and drops have been ordered, the drops should be instilled first.

References

Joanna Briggs Institute. "Strategies to Reduce Medication Errors with Reference to Older Adults," *Nursing Standard* 20(41):53-57, June 2006.

The Joint Commission. *Comprehensive Accreditation Manual for Hospitals: The Official Handbook.* Standard MM.4.30. Oakbrooke Terrace, Ill.: The Joint Commission, 2007.

The Joint Commission. *Comprehensive Accreditation Manual for Hospitals: The Official Handbook.* Standard MM.5.10. Oakbrooke Terrace, Ill.: The Joint Commission, 2007.

The Joint Commission. *Comprehensive Accreditation Manual for Hospitals: The Official Handbook.* Standard MM.5.20. Oakbrooke Terrace, Ill.: The Joint Commission, 2007.

The Joint Commission. *Comprehensive Accreditation Manual for Hospitals: The Official Handbook.* Standard MM.6.20. Oakbrooke Terrace, Ill.: The Joint Commission, 2007.

McIntyre, L.J., and Courey, T.J. "Safe Medication Administration," *Journal of Nursing Care Quality* 22(1):40-42, January-March 2007.

Taylor, C., et al. *Fundamentals of Nursing: The Art and Science of Nursing Care,* 6th ed. Philadelphia: Lippincott Williams & Wilkins, 2008.

F

Fecal occult blood test

Fecal occult blood tests are valuable for determining the presence of occult blood (hidden GI bleeding) and for distinguishing true melena from melena-like stools. Certain medications, such as iron supplements and bismuth compounds, can darken stools so that they resemble melena.

Occult blood tests are particularly important for early detection of colorectal cancer because 80% of patients with this disorder test positive. However, a single positive test result doesn't necessarily confirm GI bleeding or indicate colorectal cancer. To confirm a positive result, the test must be repeated at least three times while the patient follows a special diet. Even then, a confirmed positive test may not indicate colorectal cancer. It does, however, warrant further diagnostic studies because GI bleeding can result from many causes other than cancer, such as ulcers and diverticula.

Equipment

Test kit ◆ gloves ◆ tongue blade or other wooden applicator.

Implementation

▶ Confirm the patient's identity using two patient identifiers according to your facility's policy. **JC**
▶ Explain the procedure to the patient, and check the patient's history for medications that may interfere with the test.
▶ Put on gloves and collect a stool specimen. **CDC**
▶ Open the flap on the slide package, and use a wooden applicator to apply a thin smear of the stool specimen to the guaiac-impregnated filter paper exposed in box A. Or, after performing a digital rectal examination, wipe the finger you used for the examination on a square of the filter paper.

▶ Apply a second smear from another part of the specimen to the filter paper exposed in box B.

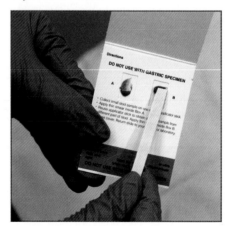

▶ Allow the specimens to dry for 3 to 5 minutes. **MFR**
▶ Open the flap on the reverse side of the slide package, and place two drops of Hemoccult developing solution on the paper over each smear. A blue reaction will appear in 30 to 60 seconds if the test is positive. **MFR**

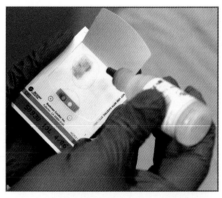

▶ Record the results, and discard the slide package.
▶ Remove and discard your gloves, and wash your hands thoroughly.

Special considerations

▶ Make sure stool specimens aren't contaminated with urine, soap solution, or toilet tissue, and test them as soon as possible after collection.
▶ Test samples from several portions of the same specimen because occult

blood isn't always evenly dispersed throughout the formed stool.

▶ Check the expiration date on the Hemoccult slides and developer, and protect the unused slides from heat, moisture, light, and chemicals.

▶ Don't collect samples during or until 3 days after a female's menstrual period to avoid a false-positive test from contamination of the specimen.

▶ Ingestion of 2 to 5 ml of blood, such as from bleeding gums or active bleeding from hemorrhoids, may produce a false positive.

▶ As ordered, have the patient discontinue the use of iron preparations, bromides, iodides, rauwolfia derivatives, indomethacin, colchicine, salicylates, potassium, phenylbutazone, bismuth compounds, steroids, and ascorbic acid for 48 to 72 hours before the test and during it to ensure accurate test results and to avoid possible bleeding, which some of these compounds may cause.

▶ If the patient will be using the Hemoccult slide package at home, advise him to complete the label on the slide package before specimen collection. Tell him that he won't have to obtain a stool specimen to perform the test but that he should follow your instructions carefully.

References

Fischbach, F. *A Manual of Laboratory and Diagnostic Tests,* 7th ed. Philadelphia: Lippincott Williams & Wilkins, 2003.

Greenwald, B. "A Comparison of Three Stool Tests for Colorectal Cancer Screening," *MedSurg Nursing* 14(5):292-99, October 2005.

Greenwald, B. "A Pilot Study Evaluating Two Alternate Methods of Stool Collection for the Fecal Occult Blood Test," *MedSurg Nursing* 15(2):89-94, April 2006.

Lastella, V.P. "Fecal Occult Blood Test," *Gastroenterology* 130(1):285, January 2006.

National Cancer Institute. "Screening for Colorectal Cancer." Available at *http://cis.nci.nih.gov/fact/5_31.htm.*

"Review Criteria for Assessment of Qualitative Fecal Occult Blood In Vitro Diagnostic Devices," U.S. Department of Health and Human Services, Food and Drug Administration, August 8, 2007.

Feeding

A patient's inability to feed herself may result from such conditions as confusion, arm or hand immobility, injury, weakness, or restrictions on activities or positions. Feeding the patient then becomes the nurse's key responsibility.

Equipment

Meal tray ♦ overbed table ♦ linen-saver pad or towels ♦ clean linens ♦ flexible straws ♦ basin of water ♦ feeding syringe ♦ assistive feeding devices, if necessary.

Implementation

▶ Allow the patient some control over mealtime, such as letting her set the pace of the meal or deciding the order in which she eats various foods.

▶ Raise the head of the bed, if allowed. Helping the patient into Fowler's or semi-Fowler's position makes swallowing easier and reduces the risk of aspiration and choking.

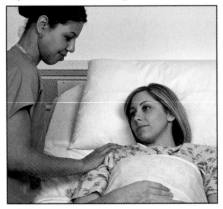

▶ Before the meal tray arrives, give the patient soap, a basin of water or a wet washcloth, and a hand towel to clean her hands. If necessary, you may wash her hands for her (as shown at the top of the next column).

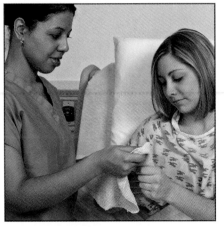

▶ Wipe the overbed table with soap and water or alcohol, especially if a urinal or bedpan was on it.

▶ When the meal tray arrives, confirm the patient's identity using two patient identifiers according to your facility's policy; make sure it matches the name on the tray. Check the tray to make sure it contains foods appropriate for the patient's condition. **JC**

▶ Encourage the patient to feed herself if she can. If she's restricted to the prone or the supine position but can use her arms and hands, encourage her to try foods she can pick up such as sandwiches. If she can assume Fowler's or semi-Fowler's position but has limited use of her arms or hands, teach her how to use assistive feeding devices. (See *Using assistive feeding devices.*)

▶ If necessary, tuck a napkin or towel under her chin to protect her gown from spills. Use a linen-saver pad or towel to protect bed linens.

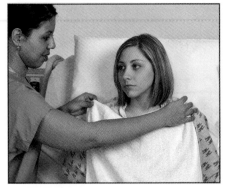

▶ Position a chair next to the patient's bed so you can sit comfortably if you need to feed her yourself.

▶ Set up the patient's tray, remove the plate from the tray warmer, and discard all plastic wrappings. Then cut the food into bite-sized pieces. Season the food according to the patient's request, as appropriate.

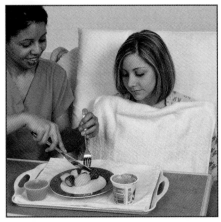

▶ To help the blind or vision-impaired patient feed herself, tell her that the placement of various foods on her plate corresponds to the hours on a

Using assistive feeding devices

Various feeding devices, available through consulting occupational therapy, can help the patient who has limited arm mobility, grasp, range of motion (ROM), or coordination. Before introducing your patient to an assistive feeding device, assess his ability to master it. Don't introduce a device he can't manage. If his condition is progressively disabling, encourage him to use the device only until his mastery of it falters.

Introduce the assistive feeding device before mealtime, with the patient seated in a natural position. Explain its purpose, show the patient how to use it, and encourage him to practice. After meals, wash the device thoroughly, and store it in the patient's bedside stand. Document the patient's progress, and share it with staff and family members to help reinforce the patient's independence. Specific devices include the following:

Plate guard

This device prevents food from spilling off the plate. Attach the guard to the side of the plate opposite the hand the patient uses to feed himself. Guiding the patient's hand, show him how to push food against the guard to secure it on the utensil. Then have him try again with food of a different consistency. When the patient tires, feed him the rest of the meal. At subsequent meals, encourage the patient to feed himself for progressively longer periods until he can feed himself an entire meal.

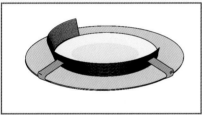

Swivel spoon

This utensil helps the patient with limited ROM in his forearm and will fit in universal cuffs.

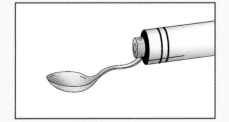

Universal cuffs

These flexible bands help the patient with flail hands or diminished grasp. Each cuff contains a slot that holds a fork or spoon. Attach the cuff to the hand the patient uses to feed himself. Then place the fork or spoon in the cuff slot. Bend the utensil to facilitate feeding.

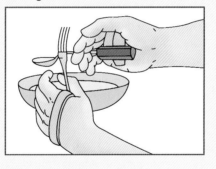

Long-handled utensils

These utensils have jointed stems to help the patient with limited ROM in his elbow and shoulder.

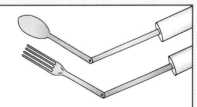

Utensils with built-up handles

These utensils (shown at the top of the next column) can help the patient with a diminished grasp. They can be purchased or can be improvised by wrapping tape around the handles.

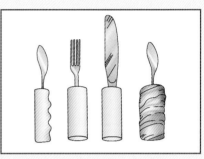

Spouted cups

These cups have a spout, which can prevent spills and burns in patients experiencing tremors or who have unsteady arms and hands.

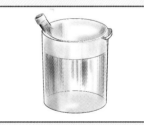

Slotted (Nosey) cups

These cups have a cut out for the nose to allow the patient to drink without bending his neck or tilting his head. Some have handles on both sides to ensure a firm grasp.

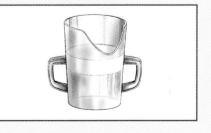

clock face. Maintain consistent placement for subsequent meals.

▶ Ask the patient which food she prefers to eat first. Some patients prefer to eat one food at a time, while others prefer to alternate foods.

▶ If the patient has difficulty swallowing, check the patient's care plan for special instructions on swallowing techniques recommended by speech therapy. Offer liquids carefully with a spoon or feeding syringe to help prevent aspiration. Pureed or soft foods, such as custard or flavored gelatin, may be easier to swallow than liquids. If the patient doesn't have difficulty swallowing, use a flexible straw to reduce the risk of spills.

▶ Ask the patient to indicate when she's ready for another mouthful. Pause between courses and whenever the patient wants to rest. During the meal, wipe the patient's mouth and chin, as needed.

▶ When the patient finishes eating, remove the tray. If necessary, clean up spills and change the bed linens. Provide mouth care.

Special considerations

▶ Don't feed the patient too quickly because this can upset her and impair digestion.

▶ If the patient is restricted to the supine position, provide foods that she can chew easily, and give liquids carefully, and only after she has swallowed her food to reduce the risk of aspiration.

▶ If the patient won't eat, try to find out the reason. For example, confirm her food preferences. Also, make sure the patient isn't in pain at mealtimes or that she hasn't received any treatments immediately before a meal that could upset or nauseate her. Find out if any medications cause anorexia, nausea, or sedation. Of course, clear the bedside of emesis basins, urinals, bedpans, and similar distractions at mealtimes.

▶ Establish a pattern for feeding the patient; share this information with the rest of the staff to maintain consistency of care.

▶ If the patient and her family are willing, suggest that family members assist with feeding. This will make the patient feel more comfortable at mealtimes and may ease discharge planning.

▶ If the patient has swallowing difficulties (such as in a stroke or head injury), consult with speech therapy before feeding to best determine the type of foods the patient requires (thickened, etc.).

References

Bownam, A., et al. "Implementation of an Evidence-Based Feeding Protocol and Aspiration Risk Reduction Algorithm," *Critical Care Nursing Quarterly* 28(4):324-33, October-December 2005.

Carlsson, E., et al. "Stroke and Eating Difficulties: Long-term Experiences," *Journal of Clinical Nursing* 13(7):824-34, October 2004.

DiBartolo, M.C. "Careful Hand Feeding: A Reasonable Alternative to PEG Tube Placement in Individuals with Dementia," *Journal of Gerontologic Nursing* 32(5):25-33, May 2006.

Hung, J.W., and Wu, Y.H. "Fitting a Bilateral Transhumeral Amputee with Utensil Prostheses and Their Functional Assessment 10 Years Later: A Case Report," *Archives of Physical Medicine and Rehabilitation* 86(11):2211-213, November 2005.

Feeding tube insertion and removal

Inserting a feeding tube nasally or orally into the stomach or duodenum allows a patient who can't or won't eat to receive nourishment. The feeding tube also permits administration of supplemental feedings to a patient who has very high nutritional requirements, such as an unconscious patient or one with extensive burns. The preferred route is nasal, but the oral route may be used for patients with such conditions as a deviated septum or a head or nose injury. Absence of bowel sounds or possible intestinal obstruction contraindicates using a feeding tube.

Equipment

For insertion: Feeding tube (#6 to #18 French, with or without guide wire) ◆ linen-saver pad ◆ gloves ◆ hypoallergenic tape ◆ water-soluble lubricant ◆ cotton-tipped applicators ◆ skin preparation (such as compound benzoin tincture) ◆ facial tissues ◆ penlight ◆ small cup of water with straw or ice chips ◆ emesis basin ◆ 60-ml syringe ◆ pH test strip.

During use: Mouthwash or normal saline solution ◆ toothbrush.

For removal: Linen-saver pad or towel ◆ bulb syringe.

Implementation

▶ Examine the tube to make sure it's free from such defects as cracks or rough or sharp edges. Next, run water through the tube to check for patency, activate the coating, and facilitate removal of the guide. **MFR**

▶ Confirm the patient's identity using two patient identifiers according to your facility's policy. **JC**

▶ Explain the procedure to the patient.

▶ Provide privacy. Wash your hands and put on gloves. **CDC**

▶ Assist the patient into semi-Fowler's or high Fowler's position. **CDC** **AACN**

▶ Place a linen-saver pad across the patient's chest.

▶ To determine the tube length needed to reach the stomach, extend the distal end of the tube from the tip of the patient's nose to her earlobe. Coil this portion of the tube around your fingers so that the end will remain curved until you insert it. Then extend the uncoiled portion from the earlobe to the xiphoid process. Use a small piece of hypoallergenic tape to mark the total length of the two portions.

Inserting the tube nasally

▶ Using the penlight, assess nasal patency. Inspect nasal passages for a deviated septum, polyps, or other obstructions. Occlude one nostril and then the other to determine which has the better airflow. Assess the patient's history of nasal injury or surgery.

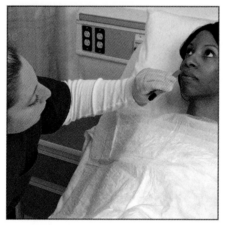

▶ Lubricate the curved tip of the tube (and the feeding tube guide, if appropriate) with a small amount of water-soluble lubricant to ease insertion and prevent tissue injury.

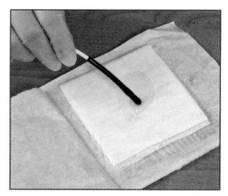

▶ Ask the patient to hold the emesis basin and facial tissues in case she needs them.

▶ Insert the curved, lubricated tip into the more patent nostril and direct it along the nasal passage toward the ear on the same side. When it passes the nasopharyngeal junction, turn the tube 180 degrees to aim it downward into the esophagus. Tell the patient to lower her chin to her chest to close the trachea. Then give her a small cup of water with a straw or ice chips. Direct her to sip the water or suck on the ice and swallow frequently. This will ease the tube's passage. Advance the tube as she swallows.

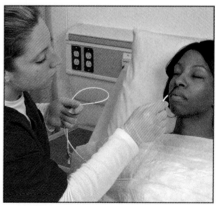

Inserting the tube orally

▶ Have the patient lower her chin to close her trachea, and ask her to open her mouth.

▶ Place the tip of the tube at the back of the patient's tongue, give water, and instruct the patient to swallow, as described above. Remind her to avoid clamping her teeth down on the tube. Advance the tube as she swallows.

Positioning the tube

▶ Keep passing the tube until the tape marking the appropriate length reaches the patient's nostril or lips. Tube placement should be confirmed by X-ray. **ASPEN**

▶ After confirming proper tube placement, remove the tape marking the tube length.

▶ Tape the tube to the patient's nose and remove the guide wire.

▶ To advance the tube to the duodenum, position the patient on her right side. This allows gravity to assist with tube passage through the pylorus. Move the tube forward 2″ to 3″ (5 to 7.5 cm) hourly until X-ray studies confirm duodenal placement. (An X-ray must confirm placement before feeding begins because duodenal feeding can cause nausea and vomiting if accidentally delivered to the stomach.)

▶ Apply a skin preparation to the patient's nose before securing the tube with tape. This helps the tube adhere to the skin and also prevents irritation.

▶ Tape the tube securely to the patient's nose.

Removing the tube

▶ Protect the patient's chest with a linen-saver pad or towel.

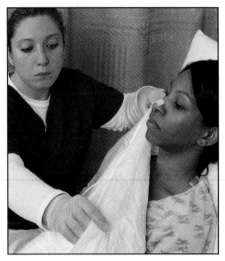

▶ Flush the tube with air, clamp or pinch it to prevent fluid aspiration during withdrawal, and withdraw it gently but quickly.

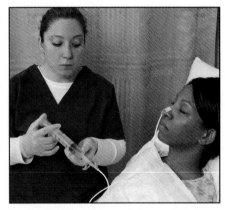

▶ Promptly cover and discard the used tube.

Special considerations

▶ Check gastric residual contents before each feeding. Feeding should be held if residual volumes are greater than 200 ml on two successive assessments. Successful aspiration also confirms correct tube placement before feeding by testing the pH of the gastric aspirate. Probability of gastric placement is increased if the aspirate has a typical gastric fluid appearance (grassy-green, clear and colorless with mucus shreds, or brown) and pH is 5.0 or less. **ASPEN** **CS**

▶ Flush the feeding tube every 4 hours with 20 to 30 ml of normal saline solution or warm water to maintain patency. Retape the tube at least daily and as needed. Alternate taping the tube toward the inner and outer side of the nose to avoid constant pressure on the same nasal area. Inspect the skin for redness and breakdown. **ASPEN**

▶ Provide nasal hygiene daily using the cotton-tipped applicators and water-soluble lubricant to remove crusted secretions. Also help the patient brush her teeth, gums, and tongue with mouthwash or saline solution at least twice daily. **CDC**

▶ Precise feeding tube placement is especially important because small-bore feeding tubes may slide into the trachea without causing immediate signs or symptoms of respiratory distress, such as coughing, choking, gasping, or cyanosis. However, the patient will usually cough if the tube enters the larynx. To be sure that the tube clears the larynx, ask the patient to speak. If she can't, the tube is in the larynx. Withdraw the tube at once and reinsert it.

▶ If you meet resistance during aspiration, stop the procedure because resistance may result simply from the tube lying against the stomach wall. If the tube coils above the stomach, you won't be able to aspirate stomach contents. To rectify this, change the patient's position or withdraw the tube a few inches, readvance it, and try to aspirate again. If the tube was inserted with a guide wire, don't use the guide wire to reposition the tube. The practitioner may do so, using fluoroscopic guidance.

References

Guenter, P., and Silkroski, M. *Tube Feeding: Practical Guidelines and Nursing Protocols.* Gaithersburg, Md.: Aspen Pubs., Inc., 2001.

Lynn-McHale Wiegand, D.J., and Carlson, K.K., eds. *AACN Procedure Manual for Critical Care,* 5th ed. Philadelphia: W.B. Saunders Co., 2005.

Metheney, N., and Titer, M. "Assessing Placement of Feeding Tubes," *AJN* 101(5):36-45, May 2001. **CS**

Metheney, N., et al. "Indicators of Tubesite During Feedings," *Journal of Neuroscience Nursing* 37(6):320-25, December 2005.

Reising, D.L., and Neal, R.S. "Enteral Tube Flushing: What You Think Are the Best Practices May Not Be," *AJN* 103(3):58-63, March 2005.

Taylor, C., et al. *Fundamentals of Nursing: The Art and Science of Nursing Care,* 6th ed. Philadelphia: Lippincott Williams & Wilkins, 2008.

Femoral compression

Femoral compression is used to maintain hemostasis at the puncture site following a procedure involving an arterial access site (such as cardiac catheterization or angiography). A femoral compression device applies direct pressure to the arterial access site. A nylon strap is placed under the patient's buttocks and is attached to the device with an inflatable plastic dome. After the dome is positioned correctly over the puncture site, it's inflated to the recommended pressure, according to the manufacturer. (See *Applying a femoral compression device*.) A physician or a specially trained nurse may apply the device.

Equipment

Femoral compression device strap ◆ compression arch with dome and three-way stopcock ◆ pressure inflation device ◆ sterile transparent dressing ◆ gloves (nonsterile and sterile) ◆ protective eyewear.

Implementation

▶ Confirm the patient's identity using two patient identifiers according to your facility's policy. **JC**
▶ Obtain a practitioner's order for the femoral compression device, including the amount of pressure to be applied and the time the device should remain in place.
▶ Explain the reason for using the device and the possible complications of the procedure. Answer any questions the patient may have.
▶ Position the patient on the stretcher or bed; don't flex the involved extremity.
▶ Assess the condition of the puncture site, obtain the patient's vital signs, perform neurovascular checks, and assess pain, according to your facility's policy for arterial access procedures.

Applying the femoral compression device

▶ Put on nonsterile gloves and protective eyewear, and place the device strap under the patient's hips before sheath removal (in cases that warrant the use of a sheath).
▶ With the assistance of another nurse, position the compression arch over the puncture site. Apply manual pressure over the dome area while the straps are secured to the arch.
▶ When the dome is properly positioned over the puncture site, connect the pressure inflation device to the stopcock that's attached to the device. Turn the stopcock to the open position, and inflate the dome with the pressure inflation device to the ordered pressure. Typically, a venous sheath is removed at 20 to 40 mm Hg and an arterial sheath is removed at 60 to 80 mm Hg. Immediately after removal of the arterial sheath, inflate the device to 10 to 20 mm Hg over the systolic blood pres-

Applying a femoral compression device

The illustration below shows the position and setup for a femoral compression device.

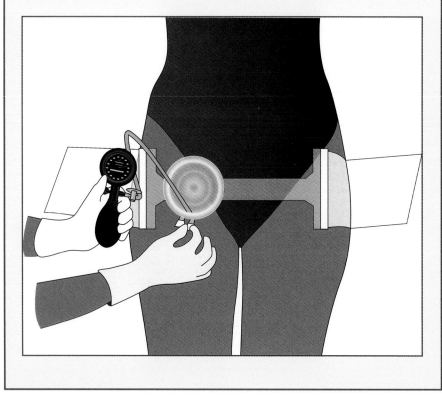

sure. After 2 to 3 minutes, a reduction in pressure, usually a value between the patient's systolic and diastolic blood pressure, is ordered. Follow specific orders for pressure changes.

▶ Assess the puncture site for proper placement of the device and for signs of bleeding or hematoma. Assess distal pulses and perform neurovascular assessments according to your facility's policy. Confirm distal pulses after any adjustments of the device.

Maintaining the device

▶ When the patient is transferred to the nursing unit, assess distal pulses, the puncture site, and placement of the device, and confirm the ordered amount of pressure.

▶ Check device placement, assess the patient's vital signs and the puncture site, and perform neurovascular checks every 2 hours or according to your facility's policy.

▶ Deflate the device hourly and assess the puncture site for bleeding or hematoma. Assess for proper placement of the dome over the puncture site. Put on gloves and protective eyewear and reposition the compression arch and dome, as necessary. Reinflate the device to the ordered pressure using the pressure inflation device.

Removing the device

▶ Explain the removal procedure to the patient.

▶ Put on nonsterile gloves and protective eyewear, and remove the air from the dome. Leave the dome in place at 0 mm Hg for at least 10 minutes, and then loosen the straps and remove the device. Assess the puncture site for bleeding or hematoma. Apply a sterile transparent dressing according to your facility's policy.

▶ Check the puncture site and distal pulses, and perform neurovascular assessments every 15 minutes for the first ½ hour and every 30 minutes for the next 2 hours. Your facility may require more frequent monitoring, however. Observe for signs of bleeding, hematoma, or infection.

▶ Dispose of the device according to your facility's policy.

Special considerations

▶ Advise the patient to use caution when moving in bed to avoid malpositioning the device. Instruct the patient not to bend the involved extremity.

▶ If you note external bleeding or signs of internal bleeding, remove the device, apply manual pressure, and notify the practitioner.

▶ Change the dressing at the puncture site every 24 to 48 hours or according to your facility's policy. (The sterile transparent dressing permits inspection of the site for bleeding, drainage, or hematoma.)

▶ The U.S. Food and Drug Administration has issued a warning to physicians about adverse events that may occur with the use of femoral compression devices following arterial access for diagnostic and therapeutic procedures. Complications include bleeding, hematoma, retroperitoneal bleeding, and pseudoaneurysm. Other potential complications may include infection and deep vein thrombosis. Tissue damage may occur if prolonged pressure is maintained.

References

Benson, L.M., et al. "Determining Best Practice: Comparison of Three Methods of Femoral Sheath Removal after Cardiac Interventional Procedures," *Heart Lung* 34(2):115-21, March-April 2005.

Chlan, L.L., et al. "Effects of Three Groin Compression Methods on Patient Discomfort, Distress, and Vascular Complications Following a Percutaneous Coronary Intervention Procedure," *Nursing Research* 54(6):391-98, November-December 2005.

Katz, S.G., and Abando, A. "The Use of Closure Devices," *Surgical Clinics of North America* 84(5):1267-280, October 2004.

U.S. Food and Drug Administration. "Complications Related to the Use of Vascular Hemostasis Devices," October 8, 1999. Available at *www.fda.gov/cdrh/safety/vashemo.html.*

Foreign body airway obstruction management

Sudden airway obstruction may occur when a foreign body lodges in the throat or bronchus; when the patient aspirates blood, mucus, or vomitus; when the tongue blocks the pharynx; or when the patient experiences traumatic injury, bronchoconstriction, or bronchospasm.

An obstructed airway causes anoxia, which in turn leads to brain damage and death in 4 to 6 minutes. The Heimlich maneuver uses an upper-abdominal thrust to create diaphragmatic pressure in the static lung below the foreign body sufficient to expel the obstruction. The Heimlich maneuver is used in conscious adult patients and in children older than age 1. However, the abdominal thrust is contraindicated in pregnant women, markedly obese patients, in patients who have recently undergone abdominal surgery, and in infants younger than age 1. For such patients, a chest thrust, which forces air out of the lungs to create an artificial cough, should be used. **AHA**

These maneuvers are contraindicated in a patient with incomplete or partial airway obstruction or when the patient can maintain adequate ventilation to dislodge the foreign body by effective coughing. However, if the patient has poor air exchange and increased breathing difficulty, a silent cough, cyanosis, or the inability to speak or breathe, immediate action to dislodge the obstruction should be taken. **AHA** (See also "Cardiopulmonary resuscitation," page 75.)

Implementation

Conscious adult with mild airway obstruction **AHA**

▶ Ask the person who's coughing or using the universal distress sign (clutching the neck between the thumb and fingers) if she's choking. If she indicates that she is but can speak and cough forcefully, she has good air exchange and should be encouraged to continue to cough. Remain with the person and monitor her.

Conscious adult with severe airway obstruction **AHA**

▶ Ask the person, "Are you choking?" If the patient nods yes and has signs of severe airway obstruction, tell her that you'll help dislodge the foreign body.
▶ Standing behind the patient, wrap your arms around her waist. Make a fist with one hand, and place the thumb side against her abdomen in the midline, slightly above the umbilicus and well below the xiphoid process.

Then grasp your fist with the other hand.

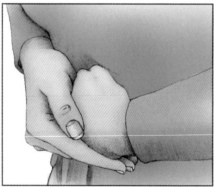

▶ Squeeze the patient's abdomen with quick inward and upward thrusts. Each thrust should be a separate and distinct movement; each should be forceful enough to create an artificial cough that will dislodge an obstruction (as shown at right).

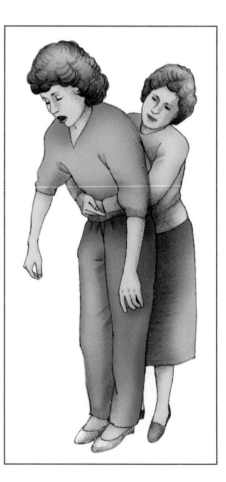

▶ Make sure you have a firm grasp on the patient because she may lose consciousness and need to be lowered to the floor. While supporting her head and neck to prevent injury, place the patient in a supine position and continue as described below.

▶ Repeat the thrusts until the foreign body is expelled or if the patient becomes unconscious. At this point, contact the emergency medical service (EMS) and follow the interventions for relieving an obstructed airway in an unconscious person.

CLINICAL ALERT

If the victim of an airway obstruction becomes unconscious, the lay rescuer should lower the patient to the ground, immediately contact the EMS, and begin cardiopulmonary resuscitation (CPR).

Unresponsive adult AHA

▶ Lower the patient to the ground and immediately contact the EMS.

▶ Begin CPR.

▶ Each time the airway is opened using a head-tilt, chin-lift maneuver, look for an object in the patient's mouth.

▶ Remove the object if present.

▶ Attempt to ventilate the patient and follow with 30 chest compressions.

CLINICAL ALERT

The blind finger-sweep is no longer recommended by the American Heart Association. A finger-sweep should only be used when a foreign body can clearly be seen in the mouth. Also, the tongue-jaw lift is no longer used. The patient's mouth should be opened using a head-tilt, chin-lift maneuver.

Obese or pregnant adult AHA

▶ If the patient is conscious, stand behind her and place your arms under her armpits and around her chest.

▶ Place the thumb side of your clenched fist against the middle of the sternum, avoiding the margins of the ribs and the xiphoid process. Grasp your fist with your other hand and perform a chest thrust with enough force to expel the foreign body. Continue until the patient expels the obstruction or loses consciousness.

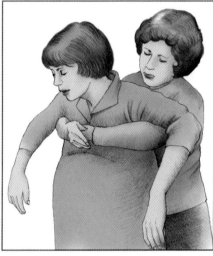

▶ If the patient loses consciousness, carefully lower her to the floor and place her in the supine position.

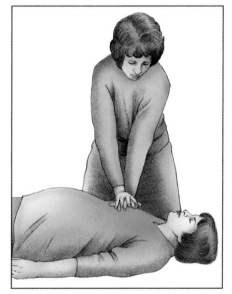

▶ Follow the same steps you would use for the unresponsive adult.

Special considerations

▶ If the patient vomits during abdominal thrusts, quickly wipe out the mouth with your fingers and resume the maneuver, as necessary.

▶ Even if your efforts to clear the airway don't seem to be effective, keep trying. As oxygen deprivation increases, smooth and skeletal muscles relax, making your maneuvers more likely to succeed.

References

American Heart Association. "2005 American Heart Association Guidelines for Cardiopulmonary Resuscitation and Emergency Cardiovascular Care," *Circulation* 112(Suppl IV):IV-19-IV-34, December 2005.

Salati, D.S. "Responding to a Foreign-Body Airway Obstruction," *Nursing* 36(12 Part 1):50-51, December 2006.

Soroudi, A., et al. "Adult Foreign Body Airway Obstruction in the Prehospital Setting," *Prehospital Emergency Care* 11(1):25-29, January-March 2007.

G

Gastric lavage

After recent poisoning or a drug overdose, especially in patients who have central nervous system depression or an inadequate gag reflex, gastric lavage flushes the stomach and removes ingested substances through a gastric lavage tube. The procedure is also used to empty the stomach in preparation for endoscopic examination. However, according to the American Academy of Clinical Toxicology, gastric lavage shouldn't be used routinely in the management of poisoned patients. Gastric lavage should be used only when the patient has ingested a *life-threatening* amount of the poison—lavage should occur within 60 minutes of ingestion. **AACT**

Gastric lavage can be continuous or intermittent. Typically, this procedure is done in the emergency department or intensive care unit by a physician, nurse, or gastroenterologist. A wide-bore lavage tube is almost always inserted by a gastroenterologist.

Gastric lavage is contraindicated after ingestion of a corrosive substance (such as lye, ammonia, or mineral acids) because the lavage tube may perforate the already compromised esophagus.

Correct lavage tube placement is essential for patient safety because accidental misplacement (in the lungs, for example) followed by lavage can be fatal. Other complications of gastric lavage include bradyarrhythmias and aspiration of gastric fluids.

Equipment

Lavage setup (two graduated containers for drainage, three pieces of large-lumen rubber tubing, Y-connector, and a clamp or hemostat) ◆ 2 to 3 L of normal saline solution or tap water, or appropriate antidote, as ordered ◆ I.V. pole ◆ basin of ice, if ordered ◆ Ewald tube or any large-lumen gastric tube, typically #36 to #40 French (see *Using wide-bore gastric tubes*) ◆ water-soluble lubricant or anesthetic ointment ◆ stethoscope ◆ 1½" hypoallergenic tape ◆ 50-ml bulb or catheter-tip syringe ◆ gloves ◆ face shield ◆ linen-saver pad or towel ◆ Yankauer or tonsil-tip suction device ◆ suction apparatus ◆ calibrated container ◆ pH strip ◆ labeled specimen container ◆ laboratory request form ◆ optional: patient restraints, charcoal tablets, norepinephrine.

Implementation

▶ Set up the lavage equipment. (See *Preparing for gastric lavage,* page 218.) If iced lavage is ordered, chill the desired irrigant (water or normal saline solution) in a basin of ice. Lubricate the end of the lavage tube with the water-soluble lubricant or anesthetic ointment.

▶ Explain the procedure to the patient, provide privacy, and wash your hands.

▶ Put on gloves and a face shield. **CDC**

▶ Drape the towel or linen-saver pad over the patient's chest.

▶ If the patient wears dentures, remove them.

▶ The physician inserts the lavage tube nasally and advances it slowly and gently because forceful insertion may injure tissues and cause epistaxis. The physician will check the placement of the tube by aspirating gastric contents and checking the pH. **CS**

▶ Because the patient may vomit when the lavage tube reaches the posterior pharynx during insertion, be prepared to suction the airway immediately with either a Yankauer or a tonsil-tip suction device.

Using wide-bore gastric tubes

If you need to deliver a large volume of fluid rapidly through a gastric tube (when irrigating the stomach of a patient with profuse gastric bleeding or poisoning, for example), a wide-bore gastric tube usually is best. Typically inserted orally, these tubes remain in place only long enough to complete the lavage and evacuate stomach contents.

Ewald tube
In an emergency, using a single-lumen tube with several openings at the distal end, such as an Ewald tube, allows you to aspirate large amounts of gastric contents quickly.

Levacuator tube
A Levacuator tube has two lumens. Use the larger lumen for evacuating gastric contents; the smaller, for instilling an irrigant.

Edlich tube
An Edlich tube is a single-lumen tube that has four openings near the closed distal tip. A funnel or syringe may be connected at the proximal end. Like the Ewald tube, the Edlich tube lets you withdraw large quantities of gastric contents quickly.

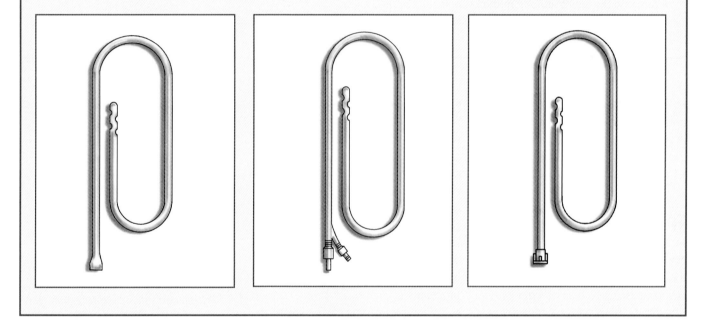

▶ When the lavage tube passes the posterior pharynx, help the patient into Trendelenburg's position and turn him toward his left side in a three-quarter prone posture.

▶ After securing the lavage tube nasally or orally and making sure the irrigant inflow tube on the lavage setup is clamped, connect the unattached end of this tube to the lavage tube. Allow the stomach contents to empty into the drainage container before instilling any irrigant. If you're using a syringe irrigation set, aspirate stomach contents with a 50-ml bulb or catheter-tip syringe before instilling the irrigant.

▶ When you confirm proper tube placement, begin gastric lavage by instilling about 250 ml of irrigant to assess the patient's tolerance and prevent vomiting. Water or normal saline solution should be used, preferably warmed to 68.4° F (20.2° C) to avoid the risk of hypothermia.

▶ Clamp the inflow tube and unclamp the outflow tube to allow the irrigant to flow out. If you're using the syringe irrigation kit, aspirate the irrigant with the syringe and empty it into a calibrated container. Measure the outflow amount to make sure it equals at least the amount of irrigant you instilled. This prevents accidental stomach distention and vomiting. If the drainage amount falls significantly short of the instilled amount, reposition the tube until sufficient solution flows out. Gently massage the abdomen over the stomach to promote outflow.

▶ Repeat the inflow-outflow cycle until returned fluids appear clear. This signals that the stomach no longer holds harmful substances or that bleeding has stopped.

Preparing for gastric lavage

Prepare the lavage setup as follows:
- Connect one of the three pieces of large-lumen tubing to the irrigant container.
- Insert the stem of the Y-connector in the other end of the tubing.
- Connect the remaining two pieces of tubing to the free ends of the Y-connector.
- Place the unattached end of one of the tubes into one of the drainage containers. (Later, you'll connect the other piece of tubing to the patient's gastric tube.)
- Clamp the tube leading to the irrigant.
- Suspend the entire setup from the I.V. pole, hanging the irrigant container at the highest level.

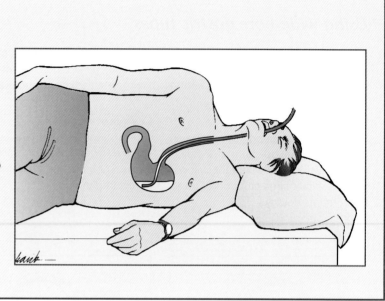

- Assess the patient's vital signs, urine output, and level of consciousness (LOC) every 15 minutes. Notify the physician of any changes.
- If ordered, remove the lavage tube.

Special considerations

- To control GI bleeding, the physician may order continuous irrigation of the stomach with an irrigant and a vasoconstrictor such as norepinephrine. Or the physician may direct you to clamp the outflow tube for a prescribed period after instilling the irrigant and the vasoconstrictive medication and before withdrawing it. This allows the mucosa time to absorb the drug.
- Never leave the patient alone during gastric lavage. Observe continuously for any changes in LOC, and monitor his vital signs frequently because the natural vagal response to intubation can depress his heart rate.

- Remember also to keep tracheal suctioning equipment nearby and watch closely for airway obstruction caused by vomiting or excess oral secretions. Throughout gastric lavage, you may need to suction the oral cavity frequently to ensure an open airway and prevent aspiration. For the same reasons, and if he doesn't exhibit an adequate gag reflex, the patient may require an endotracheal tube before the procedure.
- When performing gastric lavage to stop bleeding, keep precise intake and output records to determine the amount of bleeding. When large volumes of fluid are instilled and withdrawn, serum electrolyte and arterial blood gas levels may be measured during or at the end of lavage.

References

American Academy of Clinical Toxicology, European Association of Poison Centres and Clinical Toxicologists. "Position Paper: Gastric Lavage," *Journal of Toxicology, Clinical Toxicology* 42(7):933-43, 2004.

Heard, K. "Gastrointestinal Decontamination," *Medical Clinics of North America* 89(6):1067-1078, November 2005.

Lynn-McHale Wiegand, D.J., and Carlson, K.K., eds. *AACN Procedure Manual for Critical Care,* 5th ed. Philadelphia: W.B. Saunders Co., 2005.

Metheny, N., et al. "Effectiveness of pH Measurements in Predicting Feeding Tube Placement: An Update," *Nursing Research* 42(6):324-31, November-December 1993. CS

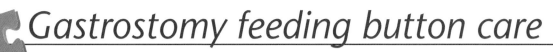

Gastrostomy feeding button care

A gastrostomy feeding button serves as an alternative feeding device for an ambulatory patient who's receiving long-term enteral feedings.

The feeding button has a mushroom dome at one end and two wing tabs and a flexible safety plug at the other. When inserted into an established stoma, the button lies almost flush with the skin, with only the top of the safety plug visible. Besides its cosmetic appeal, the device is easily maintained, reduces skin irritation and breakdown, and is less likely to become dislodged or to migrate than an ordinary feeding tube. A one-way, antireflux valve mounted just inside the mushroom dome prevents accidental leakage of gastric contents. The device should be replaced after 3 to 4 months, typically because the antireflux valve wears out.

Equipment

Gloves ◆ feeding accessories, including adapter, feeding catheter, food syringe or bag, and formula ◆ catheter clamp ◆ cleaning equipment, including water, syringe, cotton-tipped applicator, pipe cleaner, and mild soap or antiseptic solution ◆ optional: pump.

Implementation

▶ Confirm the patient's identity using two patient identifiers according to your facility's policy. **JC**
▶ Explain the insertion, reinsertion, and feeding procedure to the patient. Tell him the physician will perform the initial insertion. (See *How to reinsert a gastrostomy feeding button.*)
▶ Wash your hands and put on gloves. **CDC**
▶ Elevate the head of the bed 30 to 45 degrees.
▶ Check for residual with the syringe. If greater than 50 to 100 ml, report this to the practitioner and hold the feeding until reassessment.
▶ Attach the adapter and feeding catheter to the syringe or feeding bag. Clamp the catheter and fill the syringe or bag and catheter with formula. Refill the syringe before it's empty. These steps prevent air from entering the stomach and distending the abdomen.

How to reinsert a gastrostomy feeding button

If your patient's gastrostomy feeding button pops out (with coughing, for instance), you or he will need to reinsert the device. Here are some steps to follow.

Prepare the equipment
Collect the feeding button, an obturator, and water-soluble lubricant. If the button will be reinserted, wash it with soap and water and rinse it thoroughly.

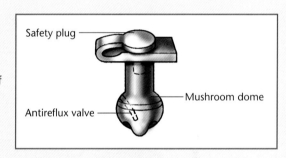

Insert the button
▶ Check the depth of the patient's stoma to make sure you have a feeding button of the correct size. Then clean around the stoma.
▶ Lubricate the obturator with a water-soluble lubricant, and distend the button several times to ensure the patency of the antireflux valve within the button.
▶ Lubricate the mushroom dome and the stoma. Gently push the button through the stoma into the stomach.

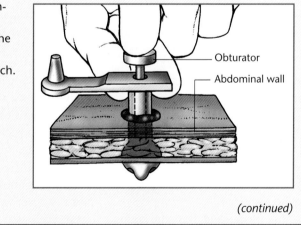

(continued)

How to reinsert a gastrostomy feeding button
(continued)

▶ Remove the obturator by gently rotating it as you withdraw it to keep the antireflux valve from adhering to it. If the valve sticks nonetheless, gently push the obturator back into the button until the valve closes.

▶ After removing the obturator, make sure the valve is closed. Then close the flexible safety plug, which should be relatively flush with the skin surface.

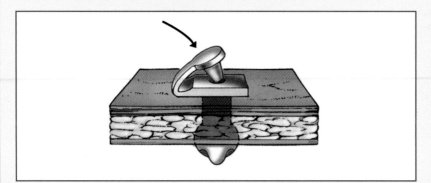

▶ If you need to administer a feeding right away, open the safety plug and attach the feeding adapter and feeding tube. Deliver the feeding, as ordered.

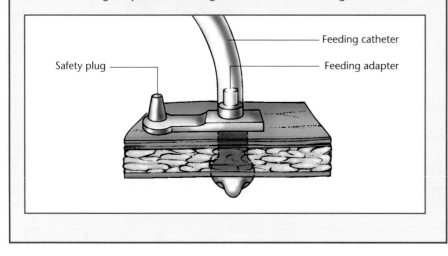

Safety plug

Feeding catheter

Feeding adapter

▶ Open the safety plug, and attach the adapter and feeding catheter to the button. Elevate the syringe or feeding bag above stomach level, and gravity-feed the formula for 15 to 30 minutes, varying the height, as needed, to alter the flow rate. Use a pump for continuous infusion or for feedings lasting several hours.

▶ After the feeding, flush the button with 10 ml of water and clean the in-side of the feeding catheter with a cotton-tipped applicator and water to preserve patency and to dislodge formula or food particles. Then, lower the syringe or bag below stomach level to allow burping. Remove the adapter and feeding catheter, and then snap the safety plug in place. If the patient feels nauseated or vomits after the feeding, vent the button with the adapter and feeding catheter to control emesis.

▶ Maintain head of bed elevation of 30 to 45 degrees for at least 1 hour after feeding.

▶ Wash the catheter and syringe or feeding bag in warm soapy water and rinse thoroughly. Clean the catheter and adapter with a pipe cleaner. Rinse well before using for the next feeding.

Special considerations

▶ If the button pops out while feeding, reinsert it, estimate the formula already delivered, and resume feeding.

▶ Once daily, clean the peristomal skin with mild soap and water or antiseptic solution, and let the skin air-dry for 20 minutes to avoid skin irritation. Also clean the site whenever spillage from the feeding bag occurs.

▶ As the patient's weight or body mass index increases, monitor the site for embedded bumper (external). Report skin irritation and increased tension between the exit site and the bumper to the practitioner.

References

"American Society for Parenteral and Enteral Nutrition Support: Hospitalized Patients," *Nutrition in Clinical Practice* 10:208-19, December 1995.

Goldberg, E., et al. "Gastrostomy Tubes: Facts, Fallacies, Fistulas, and False Tracts," *Gastroenterology Nursing* 28(6):485-93, November-December 2005.

Guenter, P., and Silkroski, M. *Tube Feeding: Practical Guidelines and Nursing Protocols.* Gaithersburg, Md.: Aspen Pubs., Inc., 2001.

Holman, C., et al. "Promoting Adequate Nutrition: Using Artificial Feeding," *Nursing Older People* 17(10):31-32, January 2006.

Smeltzer, S.C., et al. *Brunner & Suddarth's Textbook of Medical-Surgical Nursing,* 11th ed. Philadelphia: Lippincott Williams & Wilkins, 2008.

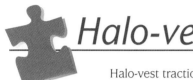

Halo-vest traction

Halo-vest traction immobilizes the head and neck after traumatic injury to the cervical vertebrae—the most common of all spinal injuries. This procedure, which can prevent further injury to the spinal cord, is performed by a neurosurgeon or an orthopedic surgeon (with nursing assistance) in the emergency department, at the patient's bedside, or in the operating room after surgical reduction of vertebral injuries. The halo-vest traction device consists of a metal ring that fits over the patient's head and metal bars that connect the ring to a plastic vest that distributes the weight of the entire apparatus around the chest. (See *Comparing halo-vest traction devices*, page 222.)

When in place, halo-vest traction allows the patient greater mobility than traction with skull tongs. It also carries less risk of infection because it doesn't require skin incisions and drill holes to position skull pins.

Equipment

Halo-vest traction unit ◆ halo ring ◆ cervical collar or sandbags (if needed) ◆ plastic vest ◆ board or padded headrest ◆ tape measure ◆ halo ring conversion chart ◆ clippers ◆ 4" × 4" gauze pads ◆ antiseptic solution ◆ sterile gloves ◆ Allen wrench ◆ four positioning pins ◆ multiple-dose vial of 1% lidocaine ◆ alcohol pads ◆ 3-ml syringe ◆ 25G needle ◆ five sterile skull pins (one more than needed) ◆ torque screwdriver ◆ sheepskin liners ◆ clean gloves ◆ cotton-tipped applicators ◆ medicated powder or cornstarch ◆ normal saline solution ◆ optional: pain medication (such as an analgesic).

Implementation

▶ Obtain a halo-vest traction unit with halo rings and plastic vests in several sizes. Vest sizes are based on the patient's head and chest measurements.
▶ Check the expiration date of the prepackaged tray, and check the outside covering for damage to ensure the sterility of the contents. Then assemble the equipment at the patient's bedside. **CDC**
▶ Check the support that was applied to the patient's neck on the way to the hospital. If necessary, apply the cervical collar immediately or immobilize the head and neck with sandbags. Keep the cervical collar or sandbags in place until the halo is applied. This support will then be carefully removed to facilitate application of the vest.
▶ Remove the headboard and any furniture at the head of the bed to provide ample working space.

> ## CLINICAL ALERT
>
> Never put the patient's head on a pillow before applying the halo to avoid further injury to the spinal cord.

▶ Elevate the bed to a working level that gives the physician easy access to the front and back of the halo unit.
▶ Stand at the head of the bed, and see if the patient's chin lines up with his midsternum, indicating proper alignment. If ordered, support the patient's head in your hands and gently rotate the neck into alignment without flexing or extending it.

Assisting with halo application

▶ Ask another nurse to help you with the procedure.
▶ Explain the procedure to the patient, wash your hands, and provide privacy.

Comparing halo-vest traction devices

TYPE	DESCRIPTION		ADVANTAGES
Low profile (standard)	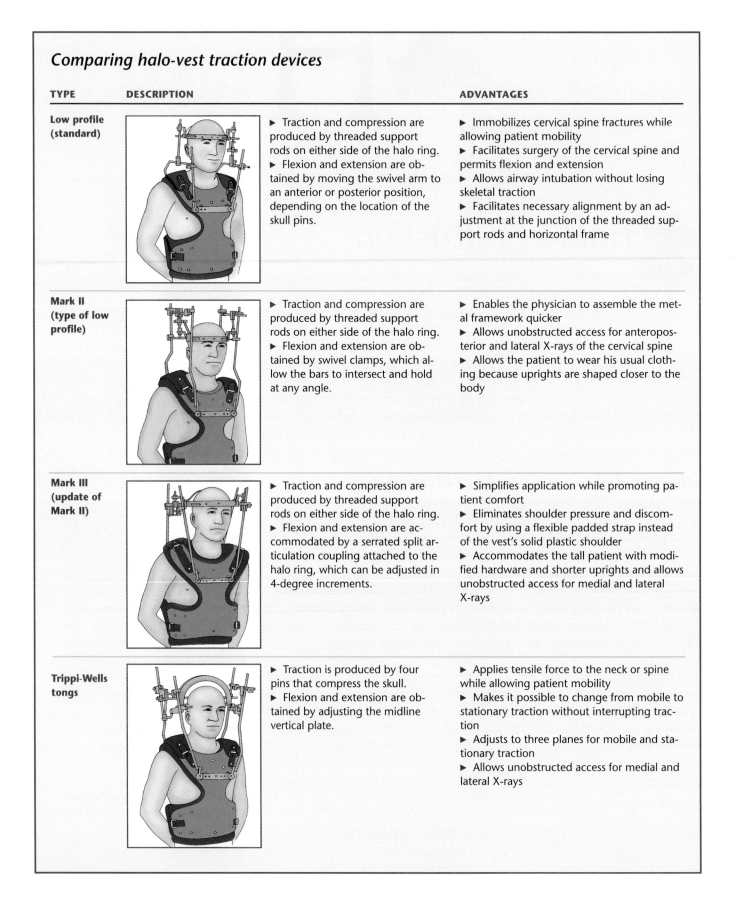	▶ Traction and compression are produced by threaded support rods on either side of the halo ring. ▶ Flexion and extension are obtained by moving the swivel arm to an anterior or posterior position, depending on the location of the skull pins.	▶ Immobilizes cervical spine fractures while allowing patient mobility ▶ Facilitates surgery of the cervical spine and permits flexion and extension ▶ Allows airway intubation without losing skeletal traction ▶ Facilitates necessary alignment by an adjustment at the junction of the threaded support rods and horizontal frame
Mark II (type of low profile)		▶ Traction and compression are produced by threaded support rods on either side of the halo ring. ▶ Flexion and extension are obtained by swivel clamps, which allow the bars to intersect and hold at any angle.	▶ Enables the physician to assemble the metal framework quicker ▶ Allows unobstructed access for anteroposterior and lateral X-rays of the cervical spine ▶ Allows the patient to wear his usual clothing because uprights are shaped closer to the body
Mark III (update of Mark II)		▶ Traction and compression are produced by threaded support rods on either side of the halo ring. ▶ Flexion and extension are accommodated by a serrated split articulation coupling attached to the halo ring, which can be adjusted in 4-degree increments.	▶ Simplifies application while promoting patient comfort ▶ Eliminates shoulder pressure and discomfort by using a flexible padded strap instead of the vest's solid plastic shoulder ▶ Accommodates the tall patient with modified hardware and shorter uprights and allows unobstructed access for medial and lateral X-rays
Trippi-Wells tongs		▶ Traction is produced by four pins that compress the skull. ▶ Flexion and extension are obtained by adjusting the midline vertical plate.	▶ Applies tensile force to the neck or spine while allowing patient mobility ▶ Makes it possible to change from mobile to stationary traction without interrupting traction ▶ Adjusts to three planes for mobile and stationary traction ▶ Allows unobstructed access for medial and lateral X-rays

► Have the assisting nurse hold the patient's head and neck stable while the physician removes the cervical collar or sandbags. Maintain this support until the halo is secure, while you assist with pin insertion.

► The physician measures the patient's head with a tape measure and refers to the halo ring conversion chart to determine the correct ring size. (The ring should clear the head by $2/3''$ [1.7 cm] and fit $1/3''$ [0.8 cm] above the bridge of the nose.)

► The physician selects four pin sites: $1/2''$ (1.3 cm) above the lateral one-third of each eyebrow and $1/2''$ above the top of each ear in the occipital area. He also takes into account the degree and type of correction needed to provide proper cervical alignment.

► Trim the hair at the pin sites with clippers to facilitate subsequent care and help prevent infection. Then use 4" × 4" gauze pads soaked in antiseptic solution to clean the sites.

► Open the halo-vest unit using sterile technique. The physician puts on the sterile gloves and removes the halo and the Allen wrench. He then places the halo over the patient's head and inserts the four positioning pins to hold the halo in place temporarily.

► Help the physician prepare the anesthetic. First, clean the injection port of the multiple-dose vial of lidocaine with the alcohol pad. Then invert the vial so the physician can insert a 25G needle attached to the 3-ml syringe and withdraw the anesthetic.

► The physician injects the anesthetic at the four pin sites. He may change needles on the syringe after each injection.

► The physician removes four of the five skull pins from the sterile setup and firmly screws in each pin at a 90-degree angle to the skull. When the pins are in place, he removes the positioning pins. He then tightens the skull pins with the torque screwdriver.

Applying the vest

► After the physician measures the patient's chest and abdomen, he selects a vest of appropriate size.

► Place the sheepskin liners inside the front and back of the vest to make it more comfortable to wear and to help prevent pressure ulcers.

► Help the physician carefully raise the patient while the other nurse supports the head and neck. Slide the back of the vest under the patient and gently lay him down. The physician then fastens the front of the vest on the patient's chest using Velcro straps.

► The physician attaches the metal bars to the halo and vest and tightens each bolt in turn to avoid tightening any single bolt completely, causing maladjusted tension. When halo-vest traction is in place, X-rays should be taken immediately to check the depth of the skull pins and verify proper alignment.

Caring for the patient

► Take routine and neurologic vital signs at least every 2 hours for 24 hours (preferably every hour for 48 hours) and then every 4 hours until stable.

> ⭐ **CLINICAL ALERT**
>
> Notify the physician immediately if you observe a loss of motor function or decreased sensation from the baseline because these findings could indicate spinal cord trauma.

► Put on gloves. Gently clean the pin sites every 4 hours with cotton-tipped applicators. Rinse the sites with normal saline solution to remove excess cleaning solution. Then clean the pin sites with antiseptic solution. Watch for signs of infection—a loose pin, swelling or redness, purulent drainage, pain at the site—and notify the physician if these signs develop.

► The physician retightens the skull pins with the torque screwdriver 24 and 48 hours after the halo is applied. If the patient complains of a headache after the pins are tightened, obtain an order for an analgesic. If pain occurs with jaw movement or any movement of the head or neck, notify the physician immediately because this may indicate that the pins have slipped onto the thin temporal plate.

► Examine the halo-vest unit every shift to make sure that everything is secure and that the patient's head is centered within the halo. If the vest fits correctly, you should be able to insert one or two fingers under the jacket at the shoulder and chest when the patient is lying supine.

► Wash the patient's chest and back daily. First, place the patient on his back. Loosen the bottom Velcro straps so you can get to the chest and back. Then, reaching under the vest, wash and dry the skin. Check for tender, reddened areas or pressure spots that may develop into ulcers. If necessary, use a hair dryer to dry damp sheepskin because moisture predisposes the skin to pressure ulcer formation. Lightly dust the skin with medicated powder or cornstarch to prevent itching.

► Turn the patient on his side (less than 45 degrees) to wash his back. Then close the vest.

► Be careful not to put stress on the apparatus, which could knock it out of alignment and lead to subluxation of the cervical spine.

Special considerations

CLINICAL ALERT

Keep two conventional wrenches available at all times; they may be taped to the patient's halo vest on the chest area. In case of cardiac arrest, use them to remove the distal anterior bolts. Pull the two upright bars outward. Unfasten the Velcro straps, and remove the front of the vest. Use the sturdy back of the vest as a board for cardiopulmonary resuscitation (CPR). Some vests have a hinged front to raise the breast plate for CPR. Know the type of vest your patient has.

▶ Never lift the patient up by the vertical bars. This could strain or tear the skin at the pin sites or misalign the traction.

▶ To prevent falls, walk with the ambulatory patient. Remember, he'll have difficulty seeing objects at or near his feet, and the weight of the halo-vest unit (about 10 lb [4.5 kg]) may throw him off balance. If the patient is in a wheelchair, lower the leg rests to prevent the chair from tipping backward.

▶ Because the vest limits chest expansion, routinely assess pulmonary function, especially in a patient with pulmonary disease.

▶ Manipulating the patient's neck during application of halo-vest traction may cause subluxation of the spinal cord, or it could push a bone fragment into the spinal cord, possibly compressing the cord and causing paralysis below the break.

References

American Association of Neuroscience Nurses. *Core Curriculum for Neuroscience Nursing,* 4th ed. Philadelphia: W.B. Saunders Co., 2004.

Holmes, S.B., and Brown, S.J. "Skeletal Pin Site Care: National Association of Orthopaedic Nurses Guidelines for Orthopaedic Nursing," *Orthopedic Nursing* 24(2):99-107, March-April 2005.

Lynn-McHale Weigand, D.J., and Carlson, K.K., eds. *AACN Procedure Manual for Critical Care,* 5th ed. Philadelphia: W.B. Saunders Co., 2005.

Patterson, M.M. "Multicenter Pin Care Study," *Orthopedic Nursing* 24(5):349-60, September-October 2005.

Hand hygiene

The hands are the conduits for almost every transfer of potential pathogens from one patient to another, from a contaminated object to the patient, or from a staff member to the patient. Thus, hand hygiene is the single most important procedure for preventing infection. To protect the patient from healthcare acquired infections, hand hygiene must be performed routinely and thoroughly. In effect, clean and healthy hands with intact skin, short fingernails, and no rings minimize the risk of contamination. Artificial nails may serve as a reservoir for microorganisms, and microorganisms are more difficult to remove from rough or chapped hands.

Washing with soap (plain or antimicrobial) and water is appropriate when hands are visibly soiled or contaminated with infectious material. **CDC**

Equipment

Hand washing

Soap or detergent ◆ warm, running water ◆ paper towels ◆ optional: fingernail brush, antiseptic cleaning agent, disposable sponge brush, plastic cuticle stick.

Hand sanitizing

Alcohol-based hand rub.

Implementation

Hand washing

▶ Remove rings per your facility's policy because they harbor dirt and skin microorganisms. Remove your watch or wear it well above the wrist. *Note:* Artificial fingernails and nail polish must be kept in good repair to minimize their potential to harbor microorganisms; refer to your facility's policy regarding nail polish and artificial nails. Natural nails should be short (less than 1/4"). **CDC** **CS1** **CS2**

▶ Wet your hands and wrists with warm water, and apply soap from a dispenser. Don't use bar soap because it allows cross-contamination. Hold your hands below elbow level to prevent water from running up your arms and back down, thus contaminating clean areas. **CDC**

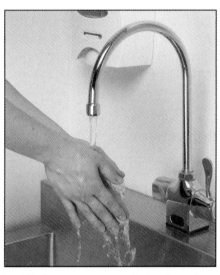

▶ Work up a generous lather by rubbing your hands together vigorously for about 10 seconds. Soap and warm water reduce surface tension and this, aided by friction, loosens surface microorganisms, which wash away in the lather. **CDC**

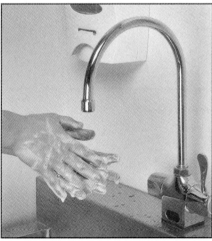

▶ Pay special attention to the areas under fingernails and around cuticles, and to the thumbs, knuckles, and sides of the fingers and hands. If you don't remove your wedding band, move it up and down your finger to clean beneath it.

▶ Avoid splashing water on yourself or the floor because microorganisms spread more easily on wet surfaces and because slippery floors are dangerous. Avoid touching the sink or faucets because they're considered contaminated.

▶ Rinse hands and wrists well because running water flushes suds, soil, soap or detergent, and microorganisms away.

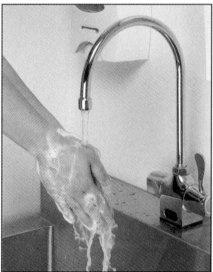

▶ Pat hands and wrists dry with a paper towel. Avoid rubbing, which can cause abrasion and chapping. **CDC**

▶ If the sink isn't equipped with knee or foot controls, turn off faucets by gripping them with a dry paper towel to avoid recontaminating your hands. **CDC**

Hand sanitizing

▶ Apply a small amount of the alcohol-based hand rub to all surfaces of your hand. **CDC**

▶ Rub your hands together.

Special considerations

▶ Follow your facility's policy concerning when to wash with soap and when to use an antiseptic cleaning agent. Typically, you'll wash with soap before coming on duty; before and after direct or indirect patient contact; before and after performing any bodily functions, such as blowing your nose or using the bathroom; before preparing or serving food; before preparing or administering medications; after removing gloves or other personal protective equipment; and after completing your shift. **CDC**

▶ Don't use an alcohol-based hand rub if contact with items contaminated with *Clostridium difficile* or *Bacillus anthracis* occurs. These organisms can form spores, and alcohol won't kill them. Rather, wash your hands with soap and water.

▶ Use an antiseptic cleaning agent before performing invasive procedures, wound care, and dressing changes and after contamination. Antiseptics are also recommended for hand washing in isolation rooms, neonatal and special care nurseries, and before caring for any highly susceptible patient. **CDC**

▶ Wash your hands before and after performing patient care or procedures or having contact with contaminated objects, even though you may have worn gloves. Always wash your hands after removing gloves. **CDC**

References

Centers for Disease Control and Prevention. "Guidelines for Hand Hygiene in Health-Care Settings," *MMWR* 51(RR-16):1-144, October 2002.

Houghton, D. "HAI Prevention: The Power Is in Your Hands," *Nursing Management* 37(Suppl):1-7, May 2006.

Hughes, N. "Handwashing: Going Back to Basics in Infection Control," *AJN* 107(7):96, July 2006.

Parry, M.F., et al. "Candida Osteomyelitis and Diskitis After Spinal Surgery: An Outbreak that Implicates Artificial Nail Use," *Clinical Infection Disease* 32(3):352-7, February 2001. **CS1**

Salisbury, D.M., et al. "The Effect of Rings on Microbial Load of Health Care Workers' Hands," *American Journal of Infection Control* 25(1):24-7, February 1997. **CS2**

Scalise, D. "Save Lives Now. 30 Things You Can Do to Eliminate Infections," *Hospital & Health Networks/AHA* 80(9):32-36, 38-40, September 2006.

Handheld oropharyngeal inhalers

Handheld inhalers include the metered-dose inhaler (or nebulizer), the turbo inhaler, and the nasal inhaler. These devices deliver topical medications to the respiratory tract, producing local and systemic effects. The mucosal lining of the respiratory tract absorbs the inhalant almost immediately. Examples of common inhalants used to decrease inflammation include bronchodilators, mucolytics, and corticosteroids.

The use of these inhalers may be contraindicated in patients who can't form an airtight seal around the device and in patients who lack the coordination or clear vision necessary to assemble a turbo inhaler. Specific inhalant drugs may also be contraindicated. For example, bronchodilators are contraindicated if the patient has tachycardia or a history of cardiac arrhythmias associated with tachycardia.

Equipment

Patient's medication record and chart ◆ metered-dose inhaler, turbo inhaler, or nasal inhaler ◆ prescribed medication ◆ normal saline solution (or another appropriate solution) for gargling ◆ optional: emesis basin. (See *Types of handheld inhalers*.)

Implementation

▶ Verify the order on the patient's medication record by checking it against the practitioner's order. **JC** **ISMP**
▶ Wash your hands.
▶ Check the label on the inhaler against the order on the medication record. Verify the expiration date.

▶ Confirm the patient's identity using two patient identifiers according to your facility's policy. **JC**
▶ If your facility uses a bar code scanning system, be sure to scan your ID badge, the patient's ID bracelet, and the medication's bar code. **JC** **ISMP**
▶ Explain the procedure to the patient.

Types of handheld inhalers

Handheld inhalers use air under pressure to produce a mist containing tiny droplets of medication. Drugs delivered in this form (such as mucolytics and bronchodilators) can travel deep into the lungs.

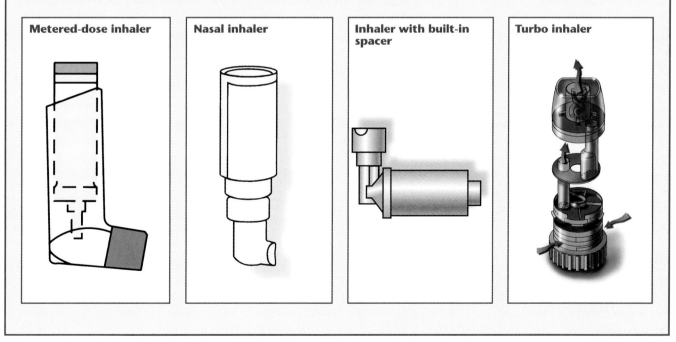

Metered-dose inhaler   **Nasal inhaler**   **Inhaler with built-in spacer**   **Turbo inhaler**

Using a metered-dose inhaler

▶ Shake the inhaler bottle to mix the medication and aerosol propellant.

▶ Remove the mouthpiece and cap. *Note:* Some metered-dose inhalers have a spacer built into the inhaler. Pull the spacer away from the section holding the medication canister until it clicks into place.

▶ Insert the metal stem on the bottle into the small hole on the flattened portion of the mouthpiece. Then, turn the bottle upside down.

▶ Have the patient exhale, and then place the mouthpiece in his mouth and close his lips around it.

▶ As you firmly push the bottle down against the mouthpiece, ask the patient to inhale slowly and to continue inhaling until his lungs feel full. This action draws the medication into his lungs. Compress the bottle against the mouthpiece only once.

▶ Remove the mouthpiece from the patient's mouth, and tell him to hold his breath for several seconds to allow the medication to reach the alveoli. Then instruct him to exhale slowly through pursed lips to keep the distal bronchioles open, allowing increased absorption and diffusion of the drug and better gas exchange.

▶ Have the patient gargle with normal saline solution, if desired, to remove medication from the mouth and back of the throat. (The lungs retain only about 10% of the inhalant; most of the remainder is exhaled, but substantial amounts may remain in the oropharynx.)

▶ Rinse the mouthpiece thoroughly with warm water to prevent accumulation of residue.

Using a turbo inhaler

▶ Hold the mouthpiece in one hand, and with the other hand, slide the sleeve away from the mouthpiece as far as possible.

▶ Unscrew the tip of the mouthpiece by turning it counterclockwise.

▶ Firmly press the colored portion of the medication capsule into the propeller stem of the mouthpiece.

▶ Screw the inhaler together again securely.

▶ Holding the inhaler with the mouthpiece at the bottom, slide the sleeve all the way down and then up again to puncture the capsule and release the medication. Do this only once.

▶ Have the patient exhale and tilt his head back. Tell him to place the mouthpiece in his mouth, close his lips around it, and inhale once—quickly and deeply—through the mouthpiece.

▶ Tell the patient to hold his breath for several seconds to allow the medication to reach the alveoli. (Instruct him not to exhale through the mouthpiece.)

▶ Remove the inhaler from the patient's mouth, and tell him to exhale as much air as possible.

▶ Repeat the procedure until all the medication in the device is inhaled.

▶ Have the patient gargle with normal saline solution, if desired, to remove medication from the mouth and back of the throat. Be sure to provide an emesis basin if the patient needs one.

▶ Discard the empty medication capsule, put the inhaler in its can, and secure the lid. Rinse the inhaler with warm water at least once per week.

Using a nasal inhaler

▶ Have the patient blow his nose to clear his nostrils.

▶ Shake the medication cartridge and then insert it in the adapter. (Before inserting a refill cartridge, remove the protective cap from the stem.)

▶ Remove the protective cap from the adapter tip.

▶ Hold the inhaler with your index finger on top of the cartridge and your thumb under the nasal adapter. The adapter tip should be pointing toward the patient.

▶ Have the patient tilt his head back. Then tell him to place the adapter tip into one nostril while occluding the other nostril with his finger.

▶ Instruct the patient to inhale gently as he presses the adapter and the cartridge together firmly to release a measured dose of medication.

▶ Tell the patient to remove the inhaler from his nostril and to hold his breath for a few seconds.

▶ Have the patient exhale through his mouth.

▶ Shake the inhaler, and have the patient repeat the procedure in the other nostril.

▶ Have the patient gargle with normal saline solution to remove medication from his mouth and throat.

▶ Remove the medication cartridge from the nasal inhaler, and wash the nasal adapter in lukewarm water. Let the adapter dry thoroughly before reinserting the cartridge.

Special considerations

▶ When using a turbo or nasal inhaler, make sure the pressurized cartridge isn't punctured or incinerated. Store the medication cartridge below 120° F (48.9° C).

▶ Teach the patient how to use the inhaler so that he can continue treatments himself after discharge, if necessary. Explain that overdosage—which is common—can cause the medication to lose its effectiveness. Tell him to record the date and time of each inhalation as well as his response to prevent overdosage and to help the practitioner determine the drug's effectiveness. Also, note whether the patient uses an unusual amount of medication—for example, more than one cartridge for a metered-dose nebulizer every 3 weeks. Inform the patient of possible adverse reactions.

▶ If more than one inhalation is ordered, advise the patient to wait at least 2 minutes before repeating the procedure.

▶ If the patient is also using a steroid inhaler, instruct him to use the bronchodilator first and then wait 5 minutes before using the steroid. This allows the bronchodilator to open the air passages for maximum effectiveness.

References

The Joint Commission. *Comprehensive Accreditation Manual for Hospitals: The Official Handbook*. Standard MM.1.10. Oakbrook Terrace, Ill.: The Joint Commission, 2007.

The Joint Commission. *Comprehensive Accreditation Manual for Hospitals: The Official Handbook*. Standard MM.2.10. Oakbrook Terrace, Ill.: The Joint Commission, 2007.

The Joint Commission. *Comprehensive Accreditation Manual for Hospitals: The Official Handbook*. Standard MM.3.10. Oakbrook Terrace, Ill.: The Joint Commission, 2007.

The Joint Commission. *Comprehensive Accreditation Manual for Hospitals: The Official Handbook*. Standard MM.4.10. Oakbrook Terrace, Ill.: The Joint Commission, 2007.

The Joint Commission. *Comprehensive Accreditation Manual for Hospitals: The Official Handbook*. Standard MM.4.20. Oakbrook Terrace, Ill.: The Joint Commission, 2007.

The Joint Commission. *Comprehensive Accreditation Manual for Hospitals: The Official Handbook*. Standard MM.5.10. Oakbrook Terrace, Ill.: The Joint Commission, 2007.

The Joint Commission. *Comprehensive Accreditation Manual for Hospitals: The Official Handbook*. Standard MM.6.10. Oakbrook Terrace, Ill.: The Joint Commission, 2007.

The Joint Commission. *Comprehensive Accreditation Manual for Hospitals: The Official Handbook*. Standard MM.6.20. Oakbrook Terrace, Ill.: The Joint Commission, 2007.

Leach, C.L. "Inhalation Aspects of Therapeutic Aerosols," *Toxicologic Pathology* 35(1):23-26, January 2007.

Maggio, E.T. "Intraval: Highly Effective Intranasal Delivery of Peptide and Protein Drugs," *Expert Opinions in Drug Delivery* 3(4):529-39, June 2006.

Newell, K., and Hume, S. "Choosing the Right Inhaler for Patients with Asthma," *Nursing Standard* 21(5):46-48, October 2006.

Taylor, C., et al. *Fundamentals of Nursing: The Art and Science of Nursing Care,* 6th ed. Philadelphia: Lippincott Williams & Wilkins, 2008.

Hearing aid care

The ability to hear properly is an anatomical function that has both health and social implications. Indeed, people may be embarrassed about hearing loss, no matter what their age. They may agree with things being said without knowing the true context of the dialogue. Further, people with hearing loss may unknowingly not be paying attention when someone is talking, perhaps offending the person speaking.

Patients who have hearing loss may benefit from the use of a hearing aid, and there are several types available. (See *Types of hearing aids*.)

Patients generally wear hearing aids during the day only. At night and at times of rest, the hearing aid is usually removed. Because of the fragile nature of the hearing aid, it's important to clean it properly and carefully to avoid damage.

Types of hearing aids

There are three common types of hearing aids.

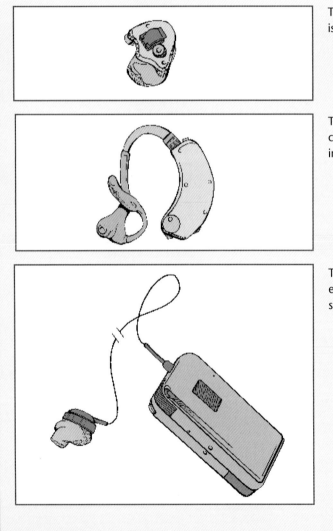

The in-the-ear device fits entirely within the patient's ear and is small and self-contained.

The behind-the-ear device is a bit larger and consists of a microphone and an amplifier. The amplifier delivers sound to an internal receiver.

The body aid device uses electrical components, which are enclosed in a case carried elsewhere on the body, to transmit sound to an ear mold receiver via a wire.

Equipment

Bath towel ◆ facial tissue ◆ cleaning brush or wire loop or soft toothbrush ◆ storage case ◆ washcloth ◆ water ◆ soap ◆ optional: spare battery, dryer for hearing aids, gloves.

Implementation

Removing the hearing aid

▶ Assess the patient's ear. If drainage is present, put on gloves.

▶ Gently turn the hearing aid off to prevent feedback during removal. Grasp the hearing aid and remove it from the ear.

▶ Hold the hearing aid over a towel to prevent damaging it if dropped. Wipe the outside of the hearing aid with a tissue.

CLINICAL ALERT

Don't use alcohol or other solvents on the hearing aid because they may cause breakdown of the material.

▶ Carefully inspect the hearing aid and look for accumulated cerumen. Remove the cerumen using the cleaning brush or wire loop that was supplied with the hearing aid. If this isn't available, use a soft toothbrush to gently remove the cerumen. Be careful not to push the cerumen into any openings. **NIDCD**

▶ Feel along the hearing aid for any rough areas that may irritate the ear canal.

▶ Open the battery to allow internal components exposure to air to dry.

▶ Place the hearing aid and battery in a storage container labeled with the pa-

tient's name, identification number, and room number.

▶ Place a towel under the patient's ear and generally wash the ear and ear canal with a washcloth and soap and warm water.

Inserting the hearing aid

▶ Remove the hearing aid from the storage case and close the battery door.

▶ Check the battery by slowly turning the volume up to high. Place your hand over the hearing aid and listen for feedback. Turn the volume off to prevent feedback while inserting the hearing aid.

▶ Look at the hearing aid and determine if it's for the right or left ear. Hearing aids for the right ear will be marked with an R or have a red dot, whereas hearing aids for the left ear will be marked with an L or have a blue dot.

▶ Holding the hearing aid gently, insert the shaped end into the ear canal. Avoid pulling on the ear because this may alter the shape of the ear canal and cause the hearing aid to be improperly placed.

▶ Turn the volume up slowly to a comfortable level.

Special considerations

▶ Many individuals with severe hearing loss have learned to read lips; therefore, face the patient when you speak to him and speak slowly.

▶ Keep background noise to a minimum, if possible, because white noise

can cause distractions, especially at higher frequencies.

▶ Avoid placing the hearing aid in direct sunlight or direct heat. **NIDCD**

AGE FACTOR

The elderly patient may have difficulty manipulating the hearing aid to correctly clean and insert it. If this is the case, refer the patient to an audiologist who can recommend a hearing aid that will better fit his lifestyle.

▶ Tell the patient to keep the hearing aid in the storage case when not in use to avoid damaging it. Instruct the patient to keep the batteries away from pets and children to avoid accidental ingestion. **NIDCD**

References

Cook, J.A., and Hawkins, D.B. "Hearing Loss and Hearing Aid Treatment Options," *Mayo Clinic Proceedings* 81(2):234-37, February 2006.

Pothier, D.D., and Brendenkamp, C. "Hearing Aid Insertion: Correlation between Patients' Confidence and Ability," *Journal of Laryngology and Otology* 120(5):378-80, May 2006.

Wallhagen, M.I., et al. "Sensory Impairment in Older Adults: Part 1: Hearing Loss," *AJN* 106(10):40-48, October 2006.

Height and weight

Height and weight are routinely measured during admission to a health care facility. An accurate record of the patient's height and weight is essential for calculating dosages of drugs, anesthetics, and contrast agents; assessing the patient's nutritional status; and determining the height-weight ratio.

Height can be measured with the measuring bar on a standing scale, using a ruler, or with a tape measure for a supine patient. (See *Types of scales*.) Weight can be measured with a standing scale, chair scale, or bed scale.

Equipment

Standing scale or chair or bed scale ◆ ruler (if scale doesn't have measuring bar) ◆ wheelchair (if needed to transport patient) ◆ tape measure, if needed.

Implementation

Measuring height

▶ If you're using a standing scale to measure height, tell the patient to stand erect on the platform of the scale. Raise the measuring bar beyond the top of the patient's head, extend the horizontal arm, and lower the bar until it touches the top of the patient's head. Then read the patient's height.

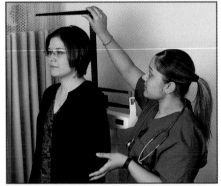

▶ Without a scale, have the patient remove his shoes. Have him stand against a wall with his back and heels touching the wall. Using a straight, level object (such as a ruler), place it on top of the patient's head parallel to the floor. Mark the location of the ruler on the wall. Measure the distance between the mark and the floor.

AGE FACTOR

When measuring the height of a child younger than age 2, measure the length of the child in a supine position, while holding the head in the midline position and gently holding the legs in full extension.

Measuring weight

▶ Select the appropriate scale—usually, a standing scale for an ambulatory patient or a chair or bed scale for an acutely ill or debilitated patient. Then, check to make sure the scale is balanced.

▶ Confirm the patient's identity using two patient identifiers according to your facility's policy. **JC**

▶ Explain the procedure to the patient.

Using a standing scale

▶ Place a paper towel on the scale's platform.

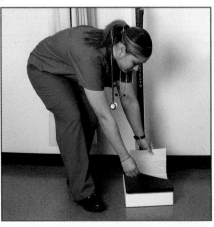

▶ Ask the patient to remove her robe and slippers or shoes. If the scale has wheels, lock them before the patient steps on. Assist the patient onto the scale, and remain close to her to prevent falls.

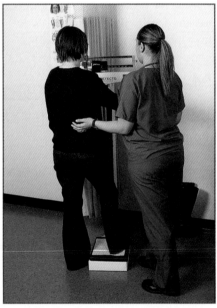

▶ If you're using an upright balance (gravity) scale, slide the lower rider to the groove representing the largest increment below the patient's estimated weight. Grooves represent 50, 100, 150, and 200 lb. Then slide the small upper rider until the beam balances.

Types of scales

Selection of scales varies, and the selection is influenced by the status of the patient.

For ambulatory patients

Standing scale

For acutely ill or debilitated patients

Chair scale   **Bed scale**

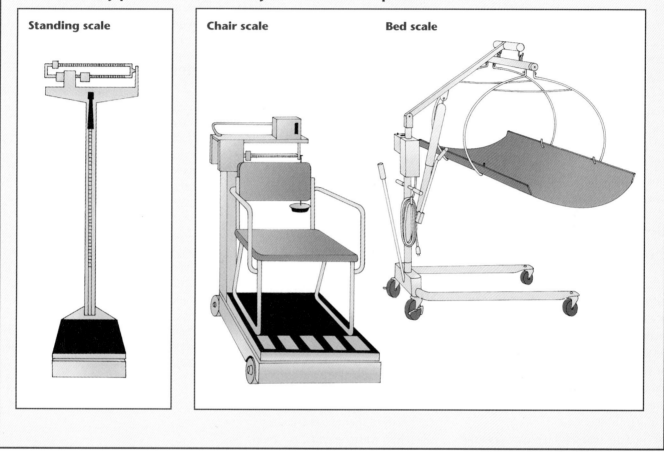

Add the upper and lower rider figures to determine the weight. (The upper rider is calibrated to eighths of a pound.)

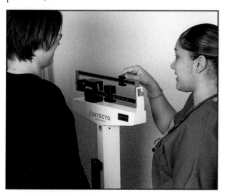

▶ Return the weight holder to its proper place.

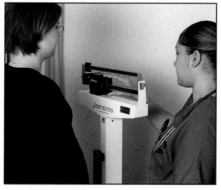

▶ If you're using a digital scale, make sure the display reads 0 before use.

Read the display with the patient standing as still as possible.
▶ Help the patient off the scale, and return her robe and slippers or shoes.

Using a chair scale
▶ Transport the patient to the weighing area or the scale to the patient's bedside.
▶ Lock the scale in place to prevent it from moving accidentally.
▶ If you're using a scale with a swing-away chair arm, unlock the arm. When unlocked, the arm swings back 180 degrees to permit easy access.

▶ Position the scale beside the patient's bed or wheelchair with the chair arm open. Transfer the patient onto the scale, swing the chair arm to the front of the scale, and lock it in place.

▶ If the chair scale is digital, make sure the display reads 0 before use. Press the button and record the weight. If using a multiple-weight chair scale, use the same process as a standing scale to determine the weight.

▶ Unlock the swing-away chair arm as before, and transfer the patient back to the bed or to a wheelchair.

▶ Lock the main beam to avoid damaging the scale during transport. Then unlock the wheels and remove the scale from the patient's room.

Using a digital bed scale

▶ Provide privacy, and tell the patient that you're going to weigh him on a special bed scale. Demonstrate its operation, if appropriate.

▶ Place the protective plastic covering over the stretcher, and confirm that the scale is balanced.

▶ Release the stretcher to the horizontal position, and then lock it in place. Turn the patient on his side, facing away from the scale.

▶ Roll the base of the scale under the patient's bed. Adjust the lever to widen the base of the scale, providing stability. Then lock the scale's wheels.

▶ Center the stretcher above the bed, lower it onto the mattress, and roll the patient onto the stretcher. Then position the circular weighing arms of the scale over the patient, and attach them securely to the stretcher bars.

▶ Pump the handle with long, slow strokes to raise the patient a few inches off the bed. Make sure the patient doesn't lean on or touch the headboard, side rails, or other bed equipment, and that nothing is pulling on the scale (such as I.V. or catheter tubing) because these types of pressure will affect the weight measurement.

▶ Depress the operate button, and read the patient's weight on the digital display panel. Then press in the scale's handle to lower the patient.

▶ Detach the circular weighing arms from the stretcher bars, roll the patient off the stretcher and remove it, and position him comfortably in bed.

▶ Release the wheel lock and withdraw the scale. Dispose of the protective plastic covering and return the stretcher to its vertical position.

Special considerations

▶ Reassure and steady patients who are at risk for losing their balance on a scale.

▶ Weigh the patient at the same time each day (usually before breakfast), in similar clothing, and using the same scale. If the patient uses crutches, weigh him with the crutches. Then weigh the crutches and any heavy clothing, and subtract their weight from the total to determine the patient's weight.

▶ Before using a bed scale, cover its stretcher with a drawsheet. Balance the scale with the drawsheet in place to ensure accurate weighing.

▶ When rolling the patient onto the stretcher, be careful not to dislodge I.V. lines, indwelling catheters, and other supportive equipment.

References

Craven, R.F., and Hirnle, C.J. *Fundamentals of Nursing: Human Health and Function,* 6th ed. Philadelphia: Lippincott Williams & Wilkins, 2009.

Fransozi, F.G. "Should We Continue to Use BMI as a Cardiovascular Risk Factor?" *Lancet* 368(9536):624-25, August 2006.

Hendershot, K.M., et al. "Estimated Height, Weight, and Body Mass Index: Implications for Research and Patient Safety," *Journal of the American College of Surgeons* 203(6):887-93, December 2006.

Stoner, A., and Walker, J. "Growth Assessment: How Do We Measure Up?" *Paediatric Nursing* 18(7):26-28, September 2006.

Hemodialysis

Hemodialysis is performed to remove toxic wastes from the blood of patients in renal failure. This potentially lifesaving procedure removes blood from the body, circulates it through a purifying dialyzer, and then returns the blood to the body. Various access sites can be used for this procedure. (See *Hemodialysis access sites,* page 236.)

The underlying mechanism in hemodialysis is differential diffusion across a semipermeable membrane, which extracts by-products of protein metabolism, such as urea and uric acid, as well as creatinine and excess body water. This process restores or maintains the balance of the body's buffer system and electrolyte level.

Hemodialysis provides temporary support for patients with acute reversible renal failure. It's also used for regular long-term treatment of patients with chronic end-stage renal disease. Hemodialysis may also be necessary to remove toxic substances from the blood in patients suffering from various acute poisoning or barbiturate or analgesic overdose. The patient's condition (rate of creatinine generation, weight gain) determines the number and duration of hemodialysis treatments.

Specially prepared personnel usually perform this procedure in a hemodialysis unit. However, if the patient is acutely ill and unstable, hemodialysis can be done at the bedside in the intensive care unit. In addition, special hemodialysis units are available for use at home.

Equipment

Preparing the hemodialysis machine: Hemodialysis machine with appropriate dialyzer ♦ I.V. solution, administration sets, lines, and related equipment ♦ dialysate ♦ optional: heparin, 3-ml syringe with needle, medication label, hemostats.

Beginning hemodialysis with a double-lumen catheter: Sterile gloves ♦ clean gloves ♦ gown ♦ sterile drape ♦ sterile 4″ × 4″ gauze pads ♦ antiseptic swabs ♦ stethoscope ♦ sphygmomanometer ♦ two 3-ml syringes ♦ two 5-ml syringes with prescribed anticoagulant flush.

Beginning hemodialysis with arteriovenous (AV) access: Two 19G winged fistula needles ♦ two 10-ml syringes ♦ prescribed anticoagulant flush solution ♦ linen-saver pad ♦ antiseptic swabs ♦ sterile 4″ × 4″ gauze pads ♦ sterile drape ♦ tourniquet ♦ sterile gloves ♦ clean gloves ♦ gown ♦ stethoscope ♦ two pairs of hemostats ♦ adhesive tape.

Discontinuing dialysis with a double-lumen catheter: Two 10-ml syringes with normal saline solution ♦ two 5-ml syringes with prescribed anticoagulant flush solution ♦ two sterile luer-lock caps ♦ antiseptic swabs ♦ stethoscope ♦ sphygmomanometer ♦ supplies for catheter site care ♦ antiseptic solution ♦ sterile drape ♦ sterile 4″ × 4″ gauze pads ♦ optional: supplies for drainage culture.

Discontinuing dialysis with AV access: Clean gloves ♦ two pairs of hemostats ♦ 4″ × 4″ gauze pads ♦ dry, sterile dressing ♦ stethoscope ♦ sphygmomanometer.

Implementation

▶ Prepare the hemodialysis equipment following the manufacturer's instructions and your facility's policy. Maintain strict sterile technique to prevent introducing pathogens into the patient's bloodstream during dialysis. Be sure to test the dialyzer and dialysis machine for residual disinfectant after rinsing, and test all the alarms. **MFR CDC**

▶ Gather the appropriate equipment.

▶ Confirm the patient's identity using two patient identifiers according to your facility's policy. **JC**

▶ Explain the procedure to the patient.

▶ Weigh the patient. To determine ultrafiltration requirements, compare his present weight to his weight after the last dialysis and his target weight. Record his baseline vital signs.

▶ Help the patient into a comfortable position (supine or sitting in a recliner chair with his feet elevated). Make sure the access site is well supported and resting on a clean drape.

▶ Wash your hands. **CDC**

Beginning hemodialysis with a double-lumen catheter

▶ Clamp the catheter tubing to prevent air from entering either lumen of the catheter.

▶ Prepare a sterile field with the sterile drapes and place the sterile 4″ × 4″ gauze pads on it.

▶ Identify the red and blue ports and place them near the sterile field. Place

Hemodialysis access sites

Hemodialysis requires vascular access. The site and type of access may vary, depending on the expected duration of dialysis, the surgeon's preference, and the patient's condition.

Subclavian vein catheterization

Using the Seldinger technique, the physician or surgeon inserts an introducer needle into the subclavian vein. He then inserts a guide wire through the introducer needle and removes the needle. Using the guide wire, he then threads a 5″ to 12″ (12.7- to 30.5-cm) plastic or Teflon catheter (with a Y-hub) into the patient's vein.

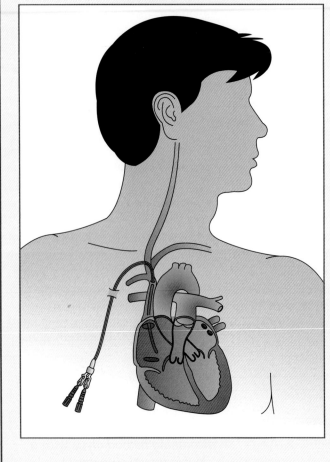

Arteriovenous fistula

To create a fistula, the surgeon makes an incision into the patient's wrist or lower forearm and then a small incision in the side of an artery and another in the side of a vein. He sutures the edges of the incisions together to make a common opening 3 to 7 mm long.

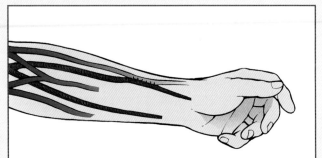

Arteriovenous graft

To create a graft, the surgeon makes an incision in the patient's forearm, upper arm, or thigh. He then tunnels a natural or synthetic graft under the skin and sutures the distal end to an artery and the proximal end to a vein.

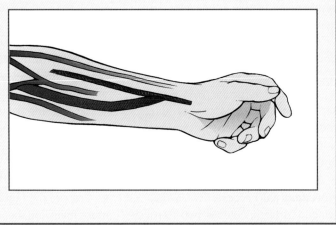

the dialyzer arterial and venous blood lines near the field.

▶ Put on sterile gloves and clean each catheter extension tube, clamp, and luer-lock injection cap with antiseptic. Place a sterile drape beneath the catheter tubing.

▶ Remove and discard the luer-lock cap on the red port and replace it with a 3-ml syringe. Unclamp the red port, aspirate 1.5 to 3 ml of blood, and reclamp the port. Remove the syringe.

▶ Connect one 5-ml syringe with anticoagulant flush to the red port, aspirate

1.5 to 3 ml of blood, and gently instill the flush. Reclamp the red port. Repeat the process with the blue port.

▶ Remove the syringe from the red port, and attach the red port to the line leading to the arterial port of the dialyzer.

▶ Remove the syringe from the blue port, and attach the blue port to the line leading to the venous port of the dialyzer.

▶ Administer the prescribed anticoagulant into the dialyzer. This prevents clotting in the extracorporeal circuit.

▶ Secure the tubing to the patient to reduce tension on the connections and prevent trauma to the catheter insertion site. Open the clamps to the arterial and venous dialyzer tubing.

▶ Begin hemodialysis treatment according to your facility's policy.

▶ Monitor the patient's condition and vital signs according to your facility's policy.

▶ Administer medications and obtain clotting times during hemodialysis, as ordered.

Beginning hemodialysis with AV access

▶ Assess the AV access site for patency. Check for the quality of the thrill and auscultate the bruit. Check for the presence of swelling, edema, erythema, or drainage.

▶ Prepare the two fistula needles by attaching a 10-ml syringe to each. Draw up the prescribed flush solution into each syringe, and prime and clamp the tubing.

▶ Place the patient's access limb on a sterile drape.

▶ Put on sterile gloves.

▶ Using sterile technique, clean a 3″ × 10″ (7.5 × 25.5 cm) area of the skin over the AV access with antiseptic swabs. Begin at the proposed needle insertion site, and swab outward in concentric circles for 1 minute. Discard the swab.

▶ Using a second antiseptic swab, repeat the previous skin cleaning procedure for a second full minute. Discard the swab.

▶ If the access is an AV fistula, apply a tourniquet above the fistula to distend the veins and facilitate the puncture. Avoid occluding the fistula.

▶ Put on clean gloves.

▶ Remove the needle guard on the first fistula needle (arterial), and squeeze the wings together. Insert the arterial needle into the fistula or graft at least 1″ (2.5 cm) from the arterial-venous anastomotic site. Be careful not to puncture the posterior wall of the access.

▶ Release the tourniquet, and flush the needle with anticoagulant solution to prevent clotting. Clamp the arterial needle tubing with a hemostat and secure the wing tips of the needle to the skin with adhesive tape to prevent accidental dislodging of the needle.

▶ Perform the second access (venous) puncture with the other fistula needle, a few inches proximal to the arterial needle. Be careful not to puncture the posterior wall of the access.

▶ Flush the needle with anticoagulant solution. Clamp the venous needle tubing with the second hemostat, and secure the wing tips of the venous needle to the patient's skin with adhesive tape.

▶ Remove the syringe from the end of the arterial needle tubing, uncap the arterial dialyzer tubing, and connect the two lines. Tape the connection securely to prevent accidental separation of the tubing.

▶ Remove the syringe from the end of the venous needle tubing, uncap the venous dialyzer tubing, and connect the two lines. Tape the connection securely to prevent accidental separation of the tubing.

▶ Remove the hemostats from the tubing and begin hemodialysis treatment.

▶ Monitor the patient's condition and vital signs according to your facility's policy.

▶ Administer medications and obtain clotting times, as ordered.

Discontinuing hemodialysis with a double-lumen catheter

▶ Wash your hands, and put on appropriate personal protective equipment.

▶ Open the syringes, luer-lock caps, and gauze pads, and place them on a sterile field.

▶ Fill the two 5-ml syringes with the prescribed amount of anticoagulant flush.

▶ Fill the two 10-ml syringes with normal saline solution. **MFR**

▶ Clamp the tubing to the red and the blue catheter ports and the blood lines to the dialyzer.

▶ Place a sterile drape beneath the ports.

▶ Clean the connection points on the catheter, the clamps, and the blood lines with antiseptic solution.

▶ Place a clean drape under the catheter and place two sterile 4″ × 4″ gauze pads beneath the catheter ports.

▶ Soak the other 4″ × 4″ gauze pads with antiseptic.

▶ Put on sterile gloves.

▶ Grasp the red port connection with the gauze pad, and disconnect it from the arterial dialyzer tubing.

▶ Attach the 10-ml syringe (with normal saline) to the red port on the catheter and slowly flush the tubing.

▶ Replace the 10-ml syringe on the red port with the 5-ml syringe filled with the prescribed anticoagulant flush and instill it. Remove the syringe, and cap the port with a sterile luer-lock cap.

▶ Grasp the blue port connection with the gauze pad and disconnect it from the venous dialyzer tubing.

▶ Attach the 10-ml syringe (with normal saline) to the blue catheter port and slowly flush the tubing.

▶ Replace the 10-ml syringe on the blue port with the 5-ml syringe filled with the prescribed anticoagulant flush and instill it. Remove the syringe, and cap the port with a sterile luer-lock cap. Clamp both ports.

▶ When catheter care is complete, redress the insertion site, apply povidone-iodine ointment to the site, and obtain a drainage sample for culture, if necessary. **CDC**

▶ Obtain the patient's post-dialysis weight, vital signs, and neurologic, respiratory, and hemodynamic parameters and compare them to his predialysis baseline.

▶ Rinse and disinfect the delivery system according to the manufacturer's instructions.

Discontinuing hemodialysis with AV access

▶ Wash your hands.

▶ Turn the blood pump on the hemodialysis machine to 50 to 100 ml/minute.

▶ Put on clean gloves.

▶ Remove the tape from the connection site of the arterial lines. Clamp the needle tubing with the hemostat and disconnect the lines. The blood in the arterial line will continue to flow toward the dialyzer, followed by a column of air. Clamp the blood line with another hemostat just before the blood reaches the point where the saline enters the line.

▶ Unclamp the saline solution to allow a small amount of saline to flow through the line. Unclamp the hemostat on the dialyzer line. This allows all blood to flow into the dialyzer where it passes through the filter and back to the patient through the venous line.

▶ After the blood is re-transfused, clamp the venous needle tubing and the dialyzer's venous line with hemostats and turn off the blood pump.

▶ Remove the tape from the connection site of the venous lines and disconnect the lines.

▶ Remove the venipuncture needle completely, and then apply pressure to

the site with a folded 4″ × 4″ gauze pad using two fingers. If inadequate pressure is used, a hematoma may develop. If excessive pressure is used, the access may thrombose. You should continue to feel a thrill above and below the compression site while holding pressure. Bleeding usually stops within 10 minutes.

▶ Apply a dry, sterile dressing to the site. Avoid circumferential taping of the dressing.

▶ Repeat the procedure on the arterial needle and site.

▶ When dialysis is complete, weigh the patient, obtain his vital signs (including blood pressure sitting and standing), and assess his mental status. Compare these to the pre-dialysis assessment data.

▶ Rinse and disinfect the delivery system according to the manufacturer's instructions.

Special considerations

▶ Obtain blood samples from the patient, as ordered. Samples are usually drawn before beginning hemodialysis.

▶ Immediately report any machine malfunction or equipment defect.

▶ Don't inject I.V. fluids or medications into either port of the double-lumen catheter.

▶ If, while instilling the anticoagulant flush into either port, you meet resistance, stop flushing immediately. Clamp the port, replace the sterile luer-lock cap, and notify the practitioner. Place a "do not use" message on the port until its patency is verified.

▶ If the patient receives meals during dialysis, make sure they're light.

▶ Bacterial endotoxins in the dialysate may cause fever. Rapid fluid removal and electrolyte changes during hemo-

dialysis can cause early dialysis disequilibrium syndrome. Signs and symptoms include headache, nausea, vomiting, restlessness, hypertension, muscle cramps, backache, and seizures.

▶ Some complications of hemodialysis can be fatal. For example, an air embolism can result if the dialyzer retains air, if tubing connections become loose, or if the saline solution container empties. Symptoms include chest pain, dyspnea, coughing, and cyanosis.

References

Hadaway, L. "Technology of Flushing Vascular Access Devices," *Journal of Infusion Nursing* 29(3):129-45, May-June 2006.

Kaveh, K., et al. "The New Arteriovenous Fistula: The Need for Earlier Intervention," *Seminars in Dialysis* 18:1, 3-7, 2005.

Konner, K. "History of Vascular Access for Haemodyalisis," *Nephrology, Dialysis, Transplantation* 20(12):2629-635, December 2005.

Lynn-McHale Wiegand, D.J., and Carlson, K.K., eds. *AACN Procedure Manual for Critical Care,* 5th ed. Philadelphia: W.B. Saunders Co., 2005.

National Kidney Foundation NKF/KDOQI Guidelines. Clinical Practice Guidelines and Clinical Practice Recommendation for Hemodialysis Adequacy, 2006 update. Available at *www.kidney.org/professionals/kdoqi/guideline_upHD_PD_VA/index.htm.*

Safdar, N., et al. "The Pathogenesis of Catheter-Related Bloodstream Infection with Non-cuffed Short-term Central Venous Catheters," *Intensive Care Medicine* 30(1):62-67, 2004.

Holter monitoring

Holter monitoring (also called *continuous electrocardiograph monitoring*) allows for the measurement of blood pressure and cardiac activity over time without confining the patient to a facility. Holter monitoring records variations in electrocardiogram (ECG) waveforms during normal activity.

Indications for Holter monitoring include evaluating the status of a patient recuperating from a myocardial infarction who has left ventricular dysfunction, evaluating arrhythmias in a patient with heart failure or idiopathic cardiomyopathy, assessing pacemaker function and assisting in optimal programming, evaluating cardiac signs and symptoms (syncope), evaluating the type and frequency of cardiac arrhythmias, assessing the effect of prescribed antiarrhythmics, and determining the relationship among cardiac events, the patient's symptoms, and associated cardiac symptoms. **ACC**

Monitoring can span over a 24-hour period, or the ECG rhythm may be recorded intermittently when the patient experiences symptoms and then triggers the device. Such intermittent monitoring may occur over 7 to 30 days, and the data may be periodically transmitted to the practitioner's office over the telephone. (See *Holter monitoring*.)

Equipment

Holter unit with new battery ◆ cable wires ◆ disposable pregelled electrodes ◆ carrying case with strap ◆ 4″ × 4″ gauze pads ◆ soap and water ◆ logbook or diary ◆ optional: clippers.

Implementation

▶ Confirm the patient's identity using two patient identifiers according to your facility's policy. **JC**

▶ Ask the patient if he's allergic to electrode gel.

▶ Place the equipment into the carrying case and connect the neck strap.

▶ As appropriate, tell the patient that you need to clip the hairs on his chest so that you can place the electrodes properly. After clipping, wash the areas with soap and water to remove body oils.

▶ Connect the wires to the electrodes and to the monitor.

▶ Apply each electrode to the patient's chest by removing the paper backing, securing the edges of the electrode, and then pressing the center to ensure proper contact.

▶ Show the patient how to reattach loosened electrodes by depressing the

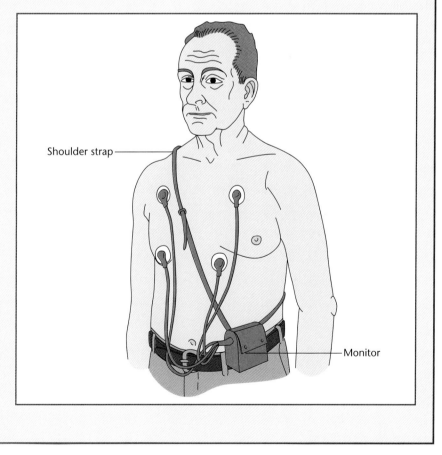

Holter monitoring

In this illustration, the monitor is attached to an over-the-shoulder strap. The monitor continuously records the electrical activity of the heart through electrodes attached to the chest.

Shoulder strap

Monitor

center; tell him to return to the office if an electrode becomes fully dislodged.

▶ Tell the patient to avoid magnets, metal detectors, high-voltage areas, and electric blankets, which may cause artifacts or interfere with monitoring.

Special considerations

▶ If the patient's skin is extremely oily, scaly, or diaphoretic, wash the patient's chest with water, and then rub dry with a 4″ × 4″ gauze pad before applying the electrodes.

▶ If the patient can't return to the office immediately after the monitoring period, show him how to remove the equipment and store the monitor and log.

▶ If the patient is wearing a patient-activated ECG, tell him that he can wear the monitor for up to 7 days. Show him how to initiate the recording manually when symptoms occur.

▶ Tell the patient that he'll need to maintain an activity log during the 24-hour monitoring period. He should record the time, activities he performs, and any symptoms (such as headache, dizziness, light-headedness, palpitations, or chest pain) that occur.

▶ Tell the patient that he can sponge bathe, but that he can't get the equipment wet.

References

American College of Cardiology and American Heart Association. "ACC/AHA Clinical Competence Statement on Electrocardiography and Ambulatory Electrocardiography," *Circulation* 104:3169-178, December 2001.

Funk, M., et al. "Feasibility of Using Ambulatory Electrocardiographic Monitors Following Discharge after Cardiac Surgery," *Home Healthcare Nurse* 23(7):441-49, July 2005.

Rockx, M.A., et al. "Is Ambulatory Monitoring for 'Community-Acquired' Syncope Economically Attractive? A Cost-Effectiveness Analysis of a Randomized Trial of External Loop Recorders Versus Holter Monitoring," *American Heart Journal* 150(5):1065, November 2005.

Hot and cold eye compresses

Whether applied hot or cold, eye compresses are soothing and therapeutic. Hot compresses may be used to relieve discomfort from trauma, injury, or infection. Because heat increases circulation, hot compresses may promote drainage of superficial infections. On the other hand, cold compresses can reduce swelling or bleeding and relieve itching. Because cold numbs sensory fibers, cold compresses may be ordered to ease periorbital discomfort between prescribed doses of pain medication. Typically, a hot or cold compress should be applied for 20-minute periods, four to six times per day. Ocular infection calls for the use of sterile technique.

Equipment

For hot compresses: Gloves ◆ prescribed solution, usually sterile water or normal saline solution ◆ sterile bowl ◆ sterile 4″ × 4″ gauze pads ◆ towel.

   For cold compresses: Small plastic bag or glove ◆ ice chips ◆ ¹/₂″ hypoallergenic tape ◆ towel ◆ sterile 4″ × 4″ gauze pads ◆ sterile water, normal saline solution, or prescribed ophthalmic irrigant ◆ gloves.

Implementation

▶ Confirm the patient's identity using two patient identifiers according to your facility's policy. **JC**

▶ Explain the procedure to the patient, ensure his comfort, and provide privacy.

Applying a hot compress

▶ Place a capped bottle of sterile water or normal saline solution in a bowl of hot water or under a stream of hot tap water. Allow the solution to become warm, not hot (no higher than 120° F [48.9° C]). Pour the warm water or saline solution into a sterile bowl, filling the bowl about halfway. Place some sterile gauze pads into the bowl.

▶ Wash your hands and put on gloves. If the patient has an eye patch, remove it. **CDC**

▶ Drape a towel around the patient's shoulder.

Applying an eye patch

With a practitioner's order, you may apply an eye patch for various reasons: to protect the eye after injury or surgery, to prevent accidental damage to an anesthetized eye, to promote healing, to absorb secretions, or to prevent the patient from touching or rubbing his eye.

   A thicker patch, called a pressure patch, may be used to help corneal abrasions heal, compress postoperative edema, or control hemorrhage from traumatic injury. Application requires an ophthalmologist's prescription and supervision.

To apply a patch, choose a gauze pad of appropriate size for the patient's face, place it gently over the closed eye (as shown), and secure it with two or three strips of tape. Extend the tape from the midforehead across the eye to below the earlobe.

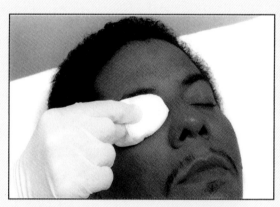

A pressure patch, which is markedly thicker than a single-thickness gauze patch, exerts extra tension against the closed eye. After placing the initial gauze pad, build it up with additional gauze pieces. Tape it firmly so that the patch exerts even pressure against the closed eye (as shown).

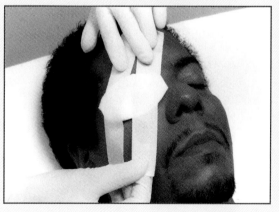

(continued)

Applying an eye patch (continued)

For increased protection of an injured eye, place a plastic or metal shield (as shown) on top of the gauze pads and apply tape over the shield.

Occasionally, you may use a head dressing to secure a pressure patch. The dressing applies additional pressure or, in burn patients, holds the patch in place without tape.

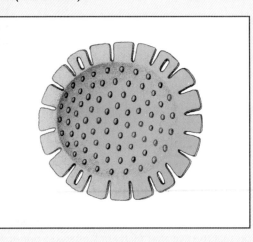

▶ Take two 4″ × 4″ gauze pads from the basin. Squeeze out the excess solution.

▶ Instruct the patient to close his eyes. Gently apply the pads to the affected eye.

▶ Change the compress every few minutes, as necessary, for the prescribed length of time. After removing each compress, check the patient's skin for signs that the compress solution is too hot.

Applying a cold compress

▶ Place ice chips in a plastic bag (or a glove, if necessary) to make an ice pack. Remove excess air from the bag or glove, and knot the open end. Cut a piece of hypoallergenic tape to secure the ice pack. Place all equipment on the bedside stand near the patient.

▶ Moisten the middle of one of the sterile 4″ × 4″ gauze pads with the sterile water, normal saline solution, or ophthalmic irrigating solution.

▶ Tell the patient to close his eyes, and then place the moist gauze pad over the affected eye.

▶ Place the ice pack on top of the gauze pad, and tape it in place. If the patient complains of pain, remove the ice pack. Some patients may have an adverse reaction to cold.

▶ After 15 to 20 minutes, remove the tape, ice pack, and gauze pad and discard them.

Concluding the procedure

▶ Use the remaining sterile 4″ × 4″ gauze pads to clean and dry the patient's face.

▶ If ordered, apply ophthalmic ointment or an eye patch. (See *Applying an eye patch*, pages 241 and 242.)

Special considerations

▶ When applying hot compresses, change the prescribed solution as frequently as necessary to maintain a constant temperature.

▶ If ordered to apply moist, cold compresses directly to the patient's eyelid, fill a bowl with ice and water and soak the 4″ × 4″ gauze pads in it. Place a compress directly on the lid; change compresses every 2 to 3 minutes.

References

Gardner, J.S. "Hospital Infection Control Practices Advisory Committee Guidelines for Isolation Precautions in Hospitals," *Infection Control and Hospital Epidemiology* 17:53-80, January 1996.

Taylor, C., et al. *Fundamentals of Nursing: The Art and Science of Nursing Care,* 6th ed. Philadelphia: Lippincott Williams & Wilkins, 2008.

Hyperthermia-hypothermia blanket

A blanket-sized aquathermia pad, the hyperthermia-hypothermia blanket raises, lowers, or maintains body temperature through conductive heat or cold transfer between the blanket and the patient. It can be operated manually or automatically.

In manual operation, the nurse or physician sets the temperature on the unit. The blanket reaches and maintains this temperature regardless of the patient's temperature. The temperature control must be adjusted manually to reach a different setting. The nurse monitors the patient's body temperature with a conventional thermometer.

In automatic operation, the unit directly and continually monitors the patient's temperature by means of a thermistor probe (rectal, skin, or esophageal) and alternates heating and cooling cycles as necessary to achieve and maintain the desired body temperature. The blanket is most commonly used to reduce high fever when more conservative measures—such as baths, ice packs, and antipyretics—are unsuccessful. Its other uses include maintaining normal temperature during surgery or shock; inducing hypothermia during surgery to decrease metabolic activity and thereby reduce oxygen requirements; reducing intracranial pressure; controlling bleeding and intractable pain in patients with amputations, burns, or cancer; and providing warmth in cases of severe hypothermia.

Equipment

Hyperthermia-hypothermia control unit ◆ fluid for the control unit (distilled water or distilled water and 20% ethyl alcohol) ◆ thermistor probe ◆ patient thermometer ◆ one or two hyperthermia-hypothermia blankets ◆ one or two disposable blanket covers (or one or two sheets or bath blankets) ◆ lanolin or a mixture of lanolin and cold cream ◆ adhesive tape ◆ towel ◆ sphygmomanometer ◆ gloves, if necessary ◆ optional: protective wraps for the patient's hands and feet.

Implementation

▶ Review the practitioner's order, and prepare one or two blankets by covering them with disposable covers (or use a sheet or bath blanket when positioning the blanket on the patient).

▶ Connect the blanket to the control unit, and set the controls for manual or automatic operation and for the desired blanket or body temperature. Make sure the machine is properly grounded before plugging it in. **MFR**

▶ Turn on the machine, and add liquid to the unit reservoir, if necessary, as fluid fills the blanket. Allow the blanket to preheat or precool so that the patient receives immediate thermal benefit. Place the control unit at the foot of the bed.

▶ Confirm the patient's identity using two patient identifiers according to your facility's policy. **JC**

▶ Assess the patient's condition, and explain the procedure to him. Provide privacy, and make sure the room is warm and free from drafts.

▶ Check your facility's policy and, if necessary, make sure the patient or a responsible family member has signed a consent form.

▶ Wash your hands thoroughly. If the patient isn't already wearing a patient gown, ask him to put one on. Use a gown with cloth ties rather than metal snaps or pins to prevent heat or cold injury.

▶ Take the patient's temperature to serve as a baseline.

▶ Keeping the bottom sheet in place and the patient recumbent, roll the patient to one side and slide the rolled

blanket halfway underneath him so that its top edge aligns with his neck. Then roll the patient back, and pull and flatten the blanket across the bed. Place a pillow under the patient's head. Make sure his head doesn't lie directly on the blanket because the blanket's rigid surface may be uncomfortable, and the heat or cold may lead to tissue breakdown. Use a sheet or bath blanket as insulation between the patient and the blanket. (See *Using a cooling system,* page 244.)

▶ Apply lanolin or a mixture of lanolin and cold cream to the patient's skin where it touches the blanket to help protect the skin from heat or cold sensation.

▶ In automatic operation, insert the thermistor probe in the patient's rectum, and tape it in place to prevent accidental dislodgment. If rectal insertion is contraindicated, tuck a skin probe deep into the axilla, and secure it with tape. Plug the other end of the probe into the correct jack on the unit's control panel.

▶ Place a sheet or, if ordered, the second hyperthermia-hypothermia blan-

Using a cooling system

A hypothermia or cooling blanket is used to lower a patient's body temperature. The pad has coils that circulate a chilled solution. While the blanket is in use, you must monitor the patient's temperature, which can be adjusted to help keep his temperature in the ordered range.

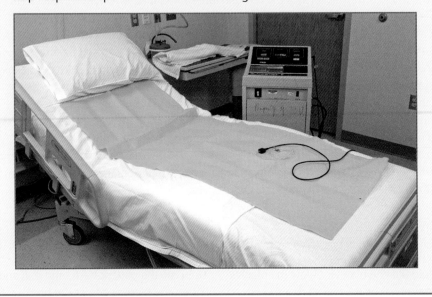

ket over the patient. This increases the thermal benefit by trapping cooled or heated air.

▶ Wrap the patient's hands and feet if he wishes to minimize chilling and promote comfort. Monitor his vital signs, and perform a neurologic assessment every 5 minutes until the desired body temperature is reached and then every 15 minutes until the temperature is stable or as ordered.

▶ Check fluid intake and output hourly or as ordered. Observe the patient regularly for color changes in skin, lips, and nail beds and for edema, induration, inflammation, pain, and sensory impairment. If they occur, discontinue the procedure and notify the practitioner.

▶ Reposition the patient every 30 minutes to 1 hour, unless contraindicated, to prevent skin breakdown. Keep the patient's skin, bedclothes, and blanket cover free from perspiration

Using a warming system

Shivering, the compensatory response to falling body temperature, may use more oxygen than the body can supply—especially in a surgical patient. In the past, patients were covered with blankets to warm their bodies. Now, health care facilities may supply a warming system, such as the Bair Hugger patient-warming system (shown below).

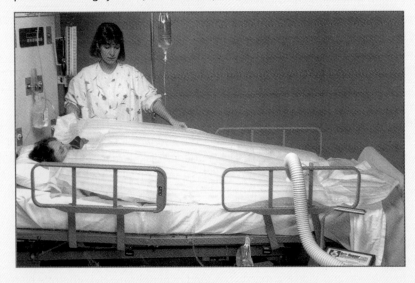

This system helps to gradually increase body temperature by drawing air through a filter, warming the air to the desired temperature, and circulating it through a hose to a warming blanket placed over the patient.

When using the warming system, follow these guidelines:
▶ Use a bath blanket in a single layer over the warming blanket to minimize heat loss.
▶ Place the warming blanket directly over the patient with the paper side facing down and the clear tubular side facing up.
▶ Make sure the connection hose is at the foot of the bed.
▶ Take the patient's temperature during the first 15 to 30 minutes and at least every 30 minutes while the warming blanket is in use.
▶ Obtain guidelines from the patient's practitioner for discontinuing use of the warming blanket.

and condensation, and reapply cream to exposed body parts, as needed.

▶ After turning off the machine, follow the manufacturer's directions. Continue to monitor the patient's temperature until it stabilizes because body temperature can fall as much as 5° F (2.8° C) after this procedure.

▶ Remove all equipment from the bed. Dry the patient and make him comfortable. Supply a fresh patient gown, if necessary. Cover him lightly.

▶ Continue to perform neurologic checks, and monitor the patient's vital signs, fluid intake and output, and his general condition every 30 minutes for 2 hours and then hourly or as ordered.

▶ Return the equipment to the central supply department for cleaning, servicing, and storage.

Special considerations

▶ If the patient shivers excessively during hypothermia treatment, discontinue the procedure, and notify the practitioner immediately. By increasing metabolism, shivering elevates body temperature.

▶ Avoid lowering the temperature more than 1° F (0.2° C) every 15 minutes to prevent premature ventricular contractions.

▶ Don't use pins to secure catheters, tubes, or blanket covers because an accidental puncture of the blanket can result in fluid leakage and burns.

▶ With hyperthermia or hypothermia therapy, the patient may experience a secondary defense reaction (vasoconstriction or vasodilation, respectively) that causes body temperature to rebound and thus defeat the treatment's purpose.

▶ To avoid bacterial growth in the reservoir or blankets, always use sterile distilled water and change it monthly. Check to see if your facility's policy calls for adding a bacteriostatic agent to the water. Avoid using deionized water because it may corrode the system. **MFR**

▶ To gradually increase body temperature, especially in postoperative patients, the practitioner may order a disposable warming system. (See *Using a warming system*.)

References

Loke, A.Y., et al. "Comparing the Effectiveness of Two Types of Cooling Blankets for Febrile Patients," *Nursing in Critical Care* 10(5):247-43, September-October 2005.

Mayer, S.A., et al. "Clinical Trial of a Novel Surface Cooling System for Fever Control in Neurocritical Care Patients," *Critical Care Medicine* 32(12):2508-515, December 2004.

I

Implanted port use

Surgically implanted under local anesthesia by a physician, an implanted port consists of a silicone catheter attached to a reservoir, which is covered with a self-sealing silicone rubber septum. It's used most commonly when an external central venous (CV) access device isn't desirable for long-term I.V. therapy. One- and two-piece ports with single or double lumens are available. (See *Understanding implanted ports.*)

Implanted ports come in two basic types: top entry—the most commonly used—and side entry. The reservoir can be made of titanium, stainless steel, or molded plastic. The type and lumen size selected depend on the patient's needs.

Implanted in a pocket under the skin, an implanted port functions much like a long-term CV access device, except that it has no external parts. The attached indwelling catheter tunnels through the subcutaneous tissue so that the catheter tip lies in a central vein—for example, the subclavian vein. An implanted

Understanding implanted ports

An implanted port is typically used to deliver intermittent infusions of medication, chemotherapy, and blood products. Implanted ports offer several advantages over external central venous therapy. Because the device is completely covered by the patient's skin, the risk of extrinsic contamination is reduced. In addition, the patient may prefer this type of central line because it doesn't alter body image and requires less routine catheter care.

The port consists of a catheter connected to a small reservoir. A septum designed to withstand multiple punctures seals the reservoir. To access the port, a special non-coring needle is inserted perpendicular to the reservoir.

Accessing an implanted port

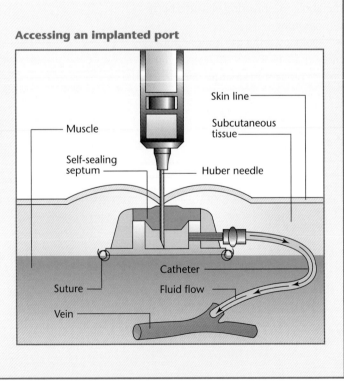

port can also be used for arterial access or can be implanted into the epidural space, peritoneum, or pericardial or pleural cavity.

Typically, implanted ports deliver intermittent infusions. They're used to deliver chemotherapy and other drugs, I.V. fluids, and blood. They can also be used to obtain blood samples.

Implanted ports offer several advantages, including minimal activity restrictions, few steps for the patient to perform, and few dressing changes (except when used to maintain continuous infusions or intermittent infusion devices). Implanted devices are easier to maintain than external devices. For instance, they require heparinization only once after each use (or periodically if not in use). They also pose less risk of infection because they have no exit site to serve as an entry for microorganisms.

Implanted ports create only a slight protrusion under the skin, so many patients find them easier to accept than external infusion devices. Because they're implanted, however, they may be harder for the patient to manage, particularly if drugs or fluids are to be administered frequently. And because accessing the device requires inserting a needle through subcutaneous tissue, patients who fear or dislike needle punctures may be uncomfortable using an implanted port and may require a local anesthetic. In addition, implantation and removal of the device require surgery and hospitalization. The cost of implanted ports makes them worthwhile only for patients who require infusion therapy for at least 6 months.

Implanted ports are contraindicated in patients who have been unable to tolerate other implanted devices and in those who may develop an allergic reaction.

Equipment

To implant a port: Noncoring needles (a noncoring needle has a deflected point, which slices the port's septum) of appropriate type and gauge with attached extension set tubing ◆ port ◆ sterile gloves ◆ mask ◆ alcohol pads ◆ chlorhexidine ◆ local anesthetic (lidocaine without epinephrine) ◆ ice pack ◆ 10- and 20-ml syringes ◆ prefilled saline flush syringe ◆ I.V. solution ◆ sterile dressings ◆ luer-lock injection cap ◆ clamp ◆ adhesive skin closures ◆ suture removal set.

To access the port: Noncoring needles of appropriate type and gauge with attached extension set tubing ◆ sterile gloves ◆ chlorhexidine ◆ local anesthetic (lidocaine without epinephrine) as needed ◆ ice pack ◆ 10-ml syringe ◆ 10 ml syringe prefilled with normal saline solution ◆ transparent semipermeable dressing ◆ luer-lock injection cap.

To administer a bolus injection: Noncoring needle of appropriate type and gauge with attached extension set tubing ◆ clamp ◆ 10-ml syringe filled with normal saline solution ◆ syringe containing the prescribed medication ◆ optional: sterile syringe filled with heparin flush solution.

To administer a continuous infusion: Prescribed I.V. solution or drug ◆ I.V. administration set ◆ filter, if ordered ◆ noncoring needle of appropriate type and gauge with attached extension set tubing ◆ clamp ◆ 10-ml syringe filled with normal saline solution ◆ adhesive tape ◆ sterile 2″ x 2″ gauze pad ◆ sterile tape ◆ transparent semipermeable dressing.

Some facilities use an implantable port access kit.

Implementation

▶ Confirm the size and type of the device and the insertion site with the physician. Prime the tubing and the noncoring needle with the extension set. All priming must be done using strict sterile technique, and all tubing must be free from air. After you've primed the tubing, recheck all connections for tightness. Make sure all open ends are covered with sealed caps.

▶ Wash your hands.

Assisting with implantation of an implanted port

▶ Reinforce to the patient the physician's explanation of the procedure, its benefit to the patient, and what's expected of him during and after implantation.

▶ Although the physician is responsible for obtaining consent for the procedure, make sure the written document is signed, witnessed, and on the chart.

▶ Allay the patient's fears and answer questions about movement restrictions, cosmetic concerns, and management regimens.

▶ Check the patient's history for hypersensitivity to local anesthetics or iodine.

▶ The physician will surgically implant the port, probably using a local anesthetic. Occasionally, a patient may receive a general anesthetic for implantation.

▶ During the implantation procedure, you may be responsible for handing equipment and supplies to the physician. First, the physician makes a small incision and introduces the catheter, typically into the superior vena cava

Managing common implanted port problems

PROBLEMS AND POSSIBLE CAUSES	NURSING INTERVENTIONS
Inability to flush the device or draw blood	
Kinked tubing or closed clamp	▶ Check the tubing or clamp.
Catheter lodged against vessel wall	▶ Reposition the patient. ▶ Teach the patient to change his position to free the catheter from the vessel wall. ▶ Raise the arm that's on the same side as the catheter. ▶ Roll the patient to his opposite side. ▶ Have the patient cough, sit up, or take a deep breath. ▶ Infuse 10 ml of normal saline solution into the catheter. ▶ Regain access to the port using a new needle.
Incorrect needle placement or needle not advanced through septum	▶ Regain access to the device. ▶ Teach the home care patient to push down firmly on the noncoring needle device in the septum and to verify needle placement by aspirating for blood return.
Clot formation	▶ Assess patency by trying to flush the port while the patient changes position. ▶ Notify the practitioner; obtain an order for instillation of a fibrinolytic agent. ▶ Teach the patient to recognize clot formation, to notify the practitioner if it occurs, and to avoid forcibly flushing the port.
Kinked catheter, catheter migration, or port rotation	▶ Notify the practitioner immediately. ▶ Tell the patient to notify the practitioner if he has trouble using the port.
Inability to palpate the device	
Deeply implanted port	▶ Note portal chamber scar. ▶ Use deep palpation technique. ▶ Ask another nurse to try locating the port. ▶ Use a ½″ or 2″ noncoring needle to gain access to the port.

through the subclavian, jugular, or cephalic vein. After fluoroscopy verifies correct placement of the catheter tip, the physician creates a subcutaneous pocket over a bony prominence in the chest wall. Then he tunnels the catheter to the pocket. Next, he connects the catheter to the reservoir, places the reservoir in the pocket, and flushes it with heparin solution. Finally, he sutures the reservoir to the underlying fascia and closes the incision.

Preparing to access the port

▶ The port can be used immediately after placement, although some edema and tenderness may persist for about 72 hours. This makes the device initially difficult to palpate and slightly uncomfortable for the patient.

▶ Prepare to access the port, following the specific steps for top-entry or side-entry ports.

▶ Using sterile technique, inspect the area around the port for signs of infection and skin breakdown.

▶ Place an ice pack over the area for several minutes to alleviate possible discomfort from the needle puncture. Alternatively, administer a local anesthetic after cleaning the area.

▶ Wash your hands thoroughly. Put on sterile gloves, and wear them throughout the procedure. **CDC**

▶ Clean the area with chlorhexidine. **INS**

▶ If your facility's policy calls for a local anesthetic, check the patient's record for possible allergies. As indicated, anesthetize the insertion site by injecting 0.1 ml of lidocaine (without epinephrine).

Accessing a top-entry port

▶ Palpate the area over the port to find the port septum.

▶ Anchor the port with your nondominant hand. Then, using your dominant hand, aim the needle at the center of the device.

▶ Insert the needle perpendicular to the port septum. Push the needle

Risks of implanted port therapy

COMPLICATION	SIGNS AND SYMPTOMS	POSSIBLE CAUSES	NURSING INTERVENTIONS
Site infection or skin breakdown	▶ Erythema and warmth at port site ▶ Oozing or purulent drainage at port site or pocket ▶ Fever	▶ Infected incision or port pocket ▶ Poor postoperative healing	▶ Assess the site daily for redness; note any drainage. ▶ Notify the practitioner. ▶ Administer antibiotics as prescribed. ▶ Apply warm soaks for 20 minutes four times per day. **Prevention** ▶ Teach the patient to inspect for and report redness, swelling, drainage, or skin breakdown at the port site.
Extravasation	▶ Burning sensation or swelling in subcutaneous tissue	▶ Needle dislodged into subcutaneous tissue ▶ Needle incorrectly placed in port ▶ Needle position not confirmed; needle pulled out of septum ▶ Use of vesicant drugs ▶ Rupture of catheter along tunnel route	▶ Stop the infusion, but don't remove the needle. ▶ Notify the practitioner; prepare to administer an antidote, if ordered. **Prevention** ▶ Teach the patient how to gain access to the device, verify its placement, and secure the needle before initiating an infusion.
Thrombosis	▶ Inability to flush port or administer infusion	▶ Frequent blood sampling ▶ Infusion of packed red blood cells (RBCs)	▶ Notify the practitioner; obtain an order to administer a fibrinolytic agent. **Prevention** ▶ Flush the port thoroughly right after obtaining a blood sample. ▶ Administer packed RBCs as a piggyback with normal saline solution and use an infusion pump; flush with saline solution between units. **INS**
Fibrin sheath formation	▶ Blocked port and catheter lumen ▶ Inability to flush port or administer infusion ▶ Possibly swelling, tenderness, and erythema in neck, chest, and shoulder	▶ Adherence of platelets to catheter	▶ Notify the practitioner; prepare to administer a thrombolytic agent. **Prevention** ▶ Use the port only to infuse fluids and medications; don't use it to obtain blood samples. ▶ Administer only compatible substances through the port.

through the skin and septum until you reach the bottom of the reservoir.
▶ Check needle placement by aspirating for blood return.
▶ If you can't obtain blood, remove the needle and repeat the procedure.

Ask the patient to raise his arms and perform Valsalva's maneuver. If you still don't get blood return, notify the physician; a fibrin sleeve on the distal end of the catheter may be occluding the opening. (See *Managing common implanted port problems* and *Risks of implanted port therapy*.)
▶ Flush the device with normal saline solution. If you detect swelling or if the patient reports pain at the site, remove the needle and notify the physician.

Continuous infusion: Securing the needle

When starting a continuous infusion, you must secure the right-angle, noncoring needle to the skin. If the needle hub is flush with the skin, apply a transparent, semipermeable dressing over the entire site. If the needle hub isn't flush with the skin, place a folded sterile dressing under the hub, as shown below. Then apply sterile adhesive skin closures across it.

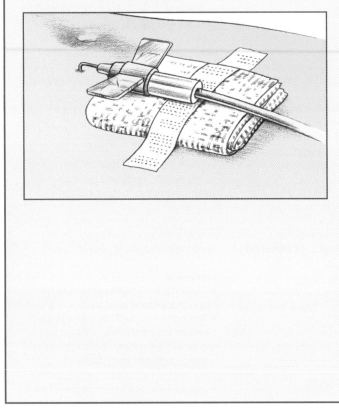

Secure the needle and tubing, using the Chevron taping technique using sterile tape.

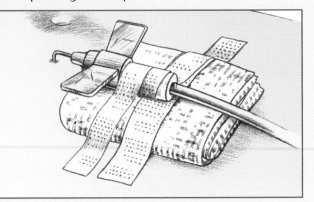

Apply a transparent semipermeable dressing over the entire site.

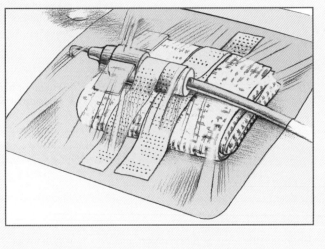

Accessing a side-entry port

▶ To gain access to a side-entry port, follow the same procedure as with a top-entry port, but insert the needle parallel to the reservoir instead of perpendicular to it.

Administering a bolus injection

▶ Attach the 10-ml syringe filled with saline solution to the end of the extension set of the noncoring needle and remove all the air. Check for blood return. Then flush the port with normal saline solution according to your facility's policy.

▶ Clamp the extension set and remove the saline syringe.

▶ Connect the medication syringe to the extension set. Open the clamp and inject the drug as ordered.

▶ Examine the skin surrounding the needle for signs of infiltration, such as swelling and tenderness. If you note these signs, stop the injection and intervene appropriately.

▶ When the injection is complete, clamp the extension set and remove the medication syringe.

▶ Open the clamp and flush with 5 ml of normal saline solution after each drug injection to minimize drug incompatibility reactions.

▶ Flush with heparin solution according to your facility's policy.

Administering a continuous infusion

▶ Remove all air from the extension set of the noncoring needle by priming it with an attached syringe of normal saline solution.

▶ Flush the port system with normal saline solution. Clamp the extension set and remove the syringe.

▶ Connect the administration set, and secure the connections with sterile tape, if necessary.

▶ Unclamp the extension set and begin the infusion.

▶ Affix the needle to the skin. Then apply a transparent semipermeable dressing. (See *Continuous infusion: Securing the needle*.)

▶ Examine the site carefully for infiltration. If the patient complains of stinging, burning, or pain at the site, discontinue the infusion and intervene appropriately.

▶ When the solution container is empty, obtain a new I.V. solution container as ordered.

▶ Flush with normal saline solution followed by heparin solution according to your facility's policy.

Special considerations

▶ After implantation, monitor the site for signs of hematoma and bleeding. Edema and tenderness may persist for about 72 hours. The incision site requires routine postoperative care for 7 to 10 days. You'll also need to assess the implantation site for signs of infection, device rotation, and skin erosion. You don't need to apply a dressing to the wound site except during infusions or to maintain an intermittent infusion device.

▶ While the patient is hospitalized, a luer-lock injection cap may be attached to the end of the extension set to provide ready access for intermittent infusions. Besides saving nursing time, a luer-lock cap reduces the discomfort of accessing the port and prolongs the life of the port septum by decreasing the number of needle punctures.

▶ If your patient is receiving a continuous or prolonged infusion, change the transparent dressing and needle every 7 days. However, any dressing should be changed immediately if its integrity is compromised. You'll also need to change the tubing and solution, as you would for a long-term CV infusion. If your patient is receiving an intermittent infusion, flush the port periodically with heparin solution. When the port isn't being used, flush it every 4 weeks. During the course of therapy, you may have to clear a clotted port as ordered. **CDC** **INS**

▶ Besides performing routine care measures, you must be prepared to handle several common problems that may arise during an infusion with a port. These common problems include an inability to flush the port, withdraw blood from it, or palpate it.

References

Centers for Disease Control and Prevention. "Guidelines for the Prevention of Intravascular Device-Related Infections," *MMWR Recommendations and Reports* 51(RR10):1-26, August 9, 2002.

Earhart, A. "Diagnostic Tools and Therapeutic Interventions that May Influence the Integrity of Vascular and Nonvascular Access Devices," *Journal of Infusion Nursing* 28(3 Suppl):S13-S17; quiz S33-S36, May-June 2005.

Jablon, L.K., et al. "Cephalic Vein Cut-Down Versus Percutaneous Access: A Retrospective Study of Complications of Implantable Venous Access Devices," *American Journal of Surgery* 192(1):63-67, July 2006.

Masoorli, S. "Legal Issues Related to Vascular Access Devices and Infusion Therapy," *Journal of Infusion Nursing* 28(3 Suppl):S18-S21; quiz S33-S36, May-June 2006.

Pieger-Mooney, S. "Innovations in Central Vascular Access Device Insertion," *Journal of Infusion Nursing* 28(3 Suppl):S7-S12; quiz S33-S36, May-June 2005.

"Standard 40. Local Anesthesia. Infusion Nursing Standards of Practice," *Journal of Infusion Nursing* 29(1S):S41, January-February 2006.

"Standard 44. Dressings. Infusion Nursing Standards of Practice," *Journal of Infusion Nursing* 29(1S):S44-S45, January-February 2006.

"Standard 45. Implanted Ports and Pumps. Infusion Nursing Standards of Practice," *Journal of Infusion Nursing* 29(1S):S44-S45, January-February 2006.

"Standard 53. Phlebitis. Infusion Nursing Standards of Practice," *Journal of Infusion Nursing* 29(1S):S58-S59, January-February 2006.

"Standard 54. Infiltration. Infusion Nursing Standards of Practice," *Journal of Infusion Nursing* 29(1S):S59-S60, January-February 2006.

Tilton, D. "Central Venous Access Device Infections in the Critical Care Unit," *Critical Care Nursing Quarterly* 29(2):117-22, April-June 2006.

Warren, D.K., et al. "A Multicenter Intervention to Prevent Catheter-Associated Bloodstream Infections," *Infection Control and Hospital Epidemiology* 27(7):662-69, July 2006.

Incentive spirometry

Incentive spirometry involves using a breathing device to help the patient achieve maximal ventilation. The device measures respiratory flow or volume and induces the patient to take a deep breath and hold it for several seconds. This deep breath increases lung volume, boosts alveolar inflation, and promotes venous return. This exercise also establishes alveolar hyperinflation for a longer time than is possible with a normal deep breath, thus preventing and reversing the alveolar collapse that causes atelectasis and pneumonitis.

Five to ten breaths are suggested per session every hour while awake (approximately 100 breaths per day). **AARC**

Devices used for incentive spirometry provide a visual incentive to breathe deeply. Some are activated when the patient inhales a certain volume of air; the device then estimates the amount of air inhaled. Others contain plastic floats, which rise according to the amount of air the patient pulls through the device when he inhales. (See *Types of incentive spirometers*.)

Equipment

Flow or volume incentive spirometer, as indicated, with sterile disposable tube and mouthpiece ◆ stethoscope ◆ watch.

The tube and mouthpiece are sterile on first use and clean on subsequent uses.

Implementation

▶ Confirm the patient's identity using two patient identifiers according to your facility's policy. **JC**
▶ Assemble the ordered equipment at the patient's bedside. Read the manufacturer's instructions for spirometer setup and operation.

▶ Remove the sterile flow tube and mouthpiece from the package, and attach them to the device. Set the flow rate or volume goal as determined by the practitioner and based on the patient's preoperative performance.
▶ Assess the patient's condition.

Types of incentive spirometers

Incentive spirometers are either flow-oriented (right) or volume-oriented (left). The type of incentive spirometer used by the patient is usually determined by the type that's available through the respiratory therapy department.

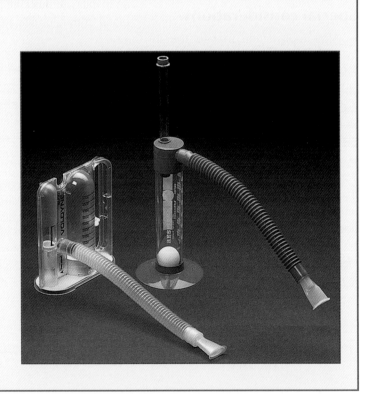

▶ Explain the procedure to the patient, making sure that she understands the importance of performing incentive spirometry regularly.

▶ Wash your hands.

▶ Help the patient into a comfortable sitting or semi-Fowler's position to promote optimal lung expansion. Instruct the patient not to tilt the incentive spirometer because doing so decreases the effort required from the patient and reduces the exercise's effectiveness.

▶ Auscultate the patient's lungs. **AARC**

▶ Instruct the patient to insert the mouthpiece and close her lips tightly around it.

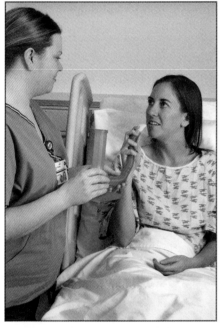

▶ Instruct the patient to exhale normally and then inhale as slowly and as deeply as possible. If she has difficulty with this step, tell her to suck as she would through a straw but more slowly. Ask the patient to retain the entire volume of air she inhaled for 3 seconds or, if you're using a device with a light indicator, until the light turns off (as shown at the top of the next column). **AARC**

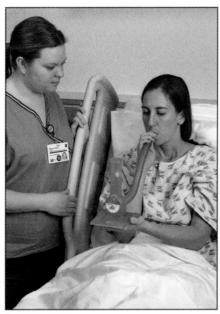

▶ Tell the patient to remove the mouthpiece and exhale normally. Allow her to relax and take several normal breaths before attempting another breath with the spirometer. Repeat this sequence 5 to 10 times during every waking hour. Note tidal volumes. **AARC**

▶ Evaluate the patient's ability to cough effectively, and encourage her to cough after each effort because deep lung inflation may loosen secretions and facilitate their removal. Observe any expectorated secretions.

▶ Auscultate the patient's lungs, and compare findings with the first auscultation. **AARC**

▶ Instruct the patient to remove the mouthpiece. Wash the device in warm water, and shake it dry.

▶ Place the mouthpiece in a plastic storage bag between exercises, and label it and the spirometer, if applicable, with the patient's name to avoid inadvertent use by another patient. **AARC**

Special considerations

▶ If the patient is scheduled for surgery, make a preoperative assessment of her respiratory pattern and capability to ensure the development of appropriate postoperative goals. Teach the patient how to use the spirometer before surgery so that she can focus on your instructions and practice the exercise. A preoperative evaluation also helps to establish a postoperative therapeutic goal.

▶ Instruct the patient to avoid exercising at mealtime to prevent nausea.

▶ If the patient has difficulty breathing only through her mouth, provide a nose clip to fully measure each breath.

▶ Immediately after surgery, monitor the exercise frequently to ensure compliance and assess progress.

▶ Adaptions for the spirometer are available to allow for use with a tracheal stoma.

▶ Premedicate the patient, as needed, for comfort and to improve effort.

References

American Association for Respiratory Care. "AARC Clinical Practice Guideline: Incentive Spirometry," *Respiratory Care* 36(12):1402-405, December 1991.

Harton, S.C., et al. "Frequency and Predictors of Return to Incentive Spirometry Volume Baseline after Cardiac Surgery," *Progress in Cardiovascular Nursing* 22(1):7-12, Winter 2007.

Pasquina, P., et al. "Respiratory Therapy to Prevent Pulmonary Complications after Abdominal Surgery: A Systematic Review," *Chest* 130(6):1887-899, December 2006.

Taylor, C., et al. *Fundamentals of Nursing: The Art and Science of Nursing Care,* 5th ed. Philadelphia: Lippincott Williams & Wilkins, 2008.

Indwelling catheter care and removal

Intended to prevent infection and other complications by keeping the catheter insertion site clean, routine catheter care typically is performed daily after the patient's morning bath and immediately after perineal care. (Bedtime catheter care may have to be performed before perineal care.)

An indwelling urinary catheter should be removed when bladder decompression is no longer necessary, when the patient can resume voiding, or when the catheter is obstructed. **CDC** Depending on the length of the catheterization, the practitioner may order bladder retraining before catheter removal.

Equipment

For catheter care: Soap and water ◆ sterile gloves ◆ sterile 4″ × 4″ gauze pads ◆ basin ◆ washcloth ◆ leg band or adhesive tape ◆ collection bag ◆ waste receptacle ◆ optional: safety pin, rubber band, adhesive remover, specimen container.

For catheter removal: Gloves ◆ 10-ml luer-lock syringe ◆ bedpan ◆ linen-saver pad ◆ optional: clamp for bladder retraining.

Implementation

▶ Confirm the patient's identity using two patient identifiers according to your facility's policy. **JC**
▶ Explain the procedure and its purpose to the patient. **SUNA**
▶ Provide the patient with the necessary equipment for self-cleaning, if possible.
▶ Provide privacy.

Catheter care

▶ Make sure the lighting is adequate so that you can see the perineum and catheter tubing clearly.
▶ Inspect the catheter for problems, and check the urine drainage for mucus, blood clots, sediment, and turbidity. Then pinch the catheter between two fingers to determine whether the lumen contains any material. If you notice any of these conditions (or if your facility's policy requires it), obtain a urine specimen from the specimen col-

lection port. Collect at least 3 ml of urine. Notify the practitioner about your findings.
▶ Inspect the outside of the catheter where it enters the urinary meatus for encrusted material and suppurative drainage. Also inspect the tissue around the meatus for irritation or swelling.
▶ Remove the leg band or, if adhesive tape was used to secure the catheter, remove the adhesive tape. Inspect the area for signs of adhesive burns—redness, tenderness, or blisters.
▶ Put on the sterile gloves. Clean the outside of the catheter and the tissue around the meatus using soap and water. To avoid contaminating the urinary tract, always clean by wiping away from—never toward—the urinary meatus using soap and water. Use a dry gauze pad to remove encrusted material. **CDC**

★ **CLINICAL ALERT**

Don't pull on the catheter while you're cleaning it. This can injure the urethra and the bladder wall. It can also expose a section of the catheter that was inside the urethra, so that when you release the catheter, the newly contaminated section will reenter the urethra, introducing potentially infectious organisms.

▶ Remove your gloves, reapply the leg band, and reattach the catheter to the leg band. If a leg band isn't available, tear a piece of adhesive tape from the roll.
▶ To prevent skin hypersensitivity or irritation, retape the catheter on the opposite side. Provide enough slack before securing the catheter to prevent tension on the tubing, which could injure the urethral lumen or bladder wall. **SUNA**
▶ Most drainage bags have a plastic clamp on the tubing to attach them to the sheet. If this isn't available, wrap a rubber band around the drainage tubing, insert the safety pin through a loop of the rubber band, and pin the tubing to the sheet below bladder level. Then attach the collection bag, below bladder level, to the bed frame.
▶ Dispose of all used supplies in a waste receptacle.

Catheter removal

▶ Wash your hands.
▶ Assemble the equipment at the patient's bedside. Explain the procedure, and tell him that he may feel slight discomfort. Tell him that you'll check him periodically during the first 6 to 24 hours after catheter removal to make sure he resumes voiding.
▶ Put on gloves. Place a linen-saver pad under the patient's buttocks. Attach the syringe to the luer-lock mechanism on the catheter.

Teaching about leg bags

A urine drainage bag attached to the leg provides the catheterized patient with greater mobility. Because the bag is hidden under clothing, it may also help him feel more comfortable about catheterization. Leg bags are usually worn during the day and are replaced at night with a standard collection device.

If your patient will be discharged with an indwelling catheter, teach him how to attach and remove a leg bag. To demonstrate, you'll need a bag with a short drainage tube, two straps, an alcohol pad, adhesive tape, and a screw clamp or hemostat.

Attaching the leg bag

▶ Provide privacy and explain the procedure. Describe the advantages of a leg bag, but caution the patient that a leg bag is smaller than a standard collection device and may have to be emptied more frequently.

▶ Remove the protective covering from the tip of the drainage tube. Then show the patient how to clean the tip with an alcohol sponge, wiping away from the opening to avoid contaminating the tube. Show him how to attach the tube to the catheter.

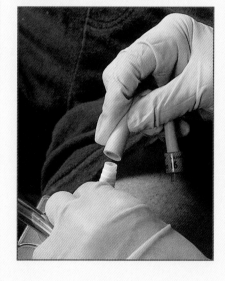

▶ Place the drainage bag on the patient's calf or thigh. Have him fasten the straps securely (as shown below), and show him how to tape the catheter to his leg. Emphasize that he must leave slack in the catheter to minimize pressure on the bladder, urethra, and related structures. Excessive pressure or tension can lead to tissue breakdown.

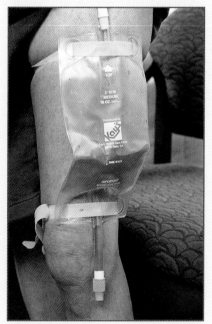

▶ Also tell him not to fasten the straps too tightly to avoid interfering with his circulation.

Avoiding complications

▶ Although most leg bags have a valve in the drainage tube that prevents urine reflux into the bladder, urge the patient to keep the drainage bag lower than his bladder at all times because urine in the bag is a perfect growth medium for bacteria. Caution him not to go to bed or take long naps while wearing the drainage bag.

▶ To prevent a full leg bag from damaging the bladder wall and urethra, encourage the patient to empty the bag when it's only half full. He should also inspect the catheter and drainage tube periodically for compression or kinking, which could obstruct urine flow and result in bladder distention.

▶ Tell the patient to wash the leg bag with soap and water or a bacteriostatic solution before each use to prevent infection.

▶ Pull back on the plunger of the syringe. This deflates the balloon by aspirating the injected fluid. The amount of fluid injected is usually indicated on the tip of the catheter's balloon lumen and in the patient's chart.

▶ Grasp the catheter and pinch it firmly with your thumb and index finger to prevent urine from flowing back into the urethra. Before doing so, offer the patient a bedpan. Gently pull the catheter from the urethra. If you meet resistance, don't apply force; instead, notify the practitioner.

▶ Measure and record the amount of urine in the collection bag before discarding it. Remove and discard gloves, and wash your hands. For the first 24 hours after catheter removal, note the time and amount of each voiding.

Special considerations

▶ Some facilities require the use of specific cleaning agents for catheter care; check your facility's policy manual before beginning this procedure.

▶ Avoid raising the drainage bag above bladder level. This prevents reflux of urine, which may contain bacteria. To avoid damaging the urethral lumen or bladder wall, always disconnect the drainage bag and tubing from the bed linen and bed frame before helping the patient out of bed. **CDC**

▶ When possible, attach a leg bag to allow the patient greater mobility. If the patient will be discharged with an indwelling catheter, teach him how to use a leg bag. (See *Teaching about leg bags,* page 255.)

▶ Encourage patients with unrestricted fluid intake to increase intake to at least 3,000 ml per day. This helps flush the urinary system and reduces sediment formation. **SUNA**

▶ After catheter removal, assess the patient for incontinence (or dribbling), urgency, persistent dysuria or bladder spasms, fever, chills, or palpable bladder distention. The patient should void within 6 to 8 hours after catheter removal.

References

Centers for Disease Control and Prevention," Guideline for Prevention of Catheter-Associated Urinary Tract Infections," Published 1981. Available at *http://www.cdc.gov/ncidod/dhqp/gl_catheter_assoc.html#.*

Clinical Practice Guidelines Task Force; Society of Urologic Nurses and Associates. "Care of the Patient with an Indwelling Catheter," *Urologic Nursing* 26(1):80-81, February 2006.

Cochran, S. "Care of the Indwelling Urinary Catheter: Is It Evidence Based?" *Journal of Wound, Ostomy and Continence Nursing* 34(3):282-88, May-June 2007.

Godfrey, H., and Fraczyk, L. "Preventing and Managing Catheter-Associated Urinary Tract Infections," *British Journal of Community Nursing* 10(5):205-206, 208-12, May 2005.

Huang, W.C., et al. "Catheter-Associated Urinary Tract Infections in Intensive Care Units Can Be Reduced by Prompting Physicians to Remove Unnecessary Catheters," *Infection Control and Hospital Epidemiology* 25(11):974-78, November 2004.

The Joanna Briggs Institute for Evidence Based Nursing and Midwifery. "Best Practice: Management of Short-Term Indwelling Urethral Catheters to Prevent Urinary Tract Infections," 4(1), 2000. Available at *www.joannabriggs.edu.au/pdf/BPISEng_4_1.pdf.*

Leaver, B. "The Evidence for Urethral Meatal Cleansing," *Nursing Standard* 21(41):39-42, June 2007.

Reilly, L., et al. "Reducing Foley Catheter Device Days in an Intensive Care Unit: Using the Evidence to Change Practice," *AACN Advances in Critical Care* 17(3):272-83, July-September 2006.

Ribby, K.J. "Decreasing Urinary Tract Infections through Staff Development, Outcomes, and Nursing Process," *Journal of Nursing Care Quality* 21(3):272-76, July-September 2006.

Robinson, J. "Removing Indwelling Urinary Catheters: Trial without Catheter in the Community," *British Journal of Community Nursing* 10(12):553-54, 556-57, December 2005.

Seymour, C. "Transferring Patients with a Urinary Catheter," *Nursing Times* 103(42):52-54, October 2007.

Taylor, C., et al. *Fundamentals of Nursing: The Art and Science of Nursing Care,* 6th ed. Philadelphia: Lippincott Williams & Wilkins, 2008.

Indwelling catheter insertion

Also known as a *Foley catheter,* an indwelling urinary catheter remains in the bladder to provide continuous urine drainage. A balloon inflated at the catheter's distal end prevents it from slipping out of the bladder after insertion.

Indwelling catheters are used most commonly to relieve bladder distention caused by urine retention and to allow continuous urine drainage when the urinary meatus is swollen from childbirth, surgery, or local trauma. Other indications for an indwelling catheter include urinary tract obstruction (by a tumor or enlarged prostate), urine retention or infection from neurogenic bladder paralysis caused by spinal cord injury or disease, and any illness in which the patient's urine output must be monitored closely.

An indwelling catheter is inserted using sterile technique and only when absolutely necessary. **CDC** Insertion should be performed with extreme care to prevent injury and infection. To avoid trauma to the urethra and decrease the risk of infection, always use the smallest-sized catheter with the smallest balloon. **CDC**

Equipment

Sterile indwelling catheter (latex or silicone #10 to #22 French [average adult sizes are #14 to #16 French]) ◆ syringe filled with 10 ml of sterile water (normal saline solution is sometimes used) ◆ washcloth ◆ towel ◆ soap and water ◆ two linen-saver pads ◆ clean gloves ◆ sterile gloves ◆ sterile drape ◆ sterile fenestrated drape ◆ sterile cotton-tipped applicators (or cotton balls and plastic forceps) ◆ antiseptic cleaning agent ◆ urine receptacle ◆ sterile water-soluble lubricant ◆ sterile drainage collection bag ◆ adhesive tape ◆ optional: urine specimen container and laboratory request form, leg band with Velcro closure, gooseneck lamp or flashlight, pillows or rolled blankets.

Prepackaged sterile disposable kits that usually contain all the necessary equipment are available. The syringes in these kits are prefilled with 10 ml of normal saline solution.

Implementation

▶ Check the order on the patient's chart to determine whether a catheter size or type has been specified. **SUNA**

▶ Wash your hands, select the appropriate equipment, and assemble it at the patient's bedside. **SUNA**

▶ Confirm the patient's identity using two patient identifiers according to your facility's policy.

▶ Explain the procedure to the patient and provide privacy. Check her chart and ask when she voided last. Percuss and palpate the bladder to establish baseline data. Ask whether she feels the urge to void. **SUNA**

▶ Have a coworker hold a flashlight or place a gooseneck lamp next to the patient's bed so that you can see the urinary meatus clearly in poor lighting.

▶ Place the female patient in the supine position, with her knees flexed and separated and her feet flat on the bed, about 2′ (61 cm) apart. If she finds this position uncomfortable, have her flex one knee and keep the other leg flat on the bed. **SUNA**

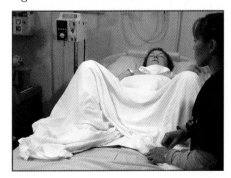

▶ Place the male patient in the supine position with his legs extended and flat on the bed.

▶ Put on clean gloves.

▶ Use the washcloth to clean the patient's genital area and perineum thoroughly with soap and water. Dry the area with the towel. Then wash your hands.

▶ Place the linen-saver pads on the bed between the patient's legs and under the hips. To create the sterile field, open the prepackaged kit or equipment tray and place it between the female patient's legs or next to the male patient's hip. If the sterile gloves are the first item on the top of the tray, put them on. Place the sterile drape under the patient's hips. Then drape the patient's lower abdomen with the sterile fenestrated drape so that only the genital area remains exposed (as shown at the top of the next column). Take care not to contaminate your gloves. **SUNA**

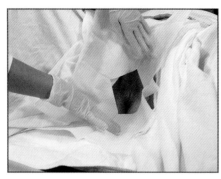

▶ Open the rest of the kit or tray. Put on the sterile gloves if you haven't already done so.

▶ Make sure the patient isn't allergic to iodine solution; if she's allergic, another antiseptic cleaning agent must be used.

▶ Tear open the packet of antiseptic cleaning agent, and use it to saturate the sterile cotton balls or applicators. Be careful not to spill the solution on the equipment.

▶ Open the packet of water-soluble lubricant and apply it to the catheter tip; attach the drainage bag to the other end of the catheter. (If you're using a commercial kit, the drainage bag may be attached.) Make sure all tubing ends remain sterile, and make sure the clamp at the emptying port of the drainage bag is closed to prevent urine leakage from the bag. **CDC** **SUNA**

▶ Before inserting the catheter, inflate the balloon with sterile water to inspect it for leaks. To do this, attach the water-filled syringe to the luer-lock; then push the plunger and check for seepage as the balloon expands. Aspirate the water to deflate the balloon. Be aware that some manufacturers recommend not inflating the balloon prior to insertion because of the risk of microtears that may cause infection. If you aren't sure, check the manufacturers instructions that are included with the kit. **MFR**

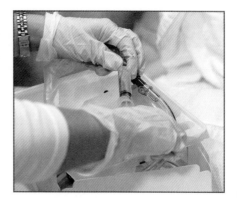

Female patient

▶ Separate the labia majora and labia minora as widely as possible with the thumb, middle, and index fingers of your nondominant hand so you have a full view of the urinary meatus. Keep the labia well separated throughout the procedure so they don't obscure the urinary meatus or contaminate the area when it's cleaned.

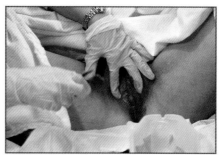

▶ With your dominant hand, use a sterile, cotton-tipped applicator (or pick up a sterile cotton ball with the plastic forceps) and wipe one side of the urinary meatus with a single downward motion. Wipe the other side with another sterile applicator or cotton ball in the same way. Then wipe directly over the meatus with still another sterile applicator or cotton ball. **SUNA**

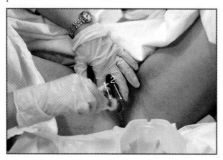

▶ Advance the catheter 2″ to 3″ (5 to 7.5 cm) while continuing to hold the labia apart until urine begins to flow. If the catheter is inadvertently inserted into the vagina, leave it there as a landmark. Then begin the procedure over again using new supplies. **SUNA**

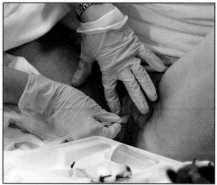

Male patient

▶ Hold the penis with your nondominant hand. If the patient is uncircumcised, retract the foreskin. Then gently lift and stretch the penis to a 60- to 90-degree angle. Hold the penis this way throughout the procedure to straighten the urethra and maintain a sterile field. **SUNA**

▶ Use your dominant hand to clean the glans with a sterile cotton-tipped applicator or a sterile cotton ball held in the forceps. Clean in a circular motion, starting at the urinary meatus and working outward. **SUNA**

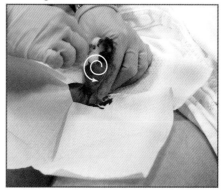

▶ Repeat the procedure, using another sterile applicator or cotton ball and taking care not to contaminate your sterile glove.

▶ Inject 5 to 10 ml of water-soluble lubricant or water-soluble 2% lidocaine jelly directly into the urethra. **SUNA**

▶ Pick up the catheter with your dominant hand, and prepare to insert the lubricated tip into the urinary meatus. To facilitate insertion by relaxing the sphincter, ask the patient to cough as you insert the catheter. Tell him to breathe deeply and slowly to further relax the sphincter and spasms. Hold the catheter close to its tip to ease insertion and control its direction. **SUNA**

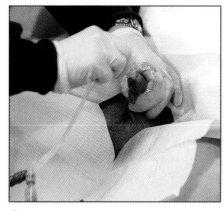

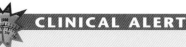

Never force a catheter during insertion. Maneuver it gently as the patient bears down or coughs. If you still meet resistance, stop and notify the practitioner.

▶ Advance the catheter to the bifurcation and check for urine flow. If the foreskin was retracted, replace it to prevent compromised circulation and painful swelling.

For male and female patients

▶ When urine stops flowing, attach the water-filled syringe to the luer-lock.

▶ Push the plunger and inflate the balloon to keep the catheter in place in the bladder. Never inflate a balloon without first establishing urine flow, which confirms that the catheter is in the bladder. **SUNA**

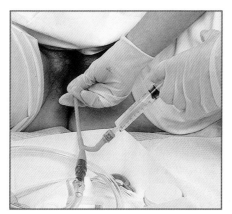

▶ Hang the collection bag below bladder level to prevent urine reflux into the bladder and to facilitate gravity drainage of the bladder. Make sure the tubing doesn't get tangled in the bed's side rails.

▶ Tape the catheter to the female patient's thigh to prevent possible tension on the urogenital trigone. **SUNA** **CDC**

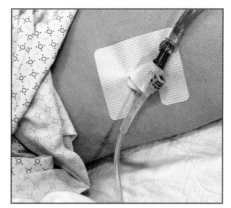

▶ Tape the catheter to the male patient's abdomen or thigh to prevent pressure on the urethra at the penoscrotal junction. Taping this way also prevents traction on the bladder and alteration in the normal direction of urine flow in males. **CDC**

▶ As an alternative, secure the catheter to the patient's thigh using a leg band with a Velcro closure. This decreases skin irritation, especially in patients with long-term indwelling catheters.

▶ Dispose of all used supplies properly.

Special considerations

▶ The balloon size determines the amount of solution or air needed for inflation, and the exact amount is usually printed on the distal extension of the catheter used for inflating the balloon.

▶ If necessary, ask the female patient to lie on her side with her knees drawn up to her chest during the catheterization procedure. This position may be especially helpful for elderly or disabled patients, such as those with severe contractures.

▶ If the practitioner orders a urine specimen for laboratory analysis, obtain it from the urine receptacle with a specimen collection container at the time of catheterization and send it to the laboratory with the appropriate laboratory request form. Connect the drainage bag when urine stops flowing.

▶ Inspect the catheter and tubing periodically while they're in place to detect compression or kinking that could obstruct urine flow.

▶ For monitoring purposes, empty the collection bag at least every 8 hours. Excessive fluid volume may require more frequent emptying to prevent traction on the catheter, which would cause the patient discomfort, and to prevent injury to the urethra and bladder wall. Some facilities encourage changing catheters at regular intervals, such as every 30 days, if the patient will have long-term continuous drainage.

EVIDENCE-BASED RESEARCH

Urinary tract infection mortality

Clec'h, C., et al. "Does Catheter-Associated Urinary Tract Infection Increase Mortality in Critically Ill Patients?" *Infection Control and Hospital Epidemiology* 28(12):1367-1373, December 2007.

Level VI
Evidence from a single descriptive or qualitative study

Description
Indwelling devices are the most common cause of hospital-acquired infection. Of those indwelling devices, urinary catheters are the most frequent cause of infection. This study was done to determine if there was an association between catheter-associated urinary tract infections (UTIs) in the intensive care unit (ICU) and mortality. The study looked at all patients who were admitted to medical or surgical ICUs between January 1997 and August 2005 who required an indwelling urinary catheter. Patients with an indwelling catheter who developed a UTI were matched against similar control patients who didn't develop a UTI. The mortality rates were then compared for both groups.

Findings
Of the 3,281 patients with an indwelling urinary catheter, 298 (9%) developed at least one catheter-associated UTI. The mortality rates of patients with catheter-associated UTIs were higher those without a UTI (32% versus 25%). However, once all factors were accounted for and adjusted, it was determined that a catheter-associated UTI wasn't associated with increased mortality.

Conclusions
Although patients with indwelling devices, such as urinary catheters, are at a higher risk for a hospital-acquired infection, patients who develop a UTI aren't at an increased risk for mortality from their infection.

Nursing practice implications
Nurses are commonly responsible for the insertion of an indwelling urinary catheter and the care of patients with such catheters. The following practice implications are important:
▶ Maintain strict sterile technique when inserting the catheter to decrease the risk of a UTI.
▶ Perform catheter care on every shift, and as needed.
▶ Monitor UTI infection rates on the unit related to indwelling urinary catheters.
▶ Educate the staff on ways to help prevent UTIs and care for patients with urinary catheters.

CLINICAL ALERT

Observe the patient carefully for adverse reactions caused by removing excessive volumes of residual urine such as hypovolemic shock. Check your facility's policy beforehand to determine the maximum amount of urine that may be drained at one time (some facilities limit the amount to 700 to 1,000 ml). Whether to limit the amount of urine drained is currently controversial. Clamp the catheter at the first sign of an adverse reaction, and notify the practitioner.

▶ Urinary tract infection can result from the introduction of bacteria into the bladder. Improper insertion can cause traumatic injury to the urethral and bladder mucosa. Bladder atony or spasms can result from rapid decompression of a severely distended bladder.

References

Bissett, L. "Reducing the Risk of Catheter-Related Urinary Tract Infection," *Nursing Times* 101(12):64-65, 67, March 2005.

Centers for Disease Control and Prevention," Guideline for Prevention of Catheter-Associated Urinary Tract Infections," Published 1981. Available at *http://www.cdc.gov/ncidod/dhqp/gl_catheter_assoc.html#*

Clinical Practice Guidelines Task Force; Society of Urologic Nurses and Associates. "Female Urethral Catheterization," *Urologic Nursing* 26(4):314, August 2006.

Clinical Practice Guidelines Task Force; Society of Urologic Nurses and Associates. "Male Urethral Catheterization," *Urologic Nursing* 26(4):315, August 2006.

Doherty, W. "Urinary Catheterization in Male Patients," *Nursing Standard* 20(35):57-63, May 2006.

Garcia, M.M., et al. "Traditional Foley Drainage Systems—Do They Drain the Bladder?" *Journal of Urology* 177(1): 203-207, January 2007.

Leaver, B. "The Evidence for Urethral Meatal Cleansing," *Nursing Standard* 21(41):39-42, June 2007.

Taylor, C., et al. *Fundamentals of Nursing: The Art and Science of Nursing Care,* 6th ed. Philadelphia: Lippincott Williams & Wilkins, 2008.

Woodward, S. "Use of Lubricant in Female Urethral Catheterization," *British Journal of Nursing* 14(19):1022-1023, October-November 2005.

Intermittent infusion device insertion

Also called a *saline lock* or *heparin lock,* an intermittent infusion device consists of a cannula with an injection cap attached. Filled with dilute heparin or saline solution to prevent blood clot formation, the device maintains venous access in patients who are receiving I.V. medication regularly or intermittently but who don't require continuous infusion. An intermittent infusion device is superior to an I.V. line that's maintained at a moderately slow infusion rate because it minimizes the risk of fluid overload and electrolyte imbalance. It also cuts costs, reduces the risk of contamination by eliminating I.V. solution containers and administration sets, increases patient comfort and mobility, reduces patient anxiety and, if inserted in a large vein, allows collection of multiple blood samples without repeated venipuncture.

Equipment

Intermittent infusion device ◆ needleless system device ◆ normal saline solution ◆ tourniquet ◆ chlorhexidine solution ◆ alcohol swab ◆ venipuncture equipment ◆ transparent semipermeable dressing ◆ tape.

Implementation

▶ Wash your hands thoroughly to prevent contamination of the venipuncture site. **CDC AACN**

▶ Confirm the patient's identity using two patient identifiers according to your facility's policy. **CDC**

▶ Explain the procedure to the patient, and describe the purpose of the intermittent infusion device.

▶ Remove the set from its packaging, wipe the port with an alcohol swab, and inject normal saline solution to fill the tubing and needleless system.

▶ Select a venipuncture site, and clean it with chlorhexidine solution, using a back-and-forth scrubbing motion. **CDC INS AACN**

▶ Perform the venipuncture, and ensure correct catheter placement in the vein. Then release the tourniquet. (See "Venipuncture," page 592, for complete instructions.)

▶ Tape the set in place or apply a commercial holder. Loop the tubing, if applicable, so that the injection port is free and easily accessible.

▶ Apply a transparent semipermeable dressing. On a dressing label, write the time, date, and your initials, and place the label on the dressing.

▶ Remove and discard your gloves.

▶ Inject normal saline solution every 8 to 24 hours or according to your facility's policy to maintain the patency of the intermittent infusion device. Inject the heparin slowly to prevent stinging.

Special considerations

▶ When accessing an intermittent infusion device, be sure to stabilize the device to prevent dislodging it from the vein.

▶ If the patient feels a burning sensation during the injection of saline, stop the injection and check cannula placement. If the cannula is in the vein, in-

---

Converting an I.V. line to an intermittent infusion device

Many types of adapter caps (shown here) allow you to convert an existing I.V. line to an intermittent infusion device. To make the conversion, follow these steps:

▶ Prime the male adapter plug with normal saline solution.
▶ Clamp the I.V. tubing, and remove the administration set from the cannula hub.
▶ Insert the male adapter cap.
▶ Flush the access with the remaining solution to prevent clot formation.

Short male adapter
This short luer-lock adapter cap twists into place.

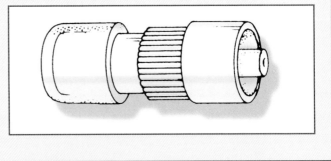

ject the saline at a slower rate to minimize irritation. If the catheter isn't in the vein, remove and discard it. Then select a new venipuncture site and, using fresh equipment, restart the procedure. **INS**

▶ Change the intermittent infusion device every 48 to 72 hours, according to your facility's policy, using a new venipuncture site. Some facilities use a transparent semipermeable dressing. This allows the patient more freedom and better observation of the injection site.

▶ If the practitioner orders an I.V. infusion discontinued and an intermittent infusion device inserted in its place, convert the existing line by disconnecting the I.V. tubing and inserting a male adapter cap into the device. (See *Converting an I.V. line to an intermittent infusion device.*)

References

Campbell, S.G., et al. "How Often Should Peripheral Intravenous Catheters in Ambulatory Patients Be Flushed?" *Journal of Infusion Nursing* 28(6):399-404, November-December 2005.

Fujita, T., et al. "Normal Saline Flushing for Maintenance of Peripheral Intravenous Sites," *Journal of Clinical Nursing* 15(1):103-104, January 2006.

Mok, E., et al. "A Randomized Controlled Trial for Maintaining Peripheral Intravenous Lock in Children," *International Journal of Nursing Practice* 13(1):33-45, February 2007.

Niesen, K.M., et al. "The Effects of Heparin versus Normal Saline for Maintenance of Peripheral Intravenous Locks in Pregnant Women," *Journal of Obstetrics, Gynecologic, and Neonatal Nursing* 32(4):503-508, July-August 2003.

"Standard 29. Add-on Devices and Junction Securement. Infusion Nursing Standards of Practice," *Journal of Infusion Nursing* 29(1S):S32, January-February 2006.

"Standard 50. Flushing. Infusion Nursing Standards of Practice," *Journal of Infusion Nursing* 29(1S):S52, January-February 2006.

Intra-abdominal pressure monitoring

Intra-abdominal pressure monitoring measures the pressure in the abdominal compartment. It can be assessed indirectly in the patient with an indwelling urinary catheter by measuring the pressure in the bladder with a needle that connects a pressure transducer to the urinary catheter or by inserting an I.V. catheter into the sampling port. Pressure in the abdomen may rise from such conditions as intraperitoneal bleeding, third space fluid resuscitation, peritonitis, ascites, gaseous bowel distention, abdominal surgery, and trauma. If pressure in the abdominal cavity becomes greater than the pressure in the capillaries that perfuse the abdominal organs, ischemia and infarction may result. Increased intra-abdominal pressure can also lead to reduced cardiac output, increased systemic vascular resistance, increased vascular resistance, and reduced venous return. By measuring intra-abdominal pressure, the nurse can detect a rise in pressure and initiate lifesaving measures.

Equipment

Indwelling single- or multi-lumen urinary catheter with drainage bag ◆ clean gloves ◆ cardiac monitor ◆ pressure cable for monitor interface ◆ 500-ml bag of normal saline solution ◆ appropriately sized pressure bag for size of saline bag ◆ I.V. tubing ◆ pressure tubing, pressure transducer with flush device, and stopcock ◆ 60-ml luer-lock syringe ◆ clamp ◆ sterile cleansing solution ◆ 16G or 18G needle or I.V. catheter or needleless adapter (when using a three-way indwelling urinary catheter, a sterile feeding Y-connector is used in place of the I.V. catheter or needleless adapter) ◆ tape ◆ I.V. pole.

Implementation

▶ Before setting up the monitoring system, wash your hands thoroughly.
▶ Connect the I.V. tubing to the transducer, the transducer to a stopcock, then the stopcock to the pressure tubing and monitor cable. Attach a 60-ml syringe to the side port of the stopcock. Place the transducer in the transducer holder attached to the I.V. pole.

▶ Hang the 500-ml I.V. normal saline bag from an I.V. pole, attach the I.V. tubing, and flush the entire line system of air. Use the pressure bag to pressurize the system to 300 mm Hg. Attach the cable from the transducer to the monitor, and select a 30 mm Hg scale for monitoring pressure.
▶ Confirm the patient's identity using two patient identifiers according to your facility's policy. **JC**
▶ Explain the procedure to the patient.
▶ Insert an indwelling urinary catheter if the patient doesn't have one in place. (See "Indwelling catheter insertion," page 257.)
▶ Place the I.V. pole with the monitoring system next to the patient.
▶ With the patient supine, level and zero the transducer to the symphysis pubis. The supine position prevents the abdominal organs from exerting pressure down onto the bladder and falsely elevating the readings.
▶ Clean the indwelling urinary catheter sampling port with antiseptic solution, and insert the needle, needleless adapter, or I.V. catheter into the port. (See *Setup for intra-abdominal pressure monitoring.*)
▶ Remove the stylet, if an I.V. catheter is used, and connect the I.V. catheter to

the pressure tubing. Secure the connection with tape.

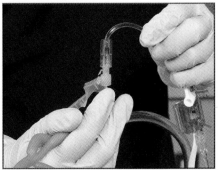

▶ When a three-way indwelling urinary catheter is used, clean the hub of the irrigation port and attach the pressure monitoring line directly into the irrigation hub using a sterile feeding tube Y-connector. Secure the connection with tape.
▶ Clamp the urinary catheter just distal to the connection of the catheter and drainage bag to keep saline from draining out of the bladder while filling the bladder.
▶ Open the stopcock from the flush line to the syringe, and fill the syringe from the I.V. normal saline solution bag.
▶ Close the stopcock to the transducer, and open it to the pressure tubing and urinary catheter; then instill 50 ml

Setup for intra-abdominal pressure monitoring

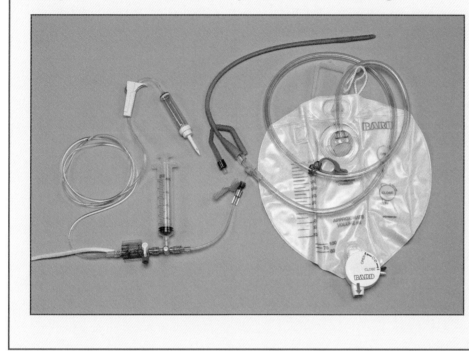

Intra-abdominal pressure monitoring can be performed through direct or indirect means. The direct method is preferred for intra-abdominal pressure monitoring and involves inserting an indwelling urinary catheter into the patient's bladder. The bladder will reflect intra-abdominal pressure when it has a volume of 100 ml or less. A needle is inserted into the sample port of the indwelling catheter. The needle is then attached to pressure tubing and a transducer, which allows the nurse to view the intra-abdominal pressure on a monitor. This photo shows a completed intra-abdominal pressure set-up.

of normal saline solution into the bladder.

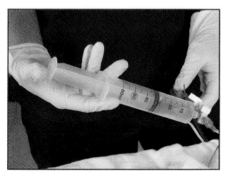

► Close the stopcock to the syringe, and open it to the pressure tubing and the transducer.
► Obtain the intra-abdominal pressure with the patient in the supine position and the point of leveling at the symphysis pubis.
► Obtain a pressure reading at the end of expiration to minimize the effects of respiration. Fluctuation should be evident in the waveform with the heartbeat or respiratory pattern.

► After the reading is obtained, turn the stopcock off to the pressure tubing and catheter, release the clamp, and allow the instilled normal saline solution to drain.

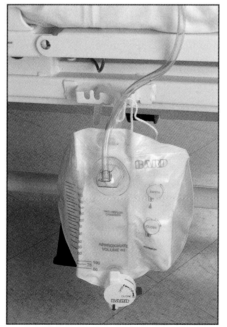

► Measure urine output after subtracting the 50 ml of instilled normal saline solution to maintain accurate intake and output.
► Remove the needle or needleless adapter from the sampling port.
► If an I.V. catheter is being left in place, tape the connection securely.

Special considerations

► Report increasing intra-abdominal pressure to the practitioner. Although intra-abdominal pressures greater than 12 to 15 mm Hg are a concern, a pressure greater than 20 mm Hg is considered intra-abdominal hypertension, and decompression surgery may be indicated.
► Patients at risk for intra-abdominal hypertension should be assessed for signs of reduced organ perfusion (such as reduced or absent urinary output), increased serum creatinine levels, hy-

potension, reduced cardiac output, increased central venous and pulmonary artery pressures, increased intracerebral pressure, increased serum lactate levels, increased peak airway pressure, decreased tidal volume, hypoxemia, hypercarbia, GI bleeding, and impaired peripheral circulation.

▶ If a patient can't lie supine to obtain a reading, take the reading with the head of the bed elevated. Document the position the patient was in for the reading, and obtain all further readings from this position.

References

Balogh, Z., et al. "Continuous Intra-abdominal Pressure Measurement Technique," *American Journal of Surgery* 188(6):679-84, December 2004.

Balogh, Z., et al. "Intra-abdominal Pressure Measurement and Abdominal Compartment Syndrome: The Opinion of the World Society of the Abdominal Compartment Syndrome," *Critical Care Medicine* 35(2):677-78, February 2007.

Lynn-McHale Wiegand, D.J., and Carlson, K.K., eds. *AACN Procedure Manual for Critical Care,* 5th ed. Philadelphia: W.B. Saunders Co., 2005.

McBeth, P.B., et al. "Effect of Patient Positioning on Intra-abdominal Pressure Monitoring," *American Journal of Surgery* 193(5):644-47, May 2007.

Sugrue, M. "Abdominal Compartment Syndrome," *Current Opinion in Critical Care* 11(4):333-38, August 2005.

Walker, J., and Criddle, L.M. "Pathophysiology and Management of Abdominal Compartment Syndrome," *American Journal of Critical Care* 12(4):367-71, July 2003.

Wittman, D.H., and Iskander, G.A. "The Compartment Syndrome of the Abdominal Cavity: A State-of-the-Art Review," *Journal of Intensive Care Medicine* 15(4):201-20, July-August 2000.

Wolfe, T., et al. "Intra-abdominal Pressure Monitoring: The Key to Avoiding Abdominal Compartment Syndrome," *AACN News* 21(9), September 2004.

World Society of Abdominal Compartment Syndrome. "Consensus Definitions." Available at *www.wsacs.org*.

Intra-aortic balloon counterpulsation

Providing temporary support for the heart's left ventricle, intra-aortic balloon counterpulsation (IABC) mechanically displaces blood within the aorta by means of an intra-aortic balloon attached to an external pump console. The balloon is usually inserted through the common femoral artery and positioned with its tip just distal to the left subclavian artery. It monitors myocardial perfusion and the effects of drugs on myocardial function and perfusion. When used correctly, IABC improves two key aspects of myocardial physiology: It increases the supply of oxygen-rich blood to the myocardium, and it decreases myocardial oxygen demand. (See *How the intra-aortic balloon pump works.*)

IABC is contraindicated in patients with severe aortic regurgitation, aortic aneurysm, or severe peripheral vascular disease.

Equipment

IABC console and balloon catheters ◆ insertion kit ◆ gas supply (usually helium) ◆ electrocardiogram (ECG) monitor ◆ two sets of ECG electrodes ◆ sedative ◆ pain medication ◆ heparin flush solution, transducer, and flush setup ◆ temporary pacemaker setup ◆ sterile drape ◆ sterile gloves ◆ gown ◆ mask ◆ sutures ◆ suction setup ◆ oxygen setup and equipment, as appropriate ◆ fluoroscope ◆ indwelling urinary catheter ◆ urinometer ◆ arterial blood gas (ABG) kits and tubes for laboratory studies ◆ antiseptic swabs ◆ dressing materials ◆ 4″ × 4″ gauze pads ◆ clippers ◆ optional: defibrillator, atropine, I.V. heparin, low-molecular-weight dextran.

Implementation

▶ Obtain the IABC console and gas supply. Make sure that the gas supply is full, and attach it to the console following the manufacturer's recommendations. (See *Parts of an IABP*, page 268.)
▶ Prepare the transducer with heparin flush solution, as appropriate. Complete any other preparation for the IABC console, as indicated by your fa-

---

How the intra-aortic balloon pump works

Made of polyurethane, the intra-aortic balloon is attached to an external pump console by means of a large-lumen catheter. The illustrations here show the direction of blood flow when the pump inflates and deflates the balloon.

Balloon inflation
The balloon inflates as the aortic valve closes and diastole begins. Diastole increases perfusion to the coronary arteries.

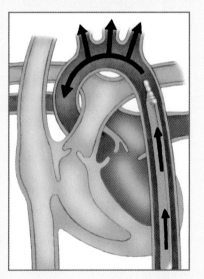

Balloon deflation
The balloon deflates before ventricular ejection, when the aortic valve opens. This permits ejection of blood from the left ventricle against a lowered resistance. As a result, aortic end-diastolic pressure and afterload decrease and cardiac output rises.

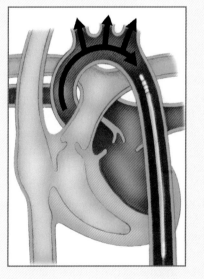

cility's policy and the instruction manual.

▶ Confirm the patient's identity using two patient identifiers according to your facility's policy. **JC**

▶ Explain to the patient that the physician will place a special balloon catheter in his aorta to help his heart pump more easily. Briefly explain the insertion procedure, and mention that the catheter will be connected to a large console next to his bed.

Preparing for intra-aortic balloon insertion

▶ Make sure the patient or a family member understands and signs a consent form. Verify that the form is attached to his chart.

▶ Obtain the patient's baseline vital signs, including pulmonary artery pressure (PAP). (A pulmonary artery [PA] line should already be in place.) Attach the patient to an ECG machine for continuous monitoring. Be sure to apply chest electrodes in a standard lead II position—or in whatever position produces the largest R wave—because the R wave triggers balloon inflation and deflation. Obtain a baseline ECG.

▶ Attach another set of ECG electrodes to the patient, unless the ECG pattern is being transmitted from the patient's bedside monitor to the balloon pump monitor through a phone cable. Administer oxygen as ordered and as needed.

▶ Make sure the patient has an arterial line, a PA line, and a peripheral I.V. line in place. The arterial line is used for withdrawing blood samples, monitoring blood pressure, and assessing the timing and effectiveness of therapy. The PA line allows measurement of PAP, aspiration of blood samples, and cardiac output studies. Increased PAP indicates increased myocardial workload and ineffective balloon pumping. Cardiac output studies are usually per-

Parts of an IABP

These illustrations show an intra-aortic balloon pump (IABP) (at right) and a close-up of the controls and screen (below).

formed with and without the balloon to check the patient's progress. The central lumen of the intra-aortic balloon, used to monitor central aortic pressure, produces an augmented pressure waveform that allows you to check for proper timing of the inflation-deflation cycle and demonstrates the effects of counterpulsation, elevated diastolic pressure, and reduced end-diastolic and systolic pressures. (See *Interpreting intra-aortic balloon waveforms*.)

Interpreting intra-aortic balloon waveforms

During intra-aortic balloon counterpulsation, you can use electrocardiogram and arterial pressure waveforms to determine whether the balloon pump is functioning properly.

Normal inflation-deflation timing

Balloon inflation occurs after aortic valve closure; deflation, during isovolumetric contraction, just before the aortic valve opens. In a properly timed waveform, like the one shown at right, the inflation point lies at or slightly above the dicrotic notch. Both inflation and deflation cause a sharp V. Peak diastolic pressure exceeds peak systolic pressure; peak systolic pressure exceeds assisted peak systolic pressure.

Early inflation

With *early inflation,* the inflation point lies before the dicrotic notch. Early inflation dangerously increases myocardial stress and decreases cardiac output.

Early deflation

With *early deflation,* a U shape appears and peak systolic pressure is less than or equal to assisted peak systolic pressure. This won't decrease afterload or myocardial oxygen consumption.

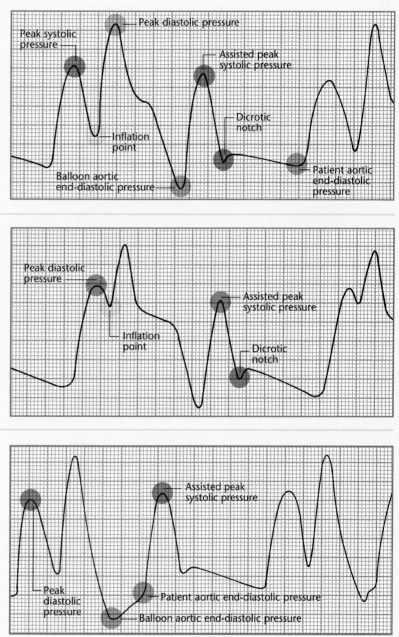

(continued)

▶ Insert an indwelling catheter with a urinometer so you can measure the patient's urine output and assess his fluid balance and renal function.

▶ Observe and record the patient's peripheral leg pulse, and document sensation, movement, color, and temperature of the legs.

▶ Administer a sedative as ordered.
▶ Have the defibrillator, suction setup, temporary pacemaker setup, and emergency medications readily avail-

Interpreting intra-aortic balloon waveforms (continued)

Late inflation

With *late inflation*, the dicrotic notch precedes the inflation point and the notch and the inflation point create a W shape. This can lead to a reduction in peak diastolic pressure, coronary and systemic perfusion augmentation time, and augmented coronary perfusion pressure.

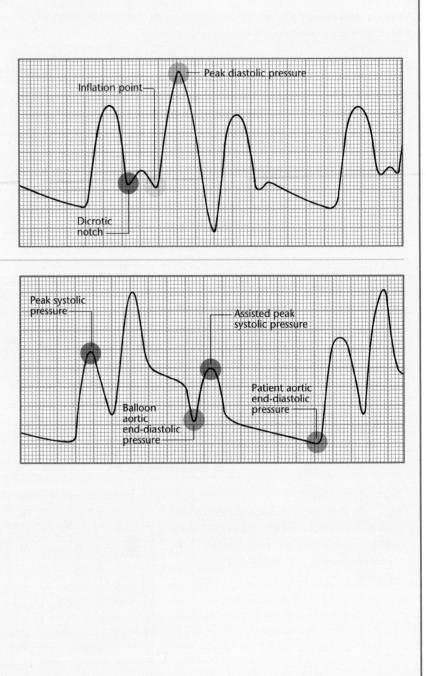

Late deflation

With *late deflation*, peak systolic pressure exceeds assisted peak systolic pressure. This threatens the patient by increasing afterload, myocardial oxygen consumption, cardiac workload, and preload. It occurs when the balloon has been inflated for too long.

able in case the patient develops complications during insertion such as an arrhythmia.

▶ Open the insertion tray using sterile technique, and place it on a bedside table within easy reach for the physician.

▶ Before the physician inserts the balloon, he puts on sterile gloves, gown, and mask. He cleans the site with antiseptic solution and drapes the area with a sterile drape.

Inserting the intra-aortic balloon percutaneously

▶ The physician may insert the balloon percutaneously through the femoral artery into the descending thoracic aorta, using a modified Seldinger technique.

▶ After the balloon is in place, the physician attaches it to the control system to initiate counterpulsation. The balloon catheter then unfurls.

▶ The physician will clean the insertion site and apply a sterile dressing.

▶ Obtain a chest X-ray to verify correct balloon placement.

Monitoring the patient with an intra-aortic balloon

CLINICAL ALERT

If the control system malfunctions or becomes inoperable, don't let the balloon catheter remain dormant for more than 30 minutes. Get another control system and attach it to the balloon; then resume pumping. In the meantime, inflate the balloon manually, using a 60-ml syringe and room air a minimum of once every 5 minutes, to prevent thrombus formation in the catheter.

▶ Assess and record pedal and posterior tibial pulses as well as color, sensation, and temperature in the affected limb every 15 minutes for 1 hour, then hourly. Notify the physician immediately if you detect circulatory changes; the balloon may need to be removed. **CS**

▶ Observe and record the patient's baseline arm pulses, arm sensation and movement, and arm color and temperature every 15 minutes for 1 hour after balloon insertion, then every

2 hours while the balloon is in place. Loss of left arm pulses may indicate upward balloon displacement. Notify the physician of any changes. **CS1**

▶ Monitor the patient's urine output every hour. Note baseline blood urea nitrogen (BUN) and serum creatinine levels, and monitor these levels daily. Changes in urine output, BUN, and serum creatinine levels may signal reduced renal perfusion from downward balloon displacement.

▶ Auscultate and record bowel sounds every 4 hours. Check for abdominal distention and tenderness as well as changes in the patient's elimination patterns.

▶ Measure the patient's temperature every 1 to 4 hours. If it's elevated, obtain blood samples for a culture, send them to the laboratory immediately, and notify the physician. Culture any drainage at the insertion site.

▶ Monitor the patient's hematologic status. Observe for bleeding gums, blood in the urine or stools, petechiae, and bleeding at the insertion site. Monitor his platelet count, hemoglobin level, and hematocrit daily. If the platelet count drops, expect to administer platelets. **CS2**

▶ Monitor partial thromboplastin time (PTT) every 6 hours while the heparin dose is adjusted to maintain PTT at $1\frac{1}{2}$ to 2 times the normal value, then every 12 to 24 hours while the balloon remains in place.

▶ Measure PAP and pulmonary artery wedge pressure (PAWP) every 1 to 2 hours as ordered. A rising PAWP reflects preload, signaling increased ventricular pressure and workload; notify the physician if this occurs. Some patients require I.V. nitroprusside during IABC to reduce preload and afterload.

▶ Obtain samples for ABG analysis as ordered.

▶ Monitor serum electrolyte levels—especially sodium and potassium—to

assess the patient's fluid and electrolyte balance and help prevent arrhythmias.

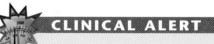

CLINICAL ALERT

Watch for signs and symptoms of a dissecting aortic aneurysm: a blood pressure differential between the left and right arms, elevated blood pressure, syncope, pallor, diaphoresis, dyspnea, a throbbing abdominal mass, a reduced red blood cell count with an elevated white blood cell count, and pain in the chest, abdomen, or back. Notify the physician immediately if you detect these complications.

Weaning the patient from IABC

▶ Assess the cardiac index, systemic blood pressure, and PAWP to help the physician evaluate the patient's readiness for weaning—usually about 24 hours after balloon insertion. The patient's hemodynamic status should be stable on minimal doses of inotropic agents, such as dopamine or dobutamine.

▶ To begin weaning, gradually decrease the frequency of balloon augmentation to 1:2 and 1:4 as ordered.

▶ Avoid leaving the patient on a low augmentation setting for more than 2 hours to prevent embolus formation.

▶ Assess the patient's tolerance of weaning. Signs and symptoms of poor tolerance include confusion and disorientation, urine output below 30 ml/ hour, cold and clammy skin, chest pain, arrhythmias, ischemic ECG changes, and elevated PAP. If the patient develops any of these problems, notify the physician at once.

(Text continues on page 274.)

Troubleshooting an IABP

When your patient has an intra-aortic balloon pump (IABP), many common problems can develop. Use this chart to help you recognize and resolve such problems.

PROBLEM	POSSIBLE CAUSES	INTERVENTIONS
High gas leak (automatic mode only)	Balloon leakage or abrasion	▶ Check for blood in the tubing. ▶ Stop pumping. ▶ Notify the physician to remove the balloon.
	Condensation in extension tubing, volume-limiter disk, or both	▶ Remove condensate from the tubing and volume-limiter disk. ▶ Refill, autopurge, and resume pumping.
	Kink in balloon catheter or tubing	▶ Check the catheter and tubing for kinks and loose connections; straighten and tighten any found. ▶ Refill and resume pumping.
	Tachycardia	▶ Change wean control to 1:2 or operate on "manual" mode. ▶ Autopurge the balloon every 1 to 2 hours, and monitor the balloon pressure waveform closely.
	Malfunctioning or loose volume-limiter disk	▶ Replace or tighten the disk. ▶ Refill, autopurge, and resume pumping.
	System leak	▶ Perform a leak test.
Balloon line block (in automatic mode only)	Kink in balloon or catheter	▶ Check the catheter and tubing for kinks and loose connections; straighten and tighten any found. ▶ Refill and resume pumping.
	Balloon catheter not unfurled; sheath or balloon positioned too high	▶ Notify the physician immediately to verify placement. ▶ Anticipate the need for repositioning or manual inflation of the balloon.
	Condensation in tubing, volume-limiter disk, or both	▶ Remove condensate from the tubing and volume-limiter disk. ▶ Refill, autopurge, and resume pumping.
	Balloon too large for aorta	▶ Decrease volume control percentage by one notch.
	Malfunctioning volume-limiter disk or incorrect volume-limiter disk size	▶ Replace the volume-limiter disk. ▶ Refill, autopurge, and resume pumping.
No electrocardiogram (ECG) trigger	Inadequate signal	▶ Adjust ECG gain, and change the lead or trigger mode.
	Lead disconnected	▶ Replace the lead.
	Improper ECG input mode (skin or monitor) selected	▶ Adjust ECG input to appropriate mode (skin or monitor).

Troubleshooting an IABP *(continued)*

PROBLEM	POSSIBLE CAUSES	INTERVENTIONS
No atrial pressure trigger	Arterial line damped	▶ Flush the line.
	Arterial line open to atmosphere	▶ Check connections on the arterial pressure line.
Trigger mode change	Trigger mode changed while pumping	▶ Resume pumping.
Irregular heart rhythm	Patient experiencing arrhythmia, such as atrial fibrillation or ectopic beats	▶ Change to R or QRS sense (to accommodate irregular rhythm, if necessary). ▶ Notify the physician of arrhythmia.
Erratic atrioventricular (AV) pacing	Demand for paced rhythm occurring when in AV sequential trigger mode	▶ Change to pacer reject trigger or QRS sense.
Noisy ECG signal	Malfunctioning leads	▶ Replace the leads. ▶ Check the ECG cable.
	Electrocautery in use	▶ Switch to atrial pressure trigger.
Internal trigger	Trigger mode set on internal 80 beats/minute	▶ Select an alternative trigger if the patient has a heartbeat or rhythm. ▶ Keep in mind that the internal trigger is used only during cardiopulmonary bypass or cardiac arrest.
Purge incomplete	OFF button pressed during autopurge; interrupted purge cycle	▶ Initiate autopurging again, or initiate pumping.
High fill pressure	Malfunctioning volume-limiter disk	▶ Replace the volume-limiter disk. ▶ Refill, autopurge, and resume pumping.
	Occluded vent line or valve	▶ Attempt to resume pumping. ▶ If unsuccessful, notify the physician and contact the manufacturer.
No balloon drive	No volume-limiter disk	▶ Insert the volume-limiter disk, and lock it securely in place.
	Tubing disconnected	▶ Reconnect the tubing. ▶ Refill, autopurge, and pump.
Incorrect timing	INFLATE and DEFLATE controls set incorrectly	▶ Place the INFLATE and DEFLATE controls at set midpoints. ▶ Reassess timing and readjust.
Low volume percentage	Volume control percentage not 100%	▶ Assess the cause of decreased volume, and reset (if necessary).

Removing the intra-aortic balloon

▶ The balloon is removed when the patient's hemodynamic status remains stable after the frequency of balloon augmentation is decreased. The control system is turned off, and the connective tubing is disconnected from the catheter to ensure balloon deflation.

▶ The physician withdraws the balloon until the proximal end of the catheter contacts the distal end of the introducer sheath.

▶ The physician then applies pressure below the puncture site and removes the balloon and introducer sheath as a unit, allowing a few seconds of free bleeding to prevent thrombus formation.

▶ To promote distal bleedback, the physician applies pressure above the puncture site.

▶ Apply direct pressure to the site for 30 minutes or until bleeding stops. (In some facilities, this is the physician's responsibility.)

▶ If the balloon was inserted surgically, the physician will close the Dacron graft and suture the insertion site. The cardiologist usually removes a percutaneous catheter.

▶ After balloon removal, provide wound care according to your facility's policy. Record the patient's pedal and posterior tibial pulses and the color, temperature, and sensation of the affected limb. Enforce bed rest as appropriate (usually for 8 hours).

▶ Check vital signs and hemodynamic parameters every 15 minutes for 1 hour, every 30 minutes for 2 hours, and then every hour, or according to your facility's policy.

Special considerations

▶ If the physician chooses not to insert the catheter percutaneously, he usually inserts it by femoral arteriotomy.

▶ Before using the IABC control system, make sure you know what the alarms and messages mean and how to respond to them.

▶ Change the dressing at the balloon insertion site every 24 hours or as needed, using strict sterile technique. Don't let povidone-iodine solution come in contact with the catheter.

▶ Make sure the head of the bed is elevated no more than 30 degrees.

▶ Watch for pump interruptions, which may result from loose ECG electrodes or leadwires, static or 60-cycle interference, catheter kinking, or improper body alignment. (See *Troubleshooting an IABP,* pages 272 and 273.)

▶ Make sure PTT is within normal limits before the balloon is removed to prevent hemorrhage at the insertion site.

▶ IABC may cause numerous complications. The most common—arterial embolism—stems from clot formation on the balloon surface. Other potential complications include extension or rupture of an aortic aneurysm, femoral or iliac artery perforation, femoral artery occlusion, and sepsis. Bleeding at the insertion site may become aggravated by pump-induced thrombocytopenia caused by platelet aggregation around the balloon.

References

American Association of Critical Care Nurses. "Standards." Available at *www.aacn.org/AACN/practice.nsf/Files/acstds/$file/130300StdsAcute.pdf.*

Arafa, O.E., et al. "Vascular Complications of the Intraaortic Balloon Pump in Patients Undergoing Open Heart Operations: 15-year Experience," *Annals of Thoracic Surgery* 67(3):645-51, March 1999. **CS1**

Field, M.L., et al. "Preoperative Intra-aortic Balloon Pumps in Patients Undergoing Coronary Artery Bypass Grafting." *Cochrane Database of Systematic Review* (1):CD004472, 2007.

Lynn-McHale Wiegand, D.J., and Carlson, K.K., eds. *AACN Procedure Manual for Critical Care,* 5th ed. Philadelphia: W.B. Saunders Co., 2005.

Reid, M.B., and Cottrell, D. "Nursing Care of Patients Receiving Intra-aortic Balloon Counterpulsation," *Critical Care Nurse* 25(5):40-44, 46-49, October 2005.

Santa-Cruz, R.A., et al. "Aortic Counterpulsation: A Review of the Hemodynamic Effects and Indications for Use," *Catheterization and Cardiovascular Interventions* 67(1):68-77, January 2006.

Trost, J.C., and Hillis, L.D. "Intra-aortic Balloon Counterpulsation," *American Journal of Cardiology* 97(9):1391-398, May 2006.

Vanderheide, R.H., et al. "Association of Thrombocytopenia with the Use of Intra-aortic Balloon Pumps," *American Journal of Medicine* 105(1):27-32, July 1998. **CS2**

Intracranial pressure monitoring

Intracranial pressure (ICP) monitoring measures pressure exerted by the brain, blood, and cerebrospinal fluid (CSF) against the inside of the skull. Normal ICP is 0 to 15 mm Hg, with the ICP threshold of 20 to 25 mm Hg as the highest acceptable limit before instituting treatment. Indications for monitoring ICP include head trauma with bleeding or edema, overproduction or insufficient absorption of CSF (hydrocephalus), cerebral hemorrhage, and space-occupying brain lesions. ICP monitoring can detect elevated ICP early, before clinical danger signs develop. **AANN** Prompt intervention can then help avert or diminish neurologic damage caused by cerebral hypoxia and shifts of brain mass.

The four basic ICP monitoring systems are intraventricular catheter, subarachnoid bolt, epidural or subdural sensor, and intraparenchymal monitoring. (See *Understanding ICP monitoring systems*.)

Understanding ICP monitoring systems

Intracranial pressure (ICP) can be monitored using one of four systems.

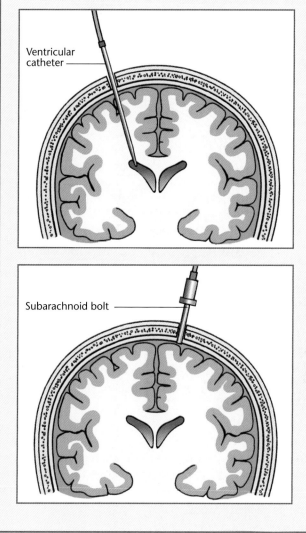

Intraventricular catheter monitoring

In intraventricular catheter monitoring, which monitors ICP directly, the physician inserts a small polyethylene or silicone rubber catheter into the lateral ventricle through a burr hole.

Although this method measures ICP most accurately and drains cerebrospinal fluid (CSF), it carries the greatest risk of infection. This is the only type of ICP monitoring that allows evaluation of brain compliance and drainage of significant amounts of CSF.

Contraindications usually include stenotic cerebral ventricles, cerebral aneurysms in the path of catheter placement, and suspected vascular lesions.

Subarachnoid bolt monitoring

Subarachnoid bolt monitoring involves insertion of a special bolt into the subarachnoid space through a twist-drill burr hole that's positioned in the front of the skull behind the hairline.

Placing the bolt is easier than placing an intraventricular catheter, especially if a computed tomography scan reveals that the cerebrum has shifted or the ventricles have collapsed. This type of ICP monitoring also carries less risk of infection and parenchymal damage because the bolt doesn't penetrate the cerebrum.

(continued)

Understanding ICP monitoring systems *(continued)*

Epidural or subdural sensor monitoring

ICP can also be monitored from the epidural or subdural space. For epidural monitoring, a fiber-optic sensor is inserted into the epidural space through a burr hole. This system's main drawback is its questionable accuracy because ICP isn't being measured directly from a CSF-filled space.

For subdural monitoring, a fiber-optic transducer-tipped catheter is tunneled through a burr hole and its tip is placed on brain tissue under the dura mater. The main drawback to this method is its inability to drain CSF.

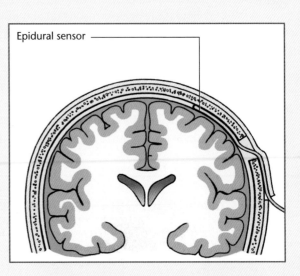

Epidural sensor

Intraparenchymal monitoring

In intraparenchymal monitoring, the physician inserts a catheter through a small subarachnoid bolt and, after puncturing the dura, advances the catheter a few centimeters into the brain's white matter. There is no need to balance or calibrate the equipment after insertion.

Although this method doesn't provide direct access to CSF, measurements are accurate because brain tissue pressures correlate well with ventricular pressures. Intraparenchymal monitoring may be used to obtain ICP measurements in patients with compressed or dislocated ventricles.

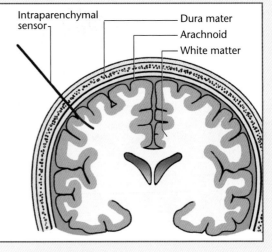

Intraparenchymal sensor

Dura mater
Arachnoid
White matter

Regardless of which system is used, the procedure is typically performed by a neurosurgeon in the operating room, emergency department (ED), or intensive care unit (ICU). Insertion of an ICP monitoring device requires sterile technique to reduce the risk of central nervous system infection. Setting up equipment for the monitoring systems also requires strict asepsis. **AANN**

Equipment

Monitoring unit and transducers as ordered ◆ 16 to 20 sterile 4″ × 4″ gauze pads ◆ linen-saver pads ◆ clippers ◆ sterile drapes ◆ povidone-iodine solution ◆ sterile gown ◆ surgical mask ◆ two pairs of sterile gloves ◆ sedation as needed ◆ sterile occlusive dressing ◆ one roll of 4″ roller gauze as needed ◆ sterile marker ◆ sterile labels ◆ 1% or 2% lidocaine with epinephrine ◆ 10 ml syringe with 18G and 23G needle ◆ sutures ◆ optional: yardstick, I.V. pole.

Implementation

▶ Confirm the patient's identity using two patient identifiers according to your facility's policy. **JC**

▶ Explain the procedure to the patient or his family. Make sure the patient or a responsible family member has signed a consent form. **AANN**

▶ Determine whether the patient is allergic to iodine preparations.

▶ Provide privacy if the procedure is being done in an open ED or ICU. Wash your hands.

▶ Obtain baseline routine and neurologic vital signs to help detect decompensation promptly during the procedure. **AANN**

▶ Place the patient in the supine position, and elevate the head of the bed 30 degrees (or as ordered). If possible, lock the bed controls after the bed is in position at the ordered height. **AANN** **CS**

▶ Place linen-saver pads under the patient's head.

▶ Clip his hair at the insertion site, as indicated by the physician, to decrease the risk of infection. Carefully fold and remove the linen-saver pads to avoid spilling loose hair onto the bed. The neurosurgeon will drape the patient with sterile drapes and scrub the insertion site for 2 minutes with povidone-iodine solution with the nurse's assistance.

▶ The physician puts on the sterile gown, mask, and sterile gloves. He then opens the interior wrap of the sterile supply tray and proceeds with insertion of the catheter or bolt. Label all medications, medication containers, and other solutions on and off the sterile field. **JC**

▶ To facilitate placement of the device, hold the patient's head in your hands or attach a long strip of 4″ roller gauze to one side rail and bring it across the patient's forehead to the opposite rail. Reassure the conscious patient, or administer reversible, quick-acting sedation to help ease his anxiety. **AANN** Talk to him frequently to assess his level of consciousness (LOC) and detect signs of deterioration. Watch for cardiac arrhythmias and abnormal respiratory patterns.

▶ After insertion, apply antiseptic solution and a sterile dressing to the site. If not done by the physician, connect the catheter to the appropriate monitoring device, depending on the system used. **AANN** (See *Setting up an ICP monitoring system,* pages 278 and 279.)

▶ If the physician has set up a drainage system, attach the drip chamber to the headboard or bedside I.V. pole as ordered.

CLINICAL ALERT

Positioning the drip chamber too high may raise ICP; positioning it too low may cause excessive CSF drainage.

▶ Inspect the insertion site at least every 4 hours (or according to your facility's policy) for redness, swelling, and drainage. Clean the site, reapply antiseptic solution, and apply a dry sterile dressing according to your facility's policy.

▶ Assess the patient's clinical status, and take routine and neurologic vital signs hourly or as ordered. Make sure you've obtained orders for pressure parameters from the physician. **AANN**

▶ Calculate cerebral perfusion pressure (CPP) hourly; use the equation:

$$CPP = MAP - ICP$$

(MAP refers to mean arterial pressure). If the CPP isn't within the specific parameters, notify the physician. **AANN**

▶ Observe digital ICP readings and waves. Remember, the trend revealed by multiple readings is more significant than any single reading. (See *Interpreting ICP waveforms,* page 280.) If you observe continually elevated ICP readings, note how long they're sustained. If they last several minutes, notify the physician immediately. Finally, record and describe any CSF drainage for color, amount, and consistency.

Special considerations

AGE FACTOR

In infants, ICP monitoring can be performed without penetrating the scalp. In this external method, a photoelectric transducer with a pressure-sensitive membrane is taped to the anterior fontanel. The transducer responds to pressure at the site and transmits readings to a bedside monitor and recording system. The external method is restricted to infants because pressure readings can be obtained only at the fontanels, the incompletely ossified areas of the skull.

▶ Monitor intake and output carefully to confirm normovolemia and to ensure adequate MAP to ensure good CPP. The patient may be on a fluid restriction of 1,200 to 1,500 ml/day to help prevent cerebral edema from worsening.

▶ Hyperventilation with oxygen from a handheld resuscitation bag or ventilator helps rid the patient of excess carbon dioxide, thereby constricting cerebral vessels and reducing cerebral blood volume and ICP. However, only normal brain tissues respond because blood vessels in damaged areas have reduced vasoconstrictive ability. Hyperventilation should be done only in an acute situation to decrease ICP until other measures can be instituted. **AANN**

▶ Because fever raises brain metabolism, which increases cerebral blood flow, fever reduction (achieved by ad-

(*Text continues on page 281.*)

Setting up an ICP monitoring system

To set up an intracranial pressure (ICP) monitoring system, follow these steps.

▶ Begin by opening a sterile towel. On the sterile field, place a 20-ml luer-lock syringe, an 18G needle, a 250-ml bag filled with normal saline solution (with outer wrapper removed), and a disposable transducer.

▶ Put on sterile gloves and gown according to your facility's policy, and fill the 20-ml syringe with normal saline solution from the I.V. bag.

▶ Remove the injection cap from the patient line, and attach the syringe. Turn the system stopcock off to the short end of the patient line, and flush through to the drip chamber. Allow a few drops to flow through the flow chamber (the manometer), the tubing, and the one-way valve into the drainage bag. (Fill the tubing and the manometer slowly to minimize air bubbles. If air bubbles surface, be sure to force them from the system.)

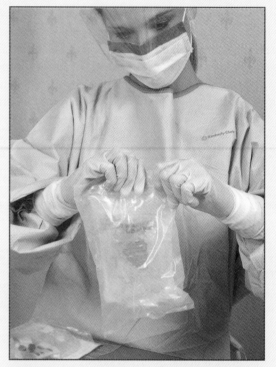

▶ Attach the manometer to the I.V. pole at the head of the bed.

▶ Slide the drip chamber onto the manometer, and align the chamber to the zero point (as shown), which should be at the inner canthus of the patient's eye.

▶ Next, connect the transducer to the monitor.

▶ Put on a clean pair of sterile gloves.

▶ Keeping one hand sterile, turn off the stopcock to the patient.

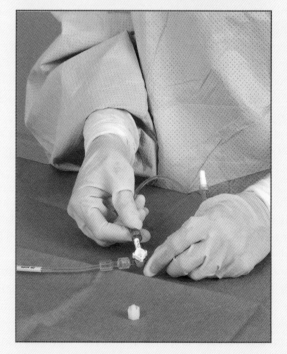

Setting up an ICP monitoring system (continued)

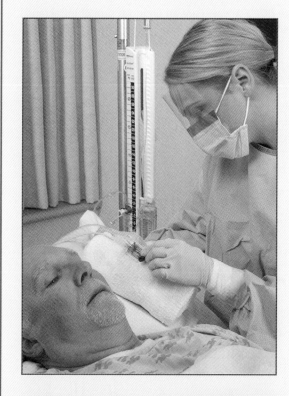

▶ Align the zero point with the center line of the patient's head, level with the middle of the ear.

▶ Lower the flow chamber to zero, and turn off the stopcock to the dead-end cap. With a clean hand, balance the system according to the monitor guidelines.

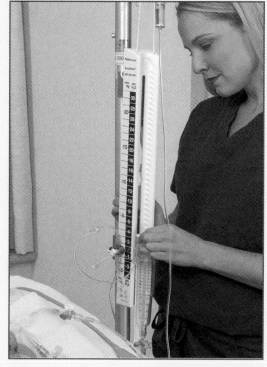

▶ Turn off the system stopcock to drainage, and raise the flow chamber to the ordered height (as shown).

▶ Return the stopcock to the ordered position, and observe the monitor for the return of ICP patterns.

Interpreting ICP waveforms

Three waveforms—A, B, and C—are used to monitor intracranial pressure (ICP). A waves are an ominous sign of intracranial decompensation and poor compliance. B waves correlate with changes in respiration, and C waves correlate with changes in arterial pressure.

Normal waveform
A normal ICP waveform typically shows a steep upward systolic slope followed by a downward diastolic slope with a dicrotic notch. In most cases, this waveform occurs continuously and indicates an ICP between 0 and 15 mm Hg—normal pressure.

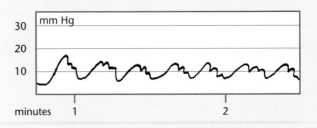

A waves
The most clinically significant ICP waveforms are A waves, which may reach elevations of 50 to 100 mm Hg, persist for 5 to 20 minutes, then drop sharply—signaling exhaustion of the brain's compliance mechanisms. A waves signify a reduction in cerebral perfusion pressure with ensuing hypoxia and decompensation. Because A waves are an ominous sign, they require emergency treatment.

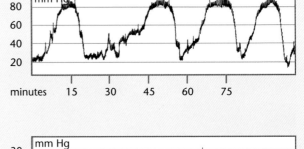

B waves
B waves, which appear sharp and rhythmic with a sawtooth pattern, occur every 30 seconds to 2 minutes and may reach elevations of 50 mm Hg. The clinical significance of B waves isn't clear, but the waves correlate with respiratory changes and may occur more frequently with decreasing compensation. Because B waves sometimes precede A waves, notify the practitioner if B waves occur frequently.

C waves
C waves are rapid and rhythmic, but not sharp, and last 1 to 2 minutes with an ICP of 20 to 50 mm Hg. Clinically insignificant, they may fluctuate with respirations or systemic blood pressure changes.

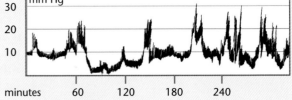

Waveform showing equipment problem
A waveform, such as the one shown at right, signals a problem with the transducer or monitor. Check for line obstruction, and determine whether the transducer needs rebalancing. If the patient has a low ICP reading, this may be a normal wave.

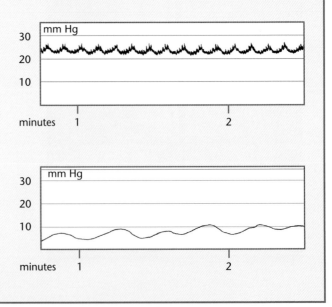

ministering acetaminophen, sponge baths, or a hypothermia blanket) also helps to reduce ICP. However, rebound increases in ICP and brain edema may occur if rapid rewarming takes place after hypothermia or if cooling measures induce shivering.

▶ Withdrawal of CSF through the drainage system reduces CSF volume and thus reduces ICP. Although less commonly used, surgical removal of a skull-bone flap provides room for the swollen brain to expand. If this procedure is performed, prevent direct trauma to the exposed tissue, keep the site clean and dry to prevent infection, and maintain sterile technique when changing the dressing.

▶ Watch for signs of impending increased ICP or overt decompensation: pupillary dilation (unilateral or bilateral); decreased pupillary response to light; decreasing LOC; rising systolic blood pressure and widening pulse pressure; bradycardia; slowed, irregular respirations; and, in late decompensation, decerebrate posturing.

References

American Association of Neuroscience Nurses. *Core Curriculum for Neuroscience Nursing,* 4th ed. Philadelphia: W.B. Saunders Co., 2004.

American Association of Neuroscience Nurses. Guide to the Care of the Patient with Intracranial Pressure Monitoring: *AANN Reference Series for Clinical Practice*. Glenview, Ill.: American Association of Neuroscience Nurses, 2005.

Cremer, O.L., et al. "Need for Intracranial Pressure Monitoring following Severe Traumatic Brain Injury," *Critical Care Medicine* 34(5):1583-584, May 2006.

Kuo, J.R., et al. "Intraoperative Applications of Intracranial Pressure Monitoring in Patients with Severe Head Injury," *Journal of Clinical Neuroscience* 12(2):218-23, February 2006.

Lynn-McHale Wiegand, D.J., and Carlson, K.K., eds. *AACN Procedure Manual for Critical Care,* 5th ed. Philadelphia: W.B. Saunders Co., 2005.

March, K. "Intracranial Pressure Monitoring: Why Monitor?" *AACN Clinical Issues* 16(4):456-75, October-December 2005.

Ng, I., et al. "Effects of Head Posture on Cerebral Hemodynamics: Its Influences on Intracranial Pressure, Cerebral Perfusion Pressure, and Cerebral Oxygenation," *Neurosurgery* 54(3): 593-97, March 2004. **CS**

Intradermal injection

Because little systemic absorption of intradermally injected agents takes place, this type of injection is used primarily to produce a local effect, as in allergy or tuberculin testing. Intradermal injections are administered in small volumes (usually 0.5 ml or less) into the outer layers of the skin.

The ventral forearm is the most commonly used site for intradermal injection because of its easy accessibility and lack of hair. In extensive allergy testing, the outer aspect of the upper arms may be used as well as the area of the back located between the scapulae. (See *Locating intradermal injection sites*.)

Equipment

Patient's medication record and chart ◆ tuberculin syringe with a 26G or 27G $1/2''$ to $3/8''$ needle ◆ prescribed medication ◆ gloves ◆ alcohol pads.

Implementation

▶ Verify the order on the patient's medication record by checking it against the practitioner's order. **JC** **ISMP**

▶ Inspect the medication to make sure it isn't abnormally discolored or cloudy and doesn't contain precipitates.

▶ Wash your hands.

▶ Check the medication label against the patient's medication record. Read the label again as you draw up the medication for injection.

▶ Confirm the patient's identity using two patient identifiers according to your facility's policy. **JC**

▶ If your facility utilizes a bar code scanning system, be sure to scan your ID badge, the patient's ID bracelet, and the medication's bar code. **JC** **ISMP**

Locating intradermal injection sites

The most common intradermal injection site is the ventral forearm. Other sites (indicated by dotted areas) include the upper chest, upper arm, and shoulder blades. Skin in these areas is usually lightly pigmented, thinly keratinized, and relatively hairless, thus aiding detection of adverse reactions.

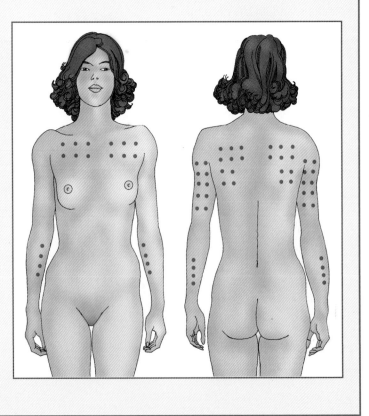

▶ Tell the patient where you'll be giving the injection.

▶ Instruct the patient to sit up and to extend his arm and support it on a flat surface, with the ventral forearm exposed.

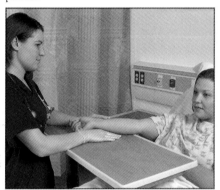

▶ Put on gloves.

▶ With an alcohol pad, clean the surface of the ventral forearm about two or three fingerbreadths distal to the antecubital space (as shown at the top of the next column). Make sure the test site you have chosen is free from hair or blemishes. Allow the skin to dry

completely before administering the injection.

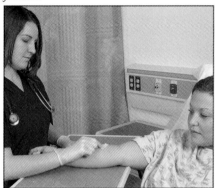

▶ While holding the patient's forearm in your hand, stretch the skin taut with your thumb.

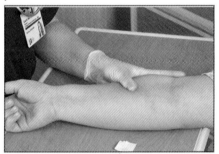

▶ With your free hand, hold the needle at a 10- to 15-degree angle to the patient's arm, with its bevel up.

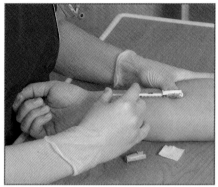

▶ Insert the needle about ¹/₈″ (0.3 cm) below the epidermis at sites 2″ (5 cm) apart. Stop when the needle's bevel tip is under the skin, and inject the antigen slowly. You should feel some resistance as you do this, and a wheal should form as you inject the antigen. (See *Giving an intradermal injection.*) If no wheal forms, you have injected the antigen too deeply; withdraw the needle, and administer another test dose

Giving an intradermal injection

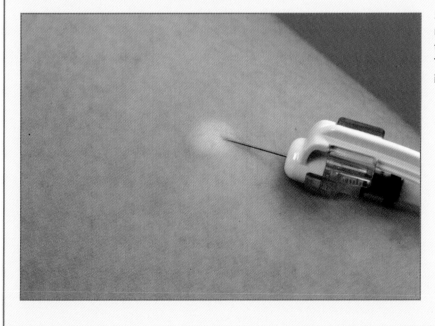

Secure the patient's forearm. Insert the needle at a 10- to 15-degree angle so that it just punctures the skin's surface. The antigen should raise a small wheal as it's injected.

at least 2″ away from the initial test site.

▶ Withdraw the needle at the same angle at which it was inserted. Don't rub the site. This could irritate the underlying tissue, which may affect test results.

▶ Circle each test site with a marking pen, and label each site according to the recall antigen given. Instruct the patient to refrain from washing off the circles until the test is completed.

▶ Dispose of needles and syringes according to your facility's policy.

▶ Remove and discard your gloves.

▶ Assess the patient's response to the skin testing in 24 to 48 hours.

Special considerations

▶ In patients who are hypersensitive to the test antigens, a severe anaphylactic response can result. This requires immediate epinephrine injection and other emergency resuscitation procedures. Be especially alert after giving a test dose of penicillin or tetanus antitoxin.

References

The Joint Commission. *Comprehensive Accreditation Manual for Hospitals: The Official Handbook*. Standard MM.4.30. Oakbrook Terrace, Ill.: The Joint Commission, 2007.

The Joint Commission. *Comprehensive Accreditation Manual for Hospitals: The Official Handbook*. Standard MM.5.10. Oakbrook Terrace, Ill.: The Joint Commission, 2007.

The Joint Commission. *Comprehensive Accreditation Manual for Hospitals: The Official Handbook*. Standard MM.5.20. Oakbrook Terrace, Ill.: The Joint Commission, 2007.

The Joint Commission. *Comprehensive Accreditation Manual for Hospitals: The Official Handbook*. Standard MM.6.20. Oakbrook Terrace, Ill.: The Joint Commission, 2007.

La Montagne, J.R., and Fauci, A.S. "Intradermal Influenza Vaccination—Can Less Be More?" *New England Journal of Medicine* 351(2):2330-332, November 2004.

Love, G.H. "Administering an Intradermal Injection," *Nursing* 36(6):20, June 2006.

Taylor, C., et al. *Fundamentals of Nursing: The Art and Science of Nursing Care,* 6th ed. Philadelphia: Lippincott Williams & Wilkins, 2008.

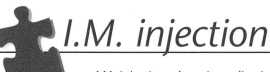

I.M. injection

I.M. injections deposit medication deep into muscle tissue. This route of administration provides rapid systemic action and absorption of relatively large doses (up to 5 ml in appropriate sites). I.M. injections are recommended for patients who are uncooperative or who can't take medication orally and for delivery of drugs that are altered by digestive juices. Because muscle tissue has few sensory nerves, I.M. injection allows less painful administration of irritating drugs.

The site for an I.M. injection must be chosen carefully, taking into account the patient's general physical status and the purpose of the injection. I.M. injections shouldn't be administered at inflamed, edematous, or irritated sites or at sites that contain moles, birthmarks, scar tissue, or other lesions. I.M. injections may also be contraindicated in patients with impaired coagulation mechanisms, occlusive peripheral vascular disease, edema, and shock; after thrombolytic therapy; and during an acute myocardial infarction (MI) because these conditions impair peripheral absorption. I.M. injections require sterile technique to maintain the integrity of muscle tissue.

Equipment

Patient's medication record and chart ◆ prescribed medication ◆ diluent or filter needle, if needed ◆ 3- or 5-ml syringe ◆ 20G to 25G 1″ to 3″ needle ◆ gloves ◆ alcohol pads ◆ 2″ × 2″ gauze pad.

The prescribed medication must be sterile.

Implementation

▶ Verify the order on the patient's medication record by checking it against the practitioner's order. Also, note whether the patient has any allergies, especially before the first dose. **JC** **ISMP**

▶ Wash your hands.

▶ Check the prescribed medication for color and clarity. Also, note the expiration date.

▶ For single-dose ampules, wrap an alcohol pad around the ampule's neck and snap off the top, directing the force away from your body. Attach a filter needle and withdraw the medication, keeping the needle's bevel tip below the level of the solution. Tap the syringe to clear air from it. Cover the needle with the needle sheath. **INS** **CS**

▶ Before discarding the ampule, check the medication label against the patient's medication record. Discard the filter needle and the ampule. Attach the appropriate needle to the syringe.

▶ For single-dose or multidose vials, reconstitute powdered drugs according to instructions. Make sure all crystals have dissolved in the solution. Warm the vial by rolling it between your palms to help the drug dissolve faster.

▶ Wipe the stopper of the medication vial with an alcohol pad, and then draw up the prescribed amount of medication. Read the medication label as you select the medication, as you draw it up, and after you've drawn it up to verify the correct dosage.

▶ Gather all necessary equipment, and proceed to the patient's room.

▶ Confirm the patient's identity using two patient identifiers according to your facility's policy. **JC**

▶ If your facility utilizes a bar code scanning system, be sure to scan your ID badge, the patient's ID bracelet, and the medication's bar code. **JC** **ISMP**

▶ Provide privacy, and explain the procedure to the patient.

▶ Select an appropriate injection site. The ventrogluteal site is used most commonly for healthy adults, although the deltoid muscle may be used for a small-volume injection (2 ml or less). Remember to rotate injection sites for patients who require repeated injections. (See *Locating I.M. injection sites,* page 286)

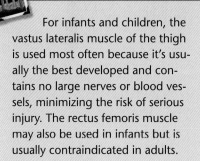

AGE FACTOR

For infants and children, the vastus lateralis muscle of the thigh is used most often because it's usually the best developed and contains no large nerves or blood vessels, minimizing the risk of serious injury. The rectus femoris muscle may also be used in infants but is usually contraindicated in adults.

▶ Position and drape the patient appropriately, making sure that the site is well exposed and that lighting is adequate.

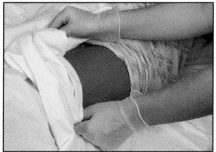

Locating I.M. injection sites

Deltoid

Find the lower edge of the acromial process and the point on the lateral arm in line with the axilla. Insert the needle 1″ to 2″ (2.5 to 5 cm) below the acromial process, usually two or three fingerbreadths, at a 90-degree angle or angled slightly toward the process. Typical injection: 0.5 ml (range: 0.5 to 2.0 ml).

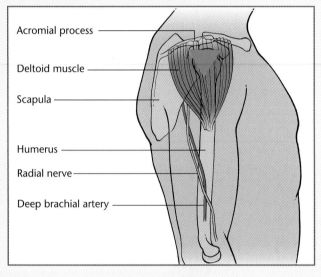

Dorsogluteal

Inject above and outside a line drawn from the posterior superior iliac spine to the greater trochanter of the femur. Or, divide the buttock into quadrants and inject in the upper outer quadrant, about 2″ to 3″ (5 to 7.5 cm) below the iliac crest. Insert the needle at a 90-degree angle. Typical injection: 1 to 4 ml (range: 1 to 5 ml).

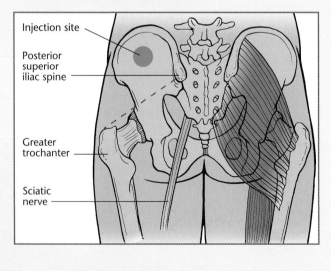

Ventrogluteal

Locate the greater trochanter of the femur with the heel of your hand. Then spread your index and middle fingers from the anterior superior iliac spine to as far along the iliac crest as you can reach. Insert the needle between the two fingers at a 90-degree angle to the muscle. (Remove your fingers before inserting the needle.) Typical injection: 1 to 4 ml (range: 1 to 5 ml).

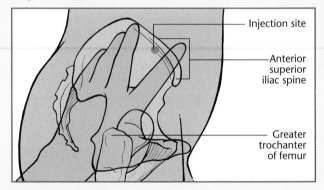

Vastus lateralis

Use the lateral muscle of the quadriceps group, from a handbreadth below the greater trochanter to a handbreadth above the knee. Insert the needle into the middle third of the muscle parallel to the surface on which the patient is lying. You may have to bunch the muscle before insertion. Typical injection: 1 to 4 ml (range: 1 to 5 ml; 1 to 3 ml for infants).

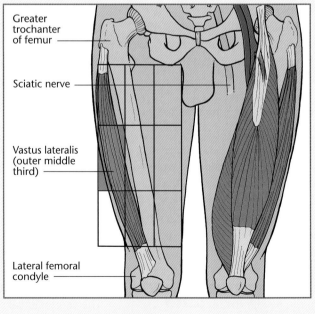

▶ Loosen the protective needle sheath, but don't remove it.

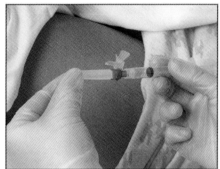

▶ After selecting the injection site, gently tap it to stimulate the nerve endings and minimize pain when the needle is inserted. Clean the skin at the site with an alcohol pad. Move the pad outward in a circular motion to a circumference of about 2″ (5 cm) from the injection site, and allow the skin to dry. Keep the alcohol pad for later use.

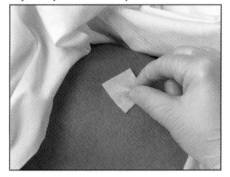

▶ Put on gloves. With the thumb and index finger of your nondominant hand, gently stretch the skin of the injection site taut.
▶ While you hold the syringe in your dominant hand, remove the needle sheath by slipping it between the free fingers of your nondominant hand and then drawing back the syringe.
▶ Position the syringe at a 90-degree angle to the skin surface, with the needle a couple of inches from the skin. Tell the patient that he'll feel a prick as you insert the needle. Then quickly and firmly thrust the needle through the skin and subcutaneous tissue, deep into the muscle.

▶ Support the syringe with your nondominant hand, if desired. Pull back slightly on the plunger with your dominant hand to aspirate for blood. If no blood appears, slowly inject the medication into the muscle. A slow, steady injection rate allows the muscle to distend gradually and accept the medication under minimal pressure. You should feel little or no resistance against the force of the injection.

CLINICAL ALERT

If blood appears in the syringe on aspiration, the needle is in a blood vessel. If this occurs, stop the injection, withdraw the needle, prepare another injection with new equipment, and inject another site. Don't inject the bloody solution.

▶ After the injection, gently but quickly remove the needle at a 90-degree angle.
▶ Using a gloved hand, cover the injection site immediately with the used alcohol pad or a 2″ × 2″ gauze pad, apply gentle pressure and, unless contraindicated, massage the relaxed muscle to help distribute the drug.

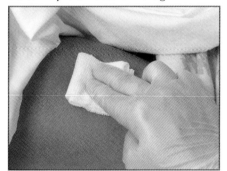

▶ Remove the alcohol pad, and inspect the injection site for signs of active bleeding or bruising. If bleeding continues, apply pressure to the site; if bruising occurs, you may apply ice.
▶ Watch for adverse reactions at the site for 10 to 30 minutes after the injection.

▶ Discard all equipment according to standard precautions and your facility's policy.

Special considerations

▶ Don't use an air bubble in the syringe. Syringes are calibrated to administer the correct dose without an air bubble. **MFR**
▶ To slow their absorption, some drugs for I.M. administration are dissolved in oil or other special solutions. Mix these preparations well before drawing them into the syringe.
▶ Never inject into sensitive muscles, especially those that twitch or tremble when you assess site landmarks and tissue depth. Injections into these trigger areas may cause sharp or referred pain such as the pain caused by nerve trauma.
▶ Keep a rotation record that lists all available injection sites, divided into various body areas, for patients who require repeated injections. Rotate from a site in the first area to a site in each of the other areas. Then return to a site in the first area that is at least 1″ (2.5 cm) away from the previous injection site in that area.
▶ Always encourage the patient to relax the muscle you'll be injecting because injections into tense muscles are more painful than usual and may bleed more readily.
▶ I.M. injections can damage local muscle cells, causing elevations in serum enzyme levels (creatine kinase [CK]) that can be confused with elevations resulting from cardiac muscle damage, as in MI. To distinguish between skeletal and cardiac muscle damage, diagnostic tests for suspected MI must identify the isoenzyme of CK specific to cardiac muscle (CK-MB) and include tests to determine lactate dehydrogenase and aspartate aminotransferase levels. If it's important to

measure these enzyme levels, suggest that the practitioner switch to I.V. administration and adjust dosages accordingly.

References

Craven, R.F., and Hirnle, C.J. *Fundamentals of Nursing: Human Health and Function,* 6th ed. Philadelphia: Lippincott Williams & Wilkins, 2009.

Donaldson, D., and Green, J. "Using the Ventrogluteal Site for Intramuscular Injections," *Nursing Times* 101(16):36-38, April 2005.

"I.M. Injections: Pick Your Site," *Nursing* 36(6):34, June 2006.

The Joint Commission. *Comprehensive Accreditation Manual for Hospitals: The Official Handbook.* Standard MM.1.10. Oakbrook Terrace, Ill.: The Joint Commission, 2007.

The Joint Commission. *Comprehensive Accreditation Manual for Hospitals: The Official Handbook.* Standard MM.2.10. Oakbrook Terrace, Ill.: The Joint Commission, 2007.

The Joint Commission. *Comprehensive Accreditation Manual for Hospitals: The Official Handbook.* Standard MM.3.10. Oakbrook Terrace, Ill.: The Joint Commission, 2007.

The Joint Commission. *Comprehensive Accreditation Manual for Hospitals: The Official Handbook.* Standard MM.4.10. Oakbrook Terrace, Ill.: The Joint Commission, 2007.

The Joint Commission. *Comprehensive Accreditation Manual for Hospitals: The Official Handbook.* Standard MM.4.20. Oakbrook Terrace, Ill.: The Joint Commission, 2007.

The Joint Commission. *Comprehensive Accreditation Manual for Hospitals: The Official Handbook.* Standard MM.5.10. Oakbrook Terrace, Ill.: The Joint Commission, 2007.

The Joint Commission. *Comprehensive Accreditation Manual for Hospitals: The Official Handbook.* Standard MM.6.10. Oakbrook Terrace, Ill.: The Joint Commission, 2007.

The Joint Commission. *Comprehensive Accreditation Manual for Hospitals: The Official Handbook.* Standard MM.6.20. Oakbrook Terrace, Ill.: The Joint Commission, 2007.

Preston, S.T., and Hegadoren, K. "Glass Contamination in Parenterally Administered Medication," *Journal of Advanced Nursing* 48(3):266-70, November 2004.

Prettyman, J. "Subcutaneous or Intramuscular? Confronting a Parenteral Administration Dilemma," *Medsurg Nursing* 14(2):93-98, April 2005.

Ramtahal, J., et al. "Sciatic Nerve Injury following Intramuscular Injection: A Case Report and Review of Literature," *Journal of Neuroscience Nursing* 38(4):238-40, 2006.

Taylor, C., et al. *Fundamentals of Nursing: The Art and Science of Nursing Care,* 6th ed. Philadelphia: Lippincott Williams & Wilkins, 2008.

Wynaden, D. "Establishing Best Practice Guidelines for Administration of Intramuscular Injections in the Adult: A Systematic Review of the Literature," *Contemporary Nurse* 20(2):267-77, December 2005.

Intrapleural injection

An intrapleural drug is injected through the chest wall into the pleural space or instilled through a chest tube placed intrapleurally for drainage. Physicians use intrapleural administration to promote analgesia, treat spontaneous pneumothorax, resolve pleural effusions, and administer chemotherapy.

Intrapleurally administered drugs diffuse across the parietal pleura and innermost intercostal muscles to affect the intercostal nerves. During intrapleural injection, the needle passes through the intercostal muscles and parietal pleura on its way to the pleural space.

Drugs commonly given by intrapleural injection include tetracycline, streptokinase, anesthetics, and chemotherapeutic agents (to treat malignant pleural effusion or lung adenocarcinoma).

Contraindications for this route include pleural fibrosis or adhesions, which interfere with diffusion of the drug to the intended site; pleural inflammation; sepsis; and infection at the puncture site. Patients with bullous emphysema and those receiving respiratory therapy using positive end-expiratory pressure also shouldn't have intrapleural injections because they may worsen an already compromised pulmonary condition.

Equipment

An intrapleural drug is given through a #16 to #20 French or #28 to #40 French chest tube if the patient has empyema, pleural effusion, or pneumothorax. Otherwise, it's given through a 16G to 18G blunt-tipped intrapleural (epidural) needle and catheter. Accessory equipment depends on the type of access device the physician uses. All equipment must be sterile.

For intrapleural catheter insertion: Gloves ◆ gauze ◆ antiseptic solution ◆ drape ◆ local anesthetic such as 1% lidocaine ◆ 3- or 5-ml syringe with 22G 1″ and 25G ⅝″ needles ◆ 18G needle or scalpel ◆ 16G to 18G blunt-tipped intrapleural needle and catheter ◆ saline-lubricated glass syringe ◆ dressings ◆ sutures ◆ tape ◆ intrapleural catheter.

For chest tube insertion: Towels ◆ gloves ◆ gauze ◆ antiseptic solution ◆ 3- or 5-ml syringe ◆ local anesthetic such as 1% lidocaine ◆ 18G needle or scalpel ◆ chest tube with or without trocar (#16 to #20 French catheter for air or serous fluid; #28 to #40 French catheter for blood, pus, or thick fluid) ◆ two rubber-tipped clamps, if neces-

sary ◆ sutures ◆ drain dressings ◆ tape ◆ thoracic drainage system and tubing.

For drug administration: Sterile gloves ◆ sterile gauze pads ◆ antiseptic solution ◆ prescribed medication ◆ appropriate-sized needles and syringes ◆ 1% lidocaine, if necessary ◆ dressings ◆ tape ◆ infusion pump ◆ two rubber-tipped clamps, if necessary.

Implementation

▶ Confirm the patient's identity using two patient identifiers according to your facility's policy. 🆘

▶ Explain the procedure to the patient to allay his fears. Encourage him to follow instructions.

Inserting an intrapleural catheter

▶ The physician inserts the intrapleural catheter at the patient's bedside with the nurse assisting.

▶ Position the patient on his side with the affected side up. The physician will insert the catheter into the fourth to eighth intercostal space, 3″ to 4″ (7.5 to 10 cm) from the posterior midline. (See *Inserting an intrapleural catheter,* page 290.)

▶ The physician puts on sterile gloves, cleans around the puncture site with antiseptic-soaked gauze, and then covers the area with a sterile drape. Next, he fills the 3- or 5-ml syringe with local anesthetic and injects it into the skin and deep tissues.

▶ The physician punctures the skin with the 18G needle or scalpel, which helps the blunt-tipped intrapleural needle penetrate the skin over the superior edge of the lower rib in the chosen interspace. Keeping the bevel tilted upward, he directs the needle medially at a 30- to 40-degree angle to the skin. When the needle tip punctures the posterior intercostal membrane, he removes the stylet and attaches a saline-lubricated glass syringe containing 2 to 4 cc of air to the needle hub.

▶ During puncture, tell the patient to hold his breath (or momentarily disconnect him from mechanical ventilation) until the needle is removed to help prevent the needle from injuring lung tissue.

▶ The physician advances the needle slowly. When the needle punctures the parietal pleura, negative intrapleural pressure moves the plunger outward. He then removes the syringe from the needle and threads the intrapleural catheter through the needle until he has advanced it about 2″ (5 cm) into the pleural space. Without removing the catheter, he carefully withdraws the needle.

▶ Tell the patient that he can breathe again (or reconnect mechanical ventilation).

▶ After inserting the catheter, the physician coils it to prevent kinking and then sutures it securely to the patient's skin. He confirms placement by aspirating the catheter. Resistance indicates correct placement in the pleural space, aspirated blood means that the catheter probably is misplaced in a blood vessel, and aspirated air means that it's probably in a lung. He will then order a chest X-ray to detect pneumothorax.

▶ Apply a sterile dressing over the insertion site to prevent catheter dislodgment. Take the patient's vital signs every 15 minutes for the 1st hour after the procedure and then as needed.

Inserting a chest tube

▶ The physician inserts the chest tube with the nurse assisting.

▶ First, position the patient with the affected side up and drape him with sterile towels.

▶ The physician puts on gloves and cleans the appropriate site with antiseptic-soaked gauze. If the patient has a pneumothorax, the physician uses the second intercostal space as the access site because air rises to the top of the pleural space. If the patient has a hemothorax or pleural effusion, the physician uses the sixth to eighth intercostal space because fluid settles to the bottom of the pleural space.

▶ The physician fills the syringe with a local anesthetic and injects it into the site. He makes a small incision with the 18G needle or scalpel, inserts the appropriate-sized chest tube, and immediately connects it to the thoracic drainage system or clamps it close to the patient's chest. He then sutures the tube to the patient's skin.

▶ Tape the chest tube to the patient's chest distal to the insertion site to help prevent accidental dislodgment. Also tape the junction of the chest tube and drainage tube to prevent their separation. Apply sterile drain dressings, and tape them to the site.

▶ After insertion, the physician checks tube placement with an X-ray. Check the patient's vital signs every 15 minutes for 1 hour and then as needed. Auscultate his lungs at least every 4 hours to assess air exchange in the affected lung. Diminished or absent breath sounds mean that the lung hasn't reexpanded.

Administering the medication

▶ The physician injects medication through the intrapleural catheter or chest tube with the nurse assisting.

▶ If the patient will receive chemotherapy, expect to give an antiemetic at least 30 minutes beforehand.

▶ Position the patient with the affected side up. Help the physician move

---

Inserting an intrapleural catheter

In intrapleural administration, the physician injects a drug into the pleural space using a catheter.

Help the patient lie on one side with the affected side up. The physician inserts a needle into the fourth to eighth intercostal space, 3″ to 4″ (7.5 to 10 cm) from the posterior midline. He then advances the needle medially over the superior edge of the patient's rib through the intercostal muscles until it tangentially penetrates the parietal pleura, as shown. The catheter is advanced into the pleural space through the needle, which is then removed.

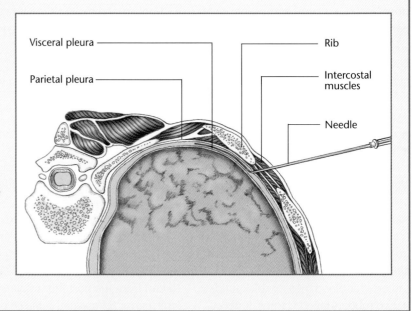

Visceral pleura

Parietal pleura

Rib

Intercostal muscles

Needle

the dressing away from the intrapleural catheter or chest tube and clamp the drainage tube, if present.

▶ The physician disinfects the access port of the catheter or chest tube with antiseptic-soaked gauze. Draw up the appropriate medication dose, and hand it to the physician with the vial for verification.

▶ The physician injects the medication. If it's an anesthetic, he gives a bolus or loading dose initially and then a continuous infusion. For tetracycline, he mixes it with an anesthetic, such as lidocaine, to alleviate pain during injection.

▶ Reapply the dressings around the catheter. Monitor the patient closely during and after drug administration to gauge the effectiveness of drug therapy and to check for complications and adverse effects.

Special considerations

▶ Make sure the patient has signed a consent form.

▶ Before catheter insertion, ask the patient to urinate to promote comfort.

▶ If the patient is receiving a continuous infusion, label the solution bag clearly. Cover all injection ports so that other drugs aren't injected into the pleural space accidentally. **JC** **ISMP**

▶ If the chest tube dislodges, cover the site at once with a sterile gauze pad and tape it in place. Stay with the patient, monitor his vital signs, and observe carefully for signs and symptoms of tension pneumothorax: hypotension, distended jugular veins, absent breath sounds, tracheal shift, hypoxemia, dyspnea, tachypnea, diaphoresis, chest pain, and weak, rapid pulse. Have another nurse call the physician and gather the equipment for reinsertion.

▶ Intrapleural chemotherapeutic drugs can irritate the pleura chemically and cause such systemic effects as neutropenia and thrombocytopenia. Administering intrapleural tetracycline without an anesthetic can cause pain.

▶ The insertion site can become infected. However, meticulous skin preparation, strict sterile technique, and sterile dressings usually prevent infection.

References

Maskell, N., et al. "Intrapleural Streptokinase for Pleural Infection," *British Medical Journal* 332(7540):552, March 2006.

Ren, S., et al. "Intrapleural Staphylococcal Superantigen Induces Resolution of Malignant Pleural Effusions and a Survival Benefit in Non-Small Cell Lung Cancer," *Chest* 126(5):1529-539, November 2004.

Tokuda, Y., et al. "Intrapleural Fibrinolytic Agents for Empyema and Complicated Parapneumonic Effusions: A Meta-Analysis," *Chest* 129(3):783-90, March 2006.

Isolation equipment use

Isolation procedures may be implemented to prevent the spread of infection from patient to patient, from the patient to health care workers, or from health care workers to the patient. They may also be used to reduce the risk of infection in immunocompromised patients. Central to the success of these procedures is the selection of the proper equipment and the adequate training of those who use it.

Equipment

Materials required for isolation typically include barrier clothing, an isolation cart or anteroom for storing equipment, and a door card announcing that isolation precautions are in effect.

Barrier clothing: Gowns ◆ gloves ◆ goggles ◆ masks. Each staff member must be trained in their proper use.

Isolation supplies: Labels ◆ tape ◆ laundry bags (and water-soluble laundry bags, if used) ◆ plastic trash bags.

An isolation cart may be used when the patient's room has no anteroom. It should include a work area (such as a pull-out shelf), drawers or a cabinet area for holding isolation supplies and, possibly, a pole on which to hang coats or jackets.

Implementation

▶ Remove the cover from the isolation cart, if necessary, and set up the work area.

▶ Check the cart or anteroom to ensure that correct and sufficient supplies are in place for the designated isolation category.

▶ Remove your watch (or push it well up your arm) and your rings according to your facility's policy. These actions help to prevent the spread of microorganisms hidden under your watch or rings. **CDC AORN**

▶ Wash your hands before putting on gloves to prevent the growth of microorganisms under gloves. **AORN**

Putting on isolation garb

▶ Put the gown on, and wrap it around the back of your uniform. Tie the strings or fasten the snaps or pressure-sensitive tabs at the neck. Make sure your uniform is completely covered to prevent contact with the patient or his environment.

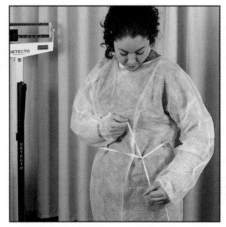

▶ Put on the gloves. Pull the gloves over the cuffs to cover the edges of the gown's sleeves.

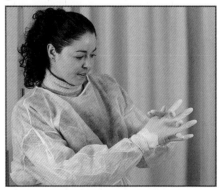

▶ Place the mask snugly over your nose and mouth. Secure ear loops around your ears or tie the strings behind your head high enough so the mask won't slip off. If the mask has a

metal strip, squeeze it to fit your nose firmly but comfortably. If you wear eyeglasses, tuck the mask under their lower edge.

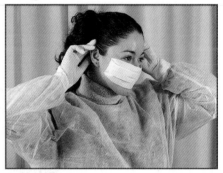

▶ If goggles are worn, put them on at this time.

Removing isolation garb

▶ Remember that the outside surfaces of your barrier clothes are contaminated.

▶ While wearing gloves, untie the gown's waist strings.

▶ With your gloved left hand, remove the right glove by pulling on the cuff, turning the glove inside out as you pull. Don't touch any skin with the outside of either glove. (See *Removing contaminated gloves*.) Then remove the left glove by wedging one or two fingers of your right hand inside the glove and pulling it off, turning it inside out as you remove it. Discard the gloves in the trash container. **AORN**

▶ Untie the neck straps of your gown. Grasp the outside of the gown at the back of the shoulders, and pull the gown down over your arms, turning it inside out as you remove it to ensure containment of the pathogens.

Removing contaminated gloves

Proper removal techniques are essential for preventing the spread of pathogens from gloves to your skin surface. Follow these steps carefully.

▶ Using your left hand, pinch the right glove near the top. Avoid allowing the glove's outer surface to buckle inward against your wrist.
▶ Pull downward, allowing the glove to turn inside out as it comes off. Keep the right glove in your left hand after removing it.

▶ Next, insert the first two fingers of your ungloved right hand under the edge of the left glove. Avoid touching the glove's outer surface or folding it against your left wrist.

▶ Pull downward so that the glove turns inside out as it comes off. Continue pulling until the left glove completely encloses the right one and its uncontaminated inner surface is facing out.

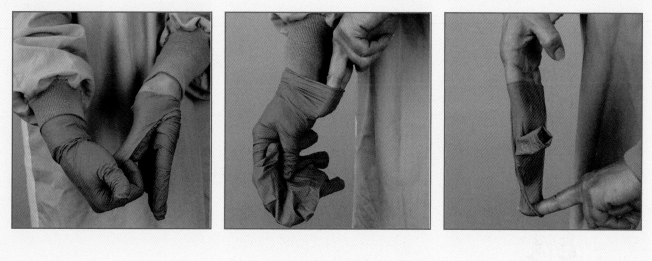

▶ Holding the gown well away from your uniform, fold it inside out. Discard it in the laundry or trash container as necessary.
▶ If the sink is inside the patient's room, wash your hands and forearms with soap or antiseptic before leaving the room. Turn off the faucet using a paper towel, and discard the towel in the room. Grasp the door handle with a clean paper towel to open it, and discard the towel in a trash container inside the room. Close the door from the outside with your bare hand. **CDC**
▶ Remove the mask last to prevent contaminating your face or hair in the process. Untie your mask, holding it only by the strings. Discard the mask in the trash container. Remove goggles.
▶ If the sink is in an anteroom, wash your hands and forearms with soap or antiseptic after leaving the room.

Special considerations

▶ If airborne precautions are required, a particulate respirator should be worn rather than a surgical mask.
▶ Use gowns, gloves, goggles, and masks only once, and discard them in the appropriate container before leaving a contaminated area. If your mask is reusable, retain it for further use unless it's damaged or damp. Be aware

that isolation garb loses its effectiveness when wet because moisture permits organisms to seep through the material. Change masks and gowns as soon as moisture is noticeable or according to the manufacturer's recommendations or your facility's policy. **MFR**
▶ At the end of your shift, restock used items for the next person. After patient transfer or discharge, return the isolation cart to the appropriate area for cleaning and restocking supplies. An isolation room or other room prepared for isolation purposes must be thoroughly cleaned and disinfected before use by another patient.

References

Centers for Disease Control and Prevention. "Guideline for Isolation Precautions: Preventing Transmission of Infections Agents in Healthcare Settings 2007." Available at *www.cdc.gov/ncidod/dhqp/g1_isolation.html.*

Perry, J., and Jagger, J. "Getting the Most from Your Personal Protective Gear," *Nursing* 34(12):72, December 2004.

Rushing, J. "Wearing Personal Protective Gear," *Nursing* 36(10):56-57, October 2006.

I.V. bolus injection

The I.V. bolus injection method allows for rapid drug administration and can be used in an emergency to provide an immediate drug effect. It can also be used to administer drugs that can't be given I.M., to achieve peak drug levels in the bloodstream, and to administer drugs that can't be diluted, such as diazepam, digoxin, and phenytoin. The term *bolus* usually refers to the concentration or amount of a drug. I.V. push is a technique for rapid I.V. injection.

Bolus doses of medication may be injected directly through an existing I.V. line or through an implanted port. The medication administered through these methods usually takes effect rapidly; therefore, the patient must be monitored for an adverse reaction, such as cardiac arrhythmia or anaphylaxis. I.V. bolus injections are contraindicated when rapid drug administration could cause life-threatening complications. For certain drugs, the safe rate of injection is specified by the manufacturer.

Equipment

Patient's medication record and chart ◆ gloves ◆ prescribed medication ◆ syringe and needleless adapter ◆ diluent, if needed ◆ tourniquet ◆ antiseptic swab ◆ tape ◆ optional: second syringe (and needleless adapter) filled with normal saline solution.

Implementation

▶ Verify the order on the patient's medication record by checking it against the practitioner's order. **JC** **ISMP**
▶ Draw up the prescribed medication in the syringe, and dilute it if necessary.
▶ Confirm the patient's identity using two patient identifiers according to your facility's policy, wash your hands, put on gloves, and explain the procedure. **JC**
▶ If your facility utilizes a bar code scanning system, be sure to scan your ID badge, the patient's ID bracelet, and the medication's bar code. **JC** **ISMP**

Giving injections through an existing I.V. line

▶ Check the compatibility of the medication with the I.V. solution.
▶ Clean the injection port of the I.V. tubing with an alcohol pad. **INS** **CDC**

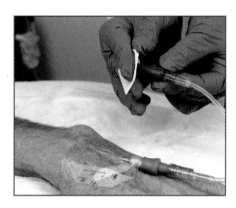

▶ Insert the syringe containing the medication into the needleless port.

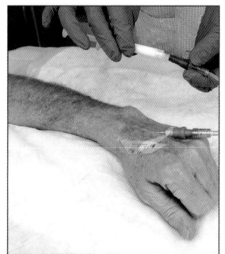

▶ Clamp the tubing above the injection port, and then inject the medication.

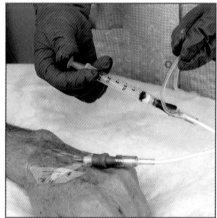

▶ Open the flow clamp, and readjust the flow rate.
▶ If the drug isn't compatible with the I.V. solution, flush the line with normal saline solution before and after the injection.

Giving a bolus injection through an implanted port

▶ Wash your hands, put on gloves, and clean the injection site with an alcohol or antiseptic pad, starting at the center of the port and working outward in a circular motion over a 4″ to 5″ (10- to 12.5-cm) diameter. Do this three times. **INS**

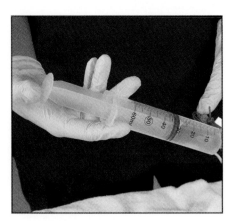

▶ Palpate the area over the port to locate the port septum.

▶ Anchor the port between the thumb and first two fingers of your nondominant hand. Then, using your dominant hand, insert the needle into the appropriate area of the device and deliver the injection. (See "Implanted port use," page 246.)

Special considerations

▶ Because drugs administered by I.V. bolus are delivered directly into the circulatory system and can produce an immediate effect, an acute allergic reaction or anaphylaxis can develop rapidly. If signs of anaphylaxis (dyspnea, cyanosis, seizures, and increasing respiratory distress) occur, notify the practitioner immediately and begin emergency procedures as necessary. Also watch for signs of extravasation (redness, swelling). If extravasation oc-

curs, stop the injection, estimate the amount of infiltration, and notify the practitioner.

References

Hatcher, I., et al. "An Intravenous Medication Safety System: Preventing High-Risk Medication Errors at the Point of Care," *Journal of Nursing Administration* 34(10):437-39, October 2004. **JC**

The Joint Commission. *Comprehensive Accreditation Manual for Hospitals: The Official Handbook.* Standard MM.1.10. Oakbrook Terrace, Ill.: The Joint Commission, 2007. **JC**

The Joint Commission. *Comprehensive Accreditation Manual for Hospitals: The Official Handbook.* Standard MM.2.10. Oakbrook Terrace, Ill.: The Joint Commission, 2007. **JC**

The Joint Commission. *Comprehensive Accreditation Manual for Hospitals: The Official Handbook.* Standard MM.3.10. Oakbrook Terrace, Ill.: The Joint Commission, 2007. **JC**

The Joint Commission. *Comprehensive Accreditation Manual for Hospitals: The Official Handbook.* Standard MM.4.10. Oakbrook Terrace, Ill.: The Joint Commission, 2007. **JC**

The Joint Commission. *Comprehensive Accreditation Manual for Hospitals: The Official Handbook.* Standard MM.4.20. Oakbrook Terrace, Ill.: The Joint Commission, 2007. **JC**

The Joint Commission. *Comprehensive Accreditation Manual for Hospitals: The Official Handbook.* Standard MM.4.30. Oakbrook Terrace, Ill.: The Joint Commission, 2007. **JC**

The Joint Commission. *Comprehensive Accreditation Manual for Hospitals: The Official Handbook.* Standard MM.4.40. Oakbrook Terrace, Ill.: The Joint Commission, 2007. **JC**

The Joint Commission. *Comprehensive Accreditation Manual for Hospitals: The Official Handbook.* Standard MM.5.10. Oakbrook Terrace, Ill.: The Joint Commission, 2007. **JC**

The Joint Commission. *Comprehensive Accreditation Manual for Hospitals: The Official Handbook.* Standard MM.6.10. Oakbrook Terrace, Ill.: The Joint Commission, 2007. **JC**

The Joint Commission. *Comprehensive Accreditation Manual for Hospitals: The Official Handbook.* Standard MM.6.20. Oakbrook Terrace, Ill.: The Joint Commission, 2007. **JC**

Paparella, S. "Avoiding Disastrous Outcomes with Rapid Intravenous Push Medications," *Journal of Emergency Nursing* 30(5):478-80, October 2004. **JC**

"Standard 68. Parenteral Medication and Solution Administration. Infusion Nursing Standards of Practice," *Journal of Infusion Nursing* 29(1S):S74-S75, January-February 2006. **JC**

I.V. pumps

Various types of I.V. pumps electronically regulate the flow of I.V. solutions or drugs with great accuracy.
Volumetric pumps, used for high-pressure infusion of drugs or for highly accurate delivery of fluids or drugs, have mechanisms to propel the solution at the desired rate under pressure. The peristaltic pump applies pressure to the I.V. tubing to force the solution through it. The piston-cylinder pump pushes the solution through special disposable cassettes. Most of these pumps operate at high pressures (up to 45 psi), delivering from 1 to 999 ml/hour with about 98% accuracy. (Some pumps operate at 10 to 25 psi.)

Pumps have various detectors and alarms that automatically signal or respond to the completion of an infusion, air in the line, low battery power, and occlusion or inability to deliver at the set rate. Depending on the problem, these devices may sound or flash an alarm, shut off, or switch to a keep-vein-open rate.

Equipment

Peristaltic pump ◆ I.V. pole ◆ I.V. solution ◆ sterile administration set ◆ sterile peristaltic tubing or cassette, if needed ◆ alcohol pads ◆ adhesive tape.

Tubing and cassettes vary among manufacturers. (See *Infusion pumps,* page 298.)

Implementation

▶ Attach the pump to the I.V. pole.

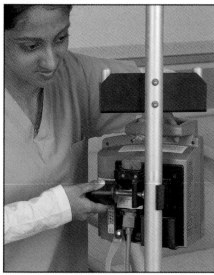

▶ Swab the port on the I.V. container with alcohol, insert the administration set spike, and fill the drip chamber completely to prevent air bubbles from entering the tubing. Next, prime the tubing and close the clamp. Follow the manufacturer's instructions for placement of tubing.

▶ If your facility utilizes a bar code automated pump, scan your ID badge, the patient's ID bracelet, and the patient ID on the medication bag. **JC** **ISMP**

▶ Position the pump on the same side of the bed as the I.V. or anticipated venipuncture site. If necessary, perform the venipuncture.

▶ Plug in the machine, and attach its tubing to the catheter hub.

▶ Depending on the machine, turn it on and press the START button. Set the appropriate dials on the front panel to the desired infusion rate and volume. Always set the volume dial at 50 ml less than the prescribed volume or 50 ml less than the volume in the container so that you can hang a new container before the old one empties.

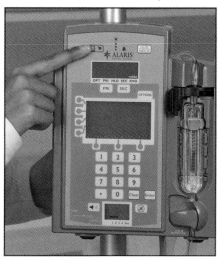

▶ Confirm that the right information is displayed on the pump, and push the RUN button.

▶ Check the patency of the I.V. line and watch for infiltration.

▶ Tape all connections. **INS**

▶ Turn on the alarm switches. Then explain the alarm system to the patient to prevent anxiety when a change in the infusion activates the alarm. **JC**

Special considerations

▶ Monitor the pump and the patient frequently to ensure the device's correct operation and flow rate and to detect infiltration and such complications as infection and air embolism. (See *Calculating flow rates,* page 298.)

▶ Keep in mind that infiltration can develop rapidly with infusion by a volumetric pump because the increased subcutaneous pressure won't slow the infusion rate until significant edema occurs.

▶ If electrical power fails, the pump automatically switches to battery power.

▶ Check the manufacturer's recommendations before administering opaque fluids, such as blood, because some pumps fail to detect such fluids and others may cause hemolysis of infused blood.

Infusion pumps

Infusion pumps electronically regulate the flow of I.V. solutions and drugs. You'll use them when a precise flow rate is needed—for example, when administering total parenteral nutrition solutions or chemotherapeutic or cardiovascular agents.

Infusion pump

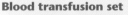

Power button

Flow rate display (ml/hr)

I.V. tubing

Flow rate control

Calculating flow rates

When calculating the flow rate of I.V. solutions, remember that the number of drops required to deliver 1 ml varies with the type and manufacturer of the administration set used. The illustration on the left shows a standard (macrodrip) set, which delivers 10 to 20 drops/ml. The illustration in the center shows a pediatric (microdrip) set, which delivers about 60 drops/ml. The illustration on the right shows a blood transfusion set, which delivers about 10 drops/ml.

To calculate the flow rate, you must know the calibration of the drip rate for each manufacturer's product. Use this formula to calculate specific drip rates:

$$\frac{\text{Volume of infusion (in ml)}}{\text{time of infusion (in minutes)}} \times \text{drip factor (in drops/ml)} = \text{drops/minute}$$

Macrodrip set

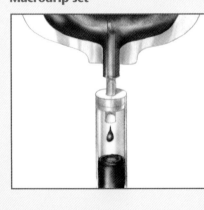

Microdrip set

Blood transfusion set

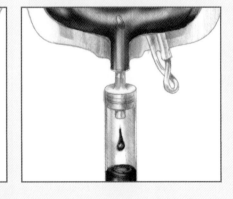

References

The Joint Commission. *Comprehensive Accreditation Manual for Hospitals: The Official Handbook.* Standard PC.6.10. Oakbrook Terrace, Ill.: The Joint Commission, 2007.

"Standard 33. Flow-Control Devices. Infusion Nursing Standards of Practice," *Journal of Infusion Nursing* 29(1S):S34-35, January-February 2006.

Weinstein, S.M. *Plummer's Principles and Practices of Intravenous Therapy,* 8th ed. Philadelphia: Lippincott Williams & Wilkins, 2007.

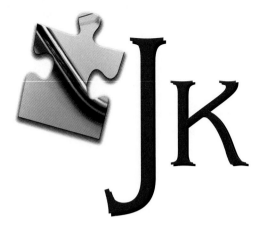

Jugular venous oxygen saturation monitoring

Jugular venous oxygen saturation (Sjvo$_2$) monitoring measures the venous oxygenation saturation of blood as it leaves the brain, reflecting the oxygen saturation of blood after cerebral perfusion has taken place. After comparing Sjvo$_2$ with the arterial venous oxygenation, you can determine whether blood flow to the brain matches the brain's metabolic demand.

The normal range for Sjvo$_2$ is from 55% to 70%. Values higher than 70% indicate hyperperfusion, whereas values between 40% and 54% indicate relative hypoperfusion. Values lower than 40% indicate ischemia. (See *Jugular venous oxygen saturation monitoring*.)

Monitoring of Sjvo$_2$ allows the nurse to maximize the balance among cerebral perfusion, oxygenation, and metabolism. Criteria for Sjvo$_2$ monitoring include any neurologic injury in which ischemia is a threat and may include intra-operative monitoring, subarachnoid hemorrhage, and post-acute head injury with increased intracranial pressure (ICP).

Equipment

For insertion of Sjvo$_2$ monitoring catheter: Sterile towels ◆ sterile drapes ◆ surgical caps ◆ gowns ◆ sterile gloves ◆ masks ◆ antiseptic solution ◆ central venous (CV) catheter insertion kit ◆ 1% or 2% lidocaine without epinephrine ◆ 5- or 10-ml syringe, with an 18G and 23G needle ◆ #5 French percutaneous introducer ◆ #4 French fiber-optic Sjvo$_2$ catheter ◆ oximetric monitor with cable ◆ 500 ml normal saline solution (heparinized or nonheparinized, according to your facility's policy) ◆ pressure tubing with continuous flush device ◆ pressure bag or device ◆ sterile occlusive dressing ◆ sterile marker ◆ sterile labels.

For removal of Sjvo$_2$ monitoring catheter: Sterile gloves ◆ suture removal set ◆ sterile hemostat ◆ sterile scissors ◆ antiseptic solution ◆ sterile occlusive dressing.

Implementation

▶ Using sterile technique, prime the pressure tubing system, removing all air bubbles and maintaining sterility of system for insertion.

Inserting the Sjvo$_2$ monitoring catheter

▶ Confirm the patient's identity using two patient identifiers according to your facility's policy. **JC**

▶ Explain the procedure to the patient and provide privacy.

▶ Wash your hands and put on sterile gloves.

▶ Position the patient with his head elevated 30 to 45 degrees and his neck in a neutral position. Document baseline ICP. **CS**

▶ Turn the patient's head laterally, away from the site chosen for catheter insertion. Note and document any change in ICP.

▶ Put on new sterile gloves. Using sterile technique, open and prepare the CV pressure insertion tray and add a #5 French sterile introducer and a #4 French fiber-optic Sjvo$_2$ catheter. Label all medications, medication containers, and other solutions on and off the sterile field.

▶ Scrub the insertion site with an antiseptic solution.

Jugular venous oxygen saturation monitoring

Juglar venous oxygen saturation ($SjvO_2$) monitoring is commonly used with other types of cerebral hemodynamic monitoring, such as intracranial pressure monitoring, to produce better information about pressure and perfusion during treatment. Treatment regimens can be titrated to enhance pressure and perfusion.

Data from monitoring can also be used to calculate cerebral extraction of oxygen (CeO_2 = oxygen saturation in arterial blood [SaO_2]- $SjvO_2$), cerebral arterial oxygen content ($CaO_2 = 1.34 \times$ hemoglobin [Hb] $\times$ $SaO_2 - 0.0031 \times$ partial pressure of arterial oxygen, the global cerebral content saturation ($CjvO_2 = 1.34 \times$ Hb $\times$ $SjvO_2 + 0.0031 \times PjvO_2$), arteriovenous jugular oxygen content ($AVjDO_2 = CaO_2 - CjVO_2$), which help determine cerebral oxygen use, metabolic demand, and adequacy of oxygen delivery.

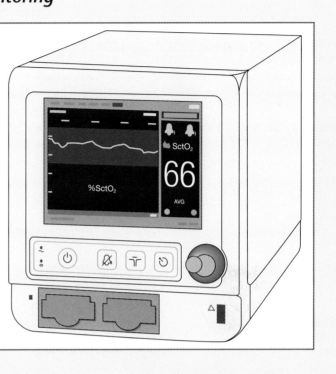

▶ Position the sterile drapes over the upper thorax and neck, exposing only the insertion site.

▶ Assist the physician during insertion as needed.

▶ Monitor neurologic status, vital signs, ICP, and pain during insertion.

▶ After the line is in place, attach the pressure tubing and confirm patency of both jugular catheter lumens by aspirating and flushing.

▶ Clean the insertion site with antiseptic solution, and apply the sterile occlusive dressing.

▶ Obtain a lateral cervical spine or lateral skull X-ray to confirm catheter placement at the level of the jugular bulb.

▶ Draw a jugular venous blood gas sample, and perform in vivo calibration according to the manufacturer's guidelines.

Monitoring and care

▶ Assess the patient's neurologic status, vital signs, and ICP immediately after insertion.

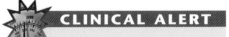

CLINICAL ALERT

Because the catheter in the jugular bulb can inhibit venous outflow, a sustained ICP of more than 5 mm Hg over preinsertion baseline may be an indication for catheter removal.

▶ Record baseline parameters for continuously monitored $SjvO_2$.

▶ Assess the patient's for a change in ICP because increased ICP of is a frequent cause of desaturation in patients with brain injury.

▶ Continuously monitor $SjvO_2$.

▶ Verify accuracy of the reading by drawing $SjvO_2$ every 8 to 12 hours. The blood sample reading should be within 4% of the monitor.

CLINICAL ALERT

A significant change in readings following sampling can signify errors related to aspiration of blood. Avoid errors by aspirating blood slowly during the sampling procedure (1 ml/minute).

▶ Record $SjvO_2$ and ICP values, and note trends. Assess ICP in relation to $SjvO_2$. Notify the physician of any deviation from the trend.

▶ Maintain a safe environment during monitoring to prevent accidental dislodgement of the catheter.

▶ Change the dressing using sterile technique if it becomes soiled or loosened and as indicated by your facility's policy for central line redressing. **INS** **CDC**

▶ Change the I.V. solution and tubing for the catheter according to your facility's policy for central lines.

▶ To prevent catheter coiling, identify rhythmic fluctuations in $SjvO_2$ trends. Obtain a lateral cervical spine or lateral skull X-ray to assess position of the catheter in the external jugular vein (compare to X-ray done on insertion). If coiling is confirmed, consider replacing the catheter.

Removing the $SjvO_2$ monitoring catheter

▶ Explain the procedure to the patient and provide privacy.

▶ Wash your hands and prepare the equipment.

▶ Deactivate alarms.

▶ Turn stopcocks off, position the patient properly, monitor his vital signs, put on sterile gloves, and assist the physician with catheter removal as needed.

▶ Apply direct pressure to the site until there are no signs of active bleeding.

▶ Put on new sterile gloves. Apply antiseptic solution and the sterile occlusive dressing to the catheter site.

▶ Assess the site for signs of bleeding every 15 minutes for 1 hour, every 30 minutes for 1 hour, and then 1 hour later.

Special considerations

▶ Use sedation or analgesia, as indicated, to maintain the monitor and enhance cerebral perfusion pressure.

▶ Replace an $Sjvo_2$ catheter with low light intensity. Check the fiber-optic catheter for obstruction or occlusion.

Aspirate the catheter until blood can be freely sampled and normal light intensity is displayed. If you can't aspirate a blood sample, the catheter needs to be replaced.

▶ For an $Sjvo_2$ catheter with high light intensity, adjust the patient's head to ensure a neutral neck position.

▶ Complications associated with $Svjo_2$ monitoring are similar to complications that can occur with any central line, the most common of which is line sepsis. Other risks include:
— pneumothorax
— carotid artery puncture
— internal jugular thrombosis
— excessive bleeding.

In rare instances, the catheter can also cause impaired cerebral venous drainage and increased ICP.

References

American Association of Neuroscience Nurses. *Core Curriculum for Neuroscience Nursing,* 4th ed. Philadelphia: W.B. Saunders Co., 2004.

Dunn, I.F., et al. "Neuromonitoring in Neurological Critical Care," *Neurocritical Care* 4(1):83-92, 2006.

Lynn-McHale Wiegand, D.J., and Carlson, K.K., eds. *AACN Procedure Manual for Critical Care,* 5th ed. Philadelphia: W.B. Saunders Co., 2005.

Ng, I., et al. "Effects of Head Posture on Cerebral Hemodynamics: It's Influences on Intracranial Pressure, Cerebral Perfusion Pressure, and Cerebral Oxygenation." *Neurosurgery* 54(3):593–97. March 2004. **CS**

Stevens, W.J. "Multimodal Monitoring: Head Injury Management Using SjvO_2 and LICOX," *Journal of Neuroscience Nursing* 36(6):332-39, December 2004.

Tobias, J.D. "Cerebral Oxygenation Monitoring: Near-Infrared Spectroscopy," *Expert Review of Medical Devices* 3(2):235-43, March 2006.

L

Laryngeal mask airway insertion

The laryngeal mask airway (LMA) is used to establish and maintain a patent airway in the unconscious patient. It's used extensively in the operating room by anesthesia personnel, and it's also appropriate for emergency airway and ventilatory support when endotracheal intubation isn't immediately possible. The LMA may also be used in place of a face mask during adult, pediatric, and neonatal resuscitation.

The LMA consists of a semirigid tube attached to a silicone mask. The mask is placed into the patient's mouth and advanced blindly until it rests above the larynx. The patient may then breathe spontaneously or be assisted with moderate positive-pressure ventilation.

The LMA doesn't protect the patient from regurgitation and aspiration; therefore, it can be used in patients with full stomachs, but only in emergency situations when intubation isn't possible or if ventilation by face mask is ineffective. In addition, the LMA should be inserted only into the patient who has lost protective cough and gag reflexes. The LMA should also be used cautiously in the patient with delayed gastric emptying because of the risk of regurgitation.

Equipment

Appropriately sized LMA based on patient's weight (reusable, disposable, or intubating) (see *LMA specifications,* page 304) ◆ syringe of appropriate size for inflating cuff ◆ water-soluble lubricant ◆ nonsterile gloves and other personal protective equipment ◆ oxygen equipment ◆ tape or device to secure tube ◆ bag-valve or mouth-to-mask device ◆ bite block ◆ stethoscope ◆ suction equipment ◆ pulse oximeter, if available ◆ capnometer, if available.

Implementation

▶ Remove the LMA from its package, and visually inspect it for discoloration, cracks, or kinks in the tube; also, make sure it's the right size. **MFR**

▶ Inspect the airway opening, and check that the aperture bars are intact. Manually tighten the connector, if needed. Test the patency of the cuff by first withdrawing all air and then over-inflating it with air injected through the pilot balloon. While inflated, visually inspect the cuff for symmetry; then deflate the cuff. **MFR**

▶ Assemble suction equipment and check that it's working properly.

▶ Confirm the patient's identity using two patient identifiers according to your facility's policy. **JC**

▶ Assess the patient's level of consciousness because the LMA shouldn't be inserted into a patient who may resist insertion.

▶ Wash your hands.

▶ Put on gloves and personal protective equipment.

▶ Teach the family about the procedure, as the patient's condition allows.

▶ Lubricate the posterior surface of the LMA, using a water-soluble lubricant. **MFR**

▶ Place the patient in the supine position with a folded towel or blanket under the head to flex the neck and extend the head (the "sniffing position") to ease insertion of the LMA. **CS**

▶ Stand behind the patient's head and place your nondominant hand under the patient's head, lifting the head slightly and keeping upward pressure.

▶ Hold the LMA in your dominant hand like a pencil, with the index finger placed at the junction of the mask

LMA specifications

The following chart will help guide you in choosing the correct size of laryngeal mask airway (LMA) for your patient. **MFR**

SIZE	PATIENT SIZE	MAXIMAL CUFF INFLATION VOLUME	OVERINFLATION VOLUME FOR CUFF TEST
1	Up to 5 kg	4 ml	8 ml
1½	5 to 10 kg	7 ml	10 ml
2	10 to 20 kg	10 ml	15 ml
2½	20 to 30 kg	14 ml	21 ml
3	30 to 50 kg	20 ml	30 ml
4	50 to 70 kg	30 ml	45 ml
5	70 to 100 kg	40 ml	60 ml
6	Greater than 100 kg	50 ml	75 ml

and the tube. The lumen of the LMA should be facing up, with the lubricated posterior surface facing the floor. Follow the steps in *Inserting the LMA*.

▶ After the LMA is in place, use the syringe to inflate the cuff to an intracuff pressure of about 60 cm H_2O. Only one-half the maximum inflation volume is required to make a seal. Don't overinflate the cuff. **MFR**

▶ Check the mouth to make sure the cuff isn't visible, and observe for minor outward movement of the tube and minor neck bulging in the area of the cricothyroid, indicating proper tube placement and cuff inflation. **MFR**

▶ Verify correct placement by auscultation of bilateral breath sounds using a stethoscope and by monitoring through pulse oximetry or capnography, if available. **AHA**

▶ Use a bag-valve device connected to an oxygen source, if indicated, to gently deliver ventilations using a peak airway pressure less than 20 cm H_2O and a tidal volume of 8 ml/kg of body weight or less. Using low-pressure ventilations avoids exceeding cuff pressure and reduces the risk of forcing air into the stomach.

▶ Insert a bite block to keep the patient from biting on the tube and causing it to become occluded or move out of proper position.

▶ Tape the LMA and bite block securely to the patient's face, or use a commercial device to secure the tube.

Special considerations

▶ If there's a risk that the patient may have neck trauma, insert the LMA with the patient's neck in a neutral position.

▶ Introducers from the manufacturer may be available to aid insertion. In that case, the introducer is used in place of the index finger. The introducer maintains contact between the posterior aspect of the tube and the pa-

tient's hard palate and should be used according to the manufacturer's instructions.

▶ Never use extreme force when inserting an LMA.

▶ Insertion of an LMA in a patient with intact or partially intact airway reflexes may result in coughing, gagging, regurgitation, or laryngospasm. Therefore, an LMA should be inserted only in controlled settings, such as when the patient is under anesthesia; in emergency settings, in which the patient has lost protective airway reflexes; or in situations where endotracheal intubation isn't readily available or possible.

▶ Monitor the patient's respiratory status continually to ensure proper ventilation, oxygenation, and tube placement while the LMA is in place.

▶ If the patient vomits, turn the patient to the side to allow for drainage of contents and then suction the airway.

Inserting the LMA

Use the following steps to correctly insert a laryngeal mask airway (LMA).

▶ Hold the LMA with your dominant hand, using the index finger and thumb to grasp the tube behind the cuff.

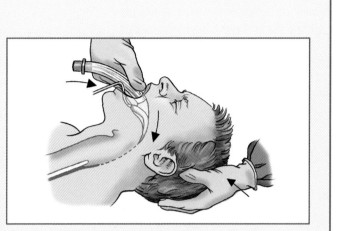

▶ Extend the patient's head while flexing the neck, and flatten the LMA against the patient's hard palate. Use your middle finger to gently press down on the patient's jaw.

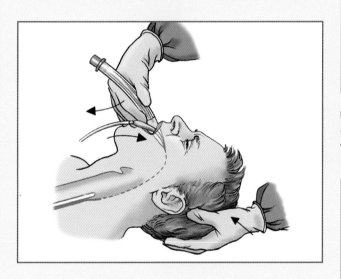

▶ Use your index finger to insert the LMA, while following the hard and soft palates (as shown at the top of the next column).

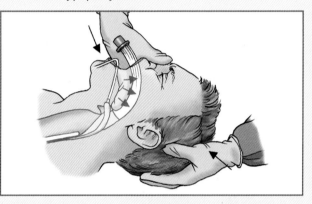

▶ Continue to gently advance the LMA until you feel resistance at the hypopharynx.

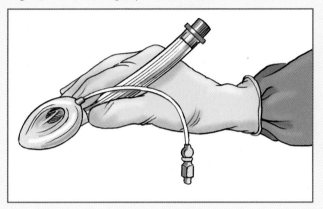

▶ After the LMA is in place, gently remove your index finger while you place gentle pressure on the patient's jaw with your opposite hand. After your index finger is removed, remove both hands.

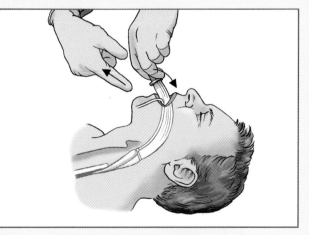

References

Baillard, C., et al. "Noninvasive Ventilation Improves Preoxygenation before Intubation of Hypoxic Patients," *American Journal of Respiratory and Critical Care Medicine* 174(2):171-77, July 2006.

Brimacombe, J., and Berry, A. "Laryngeal Mask Airway Insertion. A Comparison of the Standard Versus Neutral Position in Normal Patients With a View to Its Use in Cervical Spine Instability," *Anaesthesia* 48(8):670-71, August 1993. CS

Chmielewski, C., and Snyder-Clickett, S. "The Use of the Laryngeal Mask Airway with Mechanical Positive Pressure Ventilation," *AANA Journal* 72(5):347-51, October 2004.

Jevon, P. "Laryngeal Mask Airway," *Nursing Times* 102(36):28-29, September 2006.

Lynn-McHale Wiegand, D.J., and Carlson, K.K., eds. *AACN Procedure Manual for Critical Care,* 5th ed. Philadelphia: W.B. Saunders Co., 2005.

Lumbar puncture

Lumbar puncture involves the insertion of a sterile needle into the subarachnoid space of the spinal canal, usually between the third and fourth lumbar vertebrae. This procedure is used to determine the presence of blood in cerebrospinal fluid (CSF), to obtain CSF specimens for laboratory analysis, and to inject dyes for contrast in radiologic studies. The pressure of CSF, which flows freely between the brain and the spinal column, may be measured during the procedure. It's also used to administer drugs or anesthetics.

Performed by a physician or an advanced practice nurse, lumbar puncture requires sterile technique and careful patient positioning. This procedure is contraindicated in patients with increased intracranial pressure (ICP), lumbar deformity, or infection at the puncture site. It isn't recommended in patients with increased ICP because the rapid reduction in pressure that follows withdrawal of CSF can cause tonsillar herniation and medullary compression.

Equipment

Overbed table ◆ one or two pairs of sterile gloves for the physician ◆ sterile gloves for the nurse ◆ face masks ◆ antiseptic solution ◆ sterile gauze pads ◆ alcohol pads ◆ sterile fenestrated drape ◆ 3-ml syringe for local anesthetic ◆ 25G ³/₄″ sterile needle for injecting anesthetic ◆ local anesthetic (usually 1% lidocaine) ◆ 18G or 20G 3¹/₂″ spinal needle with stylet (22G needle for children) ◆ three-way stopcock ◆ manometer ◆ small adhesive bandage ◆ three sterile collection tubes with stoppers ◆ laboratory request forms and laboratory biohazard transport bag ◆ labels ◆ light source such as a gooseneck lamp ◆ sterile marker ◆ sterile labels ◆ optional: patient-care reminder.

Disposable lumbar puncture trays contain most of the needed sterile equipment.

Implementation

▶ Confirm the patient's identity using two patient identifiers according to your facility's policy. **JC**
▶ Explain the procedure to the patient. Make sure a consent form has been signed.

▶ Inform the patient that he may experience headache after lumbar puncture, but reassure him that his cooperation during the procedure minimizes such an effect. (*Note:* Sedatives and analgesics are usually withheld before this test if evidence of a central nervous system disorder exists because they may mask important symptoms.)
▶ Immediately before the procedure, provide privacy and instruct the patient to void.
▶ Wash your hands thoroughly.
▶ Open the equipment tray on an overbed table, being careful not to contaminate the sterile field when you open the wrapper. Label all medications, medication containers, and other solutions on and off the sterile field. **JC**
▶ Provide adequate lighting at the puncture site, and adjust the height of the patient's bed to allow the physician to perform the procedure comfortably.
▶ Position the patient, and reemphasize the importance of remaining as still as possible to minimize discomfort and trauma. (See *Positioning for lumbar puncture,* page 308.)
▶ The practitioner cleans the puncture site with sterile gauze pads soaked in antiseptic solution, wiping in a circular motion away from the puncture site. Next, he drapes the area with the fen-

estrated drape to provide a sterile field. (If the practitioner uses antiseptic solution pads instead of sterile gauze pads, he may remove his sterile gloves and put on another pair to avoid introducing antiseptic solution into the subarachnoid space with the lumbar puncture needle.)
▶ If no ampule of anesthetic is included on the equipment tray, clean the injection port of a multidose vial of anesthetic with an alcohol pad. Then invert the vial 45 degrees so that the practitioner can insert a 25G needle and syringe and withdraw the anesthetic for injection.
▶ Before the practitioner injects the anesthetic, tell the patient he'll experience a transient burning sensation and local pain. Ask him to report any other persistent pain or sensations because they may indicate irritation or puncture of a nerve root, requiring repositioning of the needle.
▶ When the practitioner inserts the sterile spinal needle into the subarachnoid space between the third and fourth lumbar vertebrae, instruct the patient to remain still and breathe normally. If necessary, hold the patient firmly in position to prevent sudden movement that may displace the needle.

Positioning for lumbar puncture

Have the patient lie on his side at the edge of the bed, with his chin tucked to his chest and his knees drawn up to his abdomen. Make sure the patient's spine is curved and his back is at the edge of the bed (as shown below, left). This position widens the spaces between the vertebrae, easing insertion of the needle.

To help the patient maintain this position, place one of your hands behind his neck and the other hand behind his knees and pull gently. Hold the patient firmly in this position throughout the procedure to prevent accidental needle displacement.

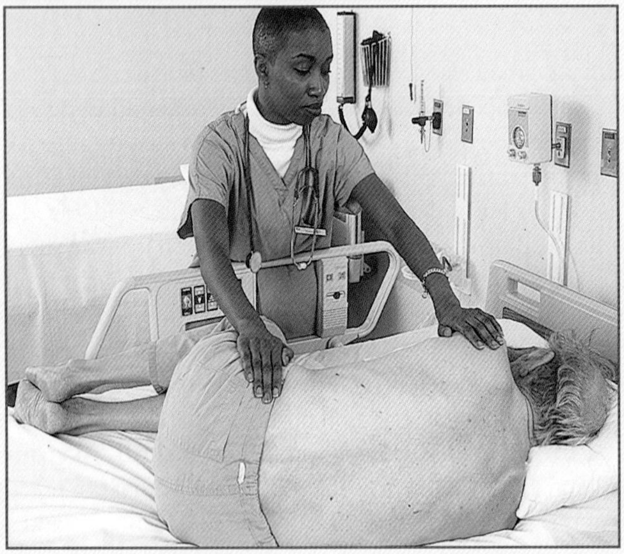

Typically, the practitioner inserts the needle between the third and fourth lumbar vertebrae (as shown below).

Patient positioning

Needle insertion

Third lumbar vertebra
Dura mater
Subarachnoid space
Cauda equina

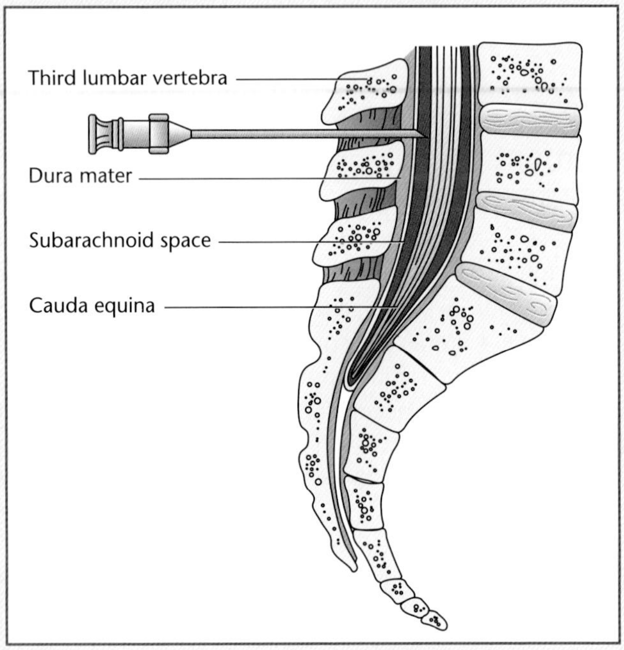

▶ If the lumbar puncture is being performed to administer contrast media for radiologic studies or spinal anesthetic, the practitioner injects the dye or anesthetic at this time.

▶ When the needle is in place, the practitioner attaches a manometer with a three-way stopcock to the needle hub to read CSF pressure. If ordered, help the patient extend his legs to provide a more accurate pressure reading.

▶ The practitioner then detaches the manometer and allows CSF to drain from the needle hub into the collection tubes. When he has collected 2 to 3 ml in each tube, mark the tubes in se-

quence, insert a stopper to secure them, and label them.

▶ If the practitioner suspects an obstruction in the spinal subarachnoid space, he may check for Queckenstedt's sign. After he takes an initial CSF pressure reading, compress the patient's jugular vein for 10 seconds as ordered. This increases ICP and, if no subarachnoid block exists, causes CSF pressure to rise as well. The practitioner then takes pressure readings every 10 seconds until the pressure stabilizes.

▶ After the practitioner collects the specimens and removes the spinal needle, clean the puncture site with anti-

septic solution and apply a small adhesive bandage.

▶ Send the CSF specimens to the laboratory immediately with completed laboratory request forms in a laboratory biohazard transport bag.

Special considerations

▶ During lumbar puncture, watch closely for signs of adverse reactions: elevated pulse rate, pallor, and clammy skin. Alert the practitioner immediately to any significant changes.

▶ The patient may be ordered to lie flat for 8 to 12 hours after the procedure to allow the restoration of spinal fluid to prevent postspinal headache. If necessary, place a patient-care reminder on his bed to this effect.

▶ Collected CSF specimens must be sent to the laboratory immediately; they can't be refrigerated for later transport.

▶ Encourage the patient to drink fluids after the procedure to reduce the risk of spinal headache.

▶ Check the puncture site for redness, swelling, and drainage every hour for the first 4 hours and then every 4 hours for the next 24 hours.

References

Armon, C., et al. "Addendum to Assessment: Prevention of Post-Lumbar Puncture Headaches: Report of the Therapeutics and Technology Assessment Subcommittee of the American Academy of Neurology," *Neurology* 65(4):510-12, August 2005.

Lenfeldt, N., et al. "CSF Pressure Assessed by Lumbar Puncture Agrees with Intracranial Pressure," *Neurology* 68(2):155-58, January 2007.

Rushing, J. "Assisting with Lumbar Puncture," *Nursing* 37(1):23, January 2007.

Straus, S.E., et al. "How Do I Perform a Lumbar Puncture and Analyze the Results to Diagnose Bacterial Meningitis?" *JAMA* 296(16):2012-2022, October 2006.

Strout, T.D., et al. "Reducing Pain in ED Patients during Lumbar Puncture: The Efficacy and Feasibility of Iontophoresis, Collaborative Approach," *Journal of Emergency Nursing* 30(5):423-30, October 2004.

M

Male incontinence device

Many patients don't require an indwelling urinary catheter to manage their incontinence. For male patients, a male incontinence device reduces the risk of urinary tract infection (UTI) from catheterization, promotes bladder retraining when possible, helps prevent skin breakdown, and improves the patient's self-image. A male incontinence device is also less likely to result in a UTI and is also associated with increased patient satisfaction compared to an indwelling urinary catheter. **CS** The device consists of a condom catheter secured to the shaft of the penis and connected to a leg bag or drainage bag. It has no contraindications but can cause skin irritation and edema.

Equipment

Condom catheter ◆ drainage bag ◆ extension tubing ◆ hypoallergenic tape or incontinence sheath holder ◆ commercial adhesive strip or skin-bond cement ◆ elastic adhesive or Velcro, if needed ◆ gloves ◆ clippers, if needed ◆ basin ◆ soap ◆ washcloth ◆ towel.

Implementation

▶ Fill the basin with lukewarm water. Then bring the basin and the remaining equipment to the patient's bedside.
▶ Confirm the patient's identity using two patient identifiers according to your facility's policy. **JC**
▶ Explain the procedure to the patient, wash your hands thoroughly, put on gloves, and provide privacy.

Applying the device

▶ If the patient is circumcised, wash the penis with soap and water, rinse well, and pat dry with a towel. If the patient is uncircumcised, gently retract the foreskin and clean beneath it. Rinse well but don't dry because moisture provides lubrication and prevents friction during foreskin replacement. Replace the foreskin to avoid penile constriction. Then, if necessary, clip hair from the base and shaft of the penis to prevent the adhesive strip or skin-bond cement from pulling pubic hair.
▶ If you're using a precut commercial adhesive strip, insert the glans penis through its opening and position the strip 1″ (2.5 cm) from the scrotal area. If you're using uncut adhesive, cut a strip to fit around the shaft of the penis. Remove the protective covering from one side of the adhesive strip, and press this side firmly to the penis to enhance adhesion. Then remove the covering from the other side of the strip. If a commercial adhesive strip isn't available, apply skin-bond cement and let it dry for a few minutes.

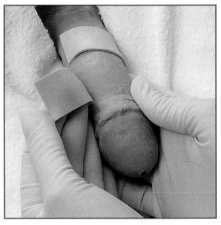

▶ Position the rolled condom catheter at the tip of the penis, leaving ¹/₂″ (1.3 cm) between the condom end and the tip of the penis, with its drainage opening at the urinary meatus.
▶ Unroll the catheter upward, past the adhesive strip on the shaft of the penis.

Then gently press the sheath against the strip until it adheres.

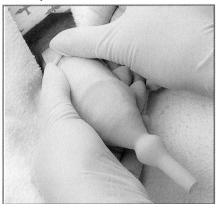

▶ After the condom catheter is in place, secure it with hypoallergenic tape or an incontinence sheath holder.
▶ Using extension tubing, connect the condom catheter to the leg bag or drainage bag. Remove and discard your gloves.

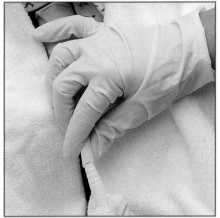

Removing the device

▶ After identifying the patient, wash your hands and put on gloves.
▶ Simultaneously roll the condom catheter and adhesive strip off the penis and discard them. If you've used skin-bond cement rather than an adhesive strip, remove it with solvent. Also remove and discard the hypoallergenic tape or incontinence sheath holder.
▶ Clean the penis with lukewarm water, rinse thoroughly, and dry. Check for swelling or signs of skin breakdown.
▶ Remove the leg bag by closing the drain clamp, unlatching the leg straps, and disconnecting the extension tubing at the top of the bag. Discard your gloves.

Special considerations

▶ If hypoallergenic tape or an incontinence sheath holder isn't available, secure the condom with a strip of elastic adhesive or Velcro. Apply the strip snugly—but not too tightly—to prevent circulatory constriction.
▶ Inspect the condom catheter for twists and the extension tubing for kinks to prevent obstruction of urine flow, which could cause the condom to balloon, eventually dislodging it.

References

Brodie, A. "A Guide to the Management of One-Piece Urinary Sheaths," *Nursing Times* 102(9):49, 51, February-March 2006.

Evans, D. "Lifestyle Solutions of Men with Continence Problems," *Nursing Times* 101(2):61-64, January 2005.

Milne, J.L., and Moore, K.N. "Factors Impacting Self-Care for Urinary Incontinence," *Urologic Nursing* 26(1):41-51, February 2006.

National Guideline Clearinghouse. "Management of Urinary Incontinence in Primary Care: A National Clinical Guideline." Available at *www.guideline. gov/summary/summary.aspx?doc_id=62 51&nbr=004011.*

Newman, O.K. "Incontinence Products and Devices for the Elderly," *Urologic Nursing* 24(4):316-33, August 2004.

Saint, S., et al. "Condom Versus Indwelling Urinary Catheters: A Randomized Trial," *Journal of the American Geriatrics Society* 54(7):1055-1061, July 2006. **CS**

Manual ventilation

A handheld resuscitation bag is an inflatable device that can be attached to a face mask or directly to an endotracheal (ET) or tracheostomy tube to allow manual delivery of oxygen or room air to the lungs of a patient who can't breathe by himself. Usually used in an emergency, manual ventilation can also be performed while the patient is disconnected temporarily from a mechanical ventilator, such as during a tubing change, during transport, or before suctioning. In such instances, use of the handheld resuscitation bag maintains ventilation. Oxygen administration with a resuscitation bag can help improve a compromised cardiorespiratory system.

Equipment

Handheld resuscitation bag ◆ mask, if needed ◆ oxygen source (wall unit or tank) ◆ oxygen tubing ◆ nipple adapter attached to oxygen flowmeter ◆ gloves ◆ goggles ◆ suction apparatus and tubing as needed ◆ oral airway, if needed ◆ optional: oxygen reservoir, positive end-expiratory pressure (PEEP) valve. (See *Using a PEEP valve*.)

Implementation

▶ Unless the patient is intubated or has a tracheostomy, select a mask that fits snugly over the mouth and nose. Attach the mask to the resuscitation bag (as shown at right).

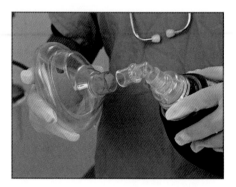

Using a PEEP valve

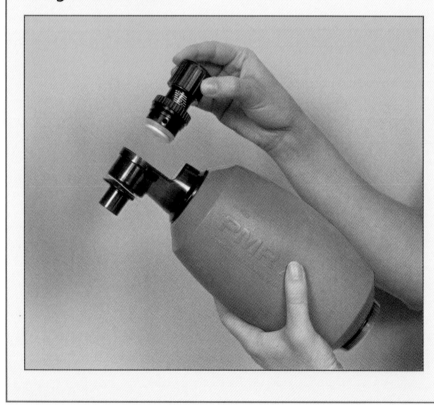

Add positive end-expiratory pressure (PEEP) to manual ventilation by attaching a PEEP valve to the resuscitation bag. This may improve oxygenation if the patient hasn't responded to increased fraction of inspired oxygen levels. Always use a PEEP valve to manually ventilate a patient who has been receiving PEEP on the ventilator.

Using a handheld resuscitation bag and mask

Bag-mask resuscitation by one rescuer
1. Circle the edges of the mask with the index and first finger of one hand while lifting the jaw with the other fingers. Make sure that there's a tight seal. Use the other hand to compress the bag. Make sure that the chest rises with each breath.

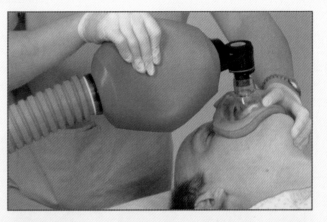

2. Make sure that the patient's mouth remains open underneath the mask. Attach the bag to the mask and to the tubing leading to the oxygen source.

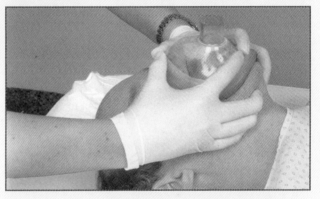

3. Alternatively, if the patient has a tracheostomy or endotracheal tube in place, remove the mask from the bag and attach the handheld resuscitation bag directly to the tube.

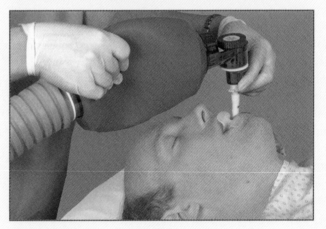

Bag-mask resuscitation by two rescuers
One rescuer stands at the victim's head and uses the thumb and the first finger of both hands to completely seal the edges of the mask. The other fingers lift the jaw and extend the victim's neck. The second rescuer squeezes the bag over 1 second until the chest rises.

▶ If oxygen is readily available, connect the handheld resuscitation bag to the oxygen. Adjust the oxygen to a minimal flow rate of 10 to 12 L/minute and oxygen greater than 40%. Ideally, an oxygen reservoir should be used. This device attaches to an adapter on the bottom of the bag and delivers 100% oxygen.

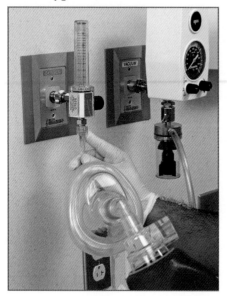

▶ Put on gloves and other personal protective equipment.
▶ Before using the handheld resuscitation bag, check the patient's upper airway for foreign objects. If present, remove them because this alone may restore spontaneous respirations in some instances. Suction the patient to remove any secretions that may obstruct the airway. If necessary, insert an oropharyngeal or nasopharyngeal airway to maintain airway patency. If the patient has a tracheostomy or ET tube in place, suction the tube.
▶ If appropriate, remove the bed's headboard and stand at the head of the bed to help keep the patient's neck extended and to free space at the side of the bed for other activities such as cardiopulmonary resuscitation.
▶ Tilt the patient's head backward, if not contraindicated, and pull his jaw forward to move the tongue away from the base of the pharynx and prevent obstruction of the airway. (See *Using a handheld resuscitation bag and mask,* page 313.)
▶ Keeping your nondominant hand on the patient's mask, exert downward pressure to seal the mask against his face. For an adult patient, use your dominant hand to compress the bag to give 8 to 10 breaths/minute.

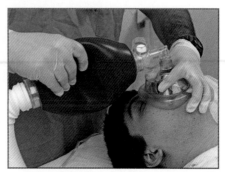

▶ Depress the 1-L bag by about one-half to two-thirds of its volume or a 2-L bag to about one-third of its volume to deliver a tidal volume sufficient to achieve a visible chest rise.
▶ Deliver each breath over 1 second. Allow the patient to exhale before giving another ventilation.

AGE FACTOR

For infants and children, deliver 20 breaths/minute, or one compression of the bag every 3 to 5 seconds. Use a pediatric handheld resuscitation bag with a volume of at least 450 to 500 ml.

▶ Deliver breaths with the patient's own inspiratory effort, if it's present. Don't attempt to deliver a breath as the patient exhales.
▶ Observe the patient's chest to ensure that it rises and falls with each compression. If ventilation fails to occur, check the fit of the mask and the patency of the patient's airway; if necessary, reposition his head and ensure patency with an oral airway.

Special considerations

▶ Avoid neck hyperextension if the patient has a possible cervical injury; instead, use the jaw-thrust technique to open the airway.
▶ If you need both hands to keep the patient's mask in place and maintain hyperextension, use the lower part of your arm to compress the bag against your side.
▶ Observe for vomiting through the clear part of the mask. If vomiting occurs, stop the procedure immediately, lift the mask, turn the patient to his side, wipe and suction the vomitus, and resume resuscitation.

References

American Heart Association. "2005 AHA Guidelines for Cardiopulmonary Resuscitation and Emergency Cardiovascular Care: International Consensus on Science," *Circulation* 112(22 Suppl):IV-1-IV-211, November 2005.

Aufderheude, T.P., et al. "Death by Hyperventilation: A Common and Life-Threatening Problem during Cardiopulmonary Resuscitation," *Critical Care Medicine* 32(9 Suppl):S345-S351, September 2004.

Lynn-McHale Wiegand, D.J., and Carlson, K.K., eds. *AACN Procedure Manual for Critical Care,* 5th ed. Philadelphia: W.B. Saunders Co., 2006.

Turki, M. "Peak Pressures during Manual Ventilation," *Respiratory Care* 50(3): 340-44, March 2005.

Mechanical debridement

Debridement involves removing necrotic tissue by mechanical, chemical, or surgical means to allow underlying healthy tissue to regenerate. Mechanical debridement procedures include irrigation, hydrotherapy, and excision of dead tissue with forceps and scissors. The procedure may be done at the bedside or in a specially prepared room.

Debridement techniques include chemical debridement (with wound-cleaning beads or topical agents that absorb exudate and debris) or surgical excision and skin grafting (usually reserved for deep burns or ulcers). Typically, the patient receives a local or general anesthetic. (See *Understanding debridement methods*.)

Ideally, the wound should be debrided daily during the dressing change. Frequent, regular debridement guards against possible hemorrhage resulting from more extensive and forceful debridement. It also reduces the need to conduct extensive debridement under anesthesia.

Equipment

Ordered pain medication ◆ two pairs of sterile gloves ◆ two gowns or aprons ◆ mask ◆ cap ◆ sterile scissors ◆ sterile forceps ◆ 4″ × 4″ sterile gauze pads ◆ sterile solutions and medications as ordered ◆ hemostatic agent as ordered ◆ #15 blade (for fine debriding) ◆ #10 or #20 blade (for thin slices of tissue).

Be sure to have the following equipment immediately available to control

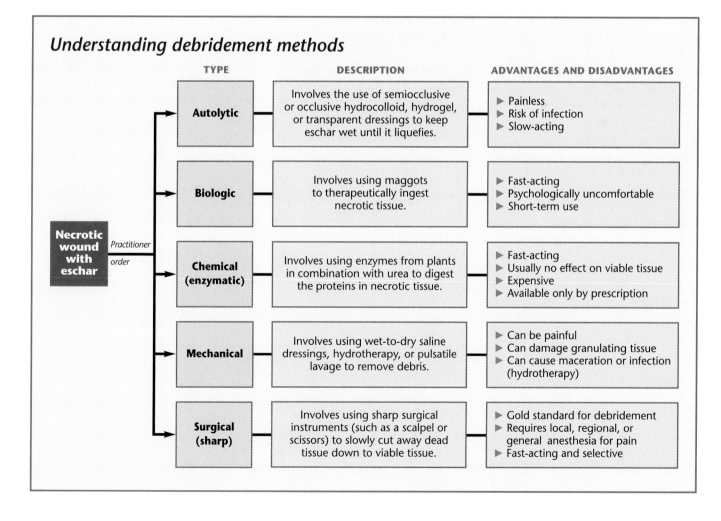

Understanding debridement methods

	TYPE	DESCRIPTION	ADVANTAGES AND DISADVANTAGES
	Autolytic	Involves the use of semiocclusive or occlusive hydrocolloid, hydrogel, or transparent dressings to keep eschar wet until it liquefies.	▶ Painless ▶ Risk of infection ▶ Slow-acting
	Biologic	Involves using maggots to therapeutically ingest necrotic tissue.	▶ Fast-acting ▶ Psychologically uncomfortable ▶ Short-term use
Necrotic wound with eschar *Practitioner order*	**Chemical (enzymatic)**	Involves using enzymes from plants in combination with urea to digest the proteins in necrotic tissue.	▶ Fast-acting ▶ Usually no effect on viable tissue ▶ Expensive ▶ Available only by prescription
	Mechanical	Involves using wet-to-dry saline dressings, hydrotherapy, or pulsatile lavage to remove debris.	▶ Can be painful ▶ Can damage granulating tissue ▶ Can cause maceration or infection (hydrotherapy)
	Surgical (sharp)	Involves using sharp surgical instruments (such as a scalpel or scissors) to slowly cut away dead tissue down to viable tissue.	▶ Gold standard for debridement ▶ Requires local, regional, or general anesthesia for pain ▶ Fast-acting and selective

hemorrhage: needle holder ◆ gut suture with needle ◆ silver nitrate sticks.

Implementation

▶ Confirm the patient's identity using two patient identifiers according to your facility's policy. **JC**

▶ Explain the procedure to the patient. Teach him distraction and relaxation techniques, if possible, to minimize his discomfort.

▶ Provide privacy. Administer an analgesic 20 minutes before debridement begins, or give an I.V. analgesic immediately before the procedure.

▶ Keep the patient warm. Expose only the area to be debrided to prevent chilling.

▶ Wash your hands, and put on a cap, mask, gown or apron, and sterile gloves. **ABA**

▶ Remove the burn dressings and clean the wound. (For detailed directions, see "Burn care," page 58.)

▶ Remove your gown or apron and dirty gloves, and change to another gown or apron and sterile gloves.

▶ Lift loosened edges of eschar with forceps. Use the blunt edge of scissors or forceps to probe the eschar. Cut the dead tissue from the wound with the scissors. Leave a $1/4''$ (0.6-cm) edge on remaining eschar to avoid cutting into viable tissue.

▶ Because debridement removes only dead tissue, bleeding should be minimal. If bleeding occurs, apply gentle pressure on the wound with sterile $4'' \times 4''$ gauze pads. Then apply the hemostatic agent or silver nitrate sticks. If bleeding persists, notify the practitioner and maintain pressure on the wound until he arrives. Excessive bleeding or spurting vessels may require ligation.

▶ Perform additional procedures, such as application of topical medications and dressing replacements, as ordered.

Special considerations

▶ Work quickly, with an assistant if possible, to complete this painful procedure as soon as possible. Try to limit the procedure time to 20 minutes.

▶ Debride no more than a $4''$ (10-cm) square area at one time.

▶ Infection may develop despite the use of sterile technique and equipment.

References

Anderson, I. "Debridement Methods in Wound Care," *Nursing Standard* 20(24):65-66, 68, February 2006.

Brem, H., and Lyder, C. "Protocol for the Successful Treatment of Pressure Ulcers," *American Journal of Surgery* 188(1 Suppl):9-17, July 2004.

Steed, D.L. "Debridement," *American Journal of Surgery* 187(5A):71S-74S, May 2004.

Mechanical traction

Mechanical traction exerts a pulling force on a part of the body—usually the spine, pelvis, or long bones of the arms and legs. It can be used to reduce fractures, treat dislocations, correct or prevent deformities, improve or correct contractures, or decrease muscle spasms. Depending on the injury or condition, an orthopedist may order either skin or skeletal traction.

Applied directly to the skin and thus indirectly to the bone, skin traction is ordered when a light, temporary, or noncontinuous pulling force is required. Contraindications for skin traction include a severe injury with open wounds, an allergy to tape or other skin traction equipment, circulatory disturbances, dermatitis, and varicose veins.

In skeletal traction, an orthopedist inserts a pin or wire through the bone and attaches the traction equipment to the pin or wire to exert a direct, constant, longitudinal pulling force. Indications for skeletal traction include fractures of the tibia, femur, and humerus. Infections, such as osteomyelitis, contraindicate skeletal traction.

After the patient is placed in the specific type of traction ordered by the orthopedist, the nurse is responsible for preventing complications from immobility, for routinely inspecting the equipment, for adding traction weights as ordered and, in patients with skeletal traction, for monitoring the pin insertion sites for signs of infection. (See *Comparing types of traction,* page 318.)

Equipment

For a claw-type basic frame: 102″ (259-cm) plain bar ♦ two 66″ (168-cm) swivel-clamp bars ♦ two upper-panel clamps ♦ two lower-panel clamps.
For an I.V.-type basic frame: 102″ plain bar ♦ 27″ (69-cm) double-clamp bar ♦ 48″ (122-cm) swivel-clamp bar ♦ two 36″ (91-cm) plain bars ♦ four 4″ (10-cm) I.V. posts with clamps ♦ cross clamp.
For an I.V.-type Balkan frame: Two 102″ plain bars ♦ two 27″ double-clamp bars ♦ two 48″ swivel-clamp bars ♦ five 36″ plain bars ♦ four 4″ I.V. posts with clamps ♦ eight cross clamps.
For all frame types: Trapeze with clamp ♦ wall bumper or roller.
For skeletal traction care: Sterile cotton-tipped applicators ♦ prescribed antiseptic solution ♦ sterile gauze pads ♦ antimicrobial solution ♦ optional: antimicrobial ointment.

Implementation

▶ Confirm the patient's identity using two patient identifiers according to your facility's policy. **JC**
▶ Explain the purpose of traction to the patient. Emphasize the importance of maintaining proper body alignment after the traction equipment is set up.

Setting up a claw-type basic frame

▶ Attach one lower-panel and one upper-panel clamp to each 66″ swivel-clamp bar.
▶ Fasten one bar to the footboard and one to the headboard by turning the clamp knobs clockwise until they're tight and then pulling back on the upper clamp's rubberized bar until it's tight.
▶ Secure the 102″ horizontal plain bar atop the two vertical bars, making sure that the clamp knobs point up.
▶ Using the appropriate clamp, attach the trapeze to the horizontal bar about 2′ (60 cm) from the head of the bed.

Setting up an I.V.-type basic frame

▶ Attach one 4″ I.V. post with clamp to each end of both 36″ horizontal plain bars.
▶ Secure an I.V. post in each I.V. holder at the bed corners. Using a cross clamp, fasten the 48″ vertical swivel-clamp bar to the middle of the horizontal plain bar at the foot of the bed.
▶ Fasten the 27″ vertical double-clamp bar to the middle of the horizontal plain bar at the head of the bed.
▶ Attach the 102″ horizontal plain bar to the tops of the two vertical bars, making sure the clamp knobs point up.
▶ Using the appropriate clamp, attach the trapeze to the horizontal bar about 2′ from the head of the bed.

Setting up an I.V.-type Balkan frame

▶ Attach one 4″ I.V. post with clamp to each end of two 36″ horizontal plain bars.
▶ Secure an I.V. post in each I.V. holder at the bed corners.

Comparing types of traction

Traction restricts movement of a patient's affected limb or body part and may confine the patient to bed rest for an extended period. The limb is immobilized by pulling with equal force on each end of the injured area—an equal mix of traction and countertraction. Weights provide the pulling force. Countertraction is produced by using other weights or by positioning the patient's body weight against the traction pull.

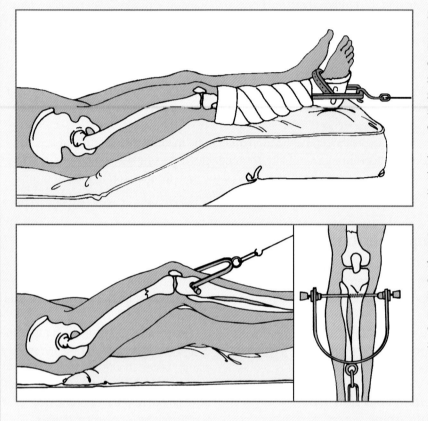

Skin traction

Skin traction immobilizes a body part intermittently over an extended period through direct application of a pulling force on the skin. The force may be applied using adhesive or nonadhesive traction tape or other skin traction devices, such as a boot, belt, or halter.

Adhesive attachment allows more continuous traction, whereas nonadhesive attachment allows easier removal for daily skin care.

Skeletal traction

Skeletal traction immobilizes a body part for prolonged periods by attaching weighted equipment directly to the patient's bones. This may be accomplished with pins, screws, wires, or tongs. The amount of weight applied is determined by body size and the extent of the injury.

▶ Attach a 48″ vertical swivel-clamp bar, using a cross clamp, to each I.V. post clamp on the horizontal plain bar at the foot of the bed.
▶ Fasten one 36″ horizontal plain bar across the midpoints of the two 48″ swivel-clamp bars using two cross clamps.
▶ Attach a 27″ vertical double-clamp bar to each I.V. post clamp on the horizontal bar at the head of the bed.
▶ Using two cross clamps, fasten a 36″ horizontal plain bar across the midpoints of two 27″ double-clamp bars.

▶ Clamp a 102″ horizontal plain bar onto the vertical bars on each side of the bed; make sure the clamp knobs point up.
▶ Use two cross clamps to attach a 36″ horizontal plain bar across the two overhead bars, about 2′ from the head of the bed.
▶ Attach the trapeze to this 36″ horizontal bar.

After setting up any frame

▶ Attach a wall bumper or roller to the vertical bar or bars at the head of the

bed. This protects the walls from damage caused by the bed or equipment.

Caring for the traction patient

▶ Show the patient how much movement he's allowed, and instruct him not to readjust the equipment. Also tell him to report any pain or pressure from the traction equipment.
▶ At least once per shift, make sure the traction equipment connections are tight and that no parts touch the bedding, the patient, or other inappropriate portions of the apparatus. Check for impingements, such as ropes rubbing

on the footboard or getting caught between pulleys.

▶ Inspect the traction equipment to ensure correct alignment.

▶ Inspect the ropes for fraying, which can eventually cause a rope to break.

▶ Make sure the ropes are positioned properly in the pulley track.

▶ To prevent tampering and aid stability and security, make sure all rope ends are taped above the knot.

▶ About every 2 hours, check the patient for proper body alignment and reposition the patient as needed.

▶ To prevent complications from immobility, assess neurovascular integrity routinely. The patient's condition, the hospital routine, and the practitioner's orders determine the frequency of neurovascular assessments.

▶ Provide skin care, encourage coughing and deep-breathing exercises, and assist with ordered range-of-motion exercises for unaffected extremities. Check elimination patterns, and provide laxatives as ordered.

▶ For the patient with skeletal traction, make sure the protruding pin or wire ends are covered with cork to prevent them from tearing the bedding or injuring the patient and staff.

▶ Check the pin site and surrounding skin regularly for signs of infection.

▶ If ordered, clean the pin site and surrounding skin. Pin-site care varies, but you'll usually follow guidelines like these: Use sterile technique; avoid digging at pin sites with the cotton-tipped applicator; if ordered, clean the pin site and surrounding skin with a cotton-tipped applicator dipped in chlorhexidine; if ordered, apply antimicrobial ointment to the pin sites; and apply a loose sterile dressing, or dress with sterile gauze pads soaked in antiseptic solution. Perform pin-site care as often as necessary, depending on the amount of drainage. **NAON**

Special considerations

▶ When using skin traction, apply ordered weights slowly and carefully to avoid jerking the affected extremity. Arrange the weights so they don't hang over the patient to avoid injury if the ropes break.

▶ When applying Buck's traction, make sure the line of pull is always parallel to the bed and not angled downward to prevent pressure on the heel. Placing a flat pillow under the extremity may help as long as it doesn't alter the line of pull.

References

Maher, A.B., et al. *Orthopaedic Nursing,* 3rd ed. Philadelphia: W.B. Saunders Co., 2002.

Mechanical ventilation

A mechanical ventilator moves air in and out of a patient's lungs. Although the equipment serves to ventilate a patient, it doesn't ensure adequate gas exchange. Mechanical ventilators may use either positive or negative pressure to ventilate patients.

Positive-pressure ventilators exert a positive pressure on the airway, which causes inspiration while increasing tidal volume. The inspiratory cycles of these ventilators may vary in volume, pressure, or time.

Negative-pressure ventilators act by creating negative pressure, which pulls the thorax outward and allows air to flow into the lungs. Examples of such ventilators are the iron lung, the cuirass (chest shell), and the body wrap. Negative-pressure ventilators are used mainly to treat neuromuscular disorders, such as Guillain-Barré syndrome, myasthenia gravis, and poliomyelitis.

Other indications for ventilator use include central nervous system disorders (such as cerebral hemorrhage and spinal cord transsection), acute respiratory distress syndrome, pulmonary edema, chronic obstructive pulmonary disease, flail chest, and acute hypoventilation.

Equipment

Oxygen source ◆ air source that can supply 50 psi ◆ mechanical ventilator ◆ humidifier ◆ ventilator circuit tubing, connectors, and adapters ◆ condensation collection trap ◆ spirometer, respirometer, or electronic device to measure flow and volume ◆ in-line thermometer ◆ gloves ◆ handheld resuscitation bag with reservoir ◆ suction equipment ◆ sterile distilled water ◆ equipment for arterial blood gas (ABG) analysis ◆ optional: oximeter, capnography device.

Implementation

▶ Verify the practitioner's order for ventilator support. If the patient isn't already intubated, prepare him for intubation. (See "Endotracheal intubation," page 170.)

▶ When possible, explain the procedure to the patient and his family to help reduce anxiety and fear. Assure the patient and his family that staff members are nearby to provide care.

▶ Perform a complete physical assessment, and draw blood for ABG analysis to establish a baseline.

▶ Make sure the patient is being adequately oxygenated.

▶ Suction the patient if necessary.

▶ Put on gloves if you haven't already done so. Connect the endotracheal tube to the ventilator. Observe for chest expansion, and auscultate for bilateral breath sounds to verify that the patient is being ventilated. **CDC**

▶ Monitor the patient's ABG values after the initial ventilator setup (usually 20 to 30 minutes), after changes in ventilator settings, and as the patient's clinical condition indicates to determine whether the patient is being adequately ventilated and to avoid oxygen toxicity. Be prepared to adjust ventilator settings based on ABG analysis.

▶ Check the ventilator tubing frequently for condensation, which can cause resistance to airflow and which may also be aspirated by the patient. As needed, drain the condensate into a collection trap or briefly disconnect the patient from the ventilator (ventilating him with a handheld resuscitation bag, if necessary), and empty the water into a receptacle. Don't drain the condensate into the humidifier because the condensate may be contaminated with the patient's secretions. Also, avoid accidental drainage of condensation into the patient's airway. **CDC AARC CS1**

▶ Inspect the humidification device regularly, and remove condensate as needed. Inspect heat and moisture exchangers, and replace if secretions contaminate the insert of the filter. Note humidifier settings. The heated humidifier should be set to deliver an inspired gas temperature of 91.4° F (33° C) plus or minus 3.6° F (2° C) and should provide a minimum of 30 mg/L of water vapor with routine use to an intubated patient. **AARC**

▶ If you're using a heated humidifier, monitor the inspired air temperature as close to the patient's airway as possible. The inspiratory gas shouldn't be greater than 98.6° F (37° C) at the opening of the airway. Check that the high temperature alarm is set no higher than 98.6° F and no lower than 86° F (30° C). Observe the amount and consistency of the patient's secretions. If the secretions are copious or increasingly tenacious when a heat and moisture exchanger is used, a heated humidifier should be used instead. **AARC**

▶ Check the in-line thermometer to make sure the temperature of the air delivered to the patient is close to body temperature.

Weaning a patient from the ventilator

Successful weaning from the ventilator depends on the patient's ability to breathe on his own. This means that he must have a spontaneous respiratory effort that can keep him ventilated, a stable cardiovascular system, and sufficient respiratory muscle strength and level of consciousness to sustain spontaneous breathing. The patient should meet some or all of the following criteria. **AACN**

Readiness criteria

▶ Arterial oxygen saturation (SaO_2) greater than 92% on fraction of inspired oxygen less than or equal to 40%; positive end-expiratory pressure less than or equal to 5 cm H_2O
▶ Hemodynamically stable, adequately resuscitated, and doesn't require vasoactive support
▶ Serum electrolyte levels and pH within normal range
▶ Hematocrit greater than 25%
▶ Core body temperature greater than 96.8° F (36° C) and less than 102.2° F (39° C)
▶ Pain adequately managed
▶ Successful withdrawal of a neuromuscular blocker
▶ Arterial blood gas values within normal limits or at patient's baseline

Weaning intervention (long term—more than 72 hours)

▶ Transfer to pressure-support ventilation (PSV) mode, and adjust support level to maintain patient's respiratory rate at fewer than 35 breaths/minute.
▶ For 30 minutes, watch for signs of early failure, such as:
– sustained respiratory rate greater than 35 breaths/minute
– SaO_2 less than 89%
– tidal volume less than or equal to 5 ml/kg
– sustained minute ventilation greater than 200 ml/kg/minute
– evidence of respiratory or hemodynamic distress: labored respiratory pattern, increased diaphoresis or anxiety or both, sustained heart rate greater than 20% higher or lower than baseline, systolic blood pressure greater than 180 mm Hg or less than 90 mm Hg higher.
▶ If tolerated, continue trial for 2 hours; then return patient to "rest" settings by adding ventilator breaths or increasing PSV to achieve a total respiratory rate of fewer than 20 breaths/minute.
▶ After 2 hours of rest, repeat trial for 2 to 4 hours at the same PSV level as the previous trial. If the patient exceeds the tolerance criteria, stop the trial and return to "rest" settings. In this case, the next trial should be performed at a higher support level than the failed trial.
▶ Record the results after each weaning episode, including specific parameters and the time frame if failure was observed.
▶ The goal is to increase trial lengths and reduce the PSV level needed in increments.
▶ With each successful trial, the PSV level may be decreased by 2 to 4 cm H_2O, the time interval may be increased by 1 to 2 hours, or both while keeping the patient within tolerable parameters.
▶ Ensure nocturnal ventilation at "rest" settings (with a respiratory rate of fewer than 20 breaths/minute) for at least 6 hours each night until the patient's weaning trials demonstrate readiness to discontinue support.

▶ When monitoring the patient's vital signs, count spontaneous breaths as well as ventilator-delivered breaths.
▶ Change, clean, or dispose of the ventilator tubing and equipment according to your facility's policy to reduce the risk of bacterial contamination. **AARC** **AACN** **CDC** **CS2**
▶ When ordered, begin to wean the patient from the ventilator. (See *Weaning a patient from the ventilator.*)

Special considerations

▶ Provide emotional support to the patient during all phases of mechanical ventilation to reduce his anxiety and promote successful treatment. Even if the patient is unresponsive, continue to explain all procedures and treatments to him.
▶ Make sure the ventilator alarms are on at all times. If an alarm sounds and the problem can't be identified easily, disconnect the patient from the ventilator and use a handheld resuscitation bag to ventilate him. (See *Responding to ventilator alarms,* page 322.) **JC**
▶ Unless contraindicated, turn the patient from side to side every 1 to 2 hours to facilitate lung expansion and removal of secretions. Perform active or passive range-of-motion exercises for all extremities. If the patient's condition permits, position him upright at regular intervals to increase lung expansion.
▶ When moving the patient or the ventilator tubing, be careful to prevent

Responding to ventilator alarms

The chart below outlines several ventilator alarms, along with their possible cause and nursing interventions.

SIGNAL	POSSIBLE CAUSE	NURSING INTERVENTIONS
Low-pressure alarm	▸ Tube disconnected from ventilator	▸ Reconnect the tube to the ventilator.
	▸ Endotracheal (ET) tube displaced above vocal cords or tracheostomy tube extubated	▸ Check tube placement and reposition, if needed. If extubation or displacement has occurred, ventilate the patient manually and call the practitioner immediately.
	▸ Leaking tidal volume from low cuff pressure (from an underinflated or ruptured cuff or a leak in the cuff or one-way valve)	▸ Listen for a whooshing sound around the tube, indicating an air leak. If you hear one, check cuff pressure. If you can't maintain pressure, call the practitioner; a new tube may need to be inserted.
	▸ Ventilator malfunction	▸ Disconnect the patient from the ventilator and ventilate him manually, if necessary. Obtain another ventilator.
	▸ Leak in ventilator circuitry (from loose connection or hole in tubing, loss of temperature-sensitive device, or cracked humidification jar)	▸ Make sure all connections are intact. Check for holes or leaks in the tubing and replace, if necessary. Check the humidification jar and replace, if cracked.
High-pressure alarm	▸ Increased airway pressure or decreased lung compliance caused by worsening disease	▸ Auscultate the lungs for evidence of increasing lung consolidation, barotrauma, or wheezing. Call the practitioner, if indicated.
	▸ Patient biting on oral ET tube	▸ Insert a bite block, if needed. ▸ Consider pain medication or sedation, if appropriate.
	▸ Secretions in airway	▸ Look for secretions in the airway. To remove them, suction the patient or have him cough.
	▸ Condensate in large-bore tubing	▸ Check tubing for condensate and remove any fluid.
	▸ Intubation of right mainstem bronchus	▸ Auscultate the lungs for evidence of diminished or absent breath sounds in the left lung fields. ▸ Check tube position. If it has slipped, call the practitioner; the tube may need to be repositioned.
	▸ Patient coughing, gagging, or attempting to talk	▸ If the patient fights the ventilator, the practitioner may order a sedative or neuromuscular blockers.
	▸ Chest wall resistance	▸ Reposition the patient to see if doing so improves chest expansion. If repositioning doesn't help, administer the prescribed analgesic.
	▸ Failure of high-pressure relief valve	▸ Have faulty equipment replaced.
	▸ Bronchospasm	▸ Assess the patient for the cause. Report to the practitioner, and treat as ordered.

Ventilator-associated pneumonia

Biancofiore, G., et al. "Nurses' Knowledge and Application of Evidence-Based Guidelines for Preventing Ventilator-Associated Pneumonia," *Minerva Anesthesiology* 73(3):129-34, March 2007.

Level VI
Evidence for a single descriptive or qualitative study

Description
Ventilator-associated pneumonia is a leading cause of mortality among patients who are mechanically ventilated. The Centers for Disease Control and Prevention have issued guidelines to help decrease the prevalence of ventilator-associated pneumonia. This study evaluated nurses' knowledge of guidelines that look to reduced ventilator-associated pneumonia as well as the causes that hinder the implementation of the guidelines. 106 nurses that worked in an ICU were given a questionnaire that listed 21 non-pharmacologic strategies for decreasing the risk of ventilator-associated pneumonia.

Findings
84 nurses responded to the questionnaire. Nineteen of the nurses (22.6%) stated that they had adequate knowledge of the guidelines and strategies to prevent ventilator-associated pneumonia. Forty-six nurses (54.8%) stated that they felt they were poorly informed about the strategies and guidelines to decrease ventilator-associated pneumonia. Sixty-eight nurses (80.9%) stated that they used one or more strategies, while 15 nurses (17.9%) stated they didn't use any of the prevention strategies. Reasons that were given for not applying the strategies included: lack of resources, high cost, disagreement with the strategy, and possibility of causing discomfort to the patient.

Conclusions
Nurses usually apply strategies to prevent ventilator-associated pneumonia but not in a responsible and informed manner.

Nursing practice implications
Nurses should receive continuous training and be involved in drawing up and updating departmental protocols and guidelines for care and behavior. The following practice implications are important:
► Provide oral care to mechanically ventilated patients according to facility protocol.
► Monitor ventilator-associated pneumonia infection rates in patients.
► Educate the staff in proper protocols for preventing ventilator-associated pneumonia.
► Discuss the risks of not providing proper oral and endotracheal tube care for patients who are mechanically ventilated.

---

condensation in the tubing from flowing into the lungs.
► Provide care for the patient's artificial airway as needed.
► Place the call light within the patient's reach, and establish a method of communication because intubation and mechanical ventilation impair the patient's ability to speak. An artificial airway may help the patient to speak by allowing air to pass through his vocal cords.
► Administer a sedative or neuromuscular blocker, as ordered, to relax the patient or eliminate spontaneous breathing efforts that can interfere with the ventilator's action. Remember that the patient receiving a neuromuscular blocker requires close observation because of his inability to breathe or communicate.
► If the patient is receiving a neuromuscular blocker, make sure he also receives a sedative. Neuromuscular blockers cause paralysis without altering the patient's level of consciousness. Reassure the patient and his family that the paralysis is temporary. Also, make sure emergency equipment is readily available in case the ventilator malfunctions or the patient is extubated accidentally.

► Make sure that the patient gets adequate rest and sleep because fatigue can delay weaning from the ventilator. Provide subdued lighting, safely muffle equipment noises, and restrict staff access to the area to promote quiet during rest periods.
► When weaning the patient, continue to observe for signs of hypoxia. Schedule weaning to fit comfortably and realistically with the patient's daily regimen. Avoid scheduling sessions after meals, baths, or lengthy therapeutic or diagnostic procedures.

References

American Association for Respiratory Care. "AARC Evidence-Based Clinical Practice Guideline: Care of the Ventilator Circuit and Its Relation to Ventilator-Associated Pneumonia," *Respiratory Care* 48(9):869-79, September 2003.

American Association for Respiratory Care. "AARC Clinical Practice Guideline: Humidification during Mechanical Ventilation," *Respiratory Care* 37(8): 887-90, August 1992.

Centers for Disease Control and Prevention. "Guidelines for Preventing Health-Care Associated Pneumonia, 2003," *MMWR Recommendations and Reports* 53(RR03):1-36, March 2004.

Chao, D.C., and Scheinhorn, D.J. "Determining the Best Threshold of Rapid Shallow Breathing Index in a Therapist-Implemented Patient-Specific Weaning Protocol," *Respiratory Care* 52(2):159-65, February 2007.

Craven, D.E., et al. "Contaminated Condensate in Mechanical Ventilator Circuits. A Risk Factor for Nosocomial Pneumonia?" *American Review of Respiratory Disease* 129(4):625-8, April 1984. **CS1**

Djedaini, K., et al. "Changing Heat and Moisture Exchangers Every 48 Hours Rather than 24 Hours Does Not Affect Their Efficacy and the Incidence of Nosocomial Pneumonia," *American Journal of Respiratory and Critical Care Medicine* 152(5 Pt 1):1562-569, November 1995. **CS2**

Happ, M.B., et al. "Family Presence and Surveillance during Weaning from Prolonged Ventilation," *Heart and Lung* 36(1):47-57, January-February 2007.

Kress, J.P., and Hall, J.B. "Sedation in the Mechanically Ventilated Patient," *Critical Care Medicine* 34(10):2541-546, October 2006.

Kress, J.P., et al. "Daily Sedative Interruption in Mechanically Ventilated Patients at Risk for Coronary Artery Disease," *Critical Care Medicine* 35(2):365-71, February 2007.

Lynn-McHale Wiegand, D.J., and Carlson, K.K., eds. *AACN Procedure Manual for Critical Care,* 5th ed. Philadelphia: W.B. Saunders Co., 2006.

Niël-Weise, B.S., et al. "Policies for Endotracheal Suctioning of Patients Receiving Mechanical Ventilation: A Systematic Review of Randomized Controlled Trials," *Infection Control and Hospital Epidemiology* 28(5):531-36, May 2007.

Rose, L., and Ed, A. "Advanced Modes of Mechanical Ventilation: Implications for Practice," *AACN Advanced Critical Care* 17(2):145-58, April-June 2006.

Shapiro, M.B., et al. "V. Guidelines for Sedation and Analgesia during Mechanical Ventilation General Overview," *The Journal of Trauma* 63(4):945-50, October 2007.

Mixed venous oxygen saturation monitoring

Mixed venous oxygen saturation (SvO_2) monitoring uses a fiber-optic thermodilution pulmonary artery (PA) catheter to continuously monitor oxygen delivery to tissues and oxygen consumption by tissues. Monitoring SvO_2 allows rapid detection of impaired oxygen delivery, as from decreased cardiac output, hemoglobin level, or arterial oxygen saturation. It also helps evaluate a patient's response to drug therapy, endotracheal tube suctioning, ventilator setting changes, positive end-expiratory pressure, and fraction of inspired oxygen. SvO_2 usually ranges from 60% to 80%; the normal value is 75%.

Equipment

Fiber-optic PA catheter ◆ co-oximeter ◆ optical module and cable ◆ gloves.

Implementation

▶ Connect the optical module and cable to the monitor. Next, peel back the wrapping covering the catheter just enough to uncover the fiber-optic connector. Attach the fiber-optic connector to the optical module while allowing the rest of the catheter to remain in its sterile wrapping. Calibrate the fiber-optic catheter by following the manufacturer's instructions (See *SvO_2 monitoring equipment*.)

SvO_2 monitoring equipment

The mixed venous oxygen saturation (SvO_2) monitoring system consists of a flow-directed pulmonary artery (PA) catheter with fiber-optic filaments, an optical module, and a co-oximeter. The co-oximeter displays a continuous digital SvO_2 value; the strip recorder prints a permanent record.

Catheter insertion follows the same technique as with any thermodilution flow-directed PA catheter. The distal lumen connects to an external PA pressure monitoring system, the proximal or central venous pressure lumen connects to another monitoring system or to a continuous-flow administration unit, and the optical module connects to the co-oximeter unit. As an alternative, many facilities have cardiac monitors that also monitor SvO_2.

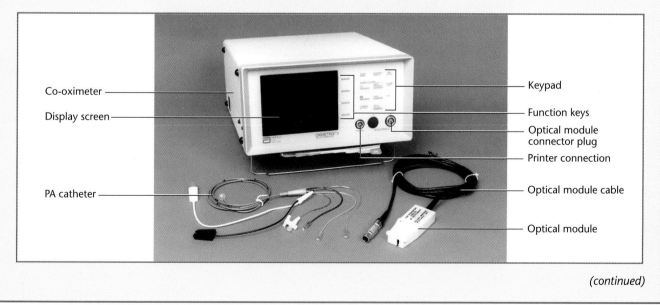

Co-oximeter

Display screen

PA catheter

Keypad

Function keys

Optical module connector plug

Printer connection

Optical module cable

Optical module

(continued)

SvO₂ *monitoring equipment* (continued)

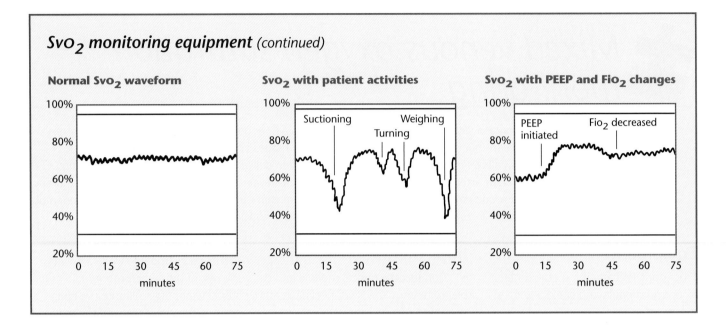

Normal SvO₂ waveform

SvO₂ with patient activities

SvO₂ with PEEP and FiO₂ changes

▶ Confirm the patient's identity using two patient identifiers according to your facility's policy. **JC**

▶ Wash your hands and put on gloves.

▶ Explain the procedure to the patient.

▶ Assist with the insertion of the fiberoptic catheter just as you would for a PA catheter. (See "PAP and PAWP monitoring," page 440.)

▶ After the catheter is inserted, confirm that the light intensity tracing on the graphic printout is within the normal range to ensure correct positioning and function of the catheter.

▶ Observe the digital readout and record the SvO₂ on graph paper. Repeat readings at least once each hour to monitor and document trends.

▶ Set the machine alarms 10% above and 10% below the patient's current SvO₂ reading.

Recalibrating the monitor

▶ Draw a mixed venous blood sample from the distal port of the PA catheter. Send it to the laboratory for analysis to compare the laboratory's SvO₂ reading with that of the fiber-optic catheter.

▶ If the catheter values and the laboratory values differ by more than 4%, follow the manufacturer's instructions to enter the SvO₂ value obtained by the laboratory into the oximeter.

▶ Recalibrate the monitor every 24 hours or whenever the catheter has been disconnected from the optical module.

Special considerations

▶ If the patient's SvO₂ drops below 60% or varies by more than 10% for 3 minutes or longer, reassess the patient. If the SvO₂ doesn't return to the baseline value after nursing interventions, notify the practitioner. A decreasing SvO₂ or a value less than 60% indicates impaired oxygen delivery, as occurs in hemorrhage, hypoxia, shock, arrhythmias, or suctioning. SvO₂ may also decrease as a result of increased oxygen demand from hyperthermia, shivering, or seizure.

▶ If the intensity of the tracing is low, make sure that all connections between the catheter and oximeter are secure and that the catheter is patent and not kinked.

▶ If the tracing is damped or erratic, try to aspirate blood from the catheter to check for patency (if allowed by your facility). If you can't aspirate blood, notify the practitioner so that the catheter can be replaced. Check the PA waveform to determine whether the catheter has wedged. If it has wedged, turn the patient from side to side and instruct him to cough. If the catheter remains wedged, notify the practitioner immediately.

References

Caille, V., and Squara, P. "Oxygen Uptake-to-Delivery Relationship: A Way to Assess Adequate Flow," *Critical Care* 10(Suppl 3):S4, 2006.

Goodrich, C. "Continuous Central Venous Oximetry Monitoring," *Critical Care Nursing Clinics of North America* 18(2):203-209, June 2006.

Lynn-McHale Wiegand, D.J., and Carlson, K.K., eds. *AACN Procedure Manual for Critical Care*, 5th ed. Philadelphia: W.B. Saunders Co., 2006.

Squara, P. "Matching Total Body Oxygen Consumption and Delivery: A Critical Objective?" *Intensive Care Medicine* 30(12):2170-179, December 2004.

Mouth care

Given in the morning, at bedtime, or after meals, mouth care entails brushing and flossing the teeth and inspecting the mouth. It removes soft plaque deposits and calculus from the teeth, cleans and massages the gums, reduces mouth odor, and helps prevent infection. By freshening the patient's mouth, mouth care also enhances appreciation of food, thereby aiding appetite and nutrition.

Although the ambulatory patient can usually perform mouth care alone, the bedridden patient may require partial or full assistance. The comatose patient requires the use of suction equipment to prevent aspiration during oral care.

Equipment

Towel or facial tissues ◆ emesis basin ◆ trash bag ◆ mouthwash ◆ toothbrush and toothpaste ◆ pitcher and glass ◆ drinking straw ◆ dental floss ◆ gloves ◆ small mirror, if necessary ◆ optional: dental floss holder, oral irrigating device.

For the comatose or debilitated patient as needed: Linen-saver pad ◆ bite block ◆ petroleum jelly ◆ hydrogen peroxide ◆ sponge-tipped mouth swab ◆ oral suction equipment or gauze pads ◆ optional: mouth-care kit, tongue blade, 4″ gauze pads, adhesive tape.

Implementation

▶ Fill a pitcher with water, and bring it and other equipment to the patient's bedside. If you'll be using oral suction equipment, connect the tubing to the suction bottle and suction catheter, insert the plug into an outlet, and check for correct operation.

▶ If necessary, devise a bite block to protect yourself from being bitten during the procedure. Wrap a gauze pad over the end of a tongue blade, fold the edge in, and secure it with adhesive tape.

▶ Wash your hands thoroughly, put on gloves, explain the procedure to the patient, and provide privacy.

Supervising mouth care

▶ For the bedridden patient capable of self-care, encourage her to perform her own mouth care.

▶ If allowed, place the patient in Fowler's position. Place the overbed table in front of the patient, and arrange the equipment on it. Open the table and set up the built-in mirror, if available, or position a small mirror on the table.

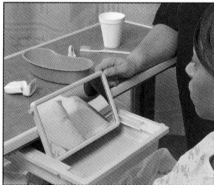

▶ Drape a towel over the patient's chest to protect her gown. Tell her to floss her teeth while looking into the mirror.

▶ Observe the patient to make sure she's flossing correctly, and correct her, if necessary. Tell her to wrap the floss around the second or third fingers of both hands. Starting with her front teeth and without injuring the gums, she should insert the floss as far as possible into the space between each pair of teeth. Then she should clean the surfaces of adjacent teeth by pulling the floss up and down against the side of each tooth. After the patient flosses a

pair of teeth, remind her to use a clean 1″ (2.5-cm) section of floss for the next pair.

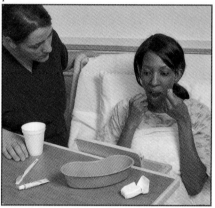

▶ After the patient flosses, mix mouthwash and water in a glass, place a straw in the glass, and position the emesis basin nearby. Then instruct the patient to brush her teeth and gums while looking into the mirror. Encourage her to rinse frequently during brushing, and provide facial tissues for her to wipe her mouth.

Performing mouth care

▶ For the comatose patient or the conscious patient incapable of self-care, you'll perform mouth care. If the patient wears dentures, clean them thoroughly. (See *Dealing with dentures,* page 328.) Some patients may benefit from using an oral irrigating device such as a Water Pik. (See *Using an oral irrigating device,* page 329.)

▶ Arrange the equipment on the overbed table or bedside stand, including the oral suction equipment, if nec-

Dealing with dentures

Prostheses made of acrylic resins, vinyl composites, or both, dentures replace some or all of the patient's natural teeth. Dentures require proper care to remove soft plaque deposits and calculus and to reduce mouth odor. Such care involves removing and rinsing dentures after meals, daily brushing and removal of tenacious deposits, and soaking in a commercial denture cleaner. Dentures must be removed from the comatose or presurgical patient to prevent possible airway obstruction.

Equipment and preparation

Start by assembling the following equipment at the patient's bedside: emesis basin ♦ labeled denture cup ♦ toothbrush or denture brush ♦ gloves ♦ toothpaste ♦ commercial denture cleaner ♦ paper towel ♦ sponge-tipped mouth swab ♦ mouthwash ♦ gauze ♦ optional: adhesive denture liner.

Wash your hands and put on gloves.

Removing dentures

▶ To remove a full upper denture, grasp the front and palatal surfaces of the denture with your thumb and forefinger. Position the index finger of your opposite hand over the upper border of the denture, and press to break the seal between denture and palate. Grasp the denture with gauze because saliva can make it slippery.

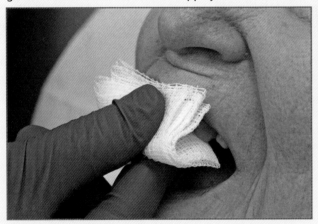

▶ To remove a full lower denture, grasp the front and lingual surfaces of the denture with your thumb and index finger and gently lift up.
▶ To remove partial dentures, first ask the patient or caregiver how the prosthesis is retained and how to remove it. If it's held in place with clips or snaps, then exert equal pressure on the border of each side of the denture. Avoid lifting the clasps, which easily bend or break.

Oral and denture care

▶ After removing dentures, place them in a properly labeled denture cup. Add warm water and a commercial denture cleaner to remove stains and hardened deposits. Follow package directions. Avoid soaking dentures in mouthwash containing alcohol because it may damage a soft liner.
▶ Instruct the patient to rinse with mouthwash to remove food particles and reduce mouth odor. Then stroke the palate, buccal surfaces, gums, and tongue with a soft toothbrush or sponge-tipped mouth swab to clean the mucosa and stimulate circulation. Inspect for irritated areas or sores because they may indicate a poorly fitting denture.
▶ Carry the denture cup, emesis basin, toothbrush, and toothpaste to the sink. After lining the basin with a paper towel, fill it with water to cushion the dentures in case you drop them. Hold the dentures over the basin, wet them with warm water, and apply toothpaste to a denture brush or long-bristled toothbrush. Clean the dentures using only moderate pressure to prevent scratches and warm water to prevent distortion.

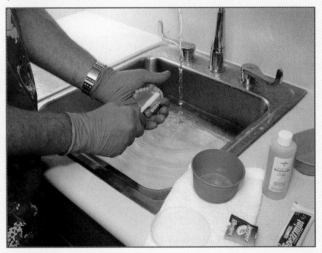

▶ Clean the denture cup, and place the dentures in it. Rinse the brush, and clean and dry the emesis basin. Return all equipment to the patient's bedside stand.

Wearing dentures

▶ If the patient desires, apply adhesive liner to the dentures. Moisten them with water, if necessary, to reduce friction and ease insertion.
▶ Encourage the patient to wear his dentures to enhance his appearance, facilitate eating and speaking, and prevent changes in the gum line that may affect denture fit.

Using an oral irrigating device

An oral irrigating device, such as the Water Pik, directs a pulsating jet of water around the teeth to massage gums and remove debris and food particles. It's especially useful for cleaning areas missed by brushing, such as around bridgework, crowns, and dental wires. Because this device enhances oral hygiene, it benefits patients undergoing head and neck irradiation, which can damage teeth and cause severe caries. The device also maintains oral hygiene in a patient with a fractured jaw or with mouth injuries that limit standard mouth care.

Equipment and preparation

To use the device, first assemble the following equipment: oral irrigating device ◆ towel ◆ emesis basin ◆ pharyngeal suction apparatus ◆ salt solution or mouthwash, if ordered ◆ soap.

Wash your hands and put on gloves.

Implementation

▶ Turn the patient to his side to prevent aspiration of water. Then place a towel under his chin and an emesis basin next to his cheek to absorb or catch drainage.

▶ Insert the oral irrigating device's plug into a nearby electrical outlet. Remove the device's cover, turn it upside down, and fill it with lukewarm water or with a mouthwash or salt solution, as ordered. When using a salt solution, dissolve the salt beforehand in a separate container. Then pour the solution into the cover. (*Note:* Salt solution shouldn't be used in patients with oral dryness or dehydration because salt exacerbates these conditions.)

▶ Secure the cover to the base of the device. Remove the water hose handle from the base, and snap the jet tip into place. If necessary, wet the grooved end of the tip to ease insertion. Adjust the pressure dial to the setting most comfortable for the patient. If his gums are tender and prone to bleed, choose a low setting.

▶ Adjust the knurled knob on the handle to direct the water jet, place the jet tip in the patient's mouth, and turn on the device. Instruct the alert patient to keep his lips partially closed to avoid spraying water.

▶ Direct the water at a right angle to the gum line of each tooth and between teeth. Avoid directing water under the patient's tongue because this may injure sensitive tissue.

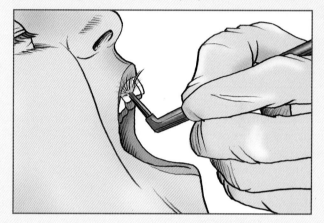

▶ After irrigating each tooth, pause briefly and instruct the patient to expectorate the water or solution into the emesis basin. If he's unable to do so, suction it from the sides of the mouth with the pharyngeal suction apparatus. After irrigating all teeth, turn off the device and remove the jet tip from the patient's mouth.

▶ Empty the remaining water or solution from the cover, remove the jet tip from the handle, and return the handle to the base. Clean the jet tip with soap and water, rinse the cover, and dry them both and return them to storage.

---

essary. Turn on the machine. If a suction machine isn't available, wipe the inside of the patient's mouth frequently with a gauze pad.

▶ Raise the bed to a comfortable working height to prevent back strain. Then lower the head of the bed, and position the patient on her side, with her face extended over the edge of the pillow to facilitate oral drainage and prevent fluid aspiration.

▶ Place a linen-saver pad under the patient's chin and an emesis basin

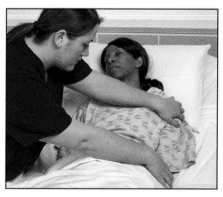

near her cheek to absorb or catch oral drainage.

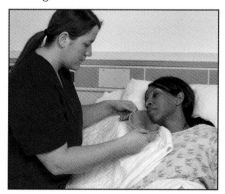

▶ Lubricate the patient's lips with petroleum jelly to prevent dryness and cracking. Reapply lubricant, as needed, during oral care.

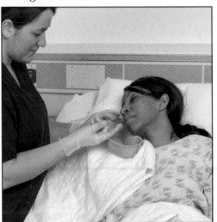

▶ If necessary, insert the bite block.

▶ Using a dental floss holder, hold the floss against each tooth and direct it as close to the gum as possible without injuring the sensitive tissues around the tooth.

▶ After flossing the patient's teeth, mix mouthwash and water in a glass and place the straw in it.

▶ Wet the toothbrush with water. If necessary, use hot water to soften the bristles. Apply toothpaste.

▶ Brush the patient's lower teeth from the gum line up; the upper teeth, from the gum line down. Place the brush at a 45-degree angle to the gum line, and press the bristles gently into the gingival sulcus. Using short, gentle strokes to prevent gum damage, brush the facial surfaces (toward the cheek) and the lingual surfaces (toward the tongue) of the bottom teeth. Use just the tip of the brush for the lingual surfaces of the front teeth. Then, using the same technique, brush the facial and lingual surfaces of the top teeth. Next, brush the biting surfaces of the bottom and top teeth, using a back-and-forth motion. If possible, ask the patient to rinse frequently during brushing by taking the mouthwash solution through the straw. Hold the emesis basin steady under the

patient's cheek, and wipe her mouth and cheeks with facial tissues as needed.

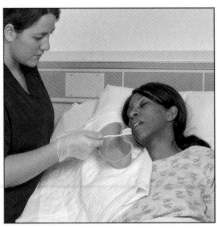

▶ After brushing the patient's teeth, dip a sponge-tipped mouth swab into the mouthwash solution. Press the swab against the side of the glass to remove excess moisture. Gently stroke the gums, buccal surfaces, palate, and tongue to clean the mucosa and stimulate circulation. Replace the swab, as necessary, for thorough cleaning. Avoid inserting the swab too deeply to prevent gagging and vomiting.

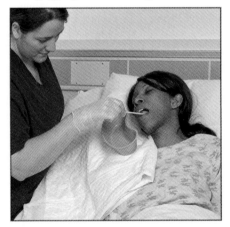

After mouth care
▶ Assess the patient's mouth for cleanliness and tooth and tissue condition.

▶ Then remove your gloves, rinse the toothbrush, and clean the emesis basin and glass. Empty and clean the suction

bottle, if used, and place a clean suction catheter on the tubing. Return reusable equipment to the appropriate storage location, and properly discard disposable equipment in the trash bag.

Special considerations
▶ Use sponge-tipped mouth swabs to clean the teeth of a patient with sensitive gums. These swabs produce less friction than a toothbrush but don't clean as well.

▶ Clean the mouth of a toothless comatose patient by wrapping a gauze pad around your index finger, moistening it with mouthwash, and gently swabbing the oral tissues.

▶ Remember that mucous membranes dry quickly in the patient breathing through the mouth or receiving oxygen therapy. Moisten the patient's mouth and lips regularly with moistened sponge-tipped swabs. **AACN**

References
Allen Furr, L., et al. "Factors Affecting Quality of Oral Care in Intensive Care Units," *Journal of Advanced Nursing* 48(5):454-62, December 2004.

Berry, A.M., and Davidson, P.M. "Beyond Comfort: Oral Hygiene as a Critical Nursing Activity in the Intensive Care Unit," *Intensive and Critical Care Nursing* 22(6):318-28, December 2006.

Kinley, J., and Brennan, S. "Changing Practice: Use of Audit to Change Oral Care Practice," *International Journal of Palliative Nursing* 10(12):580-87, December 2004.

Nasal irrigation

Irrigation of the nasal passages soothes irritated mucous membranes and washes away crusted mucus, secretions, and foreign matter. Irrigation may be done with a bulb syringe or an electronic irrigating device.

Nasal irrigation benefits patients with either acute or chronic nasal conditions, including sinusitis, rhinitis, Wegener's granulomatosis, and Sjögren's syndrome. In addition, the procedure may help people who regularly inhale toxins or allergens. Nasal irrigation is routinely recommended after some nasal surgeries to enhance healing by removal of postoperative eschar and to aid remucosolization of the sinus cavities and ostia. **AAO**

Contraindications for nasal irrigation may include advanced destruction of the sinuses, frequent nosebleeds, and foreign bodies in the nasal passages.

Equipment

Bulb syringe or oral irrigating device ◆ rigid or flexible disposable irrigation tips ◆ hypertonic saline solution ◆ plastic sheet ◆ towels ◆ facial tissue ◆ bath basin ◆ gloves.

Implementation

▶ Warm the saline solution to about 105° F (40.6° C).
▶ If you're using an oral irrigating device, plug it in so it's near the patient. Fill the reservoir of the device with warm water.
▶ Confirm the patient's identity using two patient identifiers according to your facility's policy. **JC**
▶ Wash your hands and put on gloves.
▶ Explain the procedure to the patient, and place a towel on her upper body.

▶ Have the patient sit comfortably near the equipment in a position that allows the bulb or catheter tip to enter her nose and the returning irrigant to flow into the bath basin or sink. (See *Positioning the patient for nasal irrigation,* page 332.)
▶ Remind the patient to keep her mouth open and to breath rhythmically during the procedure. This causes the soft palate to seal the throat, thus allowing the irrigant to stream out the opposite nostril and carry discharge with it.
▶ Instruct the patient not to speak or swallow during the irrigation.
▶ To avoid injuring the nasal mucosa, remove the irrigating tip from the patient's nostrils if she reports the need to sneeze or cough.

Using a bulb syringe

▶ Fill the bulb syringe with saline solution, and insert the tip about ¹/₂″ (1.3 cm) into the patient's nostril.
▶ Squeeze the bulb until a gentle stream of warm irrigant washes through the nose. Avoid forceful squeezing. Alternate the nostrils until the return irrigant runs clear.

Using an oral irrigating device

▶ Insert the irrigation tip into the nostril about ¹/₂″ to 1″ (1.3 to 2.5 cm) and turn on the device. Begin with a low pressure setting, and increase the pressure as needed. Irrigate both nostrils.
▶ Inspect returning irrigant. Changes in color, viscosity, or volume may signal an infection and should be reported to the practitioner. Also report blood or necrotic material.

Positioning the patient for nasal irrigation

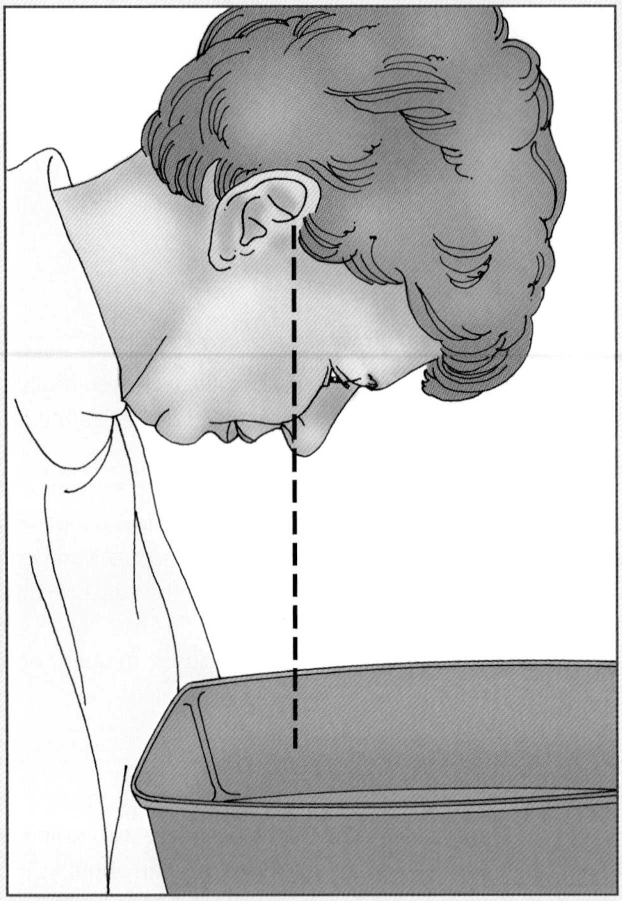

Whether you're teaching a patient to perform nasal irrigation with a bulb syringe or an oral irrigating device, the irrigation will progress more easily when the patient learns how to hold her head for optimal safety, comfort, and effectiveness.

Help the patient to sit upright with her head bent forward over the basin or sink and flexed on her chest, as shown at left. Her nose and ear should be on the same vertical plane.

Explain that she's less likely to breathe in the irrigant when holding her head in this position. This position should also keep the irrigant from entering the Eustachian tubes, which will now lie above the level of the irrigation stream.

Concluding the procedure

▶ After irrigation, have the patient wait a few minutes before blowing excess fluid from both nostrils at once. This action should help loosen and expel crusted secretions and mucus.
▶ Clean the bulb syringe or irrigating device with soap and water, and then disinfect as recommended.

Special considerations

▶ Expect fluid to drain from the patient's nose for a brief time after the irrigation and before he blows his nose.
▶ Be sure to insert the irrigation tip far enough to ensure that the irrigant cleans out the nasal membranes before draining out. A typical amount of irrigant is 500 to 1,000 ml.

References

Taylor, C., et al. *Fundamentals of Nursing: The Art and Science of Nursing Care,* 6th ed. Philadelphia: Lippincott Williams & Wilkins, 2008.

Nasal medications

Nasal medications may be instilled by means of drops, a spray (using an atomizer), or an aerosol (using a nebulizer). Most drugs instilled by these methods produce local rather than systemic effects. Drops can be directed at a specific area; sprays and aerosols diffuse medication throughout the nasal passages.

Equipment

Prescribed medication ◆ patient's medication record and chart ◆ emesis basin (with nose drops only) ◆ facial tissues ◆ optional: pillow, small piece of soft rubber or plastic tubing, gloves.

Implementation

▶ Verify the order on the patient's medication record by checking it against the practitioner's order. Note the concentration of the medication. Verify the expiration date. **JC** **ISMP**
▶ Confirm the patient's identity using two patient identifiers according to your facility's policy. **JC**
▶ If your facility utilizes a bar code scanning system, make sure to scan your ID badge, the patient's ID bracelet, and the medication's bar code. **JC** **ISMP**
▶ Explain the procedure and provide privacy.
▶ Wash your hands. Put on gloves if you notice drainage from the nostrils. **CDC**

Instilling nose drops

▶ When possible, position the patient so that the drops flow back into the nostrils, toward the affected area. (See *Positioning the patient for nose drop instillation,* page 334.)
▶ Draw up some medication into the dropper.
▶ Push up the tip of the patient's nose slightly. Position the dropper just above the nostril, and direct its tip toward the midline of the nose so that the drops flow toward the back of the nasal cavity rather than down the throat.
▶ Insert the dropper about ³/₈″ (1 cm) into the nostril. Don't let the dropper touch the sides of the nostril because this would contaminate the dropper or could cause the patient to sneeze.
▶ Instill the prescribed number of drops, observing the patient carefully for signs of discomfort.
▶ To prevent the drops from leaking out of the nostrils, ask the patient to keep his head tilted back for at least 5 minutes and to breathe through his mouth. This also allows sufficient time for the medication to constrict mucous membranes.
▶ Keep an emesis basin handy so that the patient can expectorate any medication that flows into the oropharynx and mouth. Use a facial tissue to wipe any excess medication from the patient's nostrils and face.
▶ Clean the dropper by separating the plunger and pipette and flushing them with warm water. Allow them to air-dry.

Using a nasal spray

▶ Have the patient sit upright with his head tilted back slightly. Alternatively, have the patient lie on his back with his shoulders elevated, neck hyperextended, and head tilted back over the edge of the bed. Support his head with one hand to prevent neck strain.
▶ Remove the protective cap from the atomizer.
▶ To prevent air from entering the nasal cavity and to allow the medication to flow properly, occlude one of the patient's nostrils with your finger. Insert the atomizer tip into the open nostril.
▶ Instruct the patient to inhale, and as he does so, squeeze the atomizer once, quickly and firmly. Use just enough force to coat the inside of the patient's nose with medication. Then tell the patient to exhale through his mouth.
▶ If ordered, spray the nostril again. Then repeat the procedure in the other nostril.
▶ Instruct the patient to keep his head tilted back for several minutes and to breathe slowly through his nose so that the medication has time to work. Tell him not to blow his nose for several minutes.

Using a nasal aerosol

▶ Instruct the patient to blow his nose gently to clear his nostrils.
▶ Insert the medication cartridge according to the manufacturer's directions. With some models, you'll fit the medication cartridge over a small hole in the adapter. When inserting a refill cartridge, first remove the protective cap from the stem. Spacer inhalers may be recommended. **MFR** (See "Handheld oropharyngeal inhalers," page 227.)
▶ Shake the aerosol well before each use, and remove the protective cap from the adapter tip.
▶ Hold the aerosol between your thumb and index finger, with your index finger positioned on top of the medication cartridge.
▶ Tilt the patient's head back, and carefully insert the adapter tip in one

Positioning the patient for nose drop instillation

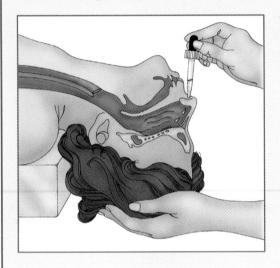

To reach the ethmoid and sphenoid sinuses, have the patient lie on her back with her neck hyperextended and her head tilted back over the edge of the bed. Support her head with one hand to prevent neck strain.

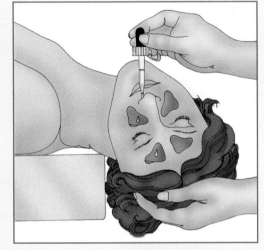

To reach the maxillary and frontal sinuses, have the patient lie on her back with her head toward the affected side and hanging slightly over the edge of the bed. Ask her to rotate her head laterally after hyperextension, and support her head with one hand to prevent neck strain.

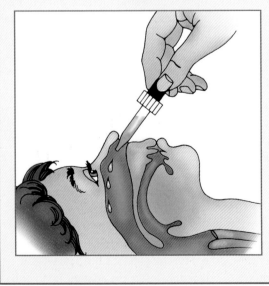

To administer drops for relief of ordinary nasal congestion, help the patient to a reclining or supine position with her head tilted slightly toward the affected side. Aim the dropper upward, toward the patient's eye, rather than downward, toward her ear.

nostril while sealing the other nostril with your finger.

▶ Press the adapter and cartridge together firmly to release one measured dose of medication.

▶ Shake the aerosol, and repeat the procedure to instill medication into the other nostril.

▶ Remove the medication cartridge, and wash the nasal adapter in lukewarm water daily. Allow the adapter to dry before reinserting the cartridge.

Special considerations

AGE FACTOR

Before instilling nose drops in a young child, attach a small piece of tubing to the end of the dropper. Do the same for an uncooperative patient.

▶ If using a metered-dose pump spray system, prime the delivery system with four sprays or until a fine mist appears. Reprime the system with two sprays or until a fine mist appears if 3 or more days have lapsed since the last use.

▶ When using an aerosol, be careful not to puncture or incinerate the pressurized cartridge.

▶ To prevent the spread of infection, label the medication bottle so that it will be used only for that patient. **JC**

▶ Teach the patient how to instill nasal medications correctly so that he can continue treatment after discharge, if necessary. Caution him against using nasal medications longer than prescribed because they may cause a rebound effect that worsens the condition. A rebound effect occurs when the medication loses its effectiveness and relaxes the vessels in the nasal turbinates, producing a stuffiness that can be relieved only by discontinuing the medication.

▶ Inform the patient of possible adverse reactions. In addition, explain that when corticosteroids are given by nasal aerosol, therapeutic effects may not appear for 2 days to 2 weeks.

▶ Teach the patient good oral and nasal hygiene.

References

DelGaudio, J.M., and Wise, S.K. "Topical Steroid Drops for the Treatment of Sinus Ostia Stenosis in the Postoperative Period," *American Journal of Rhinology* 20(6):563-67, November-December 2006.

Farkas, A., et al. "Characterization of Regional and Local Deposition of Inhaled Aerosol Drugs in the Respiratory System by Computational Fluid and Particle Dynamics Methods," *Journal of Aerosol Medications* 19(3):329-43, 2006.

The Joint Commission. *Comprehensive Accreditation Manual for Hospitals: The Official Handbook.* Standard MM.1.10. Oakbrook Terrace, Ill.: The Joint Commission, 2007.

The Joint Commission. *Comprehensive Accreditation Manual for Hospitals: The Official Handbook.* Standard MM.2.10. Oakbrook Terrace, Ill.: The Joint Commission, 2007.

The Joint Commission. *Comprehensive Accreditation Manual for Hospitals: The Official Handbook.* Standard MM.3.10. Oakbrook Terrace, Ill.: The Joint Commission, 2007.

The Joint Commission. *Comprehensive Accreditation Manual for Hospitals: The Official Handbook.* Standard MM.4.10. Oakbrook Terrace, Ill.: The Joint Commission, 2007.

The Joint Commission. *Comprehensive Accreditation Manual for Hospitals: The Official Handbook.* Standard MM.4.20. Oakbrook Terrace, Ill.: The Joint Commission, 2007.

The Joint Commission. *Comprehensive Accreditation Manual for Hospitals: The Official Handbook.* Standard MM.5.10. Oakbrook Terrace, Ill.: The Joint Commission, 2007.

The Joint Commission. *Comprehensive Accreditation Manual for Hospitals: The Official Handbook.* Standard MM.6.10. Oakbrook Terrace, Ill.: The Joint Commission, 2007.

The Joint Commission. *Comprehensive Accreditation Manual for Hospitals: The Official Handbook.* Standard MM.6.20. Oakbrook Terrace, Ill.: The Joint Commission, 2007.

Merkus, P., et al. "The 'Best Method' of Topical Nasal Drug Delivery: Comparison of Seven Techniques," *Rhinology* 44(2):102-107, June 2006.

Raghavan, U., and Jones, N.S. "A Prospective Randomized Blinded Cross-Over Trial Using Nasal Drops in Patients with Nasal Polyposis: An Evaluation of Effectiveness and Comfort Level in Two Head Positions," *American Journal of Rhinology* 20(4):397-400, July-August 2006.

Taylor, C., et al. *Fundamentals of Nursing: The Art and Science of Nursing Care,* 6th ed. Philadelphia: Lippincott Williams & Wilkins, 2008.

Nasoenteric-decompression tube insertion and removal

The nasoenteric-decompression tube is inserted nasally and advanced beyond the stomach into the intestinal tract. It's used to aspirate intestinal contents for analysis and to treat intestinal obstruction. The tube may also help to prevent nausea, vomiting, and abdominal distention after GI surgery. A physician will usually insert or remove a nasoenteric-decompression tube, but sometimes a nurse will remove it.

The nasoenteric-decompression tube may have a preweighted tip and a balloon at one end of the tube that holds air or water to stimulate peristalsis and facilitate the tube's passage through the pylorus and into the intestinal tract. (See *Common types of nasoenteric-decompression tubes*.)

Equipment

Sterile 10-ml syringe ◆ nasoenteric-decompression tube ◆ container of water ◆ 5 to 10 ml of water as ordered ◆ suction-decompression equipment ◆ gloves ◆ towel or linen-saver pad ◆ water-soluble lubricant ◆ 4″ × 4″ gauze pad ◆ ½″ hypoallergenic tape ◆ bulb syringe or 60-ml catheter-tip syringe ◆ rubber band ◆ safety pin ◆ specimen container ◆ basin of ice or warm water ◆ penlight ◆ waterproof marking pen ◆ glass of water with straw ◆ optional: ice chips, local anesthetic.

Implementation

▶ Stiffen a flaccid tube by chilling it in a basin of ice to facilitate insertion. To make a stiff tube flexible, dip it into warm water. **MFR**

▶ Air or water is added to the balloon either before or after insertion of the tube, depending on the type of tube used. Follow the manufacturer's recommendations. **MFR**

▶ Set up suction-decompression equipment, if ordered, and make sure it works properly.

▶ Confirm the patient's identity using two patient identifiers according to your facility's policy. **JC**

▶ Explain the procedure to the patient, forewarning him that he may experience some discomfort. Provide privacy and adequate lighting.

▶ Wash your hands and put on gloves.

▶ Position the patient as the physician specifies, usually in semi-Fowler's or high Fowler's position. You may also need to help the patient hold his neck in a hyperextended position.

▶ Protect the patient's chest with a linen-saver pad or towel.

▶ Agree with the patient on a signal that can be used to stop the insertion briefly if necessary.

Assisting with insertion

▶ The physician assesses the patency of the patient's nostrils.

▶ To decide how far the tube must be inserted to reach the stomach, the physician places the tube's distal end at the tip of the patient's nose and then extends the tube to the earlobe and down to the xiphoid process. He either marks the tube with a waterproof marking pen or holds it at this point.

▶ The physician applies water-soluble lubricant to the first few inches of the tube to reduce friction and tissue trauma and to facilitate insertion.

▶ If the balloon already contains water, the physician holds it so the fluid runs to the bottom. Then he pinches the balloon closed to retain the fluid as the insertion begins.

▶ Tell the patient to breathe through his mouth or to pant as the balloon enters his nostril. After the balloon begins its descent, the physician releases his grip on it, allowing the weight of the fluid or the preweighted tip to pull the tube into the nasopharynx. When the tube reaches the nasopharynx, the physician instructs the patient to lower his chin and to swallow. In some cases, the patient may sip water through a straw to facilitate swallowing as the tube advances, but not after the tube reaches the trachea. This prevents injury from aspiration. The physician continues to advance the tube slowly to prevent it from curling or kinking in the stomach.

▶ To confirm the tube's passage into the stomach, the physician aspirates stomach contents with a bulb syringe.

▶ To keep the tube out of the patient's eyes and to help avoid undue skin irritation, fold a 4″ × 4″ gauze pad in half and tape it to the patient's forehead with the fold directed toward the patient's nose. The physician can slide the tube through this sling, leaving enough slack for the tube to advance.

Common types of nasoenteric-decompression tubes

The type of nasoenteric-decompression tube chosen for your patient will depend on the size of the patient and his nostrils, the estimated duration of intubation, and the reason for the procedure. For example, to remove viscous material from the patient's intestinal tract, the physician may select a tube with a wide bore and a single lumen.

Whichever tube you use, you'll need to provide good mouth care and check the patient's nostrils often for signs of irritation. If you see any signs of irritation, retape the tube so that it doesn't cause tension and then lubricate the nostril. Or, check with the physician to see whether the tube can be inserted through the other nostril.

Most tubes are impregnated with a radiopaque mark so that placement can easily be confirmed by X-ray or other imaging technique.

Tubes such as the preweighted Miller-Abbot type intestinal tube (shown at right) have a tungsten-weighted inflatable latex balloon tip designed for temporary management of mechanical obstruction in the small or large intestines.

▶ Position the patient, as directed, to help advance the tube. He'll typically lie on his right side until the tube clears the pylorus (about 2 hours). The physician will confirm passage by X-ray.

▶ After the tube clears the pylorus, the physician may direct you to advance it 2″ to 3″ (5 to 7.5 cm) every hour and to reposition the patient until the premeasured mark reaches the patient's nostril. Gravity and peristalsis will help advance the tube. (Notify the physician if you can't advance the tube.)

▶ Keep the remaining premeasured length of tube well lubricated to ease passage and prevent irritation.

▶ Don't tape the tube while it advances to the premeasured mark unless the physician asks you to do so.

▶ After the tube progresses the necessary distance, the physician will order an X-ray to confirm tube positioning. When the tube is in place, secure the external tubing with tape to help prevent further progression.

▶ Loop a rubber band around the tube and pin the rubber band to the patient's gown with a safety pin.

▶ If ordered, attach the tube to suction.

Removing the tube

▶ Assist the patient into semi-Fowler's or high Fowler's position. Drape a linen-saver pad or towel across the patient's chest.

▶ Wash your hands and put on gloves.

▶ Clamp the tube and disconnect it from the suction. This prevents the patient from aspirating any gastric contents that leak from the tube during withdrawal.

▶ If your patient has a tube with an inflated balloon tip, attach a 10-ml syringe to the balloon port and withdraw the air or water.

▶ Slowly withdraw between 6″ and 8″ (15 and 20 cm) of the tube. Wait 10 minutes and withdraw another 6″ to 8″. Wait another 10 minutes. Continue this procedure until the tube reaches the patient's esophagus (with 18″ [46 cm] of the tube remaining inside the patient). At this point, you can gently withdraw the tube completely.

Special considerations

▶ For a double- or triple-lumen tube, note which lumen accommodates balloon inflation and which accommodates drainage.

▶ Apply a local anesthetic, if ordered, to the nostril or the back of the throat to dull sensations and the gag reflex for intubation. Letting the patient gargle with a liquid anesthetic or holding ice chips in his mouth for a few minutes serves the same purpose.

References

Smeltzer, S.C., et al. *Brunner & Suddarth's Textbook of Medical-Surgical Nursing,* 11th ed. Philadelphia: Lippincott Williams & Wilkins, 2008.

Nasogastric tube care

Providing effective nasogastric (NG) tube care requires meticulous monitoring of the patient and the equipment. Monitoring the patient involves checking drainage from the NG tube and assessing GI function. Monitoring the equipment involves verifying correct tube placement and irrigating the tube to ensure patency and to prevent mucosal damage.

Equipment

Irrigant (usually normal saline solution) ◆ irrigant container ◆ 60-ml catheter-tip syringe or bulb syringe ◆ suction equipment ◆ sponge-tipped swabs or toothbrush and toothpaste ◆ petroleum jelly ◆ ½″ or 1″ hypoallergenic tape ◆ water-soluble lubricant ◆ gloves ◆ pH test strip ◆ linen-saver pad ◆ optional: emesis basin.

Implementation

▶ Make sure the suction equipment works properly. (See *Common gastric suction devices,* page 340.) When using a Salem sump tube with suction, connect the larger, primary lumen (for drainage and suction) to suction equipment and select the appropriate setting, as ordered (usually low constant suction). If the practitioner doesn't specify the setting, follow the manufacturer's directions. A Levin tube usually calls for intermittent low suction.
▶ Confirm the patient's identity using two patient identifiers according to your facility's policy. **JC**
▶ Explain the procedure and provide privacy.
▶ Wash your hands and put on gloves.

Irrigating an NG tube

▶ Review the irrigation schedule (usually every 4 hours) if the practitioner orders this procedure.
▶ Assess tube placement by looking for discrepancies in tube markings or by measuring the external tube length and comparing it with the length documented in the chart. Have the patient open his mouth so that you can check whether the tube is coiled. **AACN**
▶ Aspirate stomach contents to check correct positioning and to prevent the patient from aspirating the irrigant. **AACN**

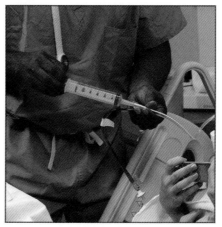

▶ Examine the aspirate, and place a small amount on the pH test strip. Probability of gastric placement is increased if the aspirate has a typical gastric fluid appearance (grassy green, clear and colorless with mucus shreds, or brown) and pH is less than or equal to 5.0. **CS** **AACN**
▶ Measure the amount of irrigant in the bulb syringe or in the 60-ml catheter-tip syringe (usually 10 to 20 ml) to maintain an accurate intake and output record.
▶ When using suction, unclamp and disconnect the tube from the suction equipment while holding it over a linen-saver pad or an emesis basin to collect any drainage.
▶ Slowly instill the irrigant into the NG tube. (When irrigating the Salem sump tube, you may instill small amounts of solution into the vent lumen without interrupting suction; however, you should instill greater amounts into the larger, primary lumen.)
▶ Gently aspirate solution with a bulb syringe or a 60-ml catheter-tip syringe, or connect the tube to suction equipment, as ordered. Report bleeding.
▶ Reconnect the tube to suction after completing irrigation.

Instilling a solution through an NG tube

▶ If the practitioner orders instillation, inject the solution and don't aspirate it. Note the amount of instilled solution as "intake" on the intake and output record.
▶ Reattach the tube to suction as ordered.
▶ After attaching the Salem sump tube's primary lumen to suction, instill 10 to 20 cc of air into the vent lumen to verify patency. Listen for a soft hiss in the vent. If you don't hear this sound, suspect a clogged tube; recheck patency by instilling 10 ml of normal saline solution and 10 to 20 cc of air into the vent.

Monitoring patient comfort and condition

▶ Provide mouth care once per shift, or as needed. Depending on the patient's condition, use sponge-tipped swabs to clean his teeth or help him brush them with a toothbrush and toothpaste. Coat the patient's lips with

Common gastric suction devices

A variety of wall-mounted suction devices are available for applying negative pressure to nasogastric (NG) and other drainage tubes. Two common types are shown here.

Portable suction machine

In the portable suction machine, a vacuum created intermittently by an electric pump draws gastric contents up the NG tube and into the collecting bottle.

Stationary suction machine

A stationary wall-unit apparatus can provide intermittent or continuous suction. On-off switches and variable power settings let you set and adjust the suction force on either machine.

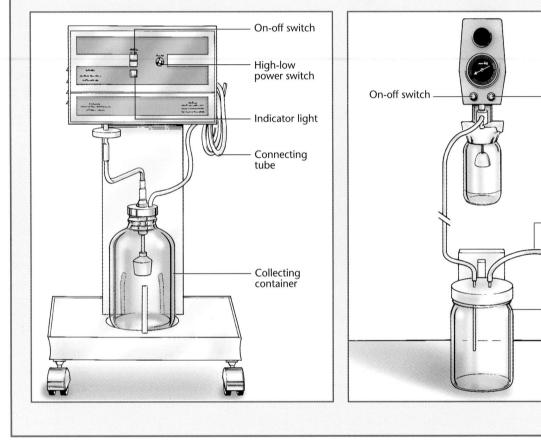

Portable suction machine labels: On-off switch · High-low power switch · Indicator light · Connecting tube · Collecting container

Stationary suction machine labels: On-off switch · Suction setting (intermittent to continuous) · Connecting tubing · Collecting container

petroleum jelly to prevent dryness from mouth breathing.

▶ Change the tape securing the tube as needed or at least daily. Clean the skin, apply fresh tape, and dab water-soluble lubricant on the nostrils, as needed.

▶ Regularly check the tape that secures the tube because sweat and nasal secretions may loosen the tape.

▶ Assess bowel sounds regularly (every 4 to 8 hours) to verify GI function.

▶ Measure the drainage amount and update the intake and output record every 8 hours. Be alert for electrolyte imbalances with excessive gastric output.

▶ Inspect gastric drainage, and note its color, consistency, odor, and amount. Normal gastric secretions have no color or appear yellow-green from bile and have a mucoid consistency. Immediately report drainage with a coffee-bean color; this may indicate bleeding. If you suspect that the drainage contains blood, use a screening test (such as Hematest) for occult blood according to your facility's policy.

Special considerations

▶ Irrigate the NG tube with 30 ml of irrigant before and after instilling medication. (See "Nasogastric tube drug administration," page 342.) Clamp the tube and wait about 30 minutes, or as ordered, after instillation before reconnecting the suction equipment to allow sufficient time for the medication to be absorbed.

▶ When no drainage appears, check the suction equipment for proper function. Then, holding the NG tube over a linen-saver pad or an emesis basin, separate the tube and the suction source. Check the suction equipment by placing the suction tubing in an irrigant container. If the apparatus draws the water, check the NG tube for proper function. Be sure to note the amount of water drawn into the suction container on the intake and output record.

▶ A dysfunctional NG tube may be clogged or incorrectly positioned. Attempt to irrigate the tube, reposition the patient, or rotate and reposition the tube. However, if the tube was inserted during surgery, avoid this maneuver to ensure that the movement doesn't interfere with gastric or esophageal sutures. Notify the practitioner.

▶ If you can ambulate the patient and interrupt suction, disconnect the NG tube from the suction equipment. Clamp the tube to prevent stomach contents from draining out of the tube.

▶ Epigastric pain and vomiting may result from a clogged or improperly placed tube. Dehydration and electrolyte imbalances may result from removing body fluids and electrolytes by suctioning.

References

Best, C. "Caring for the Patient with a Nasogastric Tube," *Nursing Standard* 20(3):59-65, September-October 2005.

McKay, L. "Nasogastric Intubation," *Nursing Standard* 20(24):63, February 2006.

Metheney, N., et al. "Effectiveness of pH Measurements in Predicting Feeding Tube Placement. An Update," *Nursing Research* 42(6):324-31, June 1993. **CS**

Richardson, D.S., et al. "An Evidence-Based Approach to Nasogastric Tube Management: Special Considerations," *Journal of Pediatric Nursing* 21(5):388-93, October 2006.

Taylor, C., et al. *Fundamentals of Nursing: The Art and Science of Nursing Care,* 6th ed. Philadelphia: Lippincott Williams & Wilkins, 2008.

Nasogastric tube drug administration

Besides providing an alternate means of nourishment, a nasogastric (NG) or gastrostomy tube allows direct instillation of medication into the GI system of patients who can't ingest the drug orally. Before instillation, the patency and positioning of the tube must be carefully checked because the procedure is contraindicated if the tube is obstructed or improperly positioned, if the patient is vomiting around the tube, or if his bowel sounds are absent.

Oily medications and enteric-coated or sustained-release tablets or capsules are contraindicated for instillation through an NG tube. Oily medications cling to the sides of the tube and resist mixing with the irrigating solution; crushing enteric-coated or sustained-release tablets to facilitate transport through the tube destroys their intended properties.

Equipment

Patient's medication record and chart ◆ prescribed medication ◆ towel or linen-saver pad ◆ 50- or 60-ml piston-type catheter-tip syringe ◆ two 4" × 4" gauze pads ◆ pH test strip ◆ gloves ◆ diluent ◆ cup for mixing medication and fluid ◆ spoon ◆ 50 ml of water ◆ rubber band ◆ gastrostomy tube and funnel, if needed (for gastrostomy tube) ◆ optional: mortar and pestle, clamp.

Implementation

▶ Verify the order on the patient's medication record by checking it against the practitioner's order. **JC ISMP**
▶ Wash your hands and put on gloves.
▶ Check the label on the medication three times before preparing it for administration to make sure you'll be giving the medication correctly. **ISMP**
▶ If your facility utilizes a bar code scanning system, be sure to scan your ID badge, the patient's ID bracelet, and the medication's bar code. **JC ISMP**
▶ If the prescribed medication is in tablet form, crush the tablets to ready them for mixing in a cup with the diluting liquid. Request liquid forms of medications, if available. Bring the medication and equipment to the patient's bedside.
▶ Explain the procedure to the patient; provide privacy.

▶ Confirm the patient's identity using two patient identifiers according to your facility's policy. **JC**
▶ Unpin the tube from the patient's gown. To avoid soiling the sheets, fold back the bed linens to the patient's waist and drape his chest with a towel or linen-saver pad.
▶ Elevate the head of the bed so that the patient is in Fowler's position, as tolerated.
▶ After unclamping the tube, take the 50- or 60-ml syringe and attach it to the end of the tube.

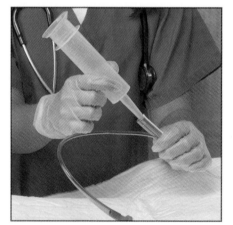

▶ Aspirate stomach contents, and place a small amount on a pH test strip. Probability of gastric placement is increased if aspirate has a typical gastric fluid appearance (grassy green, clear and colorless with mucus shreds, or brown) and pH is 5.0. If no gastric contents appear when you draw back

on the syringe, the tube may have risen into the esophagus; you'll have to advance it and confirm placement before proceeding. **AACN CS**
▶ If you meet resistance when aspirating for gastric contents, stop the procedure. Resistance may indicate a non-patent tube or improper tube placement. (Keep in mind that some smaller NG tubes may collapse when aspiration is attempted.) If the tube seems to be in the stomach, resistance probably means that the tube is lying against the stomach wall. To relieve resistance, withdraw the tube slightly or turn the patient.
▶ After you have established that the tube is patent and in the correct position, clamp the tube, detach the syringe, and lay the end of the tube on the 4" × 4" gauze pad.
▶ Mix the crushed tablets or liquid medication with the diluent. If the medication is in capsule form, open the capsules and empty their contents into the liquid. Pour liquid medications directly into the diluent. Stir well. (If the medication was in tablet form, make sure the particles are small enough to pass through the eyes at the distal end of the tube.)
▶ Reattach the syringe, without the piston, to the end of the tube and open the clamp.

Giving medications through an NG tube

Holding the nasogastric (NG) tube at a level somewhat above the patient's nose, pour up to 30 ml of diluted medication into the syringe barrel. To prevent air from entering the patient's stomach, hold the tube at a slight angle and add more medication before the syringe empties. If necessary, raise the tube slightly higher to increase the flow rate.

After you've delivered the whole dose, position the patient on her right side, head slightly elevated, to minimize esophageal reflux.

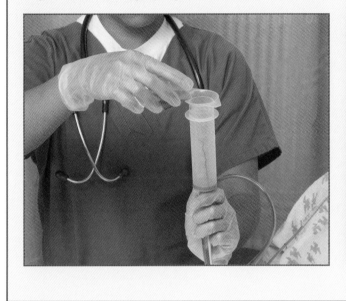
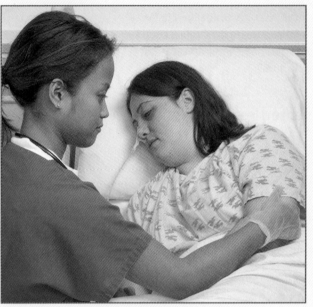

▶ Deliver the medication slowly and steadily. (See *Giving medications through an NG tube*.)

▶ If the medication flows smoothly, slowly add more until the entire dose has been given.

▶ If the medication doesn't flow properly, don't force it. If it's too thick, dilute it with water. If you suspect that tube placement is inhibiting the flow, stop the procedure and reevaluate tube placement.

▶ Watch the patient's reaction throughout the instillation. If there's any sign of discomfort, stop the procedure immediately.

▶ As the last of the medication flows out of the syringe, start to irrigate the tube by adding 30 to 50 ml of water. Irrigation clears medication from the

sides of the tube and from the distal end, reducing the risk of clogging.

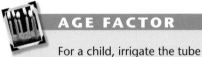
AGE FACTOR
For a child, irrigate the tube using only 15 to 30 ml of water.

▶ When the water stops flowing, quickly clamp the tube. Detach the syringe and dispose of it.

▶ Fasten the NG tube to the patient's gown.

▶ Remove the towel or linen-saver pad and replace bed linens.

▶ Leave the patient in Fowler's position, or have him lie on his right side with the head of the bed partially elevated. Tell him to maintain this position for at least 30 minutes after the proce-

dure. This position facilitates the downward flow of medication into his stomach and prevents esophageal reflux.

Special considerations

▶ To prevent instillation of too much fluid (for an adult, more than 400 ml of liquid at one time), don't schedule the drug instillation with the patient's regular tube feeding, if possible.

▶ If you must schedule a tube feeding and medication instillation simultaneously, give the medication first to ensure that the patient receives the prescribed drug therapy even if he can't tolerate an entire feeding. Remember to avoid giving foods that interact adversely with the drug.

▶ If the patient receives continuous tube feedings, stop the feeding and check the quantity of residual stomach contents. If it's more than 50% of the previous hour's intake, withhold the medication and feeding and notify the practitioner. An excessive amount of residual contents may indicate intestinal obstruction or paralytic ileus.

▶ If the NG tube is attached to suction, be sure to turn off the suction for 20 to 30 minutes after administering medication.

Selected references

Dansereau, R.J., and Crail, D.J. "Extemporaneous Procedures for Dissolving Tablets for Oral Administration and for Feeding Tubes," *Annals of Pharmacotherapy* 39(1):63-66, January 2005.

The Joint Commission. *Comprehensive Accreditation Manual for Hospitals: The Official Handbook.* Standard MM.1.10. Oakbrook Terrace, Ill.: The Joint Commission, 2007.

The Joint Commission. *Comprehensive Accreditation Manual for Hospitals: The Official Handbook.* Standard MM.2.10. Oakbrook Terrace, Ill.: The Joint Commission, 2007.

The Joint Commission. *Comprehensive Accreditation Manual for Hospitals: The Official Handbook.* Standard MM.3.10. Oakbrook Terrace, Ill.: The Joint Commission, 2007.

The Joint Commission. *Comprehensive Accreditation Manual for Hospitals: The Official Handbook.* Standard MM.4.10. Oakbrook Terrace, Ill.: The Joint Commission, 2007.

The Joint Commission. *Comprehensive Accreditation Manual for Hospitals: The Official Handbook.* Standard MM.4.20. Oakbrook Terrace, Ill.: The Joint Commission, 2007.

The Joint Commission. *Comprehensive Accreditation Manual for Hospitals: The Official Handbook.* Standard MM.5.10. Oakbrook Terrace, Ill.: The Joint Commission, 2007.

The Joint Commission. *Comprehensive Accreditation Manual for Hospitals: The Official Handbook.* Standard MM.6.10.

The Joint Commission. *Comprehensive Accreditation Manual for Hospitals: The Official Handbook.* Standard MM.6.20. Oakbrook Terrace, Ill.: The Joint Commission, 2007.

Metheney, N., et al. "Effectiveness of pH Measurements in Predicting Feeding Tube Placement. An Update," *Nursing Research* 42(6):324-31, June 1993. **CS**

Taylor, C., et al. *Fundamentals of Nursing: The Art and Science of Nursing Care,* 6th ed. Philadelphia: Lippincott Williams & Wilkins, 2008.

Nasogastric tube insertion and removal

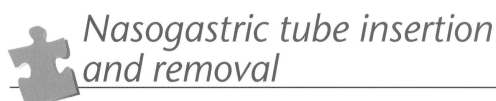

Usually inserted to decompress the stomach, a nasogastric (NG) tube can prevent vomiting after major surgery. An NG tube is typically in place for 48 to 72 hours after surgery, by which time peristalsis usually resumes. It may remain in place for shorter or longer periods, however, depending on its use. (See *Types of NG tubes,* page 346.)

The NG tube has other diagnostic and therapeutic applications, especially in assessing and treating upper GI bleeding, collecting gastric contents for analysis, performing gastric lavage, aspirating gastric secretions, and administering medications and nutrients.

Inserting an NG tube requires close observation of the patient and verification of proper placement. Removing the tube requires careful handling to prevent injury or aspiration. Most NG tubes have a radiopaque marker or strip at the distal end so that the tube's position can be verified by X-ray studies. If the position can't be confirmed, the practitioner may order fluoroscopy to verify placement.

Equipment

For inserting an NG tube: Tube (usually #12, #14, #16, or #18 French for a normal adult) ◆ towel or linen-saver pad ◆ facial tissues ◆ emesis basin ◆ penlight ◆ 1″ or 2″ hypoallergenic tape ◆ gloves ◆ water-soluble lubricant ◆ cup or glass of water with straw (if appropriate) ◆ pH test strip ◆ tongue blade ◆ catheter-tip or bulb syringe or irrigation set ◆ safety pin ◆ ordered suction equipment ◆ alcohol pad, if needed ◆ optional: ice, warm water, rubber band.

For removing an NG tube: Gloves ◆ catheter-tip syringe ◆ normal saline solution ◆ towel or linen-saver pad ◆ adhesive remover ◆ mouth care supplies.

Implementation

▶ Inspect the NG tube for defects, such as rough edges or partially closed lumens. Then check the tube's patency by flushing it with water.

▶ To ease insertion, increase a stiff tube's flexibility by coiling it around your gloved fingers for a few seconds or by dipping it into warm water. Stiffen a limp rubber tube by briefly chilling it in ice. **MFR**

▶ Whether you're inserting or removing an NG tube, be sure to provide privacy, wash your hands, and put on gloves before inserting the tube.

Inserting an NG tube

▶ Confirm the patient's identity using two patient identifiers according to your facility's policy. **JC**

▶ Explain the procedure to the patient. Inform her that she may experience some nasal discomfort, that she may gag, and that her eyes may water. Emphasize that swallowing will ease the tube's advancement.

▶ Agree on a signal that the patient can use if she wants you to stop briefly during the procedure.

▶ Gather and prepare all necessary equipment.

▶ Help the patient into high Fowler's position unless contraindicated.

▶ Stand at the patient's right side if you're right-handed or at her left side if you're left-handed to ease insertion.

▶ Drape the towel or linen-saver pad over the patient's chest to protect her gown and bed linens from spills.

▶ Have the patient gently blow her nose to clear her nostrils.

▶ Place the facial tissues and emesis basin well within the patient's reach.

▶ Help the patient face forward with her neck in a neutral position.

▶ To determine how long the NG tube must be to reach the stomach, hold the end of the tube at the tip of the patient's nose. Extend the tube to the patient's earlobe and then down to the xiphoid process.

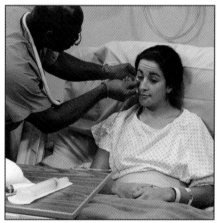

▶ Mark this distance on the tubing with the tape. (Average measurements for an adult range from 22″ to 26″ [56 to 66 cm].) It may be necessary to add 2″ (5 cm) to this measurement in tall individuals to ensure entry into the stomach.

▶ To determine which nostril will allow easier access, use a penlight and inspect for a deviated septum or other abnormalities.

Types of NG tubes

The practitioner will choose the type and diameter of nasogastric (NG) tube that best suits the patient's needs, including lavage, aspiration, enteral therapy, or stomach decompression. Choices may include the Levin and Salem sump tubes.

Levin tube
The Levin tube is a rubber or plastic tube that has a single lumen, a length of 42″ to 50″ (106.5 to 127 cm), and holes at the tip and along the side.

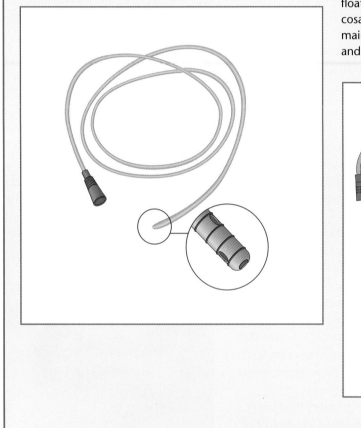

Salem sump tube
A Salem sump tube is a double-lumen tube made of clear plastic and has a blue sump port (pigtail) that allows atmospheric air to enter the patient's stomach. Thus, the tube floats freely and doesn't adhere to or damage gastric mucosa. The larger port of this 48″ (122-cm) tube serves as the main suction conduit. The tube has openings at 45, 55, 65, and 75 cm as well as a radiopaque line to verify placement.

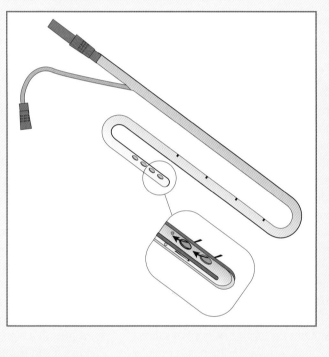

▶ Lubricate the first 3″ (7.5 cm) of the tube with a water-soluble gel to minimize injury to the nasal passages.

▶ Instruct the patient to hold her head straight and upright.

▶ Grasp the tube with the end pointing downward, curve it if necessary, and carefully insert it into the more patent nostril.

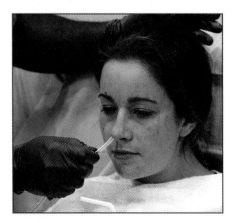

▶ Aim the tube downward and toward the ear closer to the chosen nostril. Advance it slowly to avoid pressure on the turbinates and resultant pain and bleeding.

▶ When the tube reaches the nasopharynx, you'll feel resistance. Instruct the patient to lower her head slightly to close the trachea and open the esophagus. Then rotate the tube 180 degrees toward the opposite nostril to redirect it so that the tube won't enter the patient's mouth.

▶ Unless contraindicated, offer the patient a cup or glass of water with a straw. Direct her to sip and swallow as you slowly advance the tube. This helps the tube pass to the esophagus. (If you aren't using water, ask the patient to swallow.)

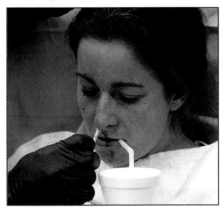

Ensuring proper tube placement

▶ Use a tongue blade and penlight to examine the patient's mouth and throat for signs of a coiled section of tubing (especially in an unconscious patient). Coiling indicates an obstruction.

▶ Keep an emesis basin and facial tissues readily available for the patient.

▶ As you carefully advance the tube and the patient swallows, watch for respiratory distress signs, which may mean the tube is in the bronchus and must be removed immediately.

▶ Stop advancing the tube when the tape mark reaches the patient's nostril.

▶ Attach a catheter-tip or bulb syringe to the tube, and try to aspirate stomach contents. If you don't obtain stomach contents, position the patient on her left side to move the contents into the stomach's greater curvature, and aspirate again. **AACN**

CLINICAL ALERT

When confirming tube placement, never place the tube's end in a container of water. If the tube should be malpositioned in the trachea, the patient may aspirate water. Water without bubbles doesn't confirm proper placement. Instead, the tube may be coiled in the trachea or the esophagus.

▶ Examine the aspirate, and place a small amount on the pH test strip. Probability of gastric placement is increased if the aspirate has a typical gastric fluid appearance (grassy green, clear and colorless with mucus shreds, or brown) and the pH is less than or equal to 5.0. **AACN** **CS**

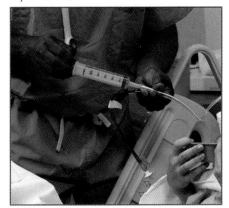

▶ Ideally, proper tube placement should be confirmed by X-ray. **AACN**

▶ Secure the NG tube to the patient's nose with hypoallergenic tape (or other designated tube holder). If the patient's skin is oily, wipe the bridge of the nose with an alcohol pad and allow to dry. You will need about 4″ (10 cm) of 1″ tape. Split one end of the tape up the center about 1½″ (3.5 cm). Make tabs on the split ends (by folding the sticky sides together). Stick the uncut tape end on the patient's nose so that the split in the tape starts about ½″ (1.3 cm) to 1½″ from the tip of her nose. Crisscross the tabbed ends

around the tube (as shown below). Then apply another piece of tape over the bridge of the nose to secure the tube.

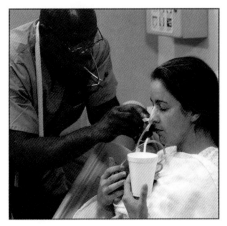

▶ Alternatively, stabilize the tube with a prepackaged product that secures and cushions it at the nose.

▶ To reduce discomfort from the weight of the tube, tie a slipknot around the tube with a rubber band and then secure the rubber band to the patient's gown with a safety pin. Or, wrap another piece of tape around the end of the tube and leave a tab; then fasten the tape tab to the patient's gown.

▶ Attach the tube to suction equipment, if ordered, and set the designated suction pressure.

▶ Provide frequent nose and mouth care while the tube is in place.

Removing an NG tube

▶ Explain the procedure to the patient, informing her that it may cause some nasal discomfort and sneezing or gagging.

▶ Assess bowel function by auscultating for peristalsis or flatus.

▶ Help the patient into semi-Fowler's position. Then drape a towel or linen-saver pad across her chest to protect her gown and bed linens from spills.

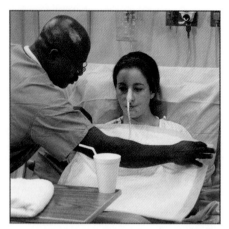

▶ Wash your hands and put on gloves.
▶ Using a catheter-tip syringe, flush the tube with 10 ml of air or normal saline solution to ensure that the tube doesn't contain stomach contents that could irritate tissues during tube removal.

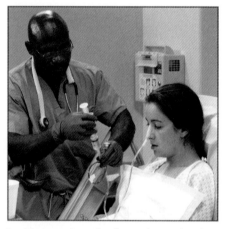

▶ Untape the tube from the patient's nose, and then unpin it from her gown.
▶ Clamp the tube by folding it in your hand.

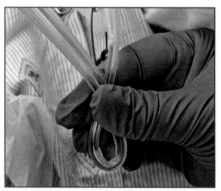

▶ Ask the patient to hold her breath to close the epiglottis. Then withdraw the tube gently and steadily. (When the distal end of the tube reaches the nasopharynx, you can pull it quickly.)
▶ When possible, immediately cover and remove the tube because its sight and odor may nauseate the patient.
▶ Assist the patient with thorough mouth care, and clean the tape residue from her nose with adhesive remover.
▶ For the next 48 hours, monitor the patient for signs of GI dysfunction, including nausea, vomiting, abdominal distention, and food intolerance. GI dysfunction may necessitate reinsertion of the tube.

Special considerations

▶ If the patient has a deviated septum or other nasal condition that prevents nasal insertion, pass the tube orally after removing any dentures, if necessary. Sliding the tube over the tongue, proceed as you would for nasal insertion.
▶ When using the oral route, remember to coil the end of the tube around your hand. This helps curve and direct the tube downward at the pharynx.
▶ If your patient is unconscious, tilt her chin toward her chest to close the trachea. Then advance the tube between respirations to ensure that it doesn't enter the trachea.
▶ While advancing the tube in an unconscious patient (or in a patient who can't swallow), stroke the patient's neck to encourage the swallowing reflex and facilitate passage down the esophagus.
▶ After tube placement, vomiting suggests tubal obstruction or incorrect position. Assess immediately to determine the cause.

References

Higgins, D. "Nasogastric Tube Insertion," *Nursing Times* 101(37):28-29, September 2005.

Jones, A.P., et al. "Insertion of a Nasogastric Tube under Direct Vision," *Anaesthesia* 61(3):305, March 2006.

Khair, J. "Guidelines for Testing the Placing of Nasogastric Tubes," *Nursing Times* 101(20):26-27, May 2006.

May, S. "Testing Nasogastric Tube Positioning in the Critically Ill: Exploring the Evidence," *British Journal of Nursing* 16(7):414-18, April 2007.

Metheney, N., et al. "Effectiveness of pH Measurements in Predicting Feeding Tube Placement. An Update," *Nursing Research* 42(6):324-31, June 1993. **CS**

Metheney, N., et al. "Visual Characteristics of Aspirates from Feeding Tubes," *AJN* 43(5):282-87, May 1994.

Metheney, N., and Titer, M. "Assessing Placement of Feeding Tubes," *AJN* 101(5):36-45, May 2001.

Taylor, C., et al. *Fundamentals of Nursing: The Art and Science of Nursing Care,* 6th ed. Philadelphia: Lippincott Williams & Wilkins, 2008.

Nasopharyngeal airway insertion and care

Insertion of a nasopharyngeal airway—a soft rubber or latex uncuffed catheter—establishes or maintains a patent airway. This airway is the typical choice for patients who have had recent oral surgery or facial trauma and for patients with loose, cracked, or avulsed teeth. It's also used to protect the nasal mucosa from injury when the patient needs frequent nasotracheal suctioning. This type of airway may also be tolerated better than an oropharyngeal airway by a patient who isn't deeply unconscious.

The airway follows the curvature of the nasopharynx, passing through the nose and extending from the nostril to the posterior pharynx. The bevel-shaped pharyngeal end of the airway facilitates insertion, and its funnel-shaped nasal end helps prevent slippage.

Insertion of a nasopharyngeal airway is preferred when an oropharyngeal airway is contraindicated or fails to maintain a patent airway. A nasopharyngeal airway is contraindicated if the patient is receiving anticoagulant therapy or has a hemorrhagic disorder, sepsis, or pathologic nasopharyngeal deformity.

Equipment

For insertion: Nasopharyngeal airway of proper size ◆ tongue blade ◆ water-soluble lubricant ◆ gloves ◆ optional: suction equipment.

For cleaning: Hydrogen peroxide ◆ water ◆ basin ◆ optional: pipe cleaner.

Implementation

▶ Measure the diameter of the patient's nostril and the distance from the tip of his nose to his earlobe. Select an airway of slightly smaller diameter than the nostril and of slightly longer length (1″ [2.5 cm]) than measured. The sizes for this type of airway are labeled according to their internal diameter.

▶ Lubricate the distal half of the airway's surface with a water-soluble lubricant to prevent traumatic injury during insertion.

▶ Put on gloves.

▶ In nonemergency situations, explain the procedure to the patient.

▶ Lubricate the airway and properly insert it. (See *Inserting a nasopharyngeal airway*.)

▶ After the airway is inserted, check it regularly to detect dislodgment or obstruction.

▶ When the patient's natural airway is patent, remove the airway in one smooth motion. If the airway sticks, apply lubricant around the nasal end of

Inserting a nasopharyngeal airway

First, hold the airway beside the patient's face to make sure it's the proper size (as shown at right). It should be slightly smaller than the patient's nostril diameter and slightly longer than the distance from the tip of his nose to his earlobe.

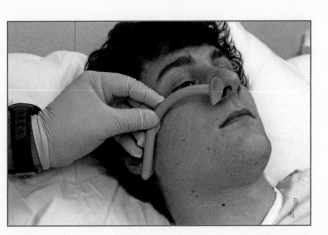

(continued)

Inserting a nasopharyngeal airway *(continued)*

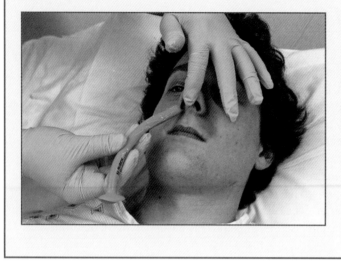

To insert the airway, hyperextend the patient's neck (unless contraindicated). Then push up the tip of his nose and pass the airway into his nostril (as shown at left). Avoid pushing against any resistance to prevent tissue trauma and airway kinking.

To check for correct airway placement, first close the patient's mouth. Then place your finger over the tube's opening to detect air exchange. Also, depress the patient's tongue with a tongue blade and look for the airway tip behind the uvula.

the tube and around the nostril; then gently rotate the airway until it's free.

Special considerations

▶ When you insert the airway, remember to use a chin-lift or jaw-thrust technique to anteriorly displace the patient's mandible. Immediately after insertion, assess the patient's respirations. If absent or inadequate, initiate artificial positive-pressure ventilation with a mouth-to-mask technique, a handheld resuscitation bag, or an oxygen-powered breathing device.
▶ If the patient coughs or gags, the tube may be too long. If so, remove the airway and insert a shorter one.
▶ At least once every 8 hours, remove the airway to check nasal mucous membranes for irritation or ulceration.

▶ Clean the airway by placing it in a basin and rinsing it with hydrogen peroxide and then with water. If secretions remain, use a pipe cleaner to remove them. Reinsert the clean airway into the other nostril (if it's patent) to avoid skin breakdown.

References

American Heart Association. "2005 American Heart Association Guidelines for Cardiopulmonary Resuscitation and Emergency Cardiovascular Care," *Circulation* 112(Suppl IV):VI-19-VI-34, December 2005.

Lynn-McHale Wiegand, D.J., and Carlson, K.K., eds. *AACN Procedure Manual for Critical Care,* 5th ed. Philadelphia: W.B. Saunders Co., 2006.

Taylor, C., et al. *Fundamentals of Nursing: The Art and Science of Nursing Care,* 5th ed. Philadelphia: Lippincott Williams & Wilkins, 2008.

Tong, J.L., and Smith, J.E. "Cardiovascular Changes following Insertion of Oropharyngeal and Nasopharyngeal Airways," *British Journal of Anaesthesiology* 93(3):339-42, September 2004.

Nephrostomy and cystostomy tube care

Two urinary diversion techniques—nephrostomy and cystostomy—ensure adequate drainage from the kidneys or bladder and help prevent urinary tract infection or kidney failure. (See *Urinary diversion techniques.*)

A nephrostomy tube drains urine directly from a kidney when a disorder inhibits the normal flow of urine. The tube is usually placed percutaneously, though sometimes it's surgically inserted through the renal cortex and medulla into the renal pelvis from a lateral incision in the flank. A cystostomy tube drains urine from the bladder, diverting it from the urethra. Inserted about 2″ (5 cm) above the symphysis pubis, a cystostomy tube may be used alone or with an indwelling urinary catheter.

Equipment

For dressing changes: Antiseptic swabs ◆ paper bag ◆ linen-saver pad ◆ clean gloves (for dressing removal) ◆ sterile gloves (for new dressing) ◆ precut 4″ × 4″ drain dressings or transparent semipermeable dressings ◆ adhesive tape (preferably hypoallergenic).

For nephrostomy-tube irrigation: 3-ml syringe ◆ antiseptic swab ◆ normal saline solution ◆ gloves ◆ optional: hemostat.

Commercially prepared sterile dressing kits may be available.

Implementation

▶ Wash your hands, and assemble all equipment at the patient's bedside.
▶ Open the antiseptic swabs, the drain dressings, and sterile gloves. If you're using a commercially packaged dressing kit, open it using sterile technique.
▶ Open the paper bag, and place it away from the other equipment to avoid contaminating the sterile field.
▶ Confirm the patient's identity using two patient identifiers according to your facility's policy. 🅙🅒
▶ Explain the procedure and provide privacy.

Urinary diversion techniques

A cystostomy or a nephrostomy can be used to create a permanent diversion, to relieve obstruction from an inoperable tumor, or to provide an outlet for urine after cystectomy. A temporary diversion can relieve obstruction from a calculus or ureteral edema.

In a *cystostomy*, a catheter is inserted percutaneously through the suprapubic area into the bladder. In a *nephrostomy*, a catheter is inserted percutaneously through the flank into the renal pelvis.

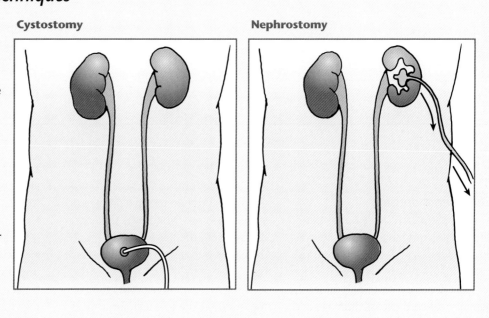

Cystostomy

Nephrostomy

Taping a nephrostomy tube

To tape a nephrostomy tube directly to the skin, cut a wide piece of hypoallergenic adhesive tape twice lengthwise to its midpoint.

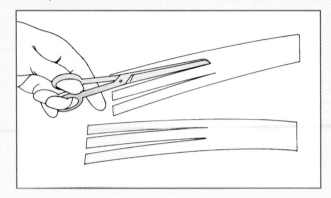

Apply the uncut end of the tape to the skin so that the midpoint meets the tube. Wrap the middle strip around the tube in a spiral fashion. Tape the other two strips to the patient's skin on both sides of the tube.

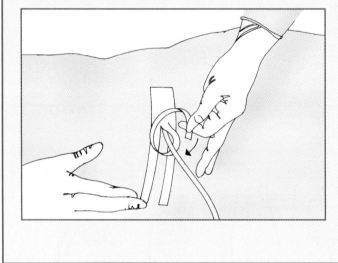

For greater security, repeat this step with a second piece of tape, applying it in the reverse direction. You may also apply two more strips of tape perpendicular to and over the first two pieces.

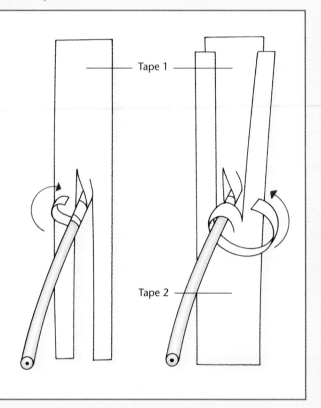

Always apply another strip of tape lower down on the tube in the direction of the drainage tube to further anchor the tube. Don't put tension on any sutures that prevent tube distention.

▶ Wash your hands.

Changing a dressing

▶ Help the patient to lie on his back (for a cystostomy tube) or on the side opposite the tube (for a nephrostomy tube).
▶ Place the linen-saver pad under the patient to absorb excess drainage and keep him dry.

▶ Put on the clean gloves.
▶ Carefully remove the tape around the tube, and then remove the wet or soiled dressing. Discard the tape and dressing into the paper bag. Remove the gloves and discard them into the bag.
▶ Note the markings on the tube at the insertion site to check for its accidental dislodging.

▶ Put on the sterile gloves. Using an antiseptic swab, clean the site from the tube site outward.
▶ Repeat the skin cleaning procedure, if needed.
▶ Pick up a sterile 4″ × 4″ drain dressing, and place it around the tube. If necessary, overlap two drain dressings to provide maximum absorption. Or, depending on your facility's policy,

apply a transparent semipermeable dressing over the site and tubing to allow observation of the site without removing the dressing.

► Secure the dressing with hypoallergenic tape. Then tape the tube to the patient's lateral abdomen to prevent tension on the tube. (See *Taping a nephrostomy tube*.)

► Dispose of all equipment appropriately. Clean the patient as necessary.

Irrigating a nephrostomy tube

► Put on gloves, and position the patient on his side opposite the tube.

► Fill the 3-ml syringe with the normal saline solution.

► Clean the junction of the nephrostomy tube and drainage tube with the antiseptic swab, and disconnect the tubes.

► Insert the syringe into the nephrostomy tube opening, and instill 2 to 3 ml of saline solution into the tube.

► Slowly aspirate the solution back into the syringe. To avoid damaging the renal pelvis tissue, never pull back forcefully on the plunger.

► If the solution doesn't return, remove the syringe from the tube and reattach it to the drainage tubing to allow the solution to drain by gravity.

► Dispose of all equipment appropriately.

Special considerations

► Change dressings once per day, or more often if needed.

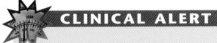

CLINICAL ALERT

Never irrigate a nephrostomy tube with more than 5 ml of solution because the capacity of the renal pelvis is usually between 4 and 8 ml.

► When necessary, irrigate a cystostomy tube as you would an indwelling urinary catheter. Be sure to perform the irrigation gently to avoid damaging any suture lines.

► Check a nephrostomy tube frequently for kinks or obstructions. Suspect an obstruction when the amount of urine in the drainage bag decreases or the amount of urine around the insertion site increases. Gently curve a cystostomy tube to prevent kinks.

► If a blood clot or mucus plug obstructs a nephrostomy or cystostomy tube, try milking the tube to restore its patency. With your nondominant hand, hold the tube securely above the obstruction to avoid pulling the tube out

of the incision. Then place the flat side of a closed hemostat under the tube (just above the obstruction), pinch the tube against the hemostat, and slide both your finger and the hemostat toward you, away from the patient.

► Typically, cystostomy tubes for postoperative urologic patients should be checked hourly for 24 hours to ensure adequate drainage and tube patency. To check tube patency, note the amount of urine in the drainage bag and check the patient's bladder for distention.

► Keep the drainage bag below the level of the kidney at all times to prevent urine reflux.

► If the tube becomes dislodged, cover the site with a sterile dressing and notify the practitioner immediately.

References

Hautman, R. "Urinary Diversion," *Urology* 29(1 Suppl):17-19, January 2007.

Taylor, C., et al. *Fundamentals of Nursing: The Art and Science of Nursing Care,* 6th ed. Philadelphia: Lippincott Williams & Wilkins, 2008.

Neurologic assessment

Neurologic assessment supplements the routine measurement of temperature, pulse rate, and respirations by evaluating the patient's level of consciousness (LOC), pupillary activity, and orientation to person, place, and date. It provides a simple, indispensable tool for quickly checking the patient's neurologic status.

If the patient's condition and circumstances of admission allow, the first neurologic assessment should occur at the time of admission to establish a baseline. The frequency and extent of the neurologic assessment will depend on the stability of the patient and the underlying condition. For a stable patient who's doing well, an assessment may be ordered every 4 to 8 hours. For an unstable patient, it may be ordered as frequently as every 5 minutes to monitor changes and the need for intervention.

LOC, a measure of environmental and self-awareness, reflects cortical function and usually provides the first sign of central nervous system deterioration. Changes in pupillary activity (pupil size, shape, equality, and response to light) may signal increased intracranial pressure (ICP) associated with a space-occupying lesion caused by an increase of fluid or tissue in the associated area. Evaluating muscle strength and tone, reflexes, and posture also may help identify nervous system damage.

Finally, changes in vital signs alone don't indicate possible neurologic compromise. Alterations in LOC or pupillary changes are the early signs that indicate neurologic problems. Therefore, any changes in vital signs should be evaluated in light of a complete neurologic assessment. Because vital signs are controlled at the medullary level, changes noted after the deterioration of neurologic status are too late, and irreversible neurologic damage should be suspected.

Equipment

Penlight ◆ thermometer ◆ sterile cotton ball or cotton-tipped applicator ◆ stethoscope ◆ sphygmomanometer ◆ pupil size chart ◆ pencil or pen.

Implementation

▶ Confirm the patient's identity using two patient identifiers according to your facility's policy. 🄹🄲
▶ Explain the procedure to the patient even if he's unresponsive. Then wash your hands and provide privacy.

Assessing LOC and orientation

▶ Assess the patient's LOC by evaluating his responses. Use standard methods, such as the Glasgow Coma Scale and the Rancho Los Amigos Cognitive Scale. (See *Using the Glasgow Coma Scale*. See also *Using the Rancho Los Amigos Cognitive Scale,* page 356.)

▶ Begin by measuring the patient's response to verbal, light tactile (touch), and painful (nail bed pressure) stimuli. First, ask the patient his full name. If he responds appropriately, assess his orientation to person, place, and date. Ask him where he is and then what day, season, and year it is. (Expect disorientation to affect the sense of date first, then time, place, caregivers and, finally, self.) When he responds verbally, assess the quality of speech to determine whether it's clear and concise. Rambling responses indicate difficulty with thought processing and organization.

▶ Assess the patient's ability to understand and follow one-step commands that require a motor response. For example, ask him to open and close his eyes or stick out his tongue. Note whether the patient can maintain his LOC. If you must gently shake him to keep him focused on your verbal commands, he may have sustained neurologic compromise.

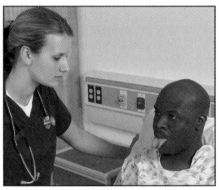

▶ If the patient doesn't respond to commands, apply a painful stimulus. With moderate pressure, squeeze the nail beds on his fingers and toes and note his response. Check motor responses bilaterally to rule out monoplegia (paralysis of a single area) and hemiplegia (paralysis of one side of the body).

A patient's response to painful stimuli should be described as one of the

Using the Glasgow Coma Scale

The Glasgow Coma Scale provides a standard reference for assessing or monitoring level of consciousness in a patient with a suspected or confirmed brain injury. This scale measures three responses to stimuli—eye opening response, motor response, and verbal response. It assigns a number to each of the possible responses within these categories.

A score of 3 is the lowest and 15 is the highest. A score of 7 or lower indicates coma. The Glasgow Coma Scale is commonly used in the emergency department, at the scene of an accident, and for evaluation of the hospitalized patient.

CHARACTERISTIC	RESPONSE	SCORE
Eye opening response	► Spontaneous	4
	► To verbal command	3
	► To pain	2
	► No response	1
Best motor response	► Obeys commands	6
	► To painful stimuli	
	– Localizes pain; pushes stimulus away	5
	– Flexes and withdraws	4
	– Abnormal flexion	3
	– Extension	2
	– No response	1
Best verbal response (Arouse the patient with painful stimuli, if necessary.)	► Oriented and converses	5
	► Disoriented and converses	4
	► Uses inappropriate words	3
	► Makes incomprehensible sounds	2
	► No response	1
		Total: 3 to 15

following: localization—the patient withdraws from the pain, attempts to push away the painful stimulus, and can localize where the pain originates; withdrawal—the patient moves slightly but makes no attempt to push the painful stimulus away; or unresponsive—the patient doesn't react to the application of painful stimulus (commonly seen in patients in a deep coma).

CLINICAL ALERT

If decorticate or decerebrate posturing develops in response to stimuli, notify the practitioner immediately. (See *Identifying warning postures*, page 357.)

Examining pupils and eye movement

► Ask the patient to open his eyes. If he doesn't respond, gently lift his upper eyelids. Inspect each pupil for size and shape, and compare the two for equality. To evaluate pupil size more precisely, use a chart showing the various pupil sizes. (See *Testing the pupils*, page 357.) Remember, pupil size varies considerably, and some patients have normally unequal pupils (anisocoria). Also check whether the pupils are positioned in, or deviate from, the midline.

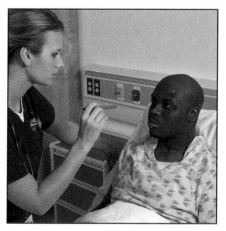

► Test the patient's direct light response. First, darken the room. Then hold each eyelid open in turn. Swing the penlight from the patient's ear toward the midline of the face. Shine the light directly into the eye. Normally, the

Using the Rancho Los Amigos Cognitive Scale

Widely used to classify brain-injured patients according to their behavior, the Rancho Los Amigos Cognitive Scale describes phases of recovery—from coma to dependent functioning—on a scale of I (unresponsive) to VIII (purposeful, appropriate, alert, and oriented). This scale is useful in assessing patients who have posttraumatic amnesia.

LEVEL	RESPONSE	CHARACTERISTIC
I	None	The patient is unresponsive to any stimulus.
II	Generalized	The patient makes limited, inconsistent, nonpurposeful responses, commonly to pain only.
III	Localized	The patient can localize and withdraw from painful stimuli, can make purposeful responses and focus on presented objects, and may follow simple commands but inconsistently and in a delayed manner.
IV	Confused and agitated	The patient is alert but agitated, confused, disoriented, and aggressive. He can't perform self-care and has no awareness of present events. Bizarre behavior is likely; agitation appears related to internal confusion.
V	Confused and inappropriate	The patient is alert and responds to commands but is easily distracted and can't concentrate on tasks or learn new information. He becomes agitated in response to external stimuli, and his behavior and speech are inappropriate. His memory is severely impaired, and he can't carry over learning from one situation to another.
VI	Confused and appropriate	The patient has some awareness of himself and others but is inconsistently oriented. He can follow simple directions consistently with cueing and can relearn some old skills, such as activities of daily living (ADLs), but he continues to have serious memory problems (especially with short-term memory).
VII	Automatic and appropriate	The patient is consistently oriented, with little or no confusion, but frequently appears robotlike when performing daily routines. His awareness of himself and his interaction with his environment increase, but he lacks insight, judgment, problem-solving skills, and the ability to plan realistically.
VIII	Purposeful and appropriate	The patient is alert and oriented, recalls and integrates past events, learns new activities, and performs ADLs independently; however, deficits in stress tolerance, judgment, and abstract reasoning persist. He may function in society at a reduced level.

pupil constricts immediately. When you remove the penlight, the pupil should dilate immediately. Wait about 20 seconds before testing the other pupil to allow it to recover from reflex stimulation.

▶ Now test consensual light response. Hold both eyelids open, but shine the light into one eye only. Watch for constriction in the other pupil, which indicates proper nerve function of the optic chiasm.

▶ Brighten the room, and have the conscious patient open his eyes. Observe the eyelids for ptosis or drooping. Then check extraocular movements. Hold up one finger, and ask the patient to follow it with his eyes alone. As you move the finger up, down, laterally,

Identifying warning postures

Decorticate and decerebrate postures are ominous signs of central nervous system deterioration.

Decorticate (abnormal flexion)

In the decorticate posture, the patient's arms are adducted and flexed, with the wrists and fingers flexed on the chest. The legs may be stiffly extended and internally rotated, with plantar flexion of the feet.

   The decorticate posture may indicate a lesion of the frontal lobe, internal capsule, or cerebral peduncles.

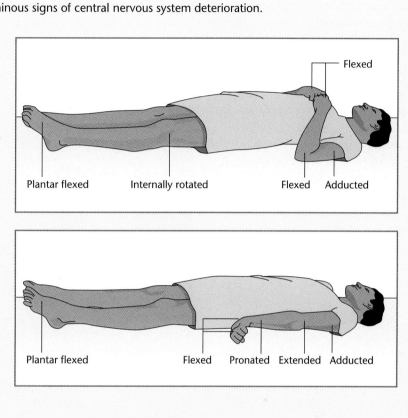

Flexed

Plantar flexed   Internally rotated   Flexed   Adducted

Decerebrate (extension)

In the decerebrate posture, the patient's arms are adducted and extended, with the wrists pronated and the fingers flexed. One or both of the legs may be stiffly extended, with plantar flexion of the feet.

   The decerebrate posture may indicate lesions of the upper brain stem.

Plantar flexed   Flexed   Pronated   Extended   Adducted

Testing the pupils

Slightly darken the room. Then test the pupils for direct response (reaction of the pupil you're testing) and consensual response (reaction of the opposite pupil) by holding a penlight about 20″ (51 cm) from the patient's eyes, directing the light at the eye from the side.

   Next, test accommodation by placing your finger about 4″ (10 cm) from the bridge of the patient's nose. Ask him to look at a fixed object in the distance and then to look at your finger. His eyes should converge, and his pupils should constrict.

Grading pupil size

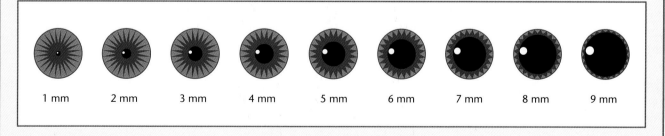

1 mm   2 mm   3 mm   4 mm   5 mm   6 mm   7 mm   8 mm   9 mm

and obliquely, see whether the patient's eyes track together to follow your finger (conjugate gaze). Watch for involuntary jerking or oscillating eye movements either laterally or vertically upon moving eyes (nystagmus).

▶ Check the patient's accommodation-convergency reflex. Hold up one finger midline to the patient's face and several feet away. Have the patient focus on your finger. Gradually move your finger toward his nose while he focuses on your finger. This should cause his eyes to converge and both pupils to constrict equally.

▶ If the patient is comatose, test the corneal reflex by touching a wisp of cotton ball to the cornea. This normally causes an immediate blink reflex. Repeat for the other eye.

▶ If the patient is unconscious, test the oculocephalic (doll's eye) reflex. Hold the patient's eyelids open. Then quickly but gently turn his head to one side and then the other. If the patient's eyes move in the opposite direction from the side to which you turn the head, the reflex is intact.

CLINICAL ALERT

Never test the doll's eye reflex on an awake, alert patient or if you know or suspect that the patient has a cervical spine injury.

Evaluating motor function

▶ Identify the patient's strength on a scale of 0 to 5, with 0 being no muscle strength and 5 being full muscle strength.

▶ If the patient is conscious, test his grip strength in both hands. Extend your hands, ask him to squeeze your fingers as hard as he can, and compare the strength of each hand. Grip

strength is usually slightly stronger in the dominant hand.

▶ Test arm strength by having the patient close his eyes and hold his arms straight out in front of him with the palms up for 20 to 30 seconds. See whether either arm drifts downward or pronates (pronator drift), indicating muscle weakness.

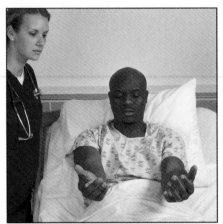

▶ Test leg strength by having the patient raise his legs, one at a time, against gentle downward pressure from your hand. Gently push down on each leg at the midpoint of the thigh to evaluate muscle strength.

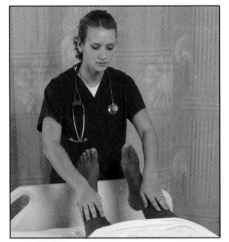

▶ Flex and extend the extremities on both sides to evaluate muscle tone.

▶ Test the plantar reflex in all patients. To do so, stroke the lateral aspect of the sole of the patient's foot with your thumbnail or another moderately

sharp object. Normally, this elicits flexion of all toes. Watch for a positive Babinski's sign—dorsiflexion of the great toe with fanning of the other toes—which indicates an upper motor neuron lesion.

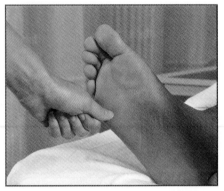

AGE FACTOR

A positive Babinski's sign is normal in patients younger than age 2.

Completing the neurologic examination

Take the patient's temperature, pulse rate, respiratory rate, and blood pressure. His pulse pressure—the difference between systolic pressure and diastolic pressure—is especially important because widening pulse pressure can indicate increasing ICP.

Special considerations

▶ A change in the LOC is one of the earliest changes that may occur with increased ICP. Changes in pulse and blood pressure also occur but are generally seen late in the course of increasing ICP. Other vital sign changes include widening pulse pressure, increase in systolic blood pressure, and bradycardia. Cushing's triad, also called *Cushing's sign,* is a late sign indicating brain stem dysfunction. Vital signs associated with Cushing's triad include hypertension (usually with widened pulse pressure), bradycardia, and abnormal or irregular respiratory patterns.

References

American Association of Neuroscience Nurses. *Core Curriculum for Neuroscience Nursing,* 4th ed. Philadelphia: W.B. Saunders Co., 2004.

Fairley, D., and Pearce, A. "Assessment of Consciousness: Part One," *Nursing Times* 102(4):26-27, January 2006.

Fairley, D., and Pearce, A. "Assessment of Consciousness: Part Two," *Nursing Times* 102(5):26-27, January-February 2006.

Iacono, L.A., and Lyones, K.A. "Making GCS as Easy as 1, 2, 3, 4, 5, 6," *Journal of Trauma Nursing* 12(3):77-81, July-September 2005.

Lynn-McHale Wiegand, D.J., and Carlson, K.K., eds. *AACN Procedure Manual for Critical Care,* 5th ed. Philadelphia: W.B. Saunders Co., 2005.

Morgan, A. "Neurological Assessment," *Nursing Standard* 20(14-16):67, December-January 2006.

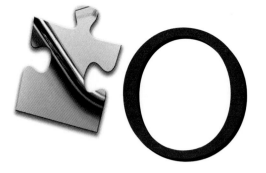

Oral drug administration

Because oral administration is usually the safest, most convenient, and least expensive method, most drugs are administered by this route. Drugs for oral administration are available in many forms: tablets, enteric-coated tablets, capsules, syrups, elixirs, oils, liquids, suspensions, powders, and granules. Some require special preparation before administration, such as mixing with juice to make them more palatable; oils, powders, and granules usually require such preparation.

Sometimes oral drugs are prescribed in higher dosages than their parenteral equivalents because after absorption through the GI system, they are immediately broken down by the liver before they reach the systemic circulation.

AGE FACTOR

Oral dosages normally prescribed for adults may be dangerous for elderly patients.

Oral administration is contraindicated for unconscious patients; it may also be contraindicated in patients with nausea and vomiting and in those unable to swallow.

Equipment

Patient's medication record and chart ◆ prescribed medication ◆ medication cup ◆ optional: appropriate vehicle, such as jelly or applesauce, for crushed pills, and juice, water, or milk for liquid medications; drinking straw; mortar and pestle for crushing pills; pill-cutting device for scored tablets.

Implementation

▶ Verify the order on the patient's medication record by checking it against the practitioner's order. **JC** **ISMP**
▶ Wash your hands.
▶ Check the label on the medication three times before administering it to make sure you'll be giving the correct prescribed medication. Check when you take the container from the shelf or drawer, again before you pour the medication into the medication cup, and again before returning the container to the shelf or drawer. If you're administering a unit-dose medication, check the label for the final time at the patient's bedside immediately after pouring the medication and before discarding the wrapper (as shown at top of nex column). **ISMP**

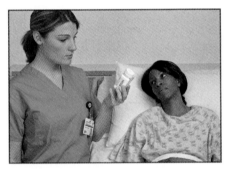

▶ Confirm the patient's identity using two patient identifiers according to your facility's policy. **JC**
▶ If your facility utilizes a bar code scanning system, be sure to scan your ID badge, the patient's ID bracelet, and the medication's bar code. **JC** **ISMP**
▶ Assess the patient's condition, including his level of consciousness and vital signs, as needed. Changes in the patient's condition may warrant withholding medication. For example, you may need to withhold a medication that will slow the patient's heart rate if his apical pulse rate is less than 60 beats/minute.

▶ Give the patient his medication and an appropriate vehicle or liquid, as needed, to aid swallowing, minimize adverse effects, or promote absorption. If appropriate, crush the medication to facilitate swallowing.

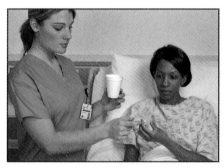

▶ Stay with the patient until he has swallowed the drug. If he seems confused or disoriented, check his mouth to make sure he has swallowed it. Return and reassess the patient's response within 1 hour after giving the medication.

Special considerations

▶ Make sure you have a written order for every medication given. Verbal orders should be signed by the practitioner within the specified time period. (Hospitals usually require a signature within 24 hours; long-term-care facilities, within 48 hours.) **JC** **ISMP**

▶ Notify the practitioner about any medication withheld, unless instructions to withhold are already written.

▶ Use care in measuring out the prescribed dose of liquid oral medication. (See *Measuring liquid medications*.)

Measuring liquid medications

To pour liquid medications, hold the medication cup at eye level. Use your thumb to mark off the correct level on the cup. Then set the cup down and read the bottom of the meniscus at eye level to ensure accuracy. If you've poured too much medication into the cup, discard the excess. Don't return it to the bottle.

Here are a few additional tips:
▶ Hold the container so that the medication flows from the side opposite the label so it won't run down the container and stain or obscure the label. Remove drips from the lip of the bottle first and then from the sides, using a clean, damp paper towel.
▶ For a liquid measured in drops, use only the dropper supplied with the medication.

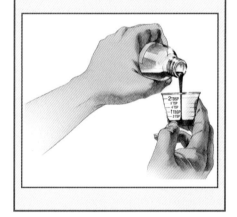

▶ Don't give medication from a poorly labeled or unlabeled container. Don't attempt to label or reinforce drug labels yourself. This must be done by a pharmacist.

▶ If the patient can't swallow a whole tablet or capsule, ask the pharmacist if the drug is available in liquid form or if it can be administered by another route. If not, ask him if you can crush the tablet or open the capsule and mix it with food. Keep in mind that many enteric-coated or time-release medications and gelatin capsules shouldn't be crushed. Remember to contact the practitioner for an order to change the administration route when necessary.

AGE FACTOR

Oral medications are relatively easy to give to infants because of infants' natural sucking instinct and, in infants younger than age 4 months, their undeveloped sense of taste.

Selected references

Craven, R. F., and Hirnle, C. J. *Fundamentals of Nursing: Human Health and Function,* 6th ed. Philadelphia: Lippincott Williams & Wilkins, 2009.

Hohenhaus, S. M. "Giving Liquid Medications to Pediatric Patients," *Journal of Emergency Nursing* 32(1):69–70, February 2006.

Joanna Briggs Institute. "Strategies to Reduce Medication Errors with Reference to Older Adults," *Nursing Standard* 209(1):53–57, June 2006.

Oronasopharyngeal suction

Oronasopharyngeal suction removes secretions from the pharynx by a suction catheter inserted through the mouth or nostril. Used to maintain a patent airway, this procedure helps the patient who can't clear his airway effectively with coughing and expectoration, such as the unconscious or severely debilitated patient. The procedure should be done as often as necessary, depending on the patient's condition.

Because the catheter may inadvertently slip into the lower airway or esophagus, oronasopharyngeal suction is a sterile procedure that requires sterile equipment.

Nasopharyngeal suctioning should be used with caution in patients who have nasopharyngeal bleeding or spinal fluid leakage into the nasopharyngeal area, in those who are receiving anticoagulant therapy, and in those who have blood dyscrasias because these conditions increase the risk of bleeding.

Equipment

Wall suction or portable suction apparatus unit ◆ connecting tubing ◆ water-soluble lubricant ◆ sterile normal saline solution ◆ disposable sterile container ◆ sterile suction catheter (a #10 to #16 French catheter for an adult, #8 or #10 French catheter for a child, or pediatric feeding tube for an infant) ◆ sterile gloves ◆ goggles ◆ clean gloves ◆ nasopharyngeal or oropharyngeal airway (optional for frequent suctioning) ◆ overbed table ◆ waterproof trash bag ◆ towel ◆ optional: tongue blade, tonsil tip suction device.

A commercially prepared kit contains a sterile catheter, disposable container, and sterile gloves.

Implementation

▶ Evaluate the patient's ability to cough and deep-breathe to determine his ability to move secretions up the tracheobronchial tree. Check his history for a deviated septum, nasal polyps, nasal obstruction, traumatic injury, epistaxis, or mucosal swelling. If no contraindications exist, gather and place the suction equipment on the patient's overbed table or bedside stand. **AARC**

▶ Position the table or stand on your preferred side of the bed to facilitate suctioning. Connect the tubing to the suctioning unit. Date and then open the bottle of normal saline solution. Open the waterproof trash bag.

▶ Confirm the patient's identity using two patient identifiers according to your facility's policy. **JC**

▶ Explain the procedure to the patient even if he's unresponsive. Inform him that suctioning may stimulate transient coughing or gagging, but tell him that coughing helps to mobilize secretions. If he has been suctioned before, just summarize the reasons for the procedure. Reassure him throughout the procedure to minimize anxiety and fear, which can increase oxygen consumption. Also, ask which nostril is more patent. **AARC**

▶ Wash your hands. Put on personal protective equipment, as appropriate. **AARC** **CDC**

▶ Place the patient in semi-Fowler's or high Fowler's position, if tolerated, to promote lung expansion and effective coughing. Consider increasing supplemental oxygen, according to your facility's policy, before suctioning. If the patient is unconscious, position him on his side facing you to help drain secretions.

▶ Place a towel across the patient's chest.

▶ Turn on the suction from the wall or portable unit, and set the pressure according to your facility's policy. The pressure is usually set between 100 and 150 mm Hg; higher pressures cause excessive trauma without enhancing secretion removal. Occlude the end of the connecting tubing to check suction pressure. **AARC**

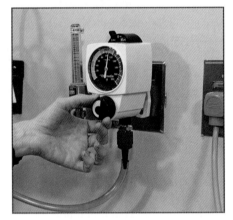

▶ Using strict sterile technique, open the suction catheter kit or the packages containing the sterile catheter, disposable container, and gloves. Put on the gloves; consider your dominant hand sterile and your nondominant hand nonsterile. Using your nondominant hand, pour the sterile saline into the sterile container.

▶ With your nondominant hand, place a small amount of water-soluble lubricant on the sterile area. The lubricant is used to facilitate passage of the catheter during nasopharyngeal suctioning.

▶ Pick up the catheter with your dominant (sterile) hand, and attach it to the connecting tubing. Use your nondominant hand to control the suction valve while your dominant hand manipulates the catheter.

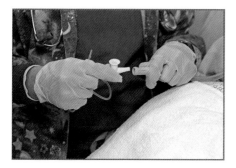

▶ Dip the catheter into the sterile saline to moisten the inside of the catheter.

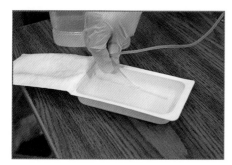

▶ Instruct the patient to cough and breathe slowly and deeply several times before beginning suction. Coughing helps loosen secretions and may decrease the amount of suctioning necessary, while deep breathing helps minimize or prevent hypoxia.

▶ To insert the catheter nasally, raise the tip of the patient's nose with your nondominant hand to straighten the passageway and facilitate insertion of the catheter. Without applying suction, gently insert the suction catheter into the patient's nares. Roll the catheter between your fingers to help it advance

through the turbinates. Continue to advance the catheter approximately 5″ to 6″ (12.5 to 15 cm) until you reach the pool of secretions or the patient begins to cough.

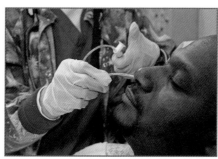

▶ To insert the catheter orally, without applying suction, gently insert the catheter into the patient's mouth. Advance it 3″ to 4″ (7.5 to 10 cm) along the side of the patient's mouth until you reach the pool of secretions or the patient begins to cough. Suction both sides of the patient's mouth and pharyngeal area.

▶ Using intermittent suction, withdraw the catheter from either the mouth or the nose with a continuous rotating motion to minimize invagination of the mucosa into the catheter's tip and side ports. Apply suction for only 10 to 15 seconds at a time to minimize tissue trauma.

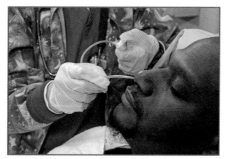

▶ Between passes, wrap the catheter around your dominant hand to prevent contamination.

▶ If secretions are thick, clear the lumen of the catheter by dipping it in water and applying suction (as shown at top of next column).

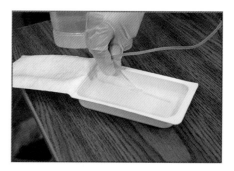

▶ Repeat the procedure up to 3 times until gurgling or bubbling sounds stop and respirations are quiet. Allow 30 seconds to 1 minute between attempts to allow reoxygenation and reventilation.

▶ Flush the connecting tubing with normal saline solution.

▶ After completing suctioning, pull off your sterile glove over the coiled catheter, and discard it and the nonsterile glove along with the container of saline.

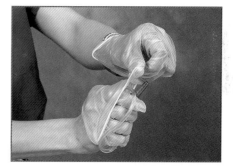

▶ Replace the used items so they're ready for the next suctioning, and wash your hands.

Special considerations

▶ If the patient has no history of nasal problems, alternate suctioning between nostrils to minimize traumatic injury. If repeated oronasopharyngeal suctioning is required, the use of a nasopharyngeal or oropharyngeal airway will help with catheter insertion, reduce traumatic injury, and promote a patent airway. To facilitate catheter insertion for oropharyngeal suctioning, depress the patient's tongue with a tongue blade, or ask another nurse to do so. This helps you to visualize the back of the throat and also prevents the patient from biting the catheter.

▶ If the patient has excessive oral secretions, consider using a tonsil tip catheter because this allows the patient to remove oral secretions independently.

▶ Let the patient rest after suctioning while you continue to observe him. Auscultate breath sounds to determine the effectiveness of the procedure. The frequency and duration of suctioning depends on the patient's tolerance of the procedure and on any complications.

Selected references

American Association for Respiratory Care. "AARC Clinical Practice Guideline: Nasotracheal Suctioning," *Respiratory Care* 49(9):1080–1084, September 2004.

Cason, C. L., et al. "Nurses' Implementation of Guidelines for Ventilator-associated Pneumonia for the Centers for Disease Control and Prevention," *American Journal of Critical Care* 16(1):28–36, January 2007.

Centers for Disease Control and Prevention. "Guidelines for the Prevention of Health-care Associated Bacterial Pneumonia," *MMWR* 53(RR-3):3–10, March 26, 2004.

Grap, M. J., and Munro, C. L. "Preventing Ventilator-associated Pneumonia: Evidence-based Care," *Critical Care Nursing Clinics of North America* 16(3):349–58, September 2004.

Lynn-McHale Wiegand, D. J., and Carlson, K. K., eds. *AACN Procedure Manual for Critical Care,* 5th ed. Philadelphia: W. B. Saunders Co., 2006.

Taylor, C., et al. *Fundamentals of Nursing: The Art and Science of Nursing Care,* 5th ed. Philadelphia: Lippincott Williams & Wilkins, 2008.

Oropharyngeal airway insertion and care

An oropharyngeal airway, a curved rubber or plastic device, is inserted into the mouth to the posterior pharynx to establish or maintain a patent airway. In an unconscious patient, the tongue usually obstructs the posterior pharynx. The oropharyngeal airway conforms to the curvature of the palate, removing the obstruction and allowing air to pass around and through the tube. It also facilitates oropharyngeal suctioning. The oropharyngeal airway is intended for short-term use, as in the postanesthesia or postictal stage. It may be left in place longer as an airway adjunct to prevent the orally intubated patient from biting the endotracheal tube.

The oropharyngeal airway isn't the airway of choice for the patient with loose or avulsed teeth or recent oral surgery. Inserting this airway in the conscious or semiconscious patient may stimulate vomiting and laryngospasm; therefore, you'll usually insert the airway only in an unconscious patient.

Equipment

For inserting: Oral airway of appropriate size ◆ tongue blade ◆ padded tongue blade ◆ gloves ◆ optional: suction equipment, handheld resuscitation bag or oxygen-powered breathing device.

For cleaning: Hydrogen peroxide ◆ water ◆ basin ◆ optional: pipe cleaner.

Implementation

▶ Select an airway of appropriate size for your patient; an oversized airway can obstruct breathing by depressing the epiglottis into the laryngeal opening. Be sure to confirm the correct size of the airway by placing the airway flange beside the patient's cheek, parallel to his front teeth. If the airway is the right size, the airway curve should reach to the angle of the jaw (as shown at top of next column). **MFR**

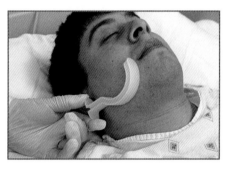

▶ Explain the procedure to the patient even though he may not appear to be alert. Provide privacy and put on gloves to prevent contact with body fluids. If the patient is wearing dentures, remove them so they don't cause further airway obstruction.
▶ Suction the patient if necessary.
▶ Place the patient in the supine position with his neck hyperextended if this isn't contraindicated.
▶ Place your thumb on the patient's lower teeth and your index finger on his upper teeth. Gently open his mouth by pushing his teeth apart.
▶ Insert the airway upside down and slide it over the tongue toward the back of the mouth (as shown at top of next column).

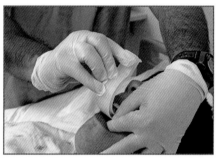

▶ Rotate the airway as it approaches the posterior wall of the pharynx so it points downward.

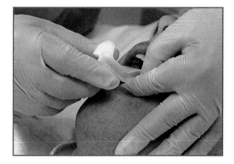

▶ Auscultate the lungs to ensure adequate ventilation. Bilateral breath sounds indicate that the airway is the proper size and in the correct position (as shown at top of next column).

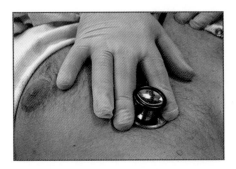

▶ After the airway is inserted, position the patient on his side to decrease the risk of aspirating vomitus.

▶ Perform mouth care every 2 to 4 hours as needed. Place the airway in a basin, and rinse it with hydrogen peroxide and then water. If secretions remain, use a pipe cleaner to remove them.

▶ While the airway is removed for mouth care, observe the mouth's mucous membranes because tissue irritation or ulceration can result from prolonged airway use.

▶ Frequently check the position of the airway to ensure correct placement.

▶ When the patient regains consciousness and can swallow, remove the airway by pulling it outward and downward, following the mouth's natural curvature. After the airway is removed, test the patient's cough and gag reflexes to ensure that removal of the airway wasn't premature and that the patient can maintain his own airway.

Special considerations

▶ Avoid taping the airway in place because untaping it could delay airway removal, thus increasing the patient's risk of aspiration.

▶ Evaluate the patient's behavior to provide the cue for airway removal. He's likely to gag or cough as he becomes more alert, indicating that he no longer needs the airway.

▶ Immediately after inserting the airway, check for respirations. If respirations are absent or inadequate, initiate artificial positive-pressure ventilation by using a mouth-to-mask technique, a handheld resuscitation bag, or an oxygen-powered breathing device. (See "Manual ventilation," page 312.)

Selected references

American Heart Association. "2005 American Heart Association Guidelines for Cardiopulmonary Resuscitation and Emergency Cardiovascular Care," *Circulation* 112(Suppl IV):IV-19-IV-34, December 2005.

Dulak, S. B. "Placing an Oropharyngeal Airway," *RN* 68(2):20ac1–20ac3, February 2005.

Lynn-McHale Wiegand, D. J., and Carlson, K. K., eds. *AACN Procedure Manual for Critical Care,* 5th ed. Philadelphia: W. B. Saunders Co., 2006.

Taylor, C., et al. *Fundamentals of Nursing: The Art and Science of Nursing Care,* 5th ed. Philadelphia: Lippincott Williams & Wilkins, 2008.

Tong, J. L., and Smith, J. E. "Cardiovascular Changes following Insertion of Oropharyngeal and Nasopharyngeal Airways," *British Journal of Anaesthesiology* 93(3):339–42, September 2004.

Oxygen administration

Oxygen therapy is warranted when hypoxemia results from a respiratory or cardiac emergency or an increase in metabolic function.

In a respiratory emergency, oxygen administration enables the patient to reduce his ventilatory effort. When such conditions as atelectasis or acute respiratory distress syndrome impair diffusion or when lung volumes are decreased from alveolar hypoventilation, this procedure boosts alveolar oxygen levels.

In a cardiac emergency, oxygen therapy helps meet the increased myocardial workload as the heart tries to compensate for hypoxemia. Oxygen administration is particularly important for the patient whose myocardium is already compromised—perhaps from a myocardial infarction or cardiac arrhythmia. **AARC**

The patient's disease, physical condition, and age will help determine the most appropriate method of oxygen administration.

Equipment

The equipment needed depends on the type of delivery system ordered. (See *Guide to oxygen delivery systems,* pages 368 to 371.)

Equipment includes selections from the following list: oxygen source (wall unit, cylinder, liquid tank, or concentrator) ◆ flowmeter ◆ adapter, if using a wall unit, or a pressure-reduction gauge, if using a cylinder ◆ sterile humidity bottle and adapter ◆ sterile distilled water ◆ oxygen precaution sign ◆ appropriate oxygen delivery system (nasal cannula, simple mask, or nonrebreather mask for low-flow and variable oxygen concentrations; a Venturi mask, aerosol mask, T tube, tracheostomy collar, tent, or oxygen hood for high-flow and specific oxygen concentrations) ◆ small-diameter and large-diameter connection tubing ◆ flashlight (for nasal cannula) ◆ water-soluble lubricant ◆ gauze pads and tape (for oxygen masks) ◆ jet adapter for Venturi mask (if adding humidity) ◆ gloves ◆ stethoscope ◆ sphygmomanometer ◆ optional: oxygen analyzer.

Implementation

▶ Check the oxygen outlet port to verify flow. Pinch the tubing near the prongs and listen for a higher pitched sound caused by the increased pressure.

▶ Gather the appropriate equipment.

▶ Confirm the patient's identity using two patient identifiers according to your facility's policy. **JC**

▶ Obtain a baseline assessment including vital signs, lung sounds, and a physical assessment. In an emergency, verify that he has an open airway before administering oxygen. **AARC**

▶ Explain the procedure to the patient, and let him know why he needs oxygen to ensure his cooperation.

▶ Check the patient's room to make sure it's safe for oxygen administration. Whenever possible, replace electrical devices with nonelectrical ones and post a "no smoking" sign in the patient's room.

AGE FACTOR

If the patient is a child and is in an oxygen tent, remove all toys that may produce a spark. Oxygen supports combustion, and the smallest spark can cause a fire.

▶ Place an oxygen precaution sign over the patient's bed and on the door to his room.

▶ Help place the oxygen delivery device on the patient. Make sure it fits properly and is stable. Pad any pressure areas to prevent skin breakdown.

▶ Monitor the patient's response to oxygen therapy. Check his ABG values during initial adjustments of oxygen flow. When the patient is stabilized, you may use pulse oximetry to monitor trends. Check the patient frequently for signs of hypoxia, such as a decreased level of consciousness, increased heart rate, arrhythmias, restlessness, perspiration, dyspnea, accessory muscle use, yawning or flared nostrils, cyanosis, and cool, clammy skin. Obtain his vital signs as needed. **AARC**

▶ Observe the patient's skin integrity to prevent skin breakdown on pressure points from the oxygen delivery device. Wipe moisture or perspiration from the patient's face and from the mask as needed.

(Text continues on page 371.)

Guide to oxygen delivery systems

Patients may receive oxygen through one of several administration systems. Each one has benefits, drawbacks, and indications for use. The advantages and disadvantages of each system are compared here.

Nasal cannula

Oxygen is delivered through plastic cannulas in the patient's nostrils.

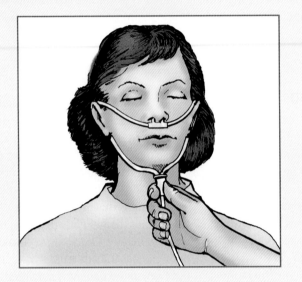

Advantages: Safe and simple; comfortable and easily tolerated; nasal prongs can be shaped to fit any face; effective for low oxygen concentrations; allows movement, eating, and talking; inexpensive and disposable.

Disadvantages: Can't deliver concentrations higher than 40%; can't be used in complete nasal obstruction; may cause headaches or dry mucous membranes; can dislodge easily.

Administration guidelines: Ensure the patency of the patient's nostrils with a flashlight. If patent, hook the cannula tubing behind the patient's ears and under the chin. Slide the adjuster upward under the chin to secure the tubing. If using an elastic strap to secure the cannula, position it over the ears and around the back of the head. Avoid applying it too tightly, *which can result in excess pressure on facial structures as well as cannula occlusion.* With a nasal cannula, oral breathers achieve the same oxygen delivery as nasal breathers. Oxygen can be administered without humidification at a flow rate of 4 L/minute or less.

Simple mask

Oxygen flows through an entry port at the bottom of the mask and exits through large holes on the sides of the mask.

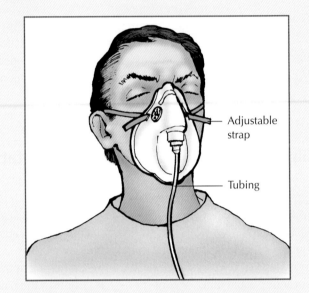

Adjustable strap

Tubing

Advantages: Can deliver concentrations of 35% to 50%.

Disadvantages: Hot and confining; may irritate the patient's skin; tight seal, which may cause discomfort, is required for higher oxygen concentration; interferes with talking and eating; impractical for long-term therapy because of imprecision.

Administration guidelines: Select the mask size that offers the best fit. Place the mask over the patient's nose, mouth, and chin, and mold the flexible metal edge to the bridge of the nose. Adjust the elastic band around the head to hold the mask firmly but comfortably over the cheeks, chin, and bridge of the nose. For an elderly patient or a cachectic patients with sunken cheeks, tape gauze pads to the mask over the cheek area to try to create an airtight seal. Without this seal, room air dilutes the oxygen, preventing delivery of the prescribed concentration. A minimum of 5 L/minute is required in all masks to flush expired carbon dioxide from the mask so that the patient doesn't rebreathe it.

Guide to oxygen delivery systems *(continued)*

Nonrebreather mask

On inhalation, the one-way inspiratory valve opens, directing oxygen from a reservoir bag into the mask. On exhalation, gas exits the mask through the one-way expiratory valves and enters the atmosphere. The patient breathes air only from the bag.

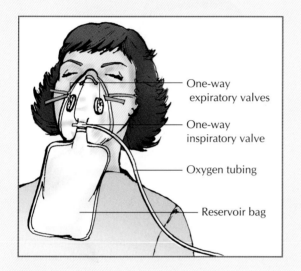

One-way expiratory valves

One-way inspiratory valve

Oxygen tubing

Reservoir bag

Advantages: Delivers the highest possible oxygen concentration (60% to 80%) short of intubation and mechanical ventilation; effective for short-term therapy; doesn't dry mucous membranes; can be converted to a partial rebreather mask, if necessary, by removing the one-way valve.

Disadvantages: Requires a tight seal, which may be difficult to maintain and may cause discomfort; may irritate the patient's skin; interferes with talking and eating; impractical for long-term therapy.

Administration guidelines: Follow the procedures listed for the simple mask. Make sure that the mask fits very snugly and that the one-way valves are secure and functioning. *Because the mask excludes room air,* a valve malfunction could cause carbon dioxide buildup and suffocate an unconscious patient. If the reservoir bag collapses more than slightly during inspiration, raise the flow rate until you see only a slight deflation. Marked or complete deflation indicates an insufficient flow rate. Keep the reservoir bag from twisting or kinking. Ensure free expansion by making sure the bag lies outside the patient's gown and bedcovers.

CPAP mask

This system allows the spontaneously breathing patient to receive continuous positive airway pressure (CPAP) with or without an artificial airway.

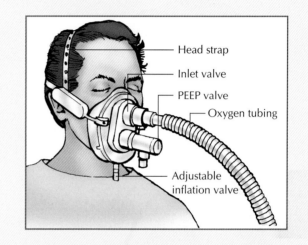

Head strap

Inlet valve

PEEP valve

Oxygen tubing

Adjustable inflation valve

Advantages: Noninvasively improves arterial oxygenation by increasing functional residual capacity; allows the patient to avoid intubation; allows the patient to talk and cough without interrupting positive pressure.

Disadvantages: Requires a tight fit, which may cause discomfort; interferes with eating and talking; heightened risk of aspiration if the patient vomits; increased risk of pneumothorax, diminished cardiac output, and gastric distention; generally contraindicated in patients with chronic obstructive pulmonary disease, bullous lung disease, low cardiac output, or tension pneumothorax.

Administration guidelines: Place one strap behind the patient's head and the other strap over his head to ensure a snug fit. Attach one latex strap to the connector prong on one side of the mask. Then use one hand to position the mask on the patient's face while using the other hand to connect the strap to the other side of the mask. After the mask is applied, assess the patient's respiratory, circulatory, and GI function every hour. Watch for signs of pneumothorax, decreased cardiac output, a drop in blood pressure, and gastric distention.

(continued)

Guide to oxygen delivery systems (continued)

Transtracheal oxygen

The patient receives oxygen through a catheter inserted into the base of his neck in a simple outpatient procedure.

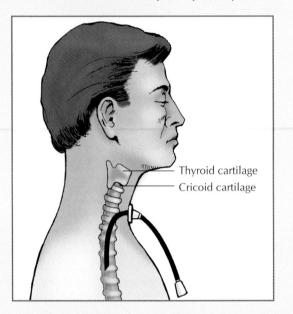

Thyroid cartilage
Cricoid cartilage

Advantages: Supplies oxygen to the lungs throughout the respiratory cycle; provides continuous oxygen without hindering mobility; doesn't interfere with eating or talking; doesn't dry mucous membranes; catheter can easily be concealed by a shirt or scarf.

Disadvantages: Not suitable for use in patients at risk for bleeding or those with severe bronchospasm, uncompensated respiratory acidosis, pleural herniation into the base of the neck, or high corticosteroid dosages.

Administration guidelines: After insertion, obtain a chest X-ray to confirm placement. Monitor the patient for bleeding, respiratory distress, pneumothorax, pain, coughing, or hoarseness. Don't use the catheter for about 1 week following insertion to decrease the risk of subcutaneous emphysema.

Venturi mask

The mask is connected to a Venturi device, which mixes a specific volume of air and oxygen.

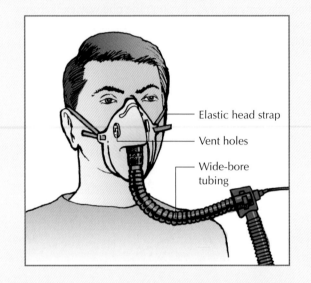

Elastic head strap
Vent holes
Wide-bore tubing

Advantages: Delivers highly accurate oxygen concentration despite the patient's respiratory pattern because the same amount of air is always entrained; dilute jets can be changed or the dial turned to change oxygen concentration; doesn't dry mucous membranes; humidity or aerosol can be added.

Disadvantages: Confining and may irritate skin; oxygen concentration may be altered if mask fits loosely, tubing kinks, oxygen intake ports become blocked, flow is insufficient, or the patient is hyperpneic; interferes with eating and talking; condensate may collect and drip on the patient if humidification is used.

Administration guidelines: Make sure that the oxygen flow rate is set at the amount specified on each mask and that the Venturi valve is set for the desired fraction of inspired oxygen.

(continued)

Guide to oxygen delivery systems *(continued)*

Aerosols

A face mask, hood, tent, or tracheostomy tube or collar is connected to wide-bore tubing that receives aerosolized oxygen from a jet nebulizer. The jet nebulizer, which is attached near the oxygen source, adjusts air entrainment in a manner similar to the Venturi device.

Advantages: Administers high humidity; gas can be heated (when delivered through an artificial airway) or cooled (when delivered through a tent).

Disadvantages: Condensate collected in the tracheostomy collar or T tube may drain into the tracheostomy; the weight of the T tube can put stress on the tracheostomy tube.

Administration guidelines: Guidelines vary with the type of nebulizer used: ultrasonic, large-volume, small-volume, and in-line types. When using a high-output nebulizer, watch for signs of overhydration, pulmonary edema, crackles, and electrolyte imbalance.

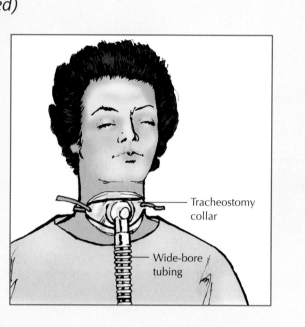

Tracheostomy collar

Wide-bore tubing

Special considerations

CLINICAL ALERT

Never administer oxygen by nasal cannula at more than 2 L/minute to a patient with chronic lung disease unless you have a specific order to do so. That's because some patients with chronic lung disease become dependent on a state of hypercapnia and hypoxia to stimulate their respirations, and supplemental oxygen could cause them to stop breathing. However, long-term oxygen therapy of 12 to 17 hours daily may help patients with chronic lung disease sleep better, survive longer, and experience a reduced incidence of pulmonary hypertension.

▶ When monitoring a patient's response to a change in oxygen flow, check the pulse oximetry monitor or measure arterial blood gas (ABG) values 20 to 30 minutes after adjusting the flow. In the interim, monitor the patient closely for any adverse response to the change in oxygen flow.

▶ If the patient will be receiving oxygen at a concentration above 60% for more than 24 hours, watch carefully for signs of oxygen toxicity.

▶ Remind the patient to cough and deep-breathe frequently to prevent atelectasis. To prevent the development of serious lung damage, measure ABG values repeatedly to determine whether high oxygen concentrations are still necessary.

Selected references

Lynn-McHale Wiegand, D. J., and Carlson, K. K., eds. *AACN Procedure Manual for Critical Care,* 5th ed. Philadelphia: W. B. Saunders Co., 2006.

Kallstrom, T. J. and American Association for Respiratory Care (AARC). "AARC Clinical Practice Guideline: oxygen therapy for adults in the acute care facility—2002 revision & update," *Respiratory Care* 47(6):717–20, June 2002.

O'Reilly, P., et al. "Long-term Continuous Oxygen Treatment in Chronic Obstructive Pulmonary Disease: Proper Use, Benefits, and Unresolved Issues," *Current Opinions in Pulmonary Medicine* 13(2):120–24, March 2007.

Slessarev, M. "Efficiency of Oxygen Administration: Sequential Gas Delivery versus Flow into a Cone Methods," *Critical Care Medicine* 34(3):829–34, March 2006.

Taylor, C., et al. *Fundamentals of Nursing: The Art and Science of Nursing Care,* 5th ed. Philadelphia: Lippincott Williams & Wilkins, 2008.

Wettstein, R. B., et al. "Delivered Oxygen Concentrations Using Low-flow and High-flow Cannulas," *Respiratory Care* 50(5):604–609, May 2005.

Pain management

Pain is defined as the sensory and emotional experience associated with actual or potential tissue damage. **ASPN** **ASPMN** Thus, pain includes not only the perception of an uncomfortable stimulus, but also the response to that perception. It's important to remember that the patient's self-report of pain is the most reliable indicator of its existence. Indeed, to assess and manage pain properly, the nurse must depend on the patient's subjective description in addition to objective tools. **ASPMN**

In health care, the practitioner's role is to identify and treat the cause of pain and prescribe medications and other interventions to relieve it, whereas nurses have traditionally been responsible for assessing and managing a patient's pain.

Several interventions can be used to manage pain, including analgesic administration, emotional support, comfort measures, and complementary and alternative therapies such as cognitive techniques. Severe pain usually requires an opioid analgesic. **ASPMN** Invasive measures, such as epidural analgesia or patient-controlled analgesia (PCA), may also be required.

Equipment

Pain assessment tool or scale ◆ oral hygiene supplies ◆ water ◆ nonopioid analgesic (acetaminophen or aspirin) ◆ optional: PCA device, mild opioid (oxycodone or codeine), strong opioid (morphine or hydromorphone).

Implementation

▶ Confirm the patient's identity using two patient identifiers according to your facility's policy. **JC**
▶ Explain to the patient how pain medications work together with other pain management therapies to provide relief. Also explain that management aims to keep pain at a low level to permit optimal bodily function. **ASPMN**
▶ Assess the patient's pain by asking key questions and noting his response to the pain. Look for physiologic or behavioral clues as to the pain's severity. **ASPMN** **ASPN** **ASIPP** (See *How to assess pain,* page 373.)
▶ Develop nursing diagnoses. Appropriate nursing diagnostic categories include pain (acute, chronic), anxiety, activity intolerance, fear, risk of injury, deficient knowledge, and powerlessness. **ASPN**
▶ Work with the patient to develop a nursing care plan using interventions appropriate to the patient's lifestyle. These may include prescribed medications; emotional support; comfort measures; complementary and alternative therapies, such as cognitive techniques; and education about pain and its management. Emphasize the importance of maintaining good bowel habits, respiratory function, and mobility because pain may exacerbate problems in these areas.
▶ Implement your care plan. Because individuals respond to pain differently, you'll find that what works for one person may not work for another.

Giving medications

▶ If the patient is allowed oral intake, begin with a nonopioid analgesic, every 4 to 6 hours, as ordered. **WHO**
▶ If the patient needs more relief than a nonopioid analgesic provides, you may give a mild opioid as ordered. **WHO**
▶ If the patient needs still more pain relief, you may administer a strong opioid as prescribed. Administer oral medications, if possible. Check the appropriate drug information for each medication given. **WHO**

How to assess pain

To assess pain properly, you'll need to consider the patient's description and your observations of the patient's physical and behavioral responses. Start by asking the following series of key questions (bearing in mind that the patient's responses will be shaped by his prior experiences, self-image, and beliefs about his condition):
▶ Where is the pain located? How long does it last? How often does it occur?
▶ Can you describe the pain?
▶ What brings the pain on?
▶ What relieves the pain or makes it worse?

Ask the patient to rank his pain on a scale of 0 to 10, with 0 denoting lack of pain and 10 denoting the worst pain. This helps the patient verbally evaluate pain therapies.

Observe the patient's behavioral and physiologic responses to pain. Physiologic responses may be sympathetic or parasympathetic.

Behavioral responses
Behavioral responses include altered body position, moaning, sighing, grimacing, withdrawal, crying, restlessness, muscle twitching, irritability, and immobility.

Sympathetic responses
Sympathetic responses are commonly associated with mild to moderate pain and include pallor, elevated blood pressure, dilated pupils, skeletal muscle tension, dyspnea, tachycardia, and diaphoresis.

Parasympathetic responses
Parasympathetic responses are commonly associated with severe, deep pain and include pallor, decreased blood pressure, bradycardia, nausea and vomiting, weakness, dizziness, and loss of consciousness.

Assess pain at least every 2 hours and during rest, during activity, and through the night when pain is usually heightened. Keep in mind that the ability to sleep doesn't indicate absence of pain.

▶ Instruct the patient to splint the incision or support abdominal and chest incisions with a pillow when he coughs or changes position to help decrease pain.
▶ Apply cold compresses, as appropriate, to decrease discomfort. **ASPN**
▶ Give the patient a back massage to help relax tense muscles. **ASPN**
▶ Perform passive range-of-motion exercises to prevent stiffness and further loss of mobility, relax tense muscles, and provide comfort.
▶ Provide oral hygiene. Keep a fresh cup of water at the bedside because many pain medications tend to dry the mouth.
▶ Wash the patient's face and hands.

Using complementary and alternative therapies
▶ Help the patient enhance the effect of analgesics by using such techniques as distraction, guided imagery, deep breathing, and relaxation. You can easily use these "mind-over-pain" techniques at the bedside. Choose the method the patient prefers. If possible, start these techniques when the patient feels little or no pain. If he feels persistent pain, begin with short, simple exercises. **ASPN**

▶ If ordered, teach the patient how to use a PCA device. Such a device can help the patient manage his pain and decrease his anxiety. (See *Understanding patient-controlled analgesia,* page 374.)

Providing emotional support
▶ Show your concern by spending time talking with the patient. Because of his pain and his inability to manage it, the patient may be anxious and frustrated. Such feelings can worsen his pain.

Performing comfort measures
▶ Periodically reposition the patient to reduce muscle spasms and tension and to relieve pressure on bony prominences. Increasing the angle of the bed can reduce pull on an abdominal incision, thus diminishing pain. If appropriate, elevate a limb to reduce swelling, inflammation, and pain.

Special considerations
▶ Evaluate your patient's response to pain management. If he's still in pain, reassess him and alter your care plan as appropriate. **ASPN** **ASPMN** **ASIPP** **JC**
▶ Culture and beliefs affect behavioral responses to pain and treatment preferences. Therefore, patient expectations regarding pain relief need to be taken into account when developing the care plan. **ASPN**

Understanding patient-controlled analgesia

In patient-controlled analgesia (PCA), the patient controls I.V. delivery of an analgesic (usually morphine) by pressing the button on a delivery device. In this way, he receives analgesia at the level he needs and at the time he needs it. The PCA device prevents the patient from accidentally overdosing by imposing a lockout time between doses— usually 6 to 10 minutes. During this interval, the patient won't receive any analgesic, even if he pushes the button.

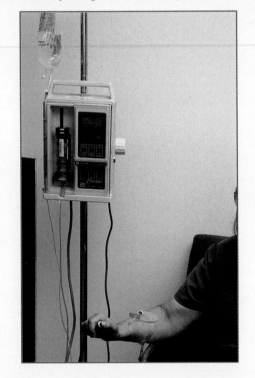

Indications and advantages
Indicated for patients who need parenteral analgesia, PCA therapy is typically given to patients postoperatively and to terminal cancer patients and others with chronic diseases. To receive PCA therapy, patients must be mentally alert and able to understand and comply with instructions and procedures and have no history of allergy to the analgesic.

Patients ineligible for therapy include those with limited respiratory reserve, a history of drug abuse or chronic sedative or tranquilizer use, or a psychiatric disorder. PCA therapy's advantages include:
► no need for I.M. analgesics
► pain relief tailored to each patient's size and pain tolerance
► a sense of control over pain
► ability to sleep at night with minimal daytime drowsiness
► lower opioid use compared with patients not on PCA
► improved postoperative deep breathing, coughing, and ambulation.

PCA setup
To set up a PCA system, the practitioner's order should include:
► medication to be dosed
► the appropriate lockout interval
► the amount the patient will receive when he activates the device
► the maximum amount the patient can receive within a specified time (if an adjustable device is used).

Occasionally the practitioner may order a loading dose and sometimes a base rate will be prescribed.

Nursing considerations
Because the primary adverse effect of analgesics is respiratory depression, monitor the patient's respiratory rate routinely. Also, check for infiltration into the subcutaneous tissues and for catheter occlusion, which may cause the drug to back up in the primary I.V. tubing. If the analgesic nauseates the patient, you may need to administer an antiemetic.

Before the patient starts using the PCA device, teach him how it works. Then have the patient practice with a sample device. Explain that he should take enough analgesic to relieve acute pain but not enough to induce drowsiness.

During therapy, monitor and record the amount of analgesic infused, the patient's respiratory rate, and the patient's assessment of pain relief. If the patient reports insufficient pain relief, notify the practitioner.

AGE FACTOR

Pain shouldn't be considered a normal part of the aging process. Provide pain relief for the elderly patient using pharmacologic and nonpharmacologic approaches. Remember that safety is a special concern, especially the risk of falls due to impaired mobility from pain and from adverse effects of opioids.

AGE FACTOR

It's important to identify age-related factors that affect assessment and pain management in elderly patients. Because of adverse effects, certain medications, such as meperidine and propoxyphene, should be avoided.

▶ Remember, children experience pain just as adults do, but developmental factors make pain assessment in children more difficult. Neonates and young children have difficulty expressing pain verbally, and it's important to look for behavioral cues (such as crying, facial grimacing, or eye closing). Pain tools, such as the Wong-Baker FACES Pain Rating Scale, are available to assess pain in children. (See *Visual pain rating*.) **ASPMN**

▶ Patients receiving opioid analgesics may be at risk for developing tolerance, dependence, or addiction. Patients with acute pain may have a smaller risk of dependence or addiction than patients with chronic pain. **ASIPP ASPMN ASPN**

▶ If a patient receiving an opioid analgesic experiences abstinence syndrome when the drug is withdrawn abruptly, suspect physical dependence. Signs and symptoms include anxiety, irritability, chills and hot flashes, excessive salivation and tearing, rhinorrhea, sweating, nausea, vomiting, and seizures. These signs and symptoms are likely to begin in 6 to 12 hours and peak in 24 to 72 hours. To reduce the risk of dependence, discontinue an opioid by decreasing the dose gradually each day. You may switch to an oral opioid and decrease its dose gradually.

▶ If a patient becomes addicted, his behavior will be characterized by compulsive drug use and a craving for the drug to experience effects other than pain relief. A patient demonstrating such behavior usually has a preexisting problem that's exacerbated by the opioid use. Discuss the patient's problem with supportive personnel, and make appropriate referrals. **ASPN**

▶ During periods of intense pain, the patient's ability to concentrate diminishes. If the patient is in severe pain, help him select a cognitive technique that's simple to use. After he selects a technique, encourage him to use it consistently.

Selected references

Assessment and Management of Acute Pain. Bloomington, Minn.: Institute for Clinical Systems Improvement, March 2006.

Assessment and Management of Chronic Pain. Bloomington, Minn.: Institute for Clinical Systems Improvement, November 2005.

Visual pain rating

You can evaluate pain in a nonverbal manner for pediatric patients age 3 and older and for adults with language difficulties. One instrument is the Wong-Baker FACES pain rating scale shown below left, and another uses two simple faces, such as the ones shown below right. Ask the patient to choose the face that describes how he's feeling—either happy because he has no pain, or sad because he has some or a lot of pain. Alternatively, to pinpoint varying levels of pain, you can ask the patient to draw a face.

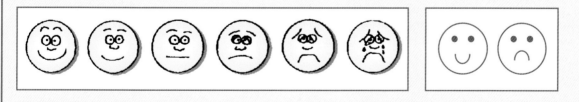

Wong-Baker FACES pain rating scale from Wong, D.L., et al. *Wong's Essentials of Pediatric Nursing*, 6th ed. St. Louis: Mosby, Inc., 2001. Reprinted with permission.

EVIDENCE-BASED RESEARCH

Determining pain reduction

Sloman, R., et al. "Determination of clinically meaningful levels of pain reduction in patients experiencing acute postoperative pain," Pain Management Nursing 7(4):153–8, December 2006.

Level VI
Evidence from a single descriptive or qualitative study

Description
Nurses who care for postoperative patients quantify and document pain by use of unidimensional scales such as the numeric rating scale, the visual analogue scale, or a verbal descriptor scale. Improvements in pain ratings on these scales are viewed as a welcome result by nurses and doctors. Pain, however, is a multidimensional phenomenon. Furthermore, pain is subjective, and therefore no objective measure of pain exists that captures every aspect of the pain experience. Given that clinical decisions are made on the basis of existing scales, it is important to know how much reduction in pain is clinically meaningful from the patient's perspective. The aim of this

study was to investigate this issue by comparing levels of postsurgical pain reduction measured by a numeric rating scale (NRS) with the patients' verbal descriptions of how meaningful they consider their pain reduction to be. A convenience sample of 150 postoperative patients was obtained. The patients' postoperative pain intensity levels before and after analgesia were measured and compared with their verbal descriptions of what constitutes a clinically meaningful pain reduction.

Findings
The results of the study showed a significant correlation between the percentage of reduction in pain severity and the patients' descriptive ratings of pain improvement. A unique finding of the study was that the degree of incremental shift on an NRS of pretreatment and posttreatment pain levels is not a good predictor of clinical relevance from the patient's perspective. A more accurate predictor was found by converting the changes on the NRS to percentages.

Conclusions
An important implication of this study is the need to include a scale in pain assessment instruments for assessing the level of clinical meaningfulness of pain reduction from the patient's perspective.

Nursing practice implications
Nurses are the ones who assess and often treat the patient's pain. The following practice implications are important:
▶ Assess the patient's pain at least every 2 hours, and before and after giving pain medication
▶ Teach the patient to request pain medication when the pain level is low; as the pain gets stronger, it also gets harder to treat
▶ Assess the patient's pain using a standard scale and document the pain using that scale so other nurses can follow the patient's progress
▶ Educate the staff on proper pain assessment and treatment

The Joint Commission. *Comprehensive Accreditation Manual for Hospitals' Pain Management Standards.* Chicago: The Joint Commission, 2007.

D'Arcy, Y. "Managing Pain in a Patient Who's Drug Dependent," *Nursing* 37(3):37–41, March 2007.

Lewandowski, W., et al. "Changes in the Meaning of Pain with the Use of

Guided Imagery," *Pain Management Nursing* 6(2):58–67, June 2005.

Liu, S. S., and Wu, C. L. "The Effect of Analgesic Technique on Postoperative Patient-reported Outcomes Including Analgesia: A Systematic Review," *Anesthesiology and Analgesia* 105(3):789–808, September 2007.

Mackintosh, C. "Assessment and Management of Patients with Post-operative Pain," *Nursing Standard* 22(5):49–55, October 2007.

Plaisance, L. "Is Your Patient's Cancer Pain under Control?" *Nursing* 25(5)52–55, May 2005.

Passive range-of-motion exercises

Used to move the patient's joints through as full a range of motion (ROM) as possible, passive ROM exercises improve or maintain joint mobility and help prevent contractures. Performed by a nurse, physical therapist, or caregiver of the patient's choosing, these exercises are indicated for the patient with temporary or permanent loss of mobility, sensation, or consciousness. Performed properly, passive ROM exercises require recognition of the patient's limits of motion and support of all joints during movement.

Exercises performed in the bed help with joint mobility, strength, and endurance, and they prepare the patient for ambulating. During passive ROM exercises, another person moves the patient's extremities so that the joints move through a complete range of movement, maximally stretching all muscle groups within each plane over each joint.

Passive ROM exercises are contraindicated in patients with septic joints, acute thrombophlebitis, severe arthritic joint inflammation, or recent trauma with possible hidden fractures or internal injuries.

Implementation

▶ Determine the joints that need ROM exercises, and consult the practitioner or physical therapist about limitations or precautions for specific exercises. The exercises described below treat all joints, but they don't have to be performed in the order given or all at once. You can schedule them over the course of a day, whenever the patient is in the most convenient position. Remember to perform all exercises slowly, gently, and to the end of the normal ROM or to the point of pain, but no further. Hold this position for 1 to 2 seconds, and then slowly release. (See *Glossary of joint movements,* page 378.)

▶ Before you begin, raise the bed to a comfortable working height, and provide privacy for the patient.

▶ Confirm the patient's identity using two patient identifiers according to your facility's policy. **JC**

Exercising the neck

▶ Support the patient's head with your hands and extend the neck, flex the chin to the chest, and tilt the head laterally toward each shoulder (as shown top of next column).

▶ Rotate the head from right to left.

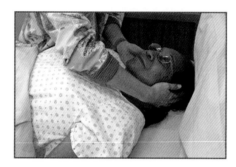

Exercising the shoulders

▶ Support the patient's arm in an extended, neutral position, and then extend the forearm and flex it back. Abduct the arm outward from the side of the body, and adduct it back to the side.

▶ Rotate the shoulder so that the arm crosses the midline, and bend the elbow so that the hand touches the opposite shoulder and then touches the mattress of the bed for complete internal rotation.

▶ Return the shoulder to a neutral position and, with the elbow bent, push the arm backward so that the back of the hand touches the mattress for complete external rotation (as shown top of next column).

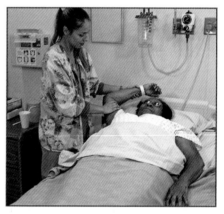

Exercising the elbow

▶ Place the patient's arm at her side with her palm facing up.

▶ Flex and extend the arm at the elbow.

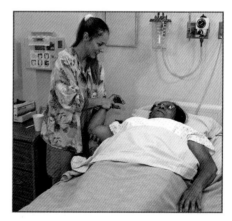

Glossary of joint movements

Joints should be exercised to the point of discomfort, but not pain. Joints should also be moved in the intended direction of function, holding the position for a few seconds, and then returning to the rest position.

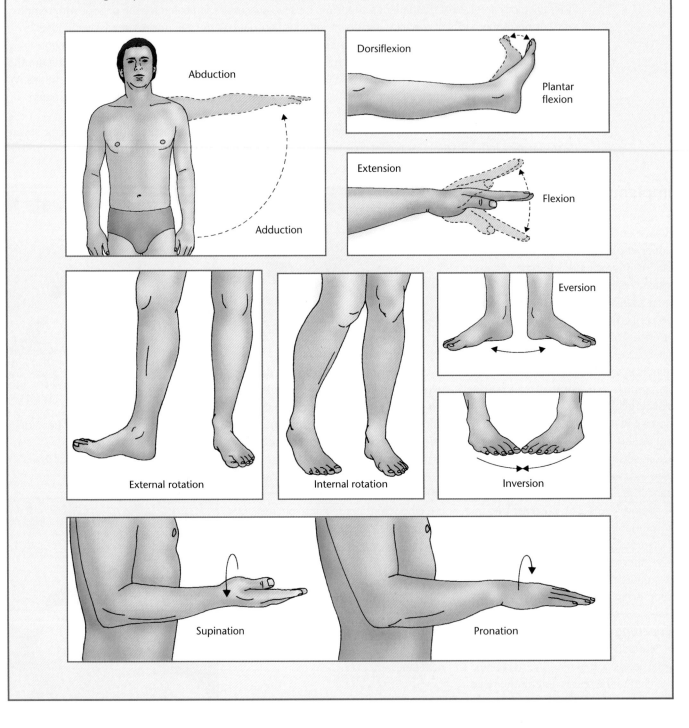

Exercising the forearm
▶ Stabilize the patient's elbow, and then twist the hand to bring the palm up (supination).

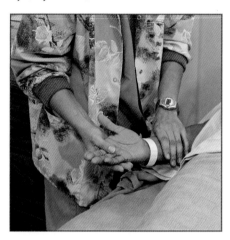

▶ Twist it back again to bring the palm down (pronation).

Exercising the wrist
▶ Stabilize the forearm, and flex and extend the wrist. Then rock the hand sideways for lateral flexion, and rotate the hand in a circular motion.

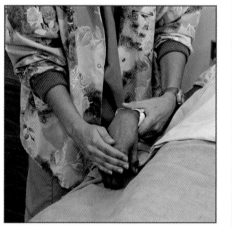

Exercising the fingers and thumb
▶ Extend the patient's fingers, and then flex the hand into a fist; repeat extension and flexion of each joint of each finger and thumb separately.
▶ Spread two adjoining fingers apart (abduction), and then bring them together (adduction), as shown at top of next column.

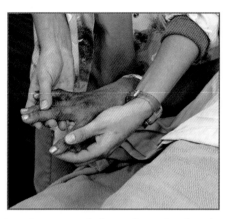

▶ Oppose each fingertip to the thumb, and rotate the thumb and each finger in a circle.

Exercising the hip and knee
▶ Fully extend the patient's leg, bend the hip and knee toward the chest, allowing full joint flexion, and then return to the extended position.
▶ Move the straight leg sideways, out and away from the other leg (abduction), and then back, over, and across it (adduction).

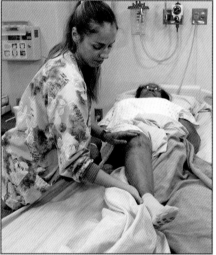

▶ Rotate the straight leg internally toward the midline, and then externally away from the midline.

Exercising the ankle
▶ Bend the patient's foot so that the toes push upward (dorsiflexion), and then bend the foot so that the toes push downward (plantar flexion).
▶ Rotate the ankle in a circular motion.
▶ Invert the ankle so that the sole of the foot faces the midline, and then evert the ankle so that the sole faces away from the midline.

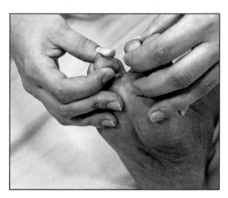

Exercising the toes
▶ Flex the patient's toes toward the sole, and then extend them back toward the top of the foot.
▶ Spread two adjoining toes apart (abduction), and then bring them together (adduction).

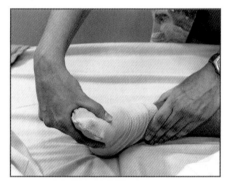

Special considerations

▶ Because joints begin to stiffen within 24 hours of disuse, start passive ROM exercises as soon as possible, and perform them at least every 4 hours. Passive ROM exercises can be performed while bathing or turning the patient. Use proper body mechanics, and repeat each exercise at least three times.

▶ If a disabled patient requires long-term rehabilitation after discharge, consult with a physical therapist and teach a family member or caregiver to perform passive ROM exercises.

Selected references

Craven, R. F., and Hirnle, C. J. *Fundamentals of Nursing: Human Health and Function,* 6th ed. Philadelphia: Lippincott Williams & Wilkins, 2009.

"Performing Passive Range-of-motion Exercises," *Nursing* 36(3):50–51, March 2006.

Winkleman, C., et al. "Activity in the Chronically Critically Ill," *Dimensions in Critical Care Nursing* 24(6):281–90, November–December 2005.

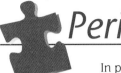

Pericardiocentesis

In pericardiocentesis, a needle is used to aspirate pericardial fluid for analysis. The procedure is both therapeutic and diagnostic and is most useful as an emergency measure to relieve cardiac tamponade. It can also provide a fluid sample to confirm and identify the cause of pericardial effusion (excess pericardial fluid) and help determine appropriate therapy. In many cases, a pericardiocentesis is done at the same time as an echocardiogram to help the physician correctly insert the needle into the pericardium.

The pericardium normally contains 10 to 50 ml of sterile fluid. Pericardial fluid is clear and straw-colored without evidence of pathogens, blood, or malignant cells. The white blood cell count in the fluid is usually less than 1,000/µl. Its glucose concentration should approximate glucose levels in the blood.

Equipment

Prepackaged pericardiocentesis tray ◆ antiseptic solution ◆ 7-ml sterile test tubes ◆ sterile specimen container for culture ◆ sterile 4″ × 4″ gauze pads ◆ sterile bandage ◆ electrocardiogram (ECG) or bedside monitor ◆ pulse oximeter ◆ defibrillator and emergency drugs ◆ gloves ◆ protective eyewear ◆ sterile gloves ◆ sterile marker ◆ sterile label.

If a prepackaged tray isn't available, obtain the following: 1% procaine or 1% lidocaine for local anesthetic ◆ sterile needles (25G for anesthetic and 14G, 16G, and 18G 4″ or 5″ cardiac needles) ◆ 50-ml syringe with luer-lock tip ◆ Kelly clamp ◆ alligator clip ◆ three-way stopcock ◆ sterile syringe for anesthetic.

Implementation

▶ Connect the patient to the bedside monitor, which is set to read lead V_1 and the pulse oximeter. Make sure the defibrillator and emergency drugs are nearby.

▶ Confirm the patient's identity using two patient identifiers according to your facility's policy. **JC**

▶ Explain the procedure to the patient to ease his anxiety and ensure his cooperation. Answer any questions he may have. Make sure an informed consent form has been signed.

▶ Inform the patient that he will feel some pressure when the needle is inserted into the pericardial sac.

▶ Wash your hands.

▶ Open the equipment tray on an overbed table, being careful not to contaminate the sterile field when you open the wrapper.

▶ Label all medications, medication containers, and other solutions on and off the sterile field. **JC**

▶ Provide adequate lighting at the puncture site, and adjust the height of the patient's bed to allow the physician to perform the procedure comfortably.

▶ Position the patient in the supine position with the thorax elevated 60 degrees.

▶ Wash your hands again and put on gloves and protective eyewear.

▶ The physician cleans the skin with sterile gauze pads soaked in antiseptic solution from the left costal margin to the xiphoid process.

▶ If no ampule of anesthetic is included on the equipment tray, clean the injection port of a multidose vial of anesthetic with an alcohol pad. Then invert the vial 45 degrees so that the physician can insert a 25G needle attached to a syringe and withdraw the anesthetic for injection.

▶ Before the physician injects the anesthetic, tell the patient he'll experience a transient burning sensation and local pain.

▶ The physician attaches a 50-ml syringe to one end of a three-way stopcock and the cardiac needle to the other. Using the alligator clip, the V_1 lead (precordial lead wire) of the ECG may be attached to the hub of the aspirating needle to help determine whether the needle has come in contact with the epicardium during the procedure.

▶ The physician inserts the needle through the chest wall into the pericardial sac, maintaining gentle aspiration until fluid appears in the syringe.

▶ When the needle is positioned properly, the physician attaches a Kelly clamp to the skin surface so that the needle won't advance farther.

▶ Assist the physician during aspiration of the pericardial fluid, and label and number the specimen tubes. (See *Aspirating pericardial fluid,* page 382.)

▶ Clean the top of the culture and sensitivity tube with antiseptic solution. If bacterial culture and sensitivity tests are scheduled, record on the laboratory request any antimicrobial drugs the patient is receiving. If anaerobic organisms are suspected, consult the laboratory about the proper collection technique to avoid exposing the aspirate to air. Send all specimens to the laboratory immediately.

▶ When the needle is withdrawn, apply pressure to the site immediately with sterile gauze pads for 3 to 5 minutes. Then apply a sterile bandage.

Aspirating pericardial fluid

In pericardiocentesis, a needle and syringe are inserted through the chest wall into the pericardial sac (as shown below). Electrocardiogram (ECG) monitoring, with a leadwire attached to the needle and electrodes placed on the limbs (right arm [RA], left arm [LA], and left leg [LL]), helps ensure proper needle placement and avoids damage to the heart.

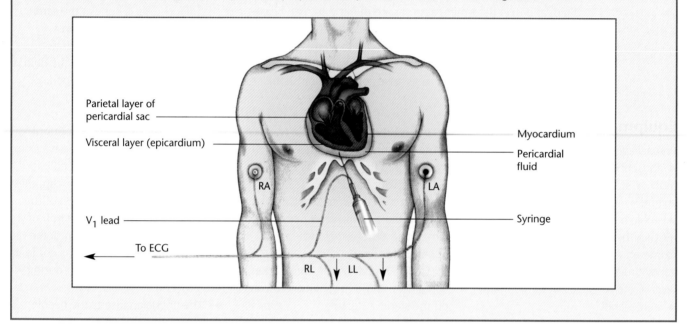

- Obtain a portable chest X-ray immediately after the procedure.
- Assess for complications and check blood pressure, pulse, respirations, oxygen saturation, and heart sounds every 15 minutes until stable, every 30 minutes for 2 hours, every hour for 4 hours, and every 4 hours thereafter. Your facility may require more frequent monitoring. Reassure the patient that such monitoring is routine.
- Monitor continually for cardiac arrhythmias, and document rhythm strips according to your facility's policy.
- Return all equipment to the proper location, and dispose of equipment according to your facility's policy.

Special considerations

- Carefully observe the ECG tracing when the cardiac needle is being inserted because ST-segment elevation indicates that the needle has reached the epicardial surface and should be retracted slightly. Likewise, an abnormally shaped QRS complex may indicate perforation of the myocardium. Premature ventricular contractions usually indicate that the needle has touched the ventricular wall.
- Watch for grossly bloody fluid aspirate, which may indicate inadvertent puncture of a cardiac chamber.
- After the procedure, be alert for respiratory and cardiac distress. Watch especially for signs of cardiac tamponade, including muffled and distant heart sounds, distended neck veins, paradoxical pulse, and shock. Cardiac tamponade may result from rapid accumulation of pericardial fluid or puncture of a coronary vessel, causing bleeding into the pericardial sac.

Selected references

Ben-Horin, S., et al. "The Composition of Normal Pericardial Fluid and its Implications for Diagnosing Pericardial Effusions," *American Journal of Medicine* 118(6):636–40, June 2005.

Cubero, G. I., et al. "Pericardial Effusion: Clinical and Analytical Parameters Clues," *International Journal of Cardiology* 108(3):404–405, April 2006.

Humphreys, M. "Pericardial Conditions: Signs, Symptoms, and Electrocardiogram Changes," *Emergency Nursing* 14(1):30–36, April 2006.

Little, W. C., and Freeman, G. L. "Pericardial Disease," *Circulation* 113(12):1622–632, March 2006.

Lynn-McHale Wiegand, D. J., and Carlson, K. K., eds. *AACN Procedure Manual for Critical Care,* 5th ed. Philadelphia: W. B. Saunders Co., 2005.

Perineal care

Perineal care, which includes care of the external genitalia and the anal area, should be performed during the daily bath and, if necessary, at bedtime and after urination and bowel movements. The procedure promotes cleanliness and prevents infection. It also removes irritating and odorous secretions, such as smegma, a cheeselike substance that collects under the foreskin of the penis and on the inner surface of the labia. For the patient with perineal skin breakdown, frequent bathing followed by application of an ointment or cream aids healing.

Standard precautions must be followed when providing perineal care, with due consideration given to the patient's privacy. CDC

Equipment

Gloves ◆ washcloths ◆ clean basin ◆ mild soap ◆ bath towel ◆ bath blanket ◆ toilet tissue ◆ linen-saver pad ◆ trash bag ◆ optional: bedpan, peri bottle, antiseptic soap, petroleum jelly, zinc oxide cream, vitamin A and D ointment, abdominal pad.

Following genital or rectal surgery, you may need to use sterile supplies, including sterile gloves, gauze, and cotton balls.

Implementation

▶ Obtain ointment or cream as needed. Fill the basin two-thirds full with warm water. Also fill the peri bottle with warm water if needed.
▶ Assemble equipment at the patient's bedside and provide privacy.
▶ Wash your hands thoroughly, put on gloves, and explain to the patient what you're about to do. CDC
▶ Adjust the bed to a comfortable working height to prevent back strain, and lower the head of the bed, if allowed.
▶ Help the patient to a supine position. Place a linen-saver pad under the patient's buttocks to protect the bed from stains and moisture.

Perineal care for the female patient

▶ To minimize the patient's exposure and embarrassment, place the bath blanket over her with corners head to foot and side to side. Wrap each leg with a side corner, tucking it under her hip. Then fold back the corner between her legs to expose the perineum.
▶ Ask the patient to bend her knees slightly and to spread her legs. Separate her labia with one hand and wash with the other, using gentle downward strokes from the front to the back of the perineum to prevent intestinal organisms from contaminating the urethra or vagina. Avoid the area around the anus, and use a clean section of washcloth for each stroke by folding each used section inward.

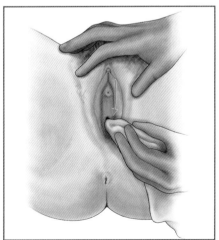

▶ Using a clean washcloth, rinse thoroughly from front to back because soap residue can cause skin irritation. Pat the area dry with a bath towel.
▶ Apply ordered ointments or creams.
▶ Turn the patient on her side to Sims' position, if possible, to expose the anal area.
▶ Clean, rinse, and dry the anal area, starting at the posterior vaginal opening and wiping from front to back.

Perineal care for the male patient

▶ Drape the patient's legs to minimize exposure and embarrassment and expose the genital area.
▶ Hold the shaft of the penis with one hand, and wash with the other, beginning at the tip and working in a circular motion from the center to the periphery to avoid introducing microorganisms into the urethra (as shown at top of next page). Use a clean section of washcloth for each stroke to prevent the spread of contaminated secretions or discharge.

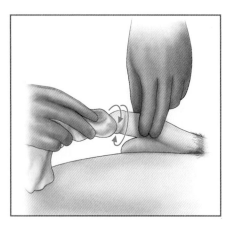

▶ Rinse thoroughly, using the same circular motion.

▶ For the uncircumcised patient, gently retract the foreskin and clean beneath it. Rinse well but don't dry because moisture provides lubrication and prevents friction when replacing the foreskin. Replace the foreskin to avoid constriction of the penis, which causes edema and tissue damage.

▶ Wash the rest of the penis, using downward strokes toward the scrotum. Rinse well and pat dry with a towel.

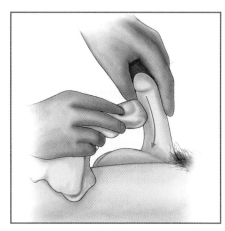

▶ Clean the top and sides of the scrotum; rinse thoroughly and pat dry. Handle the scrotum gently to avoid causing discomfort.

▶ Turn the patient on his side. Clean the bottom of the scrotum and the anal area. Rinse well and pat dry.

After providing perineal care

▶ Reposition the patient for comfort. Remove the bath blanket and linen-saver pad, and then replace the bed linens.

▶ Clean and return the basin and dispose of soiled articles, including gloves.

Special considerations

▶ Give perineal care to a patient of the opposite sex in a matter-of-fact way to minimize embarrassment.

▶ If the patient is incontinent, first remove excess feces with toilet tissue. Then position him on a bedpan, and add a small amount of antiseptic soap to a peri bottle to eliminate odor. Irrigate the perineal area to remove any remaining fecal matter.

▶ After cleaning the perineum, apply ointment or cream (petroleum jelly, zinc oxide cream, or vitamin A and D ointment) to prevent skin breakdown by providing a barrier between the skin and excretions.

▶ To reduce the number of linen changes, tuck an abdominal pad between the patient's buttocks to absorb oozing feces.

Selected references

Grant, B. M., et al. "Vulnerable Bodies: Competing Discourses of Intimate Bodily Care," *Journal of Nursing Education* 44(11):498–504, November 2005.

Hansen, D., et al. "Perineal Dermatitis: A Consequence of Incontinence," *Advances in Skin and Wound Care* 19(5):246–50, June 2006.

Holloway, S., and Jones, V. "The Importance of Skin Care and Assessment," *British Journal of Nursing* 14(22):1172–176, December 2005–January 2006.

Kettle, C. "Perineal Care," *Clinical Evidence* 15:1905–918, June 2006.

Nix, D. "Prevention and Treatment of Perineal Skin Breakdown Due to Incontinence," *Ostomy/Wound Management* 52(4):26–28, April 2006.

Nix, D., and Ermer-Seltun, J. "A Review of Perineal Skin Care Protocols and Skin Barrier Product Use," *Ostomy/Wound Management* 50(12):59–67, December 2004.

Rader, J., et al. "The Bathing of Older Adults with Dementia," *AJN* 106(4):40–48, April 2006.

Peripheral I.V. catheter insertion

Peripheral I.V. catheter insertion involves selection of a venipuncture device and an insertion site, application of a tourniquet, preparation of the site, and venipuncture. Selection of a venipuncture device and site depends on the type of solution to be used; frequency and duration of infusion; patency and location of accessible veins; the patient's age, size, and condition; and, when possible, the patient's preference. **INS**

If possible, choose a vein in the nondominant arm or hand. Preferred venipuncture sites are the cephalic and basilic veins in the lower arm and the veins in the dorsum of the hand; least favorable are the leg and foot veins because of the increased risk of thrombophlebitis. Antecubital veins can be used if no other venous access is available. Subsequent venipunctures should be performed proximal to a previously used or injured vein. **INS**

A peripheral catheter allows administration of fluids, medication, blood, and blood components and maintains I.V. access to the patient. Insertion is contraindicated in a sclerotic vein, an edematous or impaired arm or hand, or in a postmastectomy arm and in patients with burns or an arteriovenous fistula. If the catheter has to be inserted in the postmastectomy arm or one with impaired circulation, the practitioner should be contacted and an order written before starting therapy. **INS**

Equipment

Chlorhexidine solution ◆ gloves ◆ tourniquet (rubber tubing or a blood pressure cuff) ◆ I.V. access devices ◆ I.V. solution with attached and primed administration set ◆ I.V. pole ◆ sharps container ◆ sterile 2″ × 2″ gauze pads, transparent semipermeable dressing, or catheter securement device ◆ hypoallergenic tape ◆ optional: arm board, roller gauze, tube gauze, warm packs, scissors.

Commercial venipuncture kits come with or without an I.V. access device. (See *Comparing venous access devices,* page 386.)

Implementation

▶ Check the information on the label of the I.V. solution container, including the patient's name and room number, type of solution, time and date of its preparation, preparer's name, and ordered infusion rate. Compare the practitioner's orders with the solution label to verify that the solution is the correct one. **JC** **ISMP**

▶ Select the smallest-gauge device that's appropriate for the infusion (unless subsequent therapy will require a larger one). Smaller gauges cause less trauma to veins, allow greater blood flow around their tips, and reduce the risk of phlebitis. **INS**

▶ If you're using a winged infusion set, connect the adapter to the administration set, and unclamp the line until fluid flows from the open end of the needle cover. Then close the clamp and place the needle on a sterile surface, such as the inside of its packaging. If you're using a catheter device, open its package to allow easy access.

▶ Confirm the patient's identity using two patient identifiers according to your facility's policy. **JC**

▶ Place the I.V. pole in the proper slot in the patient's bed frame. If you're using a portable I.V. pole, position it close to the patient.

▶ Hang the I.V. solution with attached primed administration set on the I.V. pole.

▶ Wash your hands thoroughly. **INS** **CDC** **AACN**

▶ Explain the procedure to the patient to ensure his cooperation and reduce anxiety. Anxiety can cause a vasomotor response resulting in venous constriction.

Selecting the site

▶ Select the puncture site. If long-term therapy is anticipated, start with a vein at the most distal site so that you can move proximally as needed for subsequent I.V. insertion sites. For infusion of an irritating medication, choose a large vein distal to any nearby joint. Make sure the intended vein can accommodate the cannula. **INS**

▶ Place the patient in a comfortable, reclining position, leaving the arm in a dependent position to increase venous fill of the lower arms and hands. If the patient's skin is cold, warm it by rubbing and stroking the arm, or cover the entire arm with warm packs or submerge in warm water for 5 to 10 minutes.

Comparing venous access devices

Most I.V. infusions are delivered through one of two basic types of venous access devices: an over-the-needle cannula, or a winged infusion set. To improve I.V. therapy and guard against accidental needle sticks, use a needle-free system and shielded or retracting peripheral I.V. catheters.

Over-the-needle cannula

Purpose: Long-term therapy for an active or agitated patient

Advantages: More comfortable for the patient when it's in place; contains radiopaque thread for easy location. Some units come with a syringe that permits easy check of blood return; some units include wings. Activity-restricting devices such as arm board rarely needed.

Disadvantage: More difficult to insert than other devices.

Winged infusion set

Purpose: Short-term therapy for cooperative adult patient; therapy of any duration for a neonate or a child or for an elderly patient with fragile or sclerotic veins

Advantages: Less painful to insert; ideal for nonirritating I.V. push drugs.

Disadvantage: May easily cause infiltration. Not ideal for longer therapy.

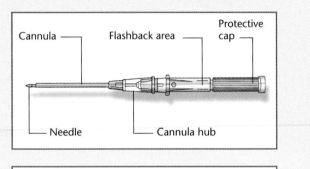

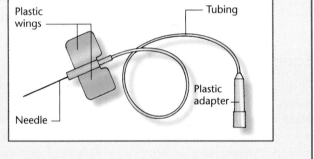

Applying the tourniquet

▶ Apply a tourniquet about 6″ (15 cm) above the intended puncture site to dilate the vein. Check for a radial pulse. If it isn't present, release the tourniquet and reapply it with less tension to prevent arterial occlusion. **INS**

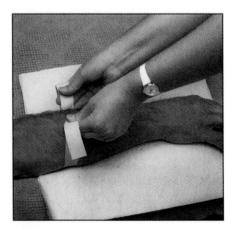

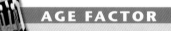

AGE FACTOR

Apply the tourniquet carefully to avoid pinching the skin. If necessary, apply it over the patient's gown.

▶ Lightly palpate the vein with the index and middle fingers of your nondominant hand. Stretch the skin to anchor the vein. If the vein feels hard or ropelike, select another.

▶ If the vein is easily palpable but not sufficiently dilated, one or more of the following techniques may help raise the vein. Place the extremity in a dependent position for several seconds, and gently tap your finger over the vein or rub or stroke the skin upward toward the tourniquet. If you have selected a vein in the arm or hand, tell the patient to open and close his fist several times.

▶ Leave the tourniquet in place for no longer than 3 minutes. If you can't find a suitable vein and prepare the site in that time, release the tourniquet for a few minutes. Then reapply it and continue the procedure.

Preparing the site

▶ If ordered, administer a local anesthetic. Make sure the patient isn't sensitive to lidocaine. **INS** **CS1**

▶ Put on gloves. Clip the hair around the insertion site if needed. Clean the site with chlorhexidine solution using a back and forth scrubbing motion. Allow the antimicrobial solution to dry (as shown at top of next column). **INS** **CDC** **AACN** **CS2**

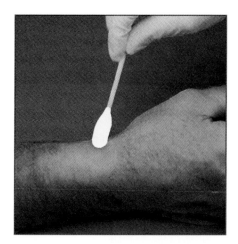

► Lightly press the vein with the thumb of your nondominant hand about 1¹/₂" (4 cm) from the intended insertion site. The vein should feel round, firm, fully engorged, and resilient.

► Grasp the access cannula. If you're using a winged infusion set, hold the short edges of the wings (with the needle's bevel facing upward) between the thumb and forefinger of your dominant hand. Then squeeze the wings together. If you're using an over-the-needle cannula, grasp the plastic hub with your dominant hand, remove the cover, and examine the cannula tip. If the edge isn't smooth, discard and replace the device.

► Using the thumb of your nondominant hand, stretch the skin taut below the puncture site to stabilize the vein.

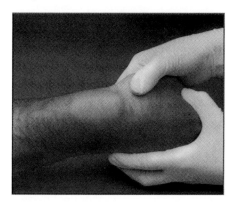

► Tell the patient that you are about to insert the device.

► Hold the needle bevel up and enter the skin directly over the vein at a 15- to 25-degree angle.

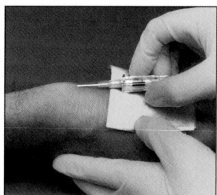

► Aggressively push the needle directly through the skin and into the vein in one motion. Check the flashback chamber behind the hub for blood return, signifying that the vein has been properly accessed. (You may not see blood return in a small vein.)

► Then level the insertion device slightly by lifting the tip of the device up to prevent puncturing the back wall of the vein with the access device.

► If you're using a winged infusion set, advance the needle fully, if possible, and hold it in place. Release the tourniquet, open the administration set clamp slightly, and check for free flow or infiltration.

► If you're using an over-the-needle cannula, advance the device to at least half its length to ensure that the cannula itself—not just the introducer needle—has entered the vein. Then remove the tourniquet.

► Grasp the cannula hub to hold it in the vein, and withdraw the needle. As you withdraw it, press lightly on the catheter tip to prevent bleeding (as shown at top of next column).

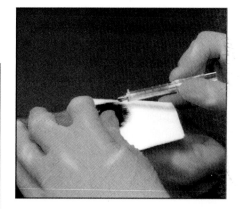

► Advance the cannula up to the hub or until you meet resistance.

► To advance the cannula while infusing I.V. solution, release the tourniquet and remove the inner needle. Using sterile technique, attach the I.V. tubing and begin the infusion. While stabilizing the vein with one hand, use the other to advance the catheter into the vein. When the catheter is advanced, decrease the I.V. flow rate. This method reduces the risk of puncturing the vein's opposite wall because the catheter is advanced without the steel needle and because the rapid flow dilates the vein.

► To advance the cannula before starting the infusion, first release the tourniquet. While stabilizing the vein and needle with one hand, use the other to advance the catheter off the needle and further into the vein up to the hub. Next, remove the inner needle and, using sterile technique, quickly attach the I.V. tubing. This method commonly results in less blood being spilled.

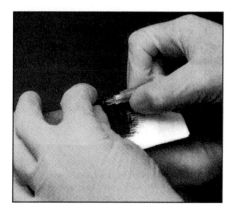

Dressing the site

▶ After the venous access device has been inserted, clean the skin completely. Dispose of the stylet in a sharps container. Then regulate the flow rate. **CDC**

▶ Secure the catheter using a commercial catheter securement device. If that isn't available, use sterile tape or sterile surgical strips to secure the catheter. Then cover the site with a sterile transparent semipermeable dressing. (See *How to apply a transparent semipermeable dressing*.) **INS** **CDC**

▶ Loop the I.V. tubing on the patient's limb, and secure the tubing with tape. The loop allows some slack to prevent dislodgment of the cannula from tension on the line. (See *Methods of taping a venous access site*.)

▶ Label the last piece of tape with the type, gauge of needle, and length of cannula; date and time of insertion; and your initials. Adjust the flow rate as ordered.

▶ If the puncture site is near a movable joint, place an arm board under the joint, and secure it with roller gauze or tape to provide stability because excessive movement can dislodge the venous access device and increase the risk of thrombophlebitis and infection.

▶ When an arm board is used, check frequently for impaired circulation distal to the infusion site.

Removing a peripheral I.V. line

▶ A peripheral I.V. line is removed on completion of therapy, for cannula site changes, and for suspected infection or infiltration; the procedure usually requires gloves, a sterile gauze pad, and an adhesive bandage. **INS** **CDC**

▶ To remove the I.V. line, first clamp the I.V. tubing to stop the flow of solution. Then gently remove the transparent dressing and all tape from the skin (as shown top of next column).

How to apply a transparent semipermeable dressing

To secure the I.V. insertion site, you can apply a transparent semipermeable dressing.

▶ Make sure the insertion site is clean and dry.

▶ Remove the dressing from the package and, using sterile technique, remove the protective seal. Avoid touching the sterile surface.

▶ Place the dressing directly over the insertion site and the hub, as shown below. Don't cover the tubing. Also, don't stretch the dressing because doing so may cause itching.

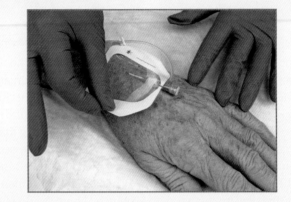

▶ Tuck the dressing around and under the cannula hub to make the site impervious to microorganisms.

▶ To remove the dressing, grasp one corner, and then lift and stretch it. If removal is difficult, try loosening the edges with alcohol or water.

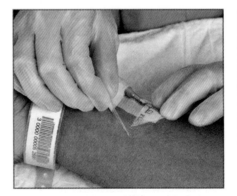

▶ Using sterile technique, open the gauze pad and adhesive bandage and place them within reach. Put on gloves. Hold the sterile gauze pad over the puncture site with one hand, and use your other hand to withdraw the cannula slowly and smoothly, keeping it parallel to the skin (as shown top of next column).

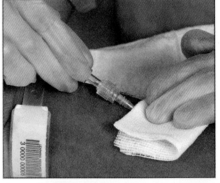

▶ Inspect the cannula tip; if it isn't smooth, assess the patient immediately, and notify the practitioner. **INS**

▶ Using the gauze pad, apply firm pressure over the puncture site for 1 to 2 minutes after removal or until bleeding has stopped. **INS**

Methods of taping a venous access site

If you'll be using tape to secure the access device to the insertion site, use one of the basic methods described below. Use sterile tape if you'll be placing a transparent dressing over the tape.

Chevron method
▶ Cut a long strip of ½" tape, and place it sticky side up under the cannula and parallel to the short strip of tape.
▶ Cross the ends of the tape over the cannula so that the tape sticks to the patient's skin (as shown below).
▶ Apply a piece of 1" tape across the two wings of the chevron.
▶ Loop the tubing, and secure it with another piece of 1" tape. When the dressing is secured, apply a label. On the label, write the date and time of insertion, type and gauge of the needle, and your initials.

U method
▶ Cut a 2" (5-cm) strip of ½" tape. With the sticky side up, place it under the hub of the cannula.
▶ Bring each side of the tape up, folding it over the wings of the cannula in a U shape (as shown below). Press it down parallel to the hub.
▶ Apply tape to stabilize the catheter.
▶ When a dressing is secured, apply a label. On the label, write the date and time of insertion, type and gauge of the needle or cannula, and your initials.

H method
▶ Cut three strips of 1" tape.
▶ Place one strip of tape over each wing, keeping the tape parallel to the cannula (as shown below).
▶ Now place the other strip of tape perpendicular to the first two. Put it either directly on top of the wings or just below the wings, directly on top of the tubing.
▶ Make sure the cannula is secure; then apply a dressing and a label. On the label, write the date and time of insertion, type and gauge of needle or cannula, and your initials.

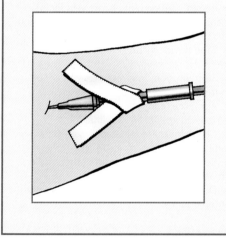

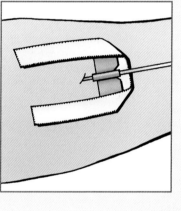

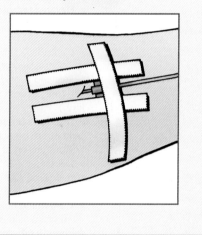

▶ Clean the site and apply the adhesive bandage or, if blood oozes, apply a pressure bandage.

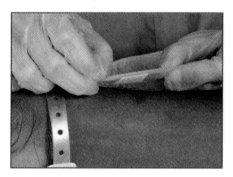

▶ If drainage appears at the puncture site, swab the tip of the device across an agar plate, or cut the tip into a sterile container using sterile scissors, and send it to the laboratory to be cultured according to your facility's policy. (A draining site may or may not be infected.) Then clean the area, apply a sterile dressing, and notify the practitioner. **INS**
▶ Instruct the patient to restrict activity for about 10 minutes and to leave the dressing in place for at least 1 hour.

If the patient experiences lingering tenderness at the site, apply warm packs and notify the practitioner.

Special considerations
▶ If you fail to see blood flashback after the needle enters the vein, pull back slightly and rotate the device. If you still fail to see flashback, remove the cannula and try again or proceed according to your facility's policy.

▶ Change a gauze or transparent dressing whenever you change the administration set (every 48 hours or according to your facility's policy). **INS** **CDC**

▶ Be sure to rotate the I.V. site every 72 hours or according to your facility's policy. **INS** **AACN** **CDC**

▶ Peripheral line complications can result from the needle or catheter (infection, phlebitis, and embolism) or from the solution (circulatory overload, infiltration, sepsis, and allergic reaction). (See *Risks of peripheral I.V. therapy.*)

(Text continues on page 395.)

Risks of peripheral I.V. therapy

COMPLICATION	SIGNS AND SYMPTOMS	POSSIBLE CAUSES	NURSING INTERVENTIONS
Local complications			
Phlebitis	▶ Tenderness at tip of and proximal to venous access device ▶ Redness at tip of cannula and along vein ▶ Puffy area over vein ▶ Vein hard on palpation ▶ Elevated temperature	▶ Poor blood flow around venous access device ▶ Friction from cannula movement in vein ▶ Venous access device left in vein too long ▶ Drug or solution with high or low pH or high osmolarity ▶ Clotting at cannula tip	▶ Remove venous access device. ▶ Apply warm packs. ▶ Notify practitioner. ▶ Document patient's condition and your interventions. **Prevention** ▶ Restart infusion using larger vein for irrigating solution, or restart with smaller-gauge device *to ensure adequate blood flow.* ▶ Tape device securely *to prevent motion.*
Infiltration	▶ Swelling at and above I.V. site (may extend along entire limb) ▶ Discomfort, burning, or pain at site (may be painless) ▶ Tight feeling at site ▶ Decreased skin temperature around site ▶ Blanching at site ▶ Continuing fluid infusion even when vein is occluded (although rate may decrease) ▶ Absent blood backflow ▶ Slower infusion rate	▶ Venous access device dislodged from vein, or perforated vein	▶ Stop infusion. Infiltrate site with an antidote, if appropriate. ▶ Apply ice (early) or warm packs (later) *to aid absorption.* Elevate limb. ▶ Check for pulse and capillary refill periodically *to assess circulation.* ▶ Restart infusion above infiltration site or in another limb. ▶ Document patient's condition and your interventions. **Prevention** ▶ Check I.V. site frequently. ▶ Don't obscure area above site with tape. ▶ Teach patient to observe I.V. site and report pain or swelling.
Cannula dislodgment	▶ Cannula partly backed out of vein ▶ Solution infiltrating	▶ Loosened tape, or tubing snagged in bed linens, resulting in partial retraction of cannula; pulled out by confused patient	▶ If no infiltration occurs, retape without pushing cannula back into vein. If pulled out, apply pressure to I.V. site with sterile dressing. **Prevention** ▶ Tape venipuncture device securely on insertion.

Risks of peripheral I.V. therapy *(continued)*

COMPLICATION	SIGNS AND SYMPTOMS	POSSIBLE CAUSES	NURSING INTERVENTIONS
Local complications *(continued)*			
Occlusion	▶ Infusion doesn't flow ▶ Infusion pump alarms indicating occlusion ▶ Discomfort at infusion site	▶ I.V. flow interrupted ▶ Saline lock not flushed ▶ Blood backflow in line when patient walks ▶ Line clamped too long ▶ Hypercoaguble patient	▶ Use mild flush injection. Don't force it. If unsuccessful, remove I.V. line and reinsert a new one. **Prevention** ▶ Maintain I.V. flow rate. ▶ Flush promptly after intermittent piggyback administration. ▶ Have patient walk with his arm bent at the elbow *to reduce risk of blood backflow.*
Vein irritation or pain at I.V. site	▶ Pain during infusion ▶ Possible blanching if vasospasm occurs ▶ Red skin over vein during infusion ▶ Rapidly developing signs of phlebitis	▶ Solution with high or low pH or high osmolarity, such as phenytoin, and some antibiotics (vancomycin and nafcillin)	▶ Decrease the flow rate. ▶ Try using an electronic flow device to achieve a steady flow. **Prevention** ▶ Dilute solutions before administration. For example, give antibiotics in 250-ml solution rather than 100-ml solution. If drug has low pH, ask pharmacist if drug can be buffered with sodium bicarbonate. (Refer to your facility's policy.) ▶ If long-term therapy of irritating drug is planned, ask practitioner to use central I.V. line.
Hematoma	▶ Tenderness at venipuncture site ▶ Bruised area around site ▶ Inability to advance or flush I.V. line	▶ Vein punctured through opposite wall at time of insertion ▶ Leakage of blood from needle displacement	▶ Remove venous access device. ▶ Apply pressure and warm packs to affected area. ▶ Recheck for bleeding. ▶ Document patient's condition and your interventions. **Prevention** ▶ Choose a vein that can accommodate the size of venous access device. ▶ Release tourniquet as soon as insertion is successful.

(continued)

Risks of peripheral I.V. therapy (continued)

COMPLICATION	SIGNS AND SYMPTOMS	POSSIBLE CAUSES	NURSING INTERVENTIONS
Local complications (continued)			
Severed cannula	▶ Leakage from cannula shaft	▶ Cannula inadvertently cut by scissors ▶ Reinsertion of needle into cannula	▶ If broken part is visible, attempt to retrieve it. If unsuccessful, notify the practitioner. ▶ If portion of cannula enters bloodstream, place tourniquet above I.V. site *to prevent progression of broken part.* ▶ Notify practitioner and radiology department. ▶ Document patient's condition and your interventions. **Prevention** ▶ Don't use scissors around I.V. site. ▶ Never reinsert needle into cannula. ▶ Remove unsuccessfully inserted cannula and needle together.
Venous spasm	▶ Pain along vein ▶ Flow rate sluggish when clamp completely open ▶ Blanched skin over vein	▶ Severe vein irritation from irritating drugs or fluids ▶ Administration of cold fluids or blood ▶ Very rapid flow rate (with fluids at room temperature)	▶ Apply warm packs over vein and surrounding area. ▶ Decrease flow rate. **Prevention** ▶ Use a blood warmer for blood or packed red blood cells.
Vasovagal reaction	▶ Sudden collapse of vein during venipuncture ▶ Sudden pallor, sweating, faintness, dizziness, and nausea ▶ Decreased blood pressure	▶ Vasospasm from anxiety or pain	▶ Lower head of bed. ▶ Have patient take deep breaths. ▶ Check vital signs. **Prevention** ▶ Prepare patient for therapy *to relieve his anxiety.* ▶ Use local anesthetic *to prevent pain.*
Thrombosis	▶ Painful, reddened, and swollen vein ▶ Sluggish or stopped I.V. flow	▶ Injury to endothelial cells of vein wall, allowing platelets to adhere and thrombi to form	▶ Remove venous access device; restart infusion in opposite limb if possible. ▶ Apply warm packs. ▶ Watch for I.V. therapy–related infection; thrombi provide an excellent environment for bacterial growth. **Prevention** ▶ Use proper venipuncture techniques *to reduce injury to vein.*
Thrombophlebitis	▶ Severe discomfort ▶ Reddened, swollen, and hardened vein	▶ Thrombosis and inflammation	▶ Same as for thrombosis. **Prevention** ▶ Check site frequently. Remove venous access device at first sign of redness and tenderness.

Risks of peripheral I.V. therapy *(continued)*

COMPLICATION	SIGNS AND SYMPTOMS	POSSIBLE CAUSES	NURSING INTERVENTIONS
Local complications *(continued)*			
Nerve, tendon, or ligament damage	▶ Extreme pain (similar to electrical shock when nerve is punctured) ▶ Numbness and muscle contraction ▶ Delayed effects, including paralysis, numbness, and deformity	▶ Improper venipuncture technique, resulting in injury to surrounding nerves, tendons, or ligaments ▶ Tight taping or improper splinting with arm board	▶ Stop procedure and remove device. **Prevention** ▶ Don't repeatedly penetrate tissues with venous access device. ▶ Don't apply excessive pressure when taping; don't encircle limb with tape. ▶ Pad arm boards and tape, securing arm boards if possible.
Systemic complications			
Systemic infection (septicemia or bacteremia)	▶ Fever, chills, and malaise for no apparent reason ▶ Contaminated I.V. site, usually with no visible signs of infection at site	▶ Failure to maintain sterile technique during insertion or site care ▶ Severe phlebitis, which can set up ideal conditions for organism growth ▶ Poor taping that permits venous access device to move, which can introduce organisms into bloodstream ▶ Prolonged indwelling time of device ▶ Weak immune system	▶ Notify practitioner. ▶ Administer medications as prescribed. ▶ Culture site and device. ▶ Monitor vital signs. **Prevention** ▶ Use scrupulous sterile technique when handling solutions and tubing, inserting venous access device, and discontinuing infusion. ▶ Secure all connections. ▶ Change I.V. solutions, tubing, and venous access device at recommended times. ▶ Use I.V. filters.
Allergic reaction	▶ Itching ▶ Watery eyes and nose ▶ Bronchospasm ▶ Wheezing ▶ Urticarial rash ▶ Edema at I.V. site ▶ Anaphylactic reaction (flushing, chills, anxiety, itching, palpitations, paresthesia, wheezing, seizures, cardiac arrest) after exposure	▶ Allergens such as medications	▶ If reaction occurs, stop infusion immediately, and infuse normal saline solution. ▶ Maintain a patent airway. ▶ Notify practitioner. ▶ Administer antihistaminic steroid, anti-inflammatory, and antipyretic drugs, as prescribed. ▶ Give epinephrine as prescribed. Repeat as needed and prescribed. ▶ Administer cortisone if prescribed. **Prevention** ▶ Obtain patient's allergy history. Be aware of crossallergies. ▶ Assist with test dosing. ▶ Monitor patient carefully during first 15 minutes of administration of a new drug.

(continued)

Risks of peripheral I.V. therapy (continued)

COMPLICATION	SIGNS AND SYMPTOMS	POSSIBLE CAUSES	NURSING INTERVENTIONS
Systemic complications (continued)			
Circulatory overload	▶ Discomfort ▶ Jugular vein engorgement ▶ Respiratory distress ▶ Increased blood pressure ▶ Crackles ▶ Increased difference between fluid intake and output	▶ Roller clamp loosened to allow run-on infusion ▶ Flow rate too rapid ▶ Miscalculation of fluid requirements	▶ Raise head of bed. ▶ Administer oxygen as needed. ▶ Slow infusion rate; don't remove I.V. line. ▶ Notify practitioner. ▶ Administer medications (probably furosemide) as prescribed. **Prevention** ▶ Use pump or rate minder for elderly or compromised patients. ▶ Recheck calculations of fluid requirements. ▶ Monitor infusion frequently.
Air embolism	▶ Respiratory distress ▶ Unequal breath sounds ▶ Weak pulse ▶ Increased central venous pressure ▶ Decreased blood pressure ▶ Loss of consciousness	▶ Solution container empty ▶ Solution container empties, and added container pushes air down the line (if line wasn't purged first) ▶ Tubing disconnected from venous access device or I.V. bag	▶ Discontinue infusion. ▶ Place patient on his left side in Trendelenburg's position *to allow air to enter right atrium.* ▶ Administer oxygen. ▶ Notify practitioner. ▶ Document patient's condition and your interventions. **Prevention** ▶ Purge tubing of air completely before starting infusion. ▶ Use air-detection device on pump or air-eliminating filter proximal to I.V. site. ▶ Secure all connections.

Selected references

Centers for Disease Control and Prevention. "Guidelines for the Prevention of Intravascular Device-related Infections," *MMWR* 51(RR-10):1–26, August 9, 2002.

Chaiyakunapruk, N, et al. "Chlorhexidine compared with povidone-iodine solution for vascular catheter-site care: a meta-analysis," *Annals of Internal Medicine* 136(11):792–801, June 2002. **CS2**

Fetzer, S. J. "Reducing venipuncture and intravenous insertion pain with eutectic mixture of local anesthetic: a meta-analysis," Nursing Research 51(2):119–24, March–April 2002. **CS1**

Rosenthal, K. "Tailor your I.V. Insertion Techniques Special Populations," *Nursing* 35(5):36–41; quiz 41-2, May 2005.

Rosenthal, K. "Get a Hold on Costs and Safety with Securement Devices," *Nursing Management* 36(5):52–54, May 2005.

"Standard 36. Tourniquet. Infusion Nursing Standards of Practice," *Journal of Infusion Nursing* 29(1S):S36, January–February 2006.

"Standard 37. Site Selection. Infusion Nursing Standards of Practice," *Journal of Infusion Nursing* 29(1S):S37–39, January–February 2006.

"Standard 38. Catheter Selection. Infusion Nursing Standards of Practice," *Journal of Infusion Nursing* 29(1S):S38–40, January–February 2006.

"Standard 39. Hair Removal. Infusion Nursing Standards of Practice," *Journal of Infusion Nursing* 29(1S):S40–41, January–February 2006.

"Standard 40. Local Anesthesia. Infusion Nursing Standards of Practice," *Journal of Infusion Nursing* 29(1S):S41, January–February 2006.

"Standard 41. Access Site Preparation. Infusion Nursing Standards of Practice," *Journal of Infusion Nursing*

29(1S):S41–42, January–February 2006.

"Standard 42. Catheter Placement. Infusion Nursing Standards of Practice," *Journal of Infusion Nursing* 29(1S):S42–44, January–February 2006.

"Standard 43. Catheter Stabilization. Infusion Nursing Standards of Practice," *Journal of Infusion Nursing* 29(1S):S44, January–February 2006.

"Standard 44. Dressings. Infusion Nursing Standards of Practice," *Journal of Infusion Nursing* 29(1S):S44–45, January–February 2006.

"Standard 49. Catheter Removal. Infusion Nursing Standards of Practice," *Journal of Infusion Nursing* 29(1S):S36, January–February 2006.

Peripheral I.V. maintenance

Routine maintenance of I.V. sites and systems includes regular assessment and rotation of the site and periodic changes of the dressing, solution, and tubing. These measures help prevent complications, such as thrombophlebitis and infection. They should be performed according to your facility's policy.

Typically, gauze I.V. dressings are changed every 48 hours or whenever the dressing becomes wet, soiled, or nonocclusive. Transparent semipermeable dressings are changed whenever I.V. tubing is changed. I.V. tubing is changed every 72 hours or according to your facility's policy, and I.V. solution is changed every 24 hours or as needed. The site should be assessed every 2 hours if a transparent semipermeable dressing is used (or with every dressing change otherwise) and should be rotated every 72 hours. Sometimes, limited venous access prevents regular site changes; if so, be sure to assess the site frequently. **INS** **CDC** **AACN**

Equipment

For dressing changes: Sterile gloves ◆ antimicrobial solution ◆ adhesive bandage, sterile 2″ × 2″ gauze pad, or transparent semipermeable dressing ◆ 1″ adhesive tape.

For solution changes: Solution container ◆ alcohol pad.

For tubing changes: I.V. administration set ◆ sterile gloves ◆ sterile 2″ × 2″ gauze pad ◆ adhesive tape for labeling ◆ optional: hemostats.

Commercial kits containing the equipment for dressing changes are available.

Implementation

▶ If you're changing the solution and tubing, attach and prime the I.V. administration set before entering the patient's room.

▶ Confirm the patient's identity using two patient identifiers according to your facility's policy. **JC**

▶ Wash your hands thoroughly to prevent the spread of microorganisms. Remember to wear sterile gloves whenever working near the venipuncture site. **CDC** **INS** **AACN**

▶ Explain the procedure to the patient to allay his fears and ensure cooperation.

Changing the dressing

▶ Open all supply packages, put on gloves, and remove the old dressing.

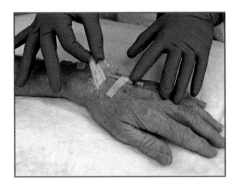

▶ Hold the cannula in place with your nondominant hand to prevent accidental movement or dislodgment.

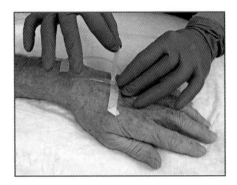

▶ Assess the venipuncture site for signs of infection (redness and pain at the puncture site), infiltration (coolness, blanching, and edema at the site), and thrombophlebitis (redness, firmness, pain along the path of the vein, and edema). If signs are present, cover the area with a sterile 2″ × 2″ gauze pad and remove the catheter. Apply pressure to the area until the bleeding stops, and apply an adhesive bandage. Then, using fresh equipment and solution, start the I.V. in another appropriate site, preferably on the opposite extremity.

▶ If the venipuncture site is intact, stabilize the cannula and carefully clean around the puncture site with antimicrobial solution. Work in a circular motion outward from the site to avoid introducing bacteria into the clean area. Allow the area to dry completely.

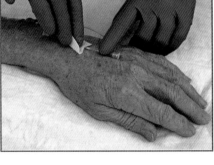

▶ Cover the site with a transparent semipermeable dressing. The transparent dressing allows visualization of the insertion site and maintains sterility. It's placed over the insertion site to halfway up the cannula (as shown at top of next column). **INS**

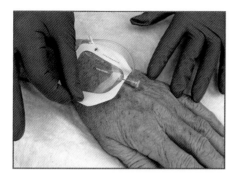

▶ Label the dressing with the date and time of the procedure.

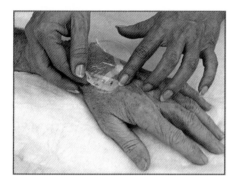

Changing the solution
▶ Wash your hands.
▶ Inspect the new solution container for cracks, leaks, and other damage. Check the solution for discoloration, turbidity, and particulates. Note the date and time the solution was mixed and its expiration date.
▶ Clamp the tubing when inverting it to prevent air from entering the tubing. Keep the drip chamber half full.
▶ If you're replacing a bag, remove the seal or tab from the new bag and remove the old bag from the pole. Remove the spike, insert it into the new bag, and adjust the flow rate.
▶ If you're replacing a bottle, remove the cap and seal from the new bottle and wipe the rubber port with an alcohol pad. Clamp the line, remove the spike from the old bottle, and insert the spike into the new bottle. Then hang the new bottle and adjust the flow rate.

Changing the tubing
▶ Reduce the I.V. flow rate, remove the old spike from the container, and hang it on the I.V. pole. Place the cover of the new spike loosely over the old one.
▶ Keeping the old spike in an upright position above the patient's heart level, insert the new spike into the I.V. container.

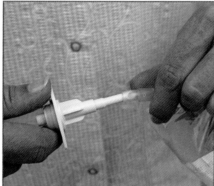

▶ Prime the system. Hang the new I.V. container and primed set on the pole, and grasp the new adapter in one hand. Then stop the flow rate in the old tubing.
▶ Put on sterile gloves.
▶ Place a sterile gauze pad under the needle or cannula hub to create a sterile field. Press one of your fingers over the cannula to prevent bleeding.
▶ Gently disconnect the old tubing, being careful not to dislodge or move the I.V. device (as shown at top of next column). (If you have trouble disconnecting the old tubing, use a hemostat to hold the hub securely while twisting the tubing to remove it. Or, use one hemostat on the venipuncture device and another on the hard plastic end of the tubing. Then pull the hemostats in opposite directions. Don't clamp the hemostats shut; this could crack the tubing adapter or the venipuncture device.)

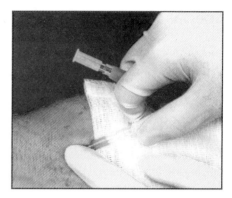

▶ Remove the protective cap from the new tubing, and connect the new adapter to the cannula. Hold the hub securely to prevent dislodging the needle or cannula tip.
▶ Observe for blood backflow into the new tubing to verify that the needle or cannula is still in place. (You may not be able to do this with small-gauge cannulas.)
▶ Adjust the clamp to maintain the appropriate flow rate.

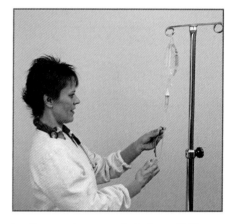

▶ Retape the cannula hub and I.V. tubing, and recheck the I.V. flow rate because taping may alter it.
▶ Label the new tubing and container with the date and time. Label the solution container with a time strip.

Special considerations

▶ Check the prescribed I.V. flow rate before each solution change to prevent errors.

▶ If you crack the adapter or hub (or if you accidentally dislodge the cannula from the vein), remove the cannula. Apply pressure and an adhesive bandage to stop any bleeding. Perform a venipuncture at another site and restart the I.V.

Selected references

Centers for Disease Control and Prevention. "Guidelines for the Prevention of Intravascular Catheter-related Infections," *MMWR* 51(RR-10):1–26, August 9, 2002.

Hindley, G. "Infection Control in Peripheral Cannulae," *Nursing Standard* 18(27):37–40, March 2004.

The Joint Commission. *Comprehensive Accreditation Manual for Hospitals: The Official Handbook*. Standard MM.3.10. Oakbrook Terrace, Ill.: The Joint Commission, 2007.

The Joint Commission. *Comprehensive Accreditation Manual for Hospitals: The Official Handbook*. Standard MM.4.20. Oakbrook Terrace, Ill.: The Joint Commission, 2007.

The Joint Commission. *Comprehensive Accreditation Manual for Hospitals: The Official Handbook*. Standard MM.4.30. Oakbrook Terrace, Ill.: The Joint Commission, 2007.

The Joint Commission. *Comprehensive Accreditation Manual for Hospitals: The Official Handbook*. Standard MM.5.10. Oakbrook Terrace, Ill.: The Joint Commission, 2007.

"Standard 14. Documentation. Infusion Nursing Standards of Practice," *Journal of Infusion Nursing* 29(1S):S22–23, January–February 2006.

"Standard 16. Product Labeling. Infusion Nursing Standards of Practice," *Journal of Infusion Nursing* 29(1S):S23–24, January–February 2006.

"Standard 23. Expiration and Beyond-use Dates. Infusion Nursing Standards of Practice," *Journal of Infusion Nursing* 29(1S):S29, January–February 2006.

"Standard 44. Dressings. Infusion Nursing Standards of Practice," *Journal of Infusion Nursing* 29(1S):S44–45, January–February 2006.

"Standard 48. Administration Set Change. Infusion Nursing Standards of Practice," *Journal of Infusion Nursing* 29(1S):S48–49, January–February 2006.

"Standard 51. Catheter Site Care. Infusion Nursing Standards of Practice," *Journal of Infusion Nursing* 29(1S):S57–56, January–February 2006.

"Standard 53. Phlebitis. Infusion Nursing Standards of Practice," *Journal of Infusion Nursing* 29(1S):S58–59, January–February 2006.

"Standard 54. Infiltration. Infusion Nursing Standards of Practice," *Journal of Infusion Nursing* 29(1S):S59–60, January–February 2006.

"Standard 55. Extravasation. Infusion Nursing Standards of Practice," *Journal of Infusion Nursing* 29(1S):S61–62, January–February 2006.

"Standard 56. Infection. Infusion Nursing Standards of Practice," *Journal of Infusion Nursing* 29(1S):S62–63, January–February 2006.

Peripheral I.V. therapy preparation

The selection and preparation of the appropriate equipment are essential for the accurate delivery of an I.V. solution. Selection of an I.V. administration set depends on the rate and type of infusion desired and the type of I.V. solution container used. Two types of drip sets are available: the macrodrip and the microdrip. The macrodrip set can deliver a solution in large quantities at rapid rates because it delivers a larger amount with each drop. The microdrip set, typically used for pediatric patients and certain adult patients who require small or closely regulated amounts of I.V. solution, delivers a smaller quantity with each drop.

Administration tubing with a secondary injection port permits separate or simultaneous infusion of two solutions; tubing with a piggyback port and a backcheck valve permits intermittent infusion of a secondary solution and, on its completion, a return to infusion of the primary solution. Vented I.V. tubing is selected for solutions in nonvented bottles; nonvented tubing is selected for solutions in bags or vented bottles. Assembly of I.V. equipment requires sterile technique to prevent contamination, which can cause local or systemic infection.

According to the Infusion Nurses Society standards, primary and secondary sets should be changed every 72 hours, using sterile technique and immediately upon suspected contamination or when the integrity of the system has been compromised. **INS** **CDC** **AACN**

Equipment

I.V. solution ◆ alcohol pad ◆ I.V. administration set ◆ in-line filter, if needed ◆ I.V. pole ◆ medication and label, if necessary.

Implementation

▶ Wash your hands thoroughly to prevent introducing contaminants during preparation. **INS** **CDC** **AACN**

▶ Verify the type, volume, and expiration date of the I.V. solution. Discard outdated solution. If the solution is contained in a glass bottle, inspect the bottle for chips and cracks; if it's in a plastic bag, squeeze the bag to detect leaks. Examine the I.V. solution for particles, abnormal discoloration, and cloudiness. If present, discard the solution and notify the pharmacy or dispensing department.

▶ If ordered, add medication to the solution, and place a completed medication-added label on the container.

▶ Remove the administration set from its box, and check for cracks, holes, and missing clamps.

▶ Slide the flow clamp of the administration set tubing down to the drip chamber or injection port, and close the clamp.

Preparing a bag

▶ Place the bag on a flat, stable surface or hang it on an I.V. pole.

▶ Remove the protective cap or tear the tab from the tubing insertion port.

▶ Remove the protective cap from the administration set spike.

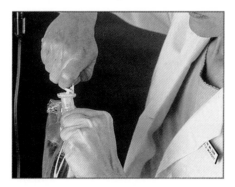

▶ Holding the port firmly with one hand, insert the spike with your other hand (as shown at top of next column).

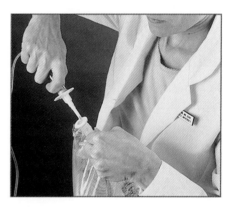

▶ Hang the bag on the I.V. pole, if you haven't already, and squeeze the drip chamber until it's half full.

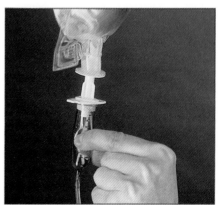

Preparing a nonvented bottle

▶ Remove the bottle's metal cap and inner disk, if present.

▶ Place the bottle on a stable surface or hang it on the I.V. pole.

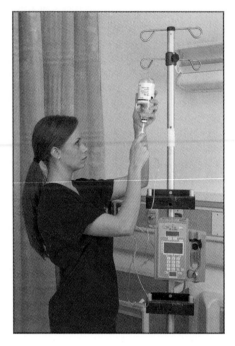

▶ Wipe the rubber stopper with an alcohol pad.

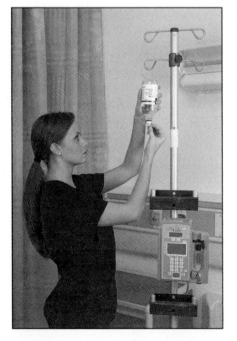

▶ Remove the protective cap from the administration set spike, and push the

spike through the center of the bottle's rubber stopper. Avoid twisting or angling the spike to prevent pieces of the stopper from breaking off and falling into the solution.

If its vacuum is intact, you'll hear a hissing sound and see air bubbles rise. (This may not occur if you've already added medication.) If the vacuum isn't intact, discard the bottle and begin again.

▶ Squeeze the drip chamber until it's half full.

Preparing a vented bottle

▶ Remove the bottle's metal cap and latex diaphragm to release the vacuum. If the vacuum isn't intact (except after medication has been added), discard the bottle and begin again.

▶ Place the bottle on a stable surface, and wipe the rubber stopper with an alcohol pad.

▶ Remove the protective cap from the administration set spike, and push the spike through the insertion port next to the air vent tube opening.

▶ Hang the bottle on the I.V. pole, and squeeze the drip chamber until it's half full.

Priming the I.V. tubing

▶ If necessary, attach a filter to the opposite end of the I.V. tubing, and follow the manufacturer's instructions for filling and priming it. Purge the tubing before attaching the filter to avoid forcing air into the filter and possibly clogging some filter channels. **INS MFR**

▶ If you aren't using a filter, aim the distal end of the tubing over a wastebasket or sink and slowly open the flow clamp. (Most distal tube coverings allow the solution to flow without having to remove the protective cover.)

▶ Leave the clamp open until the I.V. solution flows through the entire length of tubing to release trapped air bubbles and force out all the air.

▶ Invert all Y-ports and backcheck valves and tap them, if necessary, to fill them with solution.

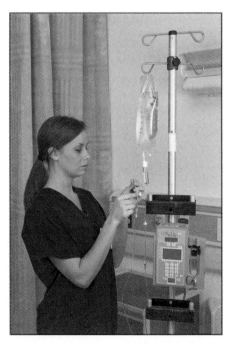

▶ After priming the tubing, close the clamp. Then loop the tubing over the I.V. pole.

▶ Label the container with the patient's name and room number, date and time, container number, ordered rate and duration of infusion, and your initials.

Special considerations

▶ Before initiating I.V. therapy, tell the patient what to expect.

▶ Always use sterile technique when preparing I.V. solutions. If you contaminate the administration set or container, replace it with a new one to prevent introducing contaminants into the system.

▶ If necessary, you can use vented tubing with a vented bottle. To do this, don't remove the latex diaphragm. Instead, insert the spike into the larger indentation in the diaphragm.

▶ Change I.V. tubing every 72 hours or according to your facility's policy or more frequently if you suspect contamination. Change the filter according to the manufacturer's recommendations or sooner if it becomes clogged. **INS**

Selected references

Hadaway, L. C. "Reopen the Pipeline for I.V. Therapy," *Nursing* 35(8):54–61; quiz 61–63, August 2005.

Higgins, D. "Priming an I.V. Infusion Set," *Nursing Times* 100(47):32–33, November 2004.

"Standard 11. Patient Education. Infusion Nursing Standards of Practice," *Journal of Infusion Nursing* 29(1S):S19–20, January–February 2006.

"Standard 14. Documentation. Infusion Nursing Standards of Practice," *Journal of Infusion Nursing* 29(1S):S22–S23, January–February 2006.

"Standard 15. Product Evaluation, Integrity, and Defect Reporting. Infusion Nursing Standards of Practice," *Journal of Infusion Nursing* 29(1S):S23, January–February 2006.

"Standard 16. Product Labeling. Infusion Nursing Standards of Practice," *Journal of Infusion Nursing* 29(1S):S23–S24, January–February 2006.

"Standard 19. Infection Control. Infusion Nursing Standards of Practice," *Journal of Infusion Nursing* 29(1S):S25–S26, January–February 2006.

"Standard 20. Hand Hygiene. Infusion Nursing Standards of Practice," *Journal of Infusion Nursing* 29(1S):S27–S28, January–February 2006.

"Standard 48. Administration Set Change. Infusion Nursing Standards of Practice," *Journal of Infusion Nursing* 29(15):S48–S51, January–February 2006.

Taylor, C., et al. *Fundamentals of Nursing: The Art and Science of Nursing Care,* 6th ed. Philadelphia: Lippincott Williams & Wilkins, 2008.

Zahourek, R. "Nursing the I.V. Tubing," *AJN* 105(10):15, October 2005.

Peripherally inserted central catheter use

Peripheral central venous (CV) therapy involves the insertion of a catheter into a peripheral vein instead of a central vein, but the catheter tip still lies in the CV circulation. A peripherally inserted central catheter (PICC) usually enters at the basilic vein and terminates in the subclavian vein or superior vena cava. A specially trained nurse may insert PICCs. (See *Understanding peripherally inserted central catheter lines*.)

For a patient who needs CV therapy for 1 to 6 months or who requires repeated venous access, a PICC may be the best option. PICCs are commonly used in home I.V. therapy, but may also be used with chest injury; chest, neck, or shoulder burns; compromised respiratory function; proximity of a surgical site to the CV line placement site; and if a practitioner isn't available to insert a CV line. With any of these conditions, a PICC helps avoid complications that may occur with a CV line.

If your state nurse practice act permits, you may insert a PICC if you show sufficient knowledge of vascular access devices. To prove your competence in PICC insertion, it's recommended that you complete an 8-hour workshop and demonstrate three successful catheter insertions. You may have to demonstrate competence every year.

Equipment

Catheter insertion kit ◆ chlorhexidine solution ◆ antiseptic ointment ◆ sterile syringes prefilled with flush solution ◆ injection port with short extension tubing ◆ sterile and clean measuring tape ◆ sterile gauze pads ◆ tape ◆ linen-saver pad ◆ sterile drapes ◆ tourniquet ◆ sterile transparent semipermeable dressing ◆ sterile marker ◆ sterile labels ◆ two pairs of sterile gloves ◆ sterile gown ◆ mask ◆ goggles ◆ clean gloves.

Understanding peripherally inserted central catheter lines

Description
▶ Silicone rubber
▶ 20″ to 24″ (51 to 61 cm) long; available in 14G, 16G, 18G, 20G, 22G, and 24G

Indications
▶ Long-term central venous (CV) access
▶ Patient with poor central access
▶ Patient at high risk for complications from insertion at CV access sites
▶ Patient who needs CV access but faces or has had head and neck surgery

Advantages
▶ Peripherally inserted
▶ Can be inserted at the bedside with minimal complications
▶ May be inserted by a trained, skilled, competent registered nurse in most states

Disadvantages
▶ May occlude smaller peripheral vessels
▶ May be difficult to keep immobile

Nursing considerations
▶ Check frequently for signs of phlebitis and thrombus formation.
▶ Insert the catheter above the antecubital fossa.
▶ Use an arm board, if necessary.
▶ The catheter may alter CV pressure measurements.

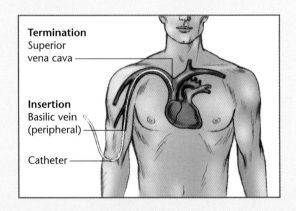

Termination
Superior vena cava

Insertion
Basilic vein (peripheral)

Catheter

Implementation

► Confirm the patient's identity using two patient identifiers according to your facility's policy. **JC**

► Describe the procedure to the patient, and answer any questions.

► Wash your hands.

► Prepare the sterile field. Label all medications, medication containers, and other solutions on and off the sterile field. **JC**

Inserting a PICC

► Select the insertion site, and place the tourniquet on the patient's arm. Assess the antecubital fossa.

► Remove the tourniquet.

► Determine catheter tip placement or the spot at which the catheter tip will rest after insertion.

► For placement in the superior vena cava, measure the distance from the insertion site to the shoulder and from the shoulder to the sternal notch. Then add 3″ (7.6 cm) to the measurement.

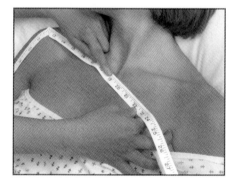

► Have the patient lie in a supine position with her arm at a 90-degree angle to her body. Place a linen-saver pad under her arm.

► Open the PICC tray and drop the rest of the sterile items onto the sterile field. Put on the sterile gown, mask, goggles, and sterile gloves. **CDC**

► Using the sterile measuring tape, cut the distal end of the catheter according to specific manufacturer's recommendations and guidelines, using

the equipment provided by the manufacturer. **MFR**

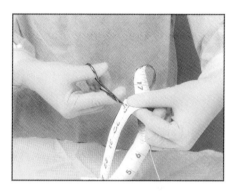

► Using sterile technique, flush the extension tubing and the cap with normal saline solution.

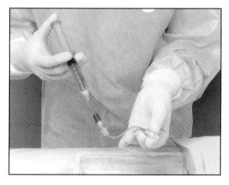

► Attach the syringe to the hub of the catheter and flush.

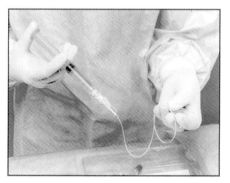

► Prepare the insertion site using chlorhexidine solution using a back and forth scrubbing motion. Allow the area to dry. Be sure not to touch the intended insertion site. **CDC** **INS** **AACN** **CS1**

► Take your gloves off. Then apply the tourniquet about 4″ (10 cm) above the antecubital fossa.

► Put on a new pair of sterile gloves. Then place a sterile drape under the patient's arm and another on top of her arm. Drop a sterile 4″ × 4″ gauze pad over the tourniquet.

► Stabilize the patient's vein. Insert the catheter introducer at a 10-degree angle, directly into the vein.

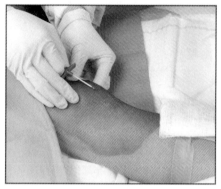

► After successful vein entry, you should see a blood return in the flashback chamber. Without changing the needle's position, gently advance the plastic introducer sheath until you're sure the tip is well within the vein.

► Carefully withdraw the needle while holding the introducer still. To minimize blood loss, try applying finger pressure on the vein just beyond the distal end of the introducer sheath.

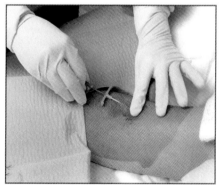

▶ Using sterile forceps, insert the catheter into the introducer sheath, and advance it into the vein 2″ to 4″ (5 to 10 cm).

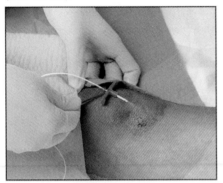

▶ Remove the tourniquet using a sterile 4″ × 4″ gauze pad to maintain sterile technique.

▶ When you have advanced the catheter to the shoulder, ask the patient to turn her head toward the affected arm and place her chin on her chest. This will occlude the jugular vein and ease the catheter's advancement into the subclavian vein.

▶ Advance the catheter until about 4″ remain. Then pull the introducer sheath out of the vein and away from the venipuncture site.

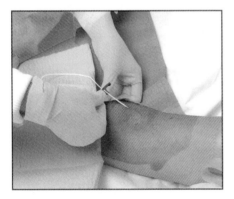

▶ Grasp the tabs of the introducer sheath, and flex them toward its distal end to split the sheath. **MFR**

▶ Pull the tabs apart and away from the catheter until the sheath is completely split. Discard the sheath. **MFR**

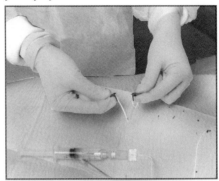

▶ Continue to advance the catheter until it's completely inserted. Flush with normal saline solution followed by heparin, according to your facility's policy.

▶ With the patient's arm below heart level, remove the syringe. Connect the capped extension set to the hub of the catheter.

▶ Apply a sterile 2″ × 2″ gauze pad directly over the site and a sterile transparent semipermeable dressing over the gauze pad. Leave this dressing in place for 24 hours.

▶ Confirm placement of the PICC with an X-ray. **INS** **CS**

▶ After the initial 24 hours, apply a new sterile transparent semipermeable dressing. The gauze pad is no longer necessary. You can place surgical strips over the catheter wings.

▶ Flush with heparin, according to your facility's policy.

Administering drugs

▶ As with any CV line, be sure to check for blood return and flush with normal saline solution before administering a drug through a PICC. **INS**

▶ Clamp the 7″ (17.8-cm) extension tubing, and connect the empty syringe to the tubing. Release the clamp and aspirate slowly to verify blood return.

Flush with 3 ml of normal saline solution, and then administer the drug.

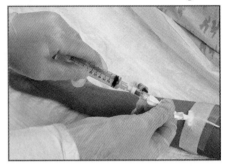

▶ After giving the drug, flush again with 3 ml of normal saline solution in a 10-ml syringe. (Remember to flush with the same solution between infusions of incompatible drugs or fluids.) Close the clamp.

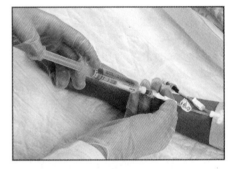

Changing the dressing

▶ Change the dressing every 2 to 7 days and more frequently if the integrity of the dressing becomes compromised. If possible, choose a transparent semipermeable dressing, which has a high moisture-vapor transmission rate. Use sterile technique. **CDC** **INS** **AACN**

▶ Wash your hands and assemble the necessary supplies. Position the patient with her arm extended away from her body at a 45- to 90-degree angle so that the insertion site is below heart level to reduce the risk of air embolism. Put on a sterile mask.

▶ Open a package of sterile gloves, and use the inside of the package as a sterile field. Then open the transparent semipermeable dressing and drop it onto the field. Put on clean gloves, and remove the old dressing by holding your left thumb on the catheter and stretching the dressing parallel to the skin. Repeat the last step with your right thumb holding the catheter. Free the remaining section of the dressing from the catheter by peeling toward the insertion site from the distal end to the proximal end to prevent catheter dislodgment. Remove the clean gloves.

▶ Put on sterile gloves. Clean the area thoroughly with chlorhexidine solution, using a back and forth scrubbing motion. Allow it to dry. **CDC** **INS** **AACN**

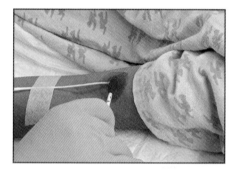

▶ Apply the dressing carefully. Secure the tubing to the edge of the dressing over the tape with ¼″ adhesive tape.

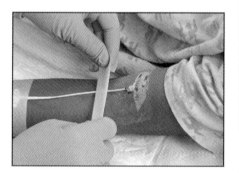

Removing a PICC

▶ You'll remove a PICC when therapy is complete, if the catheter becomes damaged or broken and can't be repaired or, possibly, if the line becomes occluded. Measure the catheter after you remove it to ensure that the line has been removed intact. **INS**

▶ Assemble the necessary equipment at the patient's bedside.

▶ Explain the procedure to the patient. Wash your hands. Place a linen-saver pad under the patient's arm.

▶ Remove the tape holding the extension tubing. Open two sterile gauze pads on a clean, flat surface. Put on clean gloves. Stabilize the catheter at the hub with one hand. Without dislodging the catheter, use your other hand to gently remove the dressing by pulling it toward the insertion site.

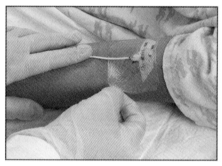

▶ Withdraw the catheter with smooth, gentle pressure in small increments. It should come out easily.

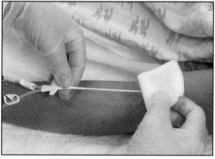

If you feel resistance, stop. Apply slight tension to the line by taping it down. Apply a warm moist pack, and then try to remove it again in a few minutes. If you still feel resistance after the second attempt, notify the practitioner for further instructions.

▶ When you successfully remove the catheter, apply manual pressure to the site with a sterile gauze pad for 1 minute. **INS**

▶ Measure and inspect the catheter. If any part has broken off during removal, notify the practitioner immediately and monitor the patient for signs of distress. **INS**

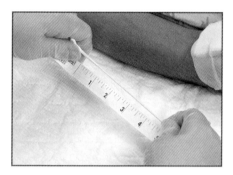

▶ Cover the site with antiseptic ointment, and tape a new folded gauze pad in place.

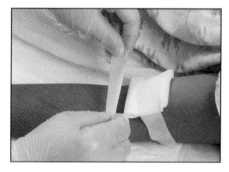

Dispose of used items properly, and wash your hands.

Special considerations

▶ For a patient receiving intermittent PICC therapy, flush the catheter with heparin flush solution at established intervals to help maintain patency. **INS**

▶ You can use a declotting agent, such as urokinase, to clear a clotted PICC, but make sure you read the manufacturer's recommendations first.

▶ Remember to add an extension set to all PICCs so you can start and stop an infusion away from the insertion site. An extension set will also make using a PICC easier for the patient who will be administering infusions herself. **INS**

▶ If a patient is to receive blood or blood products through the PICC, use at least an 18G cannula.

▶ Assess the catheter insertion site through the transparent semipermeable dressing every 24 hours. Look at the catheter and cannula pathway, and check for bleeding, redness, drainage, and swelling. Ask your patient if she's having pain associated with therapy. Although oozing is common for the first 24 hours after insertion, excessive bleeding after that should be evaluated. **INS**

CLINICAL ALERT

If a portion of the catheter breaks during removal, immediately apply a tourniquet to the upper arm, close to the axilla, to prevent advancement of the catheter piece into the right atrium. Then check the patient's radial pulse. If you don't detect the radial pulse, the tourniquet is too tight. Keep the tourniquet in place until an X-ray can be obtained, the practitioner is notified, and surgical retrieval is attempted.

Selected references

Brungs, S. M., and Render, M. L. "Using Evidence-based Practice to Reduce Central Line Infections," *Clinical Journal of Oncology Nursing* 10(6):723–25, December 2006.

Centers for Disease Control and Prevention. "Guidelines for the Prevention of Intravascular Catheter-related Infections," *MMWR* 51(RR-10):1–26, August 9, 2002.

Chaiyakunapruk, N, et al. "Chlorhexidine compared with povidone-iodine solution for vascular catheter-site care: a meta-analysis," *Annals of Internal Medicine* 136(11):792–801, June 2002. **CS**

Hadaway, L. "Keeping Central Line Infection at Bay," *Nursing* 36(4):58–63, April 2006.

Kearns, P. J., et al. "Complications of long arm-catheters: a randomized trial of central vs peripheral tip location," *Journal of Parenteral and Enteral Nutrition* 20(1):20–4, January–February 1996.

Oncology Nursing Society. *Access Device Guidelines: Recommendations for Nursing Practice and Education,* 2nd ed. Pittsburgh: Oncology Nursing Society, 2004.

Saldar, N., and Maki, D. "Risk of Catheter-related Bloodstream Infection with Peripherally Inserted Central Venous Catheters Used in Hospitalized Patients," *Chest* 128(2):489–95, August 2005.

"Standard 37. Site Selection. Infusion Nursing Standards of Practice," *Journal of Infusion Nursing* 29(1S):S37–39, January–February 2006.

"Standard 38. Catheter Selection. Infusion Nursing Standards of Practice," *Journal of Infusion Nursing* 29(1S):S39–40, January–February 2006.

"Standard 39. Hair Removal. Infusion Nursing Standards of Practice," *Journal of Infusion Nursing* 29(1S):S40–41, January–February 2006.

"Standard 40. Local Anesthesia. Infusion Nursing Standards of Practice," *Journal of Infusion Nursing* 29(1S):S41, January–February 2006.

"Standard 41. Access Site Preparation. Infusion Nursing Standards of Practice," *Journal of Infusion Nursing* 29(1S):S41–42, January–February 2006.

"Standard 44. Dressings. Infusion Nursing Standards of Practice," *Journal of Infusion Nursing* 29(1S):S44–45, January–February 2006.

"Standard 49. Catheter Removal. Infusion Nursing Standards of Practice," *Journal of Infusion Nursing* 29(1S):S51–55, January–February 2006.

"Standard 51. Catheter Site Care. Infusion Nursing Standards of Practice," *Journal of Infusion Nursing* 29(1S):S57–58, January–February 2006.

"Standard 52. Discontinuation of Therapy. Infusion Nursing Standards of Practice," *Journal of Infusion Nursing* 29(1S):S58, January–February 2006.

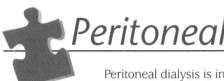

Peritoneal dialysis

Peritoneal dialysis is indicated for patients with chronic renal failure who have cardiovascular instability, vascular access problems that prevent hemodialysis, fluid overload, or electrolyte imbalances. In this procedure, dialysate—the solution instilled into the peritoneal cavity by a catheter—draws waste products, excess fluid, and electrolytes from the blood across the semipermeable peritoneal membrane. (See *How peritoneal dialysis works.*) After a prescribed period, the dialysate is drained from the peritoneal cavity, removing impurities with it. The dialysis procedure is then repeated, using a new dialysate each time, until waste removal is complete, and fluid, electrolyte, and acid-base balance has been restored.

The catheter is inserted in the operating room in an acute situation or at the patient's bedside with a nurse assisting. With special preparation, the nurse may perform dialysis, either manually or using an automatic or semiautomatic cycle machine.

Equipment

For catheter placement and dialysis:
Prescribed dialysate (in 1- or 2-L bottles or bags, as ordered) ◆ warmer, heating pad, or water bath ◆ at least three face masks ◆ medication, such as heparin, if ordered ◆ dialysis administration set with drainage bag ◆ two pairs of sterile gloves ◆ I.V. pole ◆ fenestrated sterile drape ◆ vial of 1% or 2% lidocaine ◆ antiseptic pads ◆ 3-ml syringe ◆ ordered type of multi-eyed, nylon, peritoneal catheter ◆ scalpel (with #11 blade) ◆ peritoneal stylet ◆ sutures or hypoallergenic tape ◆ antiseptic solu-

---

How peritoneal dialysis works

Peritoneal dialysis works through a combination of diffusion and osmosis.

Diffusion

In diffusion, particles move through a semipermeable membrane from an area of high-solute concentration to an area of low-solute concentration.

In peritoneal dialysis, the water-based dialysate being infused contains glucose, sodium chloride, calcium, magnesium, acetate or lactate, and no waste products. Therefore, the waste products and excess electrolytes in the blood cross through the semipermeable peritoneal membrane into the dialysate. Removing the waste-filled dialysate and replacing it with fresh solution keeps the waste concentration low and encourages further diffusion.

Osmosis

In osmosis, fluids move through a semipermeable membrane from an area of low-solute concentration to an area of high-solute concentration. In peritoneal dialysis, dextrose is added to the dialysate to give it a higher solute concentration than the blood, creating a high osmotic gradient. Water migrates from the blood through the membrane at the beginning of each infusion, when the osmotic gradient is highest.

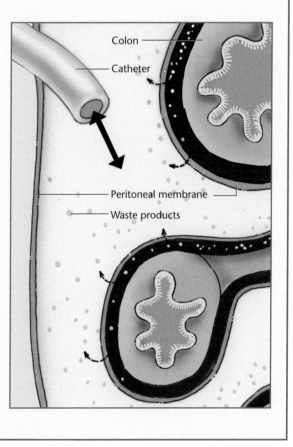

tion ◆ precut drain dressings ◆ protective cap for catheter ◆ 4″ × 4″ gauze pads ◆ small, sterile plastic clamp ◆ sterile labels ◆ sterile marker ◆ optional: 10-ml syringe with 22G ½″ needle, specimen container, label, laboratory request form.

For dressing changes: One pair of sterile gloves ◆ sterile cotton-tipped applicators or sterile 2″ × 2″ gauze pads ◆ two precut drain dressings ◆ adhesive tape ◆ antiseptic solution or normal saline solution ◆ two sterile 4″ × 4″ gauze pads.

All equipment must be sterile. Commercially packaged dialysis kits or trays are available.

Implementation

▶ Confirm the patient's identity using two patient identifiers according to your facility's policy. **JC**

▶ Bring all equipment to the patient's bedside and make sure the dialysate is at body temperature. Place the container in a warmer or a water bath, or wrap it in a heating pad set at 98.6° F (37° C) for 30 to 60 minutes to warm the solution.

▶ Explain the procedure to the patient. Assess and record his vital signs, weight, and abdominal girth to establish baseline levels.

▶ Review recent laboratory values (blood urea nitrogen, serum creatinine, sodium, potassium, and complete blood count).

Catheter placement and dialysis

▶ Have the patient try to urinate. This reduces the risk of bladder perforation during insertion of the peritoneal catheter. If he can't urinate and you suspect that his bladder isn't empty, obtain an order for straight catheterization to empty his bladder.

▶ Place the patient in the supine position, and have him put on one of the sterile face masks.

▶ Wash your hands.

▶ Inspect the warmed dialysate, which should appear clear and colorless.

▶ Put on a sterile face mask. Prepare to add any prescribed medication to the dialysate, using strict sterile technique to avoid contaminating the solution. Label all medications, medication containers, and other solutions on and off the sterile field. Medications should be added immediately before the solution will be hung and used. Disinfect multiple-dose vials by soaking them in antiseptic solution for 5 minutes. Heparin is typically added to the dialysate to prevent accumulation of fibrin in the catheter. **JC**

▶ Prepare the dialysis administration set. (See *Setup for peritoneal dialysis*.)

▶ Close the clamps on all lines. Place the drainage bag below the patient to facilitate gravity drainage, and connect the drainage line to it. Connect the dialysate infusion lines to the bottles or bags of dialysate using sterile technique. Hang the bottles or bags on the I.V. pole at the patient's bedside. To prime the tubing, open the infusion lines and allow the solution to flow until all lines are primed. Then close all clamps.

▶ At this point, the physician puts on a mask and a pair of sterile gloves. He cleans the patient's abdomen with antiseptic solution and drapes it with a sterile drape.

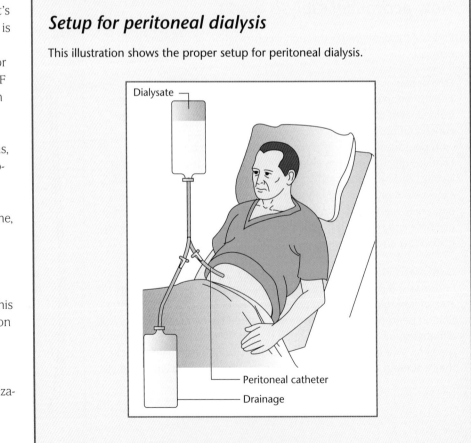

Setup for peritoneal dialysis

This illustration shows the proper setup for peritoneal dialysis.

Dialysate

Peritoneal catheter

Drainage

▶ Wipe the stopper of the lidocaine vial with antiseptic solution and allow it to dry. Invert the vial and hand it to the physician so he can withdraw the lidocaine using the 3-ml syringe.

▶ The physician anesthetizes a small area of the patient's abdomen below the umbilicus. He then makes a small incision with the scalpel, inserts the catheter into the peritoneal cavity— using the stylet to guide the catheter— and sutures or tapes the catheter in place.

▶ If the catheter is already in place, clean the site with antiseptic solution in a circular outward motion, according to your facility's policy, before each dialysis treatment.

▶ Connect the catheter to the administration set, using strict sterile technique to prevent contamination of the catheter and the solution, which could cause peritonitis.

▶ Open the drain dressing and the $4'' \times 4''$ gauze pad packages. Put on the other pair of sterile gloves. Apply the precut drain dressings around the catheter. Cover them with the gauze pads and tape them securely.

▶ Unclamp the lines to the patient. Rapidly instill 500 ml of dialysate into the peritoneal cavity to test the catheter's patency.

▶ Clamp the lines to the patient. Immediately unclamp the lines to the drainage bag to allow fluid to drain into the bag. Outflow should be brisk.

▶ Having established the catheter's patency, clamp the lines to the drainage bag and unclamp the lines to the patient to infuse the prescribed volume of solution over a period of 5 to 10 minutes. As soon as the dialysate container empties, clamp the lines to the patient immediately to prevent air from entering the tubing.

▶ Allow the solution to dwell in the peritoneal cavity for the prescribed time (10 minutes to 4 hours). This lets

excess fluid, electrolytes, and accumulated wastes move from the blood through the peritoneal membrane and into the dialysate.

▶ Warm the solution for the next infusion.

▶ At the end of the prescribed dwell time, unclamp the line to the drainage bag and allow the solution to drain from the peritoneal cavity into the drainage bag (normally 30 to 40 minutes).

▶ Repeat the infusion-dwell-drain cycle immediately after outflow until the prescribed number of fluid exchanges has been completed.

▶ If the physician (or your facility's policy) requires a dialysate specimen, you'll usually collect one after every 10 infusion-dwell-drain cycles (always during the drain phase), after every 24-hour period, or as ordered. To do this, use strict sterile technique and aspirate the drainage sample using the 10 ml syringe on the injection port of the drainage line. Transfer the sample to the specimen container, label it appropriately, and send it to the laboratory with a laboratory request form.

▶ After completing the prescribed number of exchanges, clamp the catheter and put on sterile gloves. Disconnect the administration set from the peritoneal catheter. Place the sterile protective cap over the catheter's distal end.

▶ Dispose of all used equipment appropriately.

Dressing changes

▶ Explain the procedure to the patient and wash your hands.

▶ If necessary, carefully remove the old dressings to avoid putting tension on the catheter and accidentally dislodging it and to avoid introducing bacteria into the tract through movement of the catheter.

▶ Put on the sterile gloves.

▶ Saturate the sterile applicators or the $2'' \times 2''$ gauze pads with antiseptic solution, and clean the skin around the catheter, moving in concentric circles from the catheter site outward. Remove any crusted material carefully.

▶ Inspect the catheter site for drainage and the tissue around the site for redness and swelling.

▶ Place two precut drain dressings around the catheter site. Tape the $4'' \times 4''$ gauze pads over them to secure the dressings.

Special considerations

▶ During and after dialysis, monitor the patient and his response to treatment. Peritoneal dialysis is usually contraindicated in patients who have had extensive abdominal or bowel surgery or extensive abdominal trauma.

▶ Monitor the patient's vital signs every 10 to 15 minutes for the first 1 to 2 hours of exchanges, and then every 2 to 4 hours or more frequently if necessary. Notify the practitioner of any abrupt changes in the patient's condition.

▶ To reduce the risk of peritonitis, use strict sterile technique during catheter insertion, dialysis, and dressing changes. Masks should be worn by all personnel in the room whenever the dialysis system is opened or entered. Change the dressing at least every 24 hours or whenever it becomes wet or soiled. Frequent dressing changes will also help prevent skin excoriation from any leakage.

▶ To prevent respiratory distress, position the patient for maximal lung expansion. Promote lung expansion through turning and deep-breathing exercises. In some patients, decreasing volumes may be necessary.

CLINICAL ALERT

If the patient suffers severe respiratory distress during the dwell phase of dialysis, drain the peritoneal cavity and notify the practitioner. Monitor any patient on peritoneal dialysis who is being weaned from a ventilator.

▶ To prevent protein depletion, the practitioner may order a high-protein diet or a protein supplement. He'll also monitor serum albumin levels.

▶ Patients with low serum potassium levels may require the addition of potassium to the dialysate solution to prevent further losses.

▶ Monitor fluid volume balance, blood pressure, and pulse to help prevent fluid imbalance. Assess fluid balance at the end of each infusion-dwell-drain cycle. Fluid balance is positive if less than the amount infused was recovered; it's negative if more than the amount infused was recovered. Notify the practitioner if the patient retains 500 ml or more of fluid for three consecutive cycles or if he loses at least 1 L of fluid for three consecutive cycles.

▶ Weigh the patient daily to help determine how much fluid is being removed during dialysis treatment. Note the time and any variations in the weighing technique next to his weight on his chart.

▶ If inflow and outflow are slow or absent, check the tubing for kinks. You can also try raising the I.V. pole or repositioning the patient to increase the inflow rate. Repositioning the patient or applying manual pressure to the lateral aspects of the patient's abdomen may also help increase drainage. If these maneuvers fail, notify the practitioner. Improper positioning of the catheter or an accumulation of fibrin may obstruct the catheter.

▶ Always examine outflow fluid (effluent) for color and clarity. Normally, it's clear or pale yellow, but pink-tinged effluent may appear during the first three or four cycles. If the effluent remains pink-tinged or if it's grossly bloody, suspect bleeding into the peritoneal cavity and notify the practitioner. Also notify the practitioner if the outflow contains feces, which suggests bowel perforation, or if it's cloudy, which suggests peritonitis. Obtain a sample for culture and Gram stain. Send the sample in a labeled specimen container to the laboratory with a laboratory request form.

▶ Patient discomfort at the start of the procedure is normal. If the patient experiences pain during the procedure, determine when it occurs, its quality and duration, and whether it radiates to other body parts. Then notify the practitioner.

▶ The patient undergoing peritoneal dialysis requires a great deal of assistance in his daily care. To minimize his discomfort, perform daily care during a drain phase in the cycle, when the patient's abdomen is less distended.

Selected references

Finkelstein, F. O., et al. "The Role of Chronic Peritoneal Dialysis in the Management of the Patient with Chronic Kidney Disease," *Contributions in Nephrology* 150:235–39, 2006.

Gajjar, A. H., et al. "Peritoneal Dialysis Catheters: Laparoscopic versus Traditional Placement Techniques and Outcomes," *American Journal of Surgery* 194(6):872–75, December 2007.

Hollis, J., et al. "Managing Peritoneal Dialysis (PD)—Factors that Influence Patients' Modification of Their Recommended Dialysis Regimen. A European Study of 376 Patients," *Journal of Renal Care* 32(4):202–207, October–December 2006.

Lynn-McHale Wiegand, D. J., and Carlson, K. K., eds. *AACN Procedure Manual for Critical Care,* 5th ed. Philadelphia: W. B. Saunders Co., 2005.

Saxena, R., et al. "Peritoneal Dialysis: A Viable Renal Replacement Therapy," *The American Journal of the Medical Sciences* 330(1):36–47, July 2005.

Smeltzer, S., et al. *Brunner & Suddarth's Textbook of Medical-Surgical Nursing,* 11th ed. Philadelphia: Lippincott Williams & Wilkins, 2008.

Permanent pacemaker care

Designed to operate for 3 to 20 years, a permanent pacemaker is a self-contained device. The cardiologist implants the pacemaker in a pocket beneath the patient's skin, which is usually done in the operating room or cardiac catheterization laboratory. **ASPN** Nursing responsibilities involve monitoring the electro-cardiogram (ECG) and maintaining sterile technique.

Permanent pacemakers function in the demand mode, allowing the patient's heart to beat on its own but preventing it from falling below a preset rate. Pacing electrodes can be placed in the atria, in the ventricles, or in both chambers (atrioventricular sequential, dual chamber). (See *Understanding pacemaker codes*.)

To keep the patient healthy and active, newer generation pacemakers have been specially designed to increase the heart rate with exercise.

Candidates for permanent pacemakers include patients with myocardial infarction and persistent bradyarrhythmia and patients with complete heart block or slow ventricular rates stemming from congenital or degenerative heart disease or cardiac surgery. Patients who suffer Stokes-Adams syndrome as well as those with Wolff-Parkinson-White syndrome or sick sinus syndrome may also benefit from permanent pacemaker implantation. Permanent pacemakers are also being used in patients other than those with symptomatic bradycardia. These include patients with hypertrophic cardiomyopathy, dilated cardiomyopathy, atrial fibrillation, neurocardiogenic syndrome, and long QT syndrome. A biventricular pacemaker is also available for patients with heart failure. **ACC** **ASPN** (See *Biventricular pacemaker,* page 412.)

Understanding pacemaker codes

A permanent pacemaker's three-letter (or sometimes five-letter) code simply refers to how it's programmed. The first letter represents the chamber that's paced; the second letter, the chamber that's sensed; and the third letter, how the pulse generator responds. In five-letter codes, the fourth letter denotes the pacemaker's programmability, and the fifth letter denotes the pacemaker's response to tachycardia. Typically, only the first three letters are used.

FIRST LETTER	SECOND LETTER	THIRD LETTER	FOURTH LETTER	FIFTH LETTER
A = atrium	A = atrium	I = inhibited	P = basic functions programmable	P = pacing ability
V = ventricle	V = ventricle	T = triggered	M = multiple programmable parameters	S = shock
D = dual (both chambers)	D = dual (both chambers)	D = dual (inhibited and triggered)	C = communicating functions such as telemetry	D = dual ability to shock and pace
O = not applicable	O = not applicable	O = not applicable	R = rate responsiveness	O = none

EXAMPLES OF TWO COMMON PROGRAMMING CODES

DDD
Pace: atrium and ventricle
Sense: atrium and ventricle
Response: inhibited and triggered
This is a fully automatic, or universal, pacemaker.

VVI
Pace: ventricle
Sense: ventricle
Response: inhibited
This is a demand pacemaker, inhibited.

Biventricular pacemaker

A biventricular pacemaker utilizes three leads: one to pace the right atrium, one to pace the right ventricle, and one to pace the left ventricle. The left ventricular lead is placed in the coronary sinus. Both ventricles are paced at the same time, causing them to contract simultaneously, improving cardiac output.

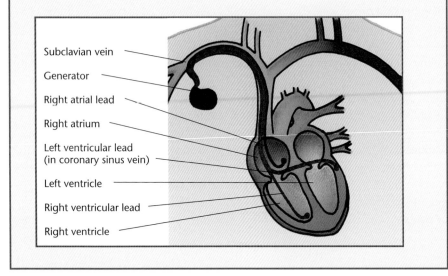

- Subclavian vein
- Generator
- Right atrial lead
- Right atrium
- Left ventricular lead (in coronary sinus vein)
- Left ventricle
- Right ventricular lead
- Right ventricle

Equipment

Sphygmomanometer ◆ stethoscope ◆ ECG monitor and strip-chart recorder ◆ sterile dressing tray ◆ antimicrobial ointment ◆ clippers ◆ sterile gauze dressing ◆ hypoallergenic tape ◆ sedatives ◆ alcohol pads ◆ emergency resuscitation equipment ◆ I.V. catheter, tubing, and I.V. solution.

Implementation

▶ Confirm the patient's identity using two patient identifiers according to your facility's policy. **JC**
▶ Explain the procedure to the patient. Provide and review literature from the manufacturer or the American Heart Association so he can learn about the pacemaker and how it works. Emphasize that the pacemaker merely augments his natural heart rate.

▶ Make sure the patient or a responsible family member signs a consent form, and ask the patient if he's allergic to anesthetics or iodine.

Preoperative care

▶ For pacemaker insertion, clip hair from the patient's chest from the axilla to the midline and from the clavicle to the nipple line on the side selected by the physician, as ordered.
▶ Establish an I.V. line at a keep-vein-open rate.
▶ Obtain baseline vital signs and a baseline ECG.
▶ Provide sedation as ordered.

Postoperative care

▶ Monitor the patient's ECG to check for arrhythmias and to ensure correct pacemaker functioning. **MFR**

▶ Monitor the I.V. flow rate; the I.V. line is usually kept in place for 24 to 48 hours postoperatively to allow for possible emergency treatment of arrhythmias.
▶ Check the dressing for signs of bleeding and infection (swelling, redness, or exudate). The practitioner may order prophylactic antibiotics for up to 7 days after the implantation. **ASPN**
▶ Change the dressing and apply antimicrobial ointment at least once every 24 to 48 hours, or according to the practitioner's orders and your facility's policy. If the dressing becomes soiled or the site is exposed to air, change the dressing immediately, regardless of when you last changed it.
▶ Check the patient's vital signs and level of consciousness (LOC) every 15 minutes for the first hour, every hour for the next 4 hours, every 4 hours for the next 48 hours, and then once every shift.

AGE FACTOR

Confused, elderly patients with second-degree heart block won't show immediate improvement in LOC.

Special considerations

▶ Provide the patient with an identification card that lists the pacemaker type and manufacturer, serial number, pacemaker rate setting, date implanted, and his cardiologist's name. **MFR**
▶ Watch for signs of pacemaker malfunction.

CLINICAL ALERT

Watch for signs and symptoms of a perforated ventricle, with resultant cardiac tamponade: persistent hiccups, distant heart sounds, pulsus paradoxus, hypotension with narrow pulse pressure, increased venous pressure, cyanosis, distended jugular veins, decreased urine output, restlessness, or complaints of fullness in the chest. If the patient develops any of these, notify the practitioner immediately.

Selected references

American College of Cardiology and the American Heart Association. "2002 Guideline Update for Implantation of Cardiac Pacemakers and Antiarrhythmia Devices." Available at *www.americanheart.org*.

American College of Cardiology and the American Heart Association. "ACC/AHA/NASPE 2002 Guideline Update for Implantation of Cardiac Pacemakers and Antiarrhythmia Devices: Summary Article," *Circulation* 106:2145–161, October 2002.

Borer, A., et al. "Prevention of Infections Associated with Permanent Cardiac Antiarrhythmic Devices by Implementation of a Comprehensive Infection Control Program," *Infection Control and Hospital Epidemiology* 25(6):492–96, June 2004.

Cotter, J., et al. "Helping Patients Who Need a Permanent Pacemaker," *Nursing* 36(8):50–54, August 2004.

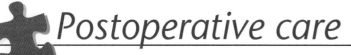

Postoperative care

This phase of care begins when the patient arrives in the postanesthesia care unit (PACU) and continues as he moves on to the short procedure unit, medical-surgical unit, or intensive care unit. Postoperative care aims to minimize postoperative complications through early detection and prompt treatment. After anesthesia, a patient may experience pain, inadequate oxygenation, or adverse physiologic effects of sudden movement.

Recovery from general anesthesia takes longer than induction because the anesthetic is retained in fat and muscle. Fat has a meager blood supply; thus, it releases the anesthetic slowly, providing enough anesthesia to maintain adequate blood and brain levels during surgery. The patient's recovery time varies with his amount of body fat, his overall condition, his premedication regimen, and the type, dosage, and duration of anesthesia.

Equipment

Thermometer ◆ watch with second hand ◆ stethoscope ◆ sphygmomanometer ◆ postoperative flowchart or other documentation tool.

Implementation

▶ Assemble the equipment at the patient's bedside.

▶ Obtain the patient's record from the PACU nurse. This should include:

— summary of operative procedures and pertinent findings

— type of anesthesia

— vital signs (preoperative, intraoperative, and postoperative)

— medical history

— medication history, including preoperative, intraoperative, and postoperative medications

— fluid therapy, including estimated blood loss, type and number of drains and catheters, and amounts and characteristics of drainage

— notes on the condition of the surgical wound. (If the patient had vascular surgery, for example, knowing the location and duration of blood vessel clamping can prevent postoperative complications.) **JC** **AORN**

▶ Transfer the patient from the PACU stretcher to the bed, and position him properly. Get a coworker to help if nec-
essary. When moving the patient, keep transfer movements smooth to minimize pain and postoperative complications and avoid back strain among team members. Use a transfer board to facilitate moving the patient.

▶ If the patient has had orthopedic surgery, always get a coworker to help transfer him. Ask the coworker to move only the affected extremity.

▶ If the patient is in skeletal traction, you may receive special orders for moving him. If you must move him, have a coworker move the weights as you and another coworker move the patient.

▶ Make the patient comfortable, and raise the bed's side rails to ensure the patient's safety.

▶ Assess the patient's level of consciousness, skin color, and mucous membranes. **AORN**

▶ Monitor the patient's respiratory status by assessing his airway. Note breathing rate and depth, and auscultate for breath sounds. Administer oxygen and initiate oximetry to monitor oxygen saturation if ordered. **AORN**

▶ Monitor the patient's pulse rate. It should be strong and easily palpable. The heart rate should be within 20% of the preoperative heart rate. **AORN**

▶ Compare postoperative blood pressure to preoperative blood pressure. It
should be within 20% of the preoperative level unless the patient suffered a hypotensive episode during surgery. **AORN**

▶ Assess the patient's temperature because anesthesia lowers body temperature. Body temperature should be at least 95° F (35° C). If it's lower, apply blankets to warm the patient or use a patient-warming system. **AORN**

▶ Assess the patient's infusion sites for redness, pain, swelling, or drainage. This indicates infiltration and requires discontinuing the I.V. line and restarting it at another site. **AORN**

▶ Assess surgical wound dressings; they should be clean and dry. If they're soiled, assess the characteristics of the drainage and outline the soiled area. Note the date and time of assessment on the dressing. Assess the soiled area frequently; if it enlarges, reinforce the dressing and alert the practitioner. Don't remove the original dressing unless specified by the physician. **AORN**

▶ Note the presence and condition of drains and tubes. Note the color, type, odor, and amount of drainage and the patient's urine output. Make sure all drains are properly connected and free from obstructions. **AORN**

▶ If the patient has had vascular or orthopedic surgery, assess the appropriate extremity—or all extremities, depending on the surgical procedure. Perform neurovascular checks and assess color, temperature, sensation, movement, and presence and quality of pulses. Notify the practitioner of any abnormalities. **AORN**

▶ Assess the patient's pain intensity using your facility's pain scale. Assess pain type, location, frequency, and duration. Also assess other sources of discomfort, such as nausea and anxiety. **AORN** **JC** **ASPMN**

▶ Provide pain medication as ordered.

▶ As the patient recovers from anesthesia, monitor his respiratory and cardiovascular status closely. Be alert for signs of airway obstruction and hypoventilation caused by laryngospasm, or for sedation, which can lead to hypoxemia. Cardiovascular complications—such as arrhythmias and hypotension—may result from the anesthetic agent or the operative procedure.

▶ Encourage coughing and deep-breathing exercises. However, don't encourage them if the patient has just had nasal, ophthalmic, or neurologic surgery to avoid increasing intracranial pressure.

▶ Administer postoperative medications, such as antibiotics, analgesics, antiemetics, or reversal agents, as ordered and appropriate.

▶ Remove all fluids from the patient's bedside until he's alert enough to eat and drink. Before giving him liquids, assess his gag reflex to prevent aspiration. To do this, lightly touch the back of his throat with a cotton swab— the patient will gag if the reflex has returned. Do this test quickly to prevent a vagal reaction. (See *PACU discharge criteria.*)

▶ Monitor the patient's intake and output.

▶ Assess the presence of bowel sounds and passage of flatus before the patient can be allowed food.

PACU discharge criteria

Typically, the patient must meet the following criteria before he can be discharged from the PACU. Make sure your documentation reflects that the patient meets discharge criteria:

▶ postanesthesia recovery score of 8 or above
▶ stable vital signs and oxygen saturation level
▶ stable respiratory and cardiac status
▶ stable fluid balance status
▶ adequate pain control
▶ adequate control of nausea and vomiting
▶ surgical site that's free from complications, with a dry, intact dressing or minimal drainage and patent drainage tubes
▶ downward progression of the level of blockade from spinal anesthesia, with return of movement and sensation.

Special considerations

▶ Fear, pain, anxiety, hypothermia, confusion, and immobility can upset the patient and jeopardize his safety and postoperative status. Offer emotional support to the patient and his family.

▶ As the patient recovers from general anesthesia, reflexes appear in reverse order to that in which they disappeared. Hearing recovers first, so avoid holding inappropriate conversations.

▶ Monitor the patient's blood pressure, heart rate, and oxygen saturation. **AORN**

▶ If the patient received spinal anesthesia, he may need to remain in a supine position with the bed adjusted at 0 to 20 degrees for at least 6 hours to reduce the risk of spinal headache from leakage of cerebrospinal fluid. Check your facility's policy and procedures for activity restriction after spinal anesthesia. The patient won't be able to move his legs, so be sure to reassure him that sensation and mobility will return. **ASPN** (See *Assessing level of blockade from spinal anesthesia,* page 416.)

▶ If the patient has an epidural analgesia infusion for postoperative pain control, monitor his respiratory status closely. Respiratory arrest may result from the respiratory depressant effects of the opioid. He may also suffer from nausea, vomiting, or itching. Epidural analgesia may also include administering a local anesthetic with the opioid. Assess the patient's lower extremity motor strength every 2 to 4 hours. If sensorimotor loss occurs (numbness or weakness of the legs), notify the physician because the dosage may need to be decreased.

▶ If the patient will be using a patient-controlled analgesia (PCA) unit, reinforce preoperative teaching and make sure he understands how to use it. Caution him to activate it only when he has pain, not when he feels sleepy or is pain-free. Review your facility's criteria for PCA use.

Assessing level of blockade from spinal anesthesia

Spinal anesthesia produces a sympathetic, sensory, and motor block. If your patient received spinal anesthesia, be sure to assess the downward progression of the level of blockade. Using a dermatome chart aids this assessment. Each dermatome represents a specific body area supplied with nerve fibers from an individual spinal root (cervical, thoracic, lumbar, or sacral). To document the patient's sensory and motor function, mentally divide his body into dermatomes, as shown here. Anatomic reference points include the nipple line at T4, xiphoid at T6, umbilicus at T10, and groin at L1.

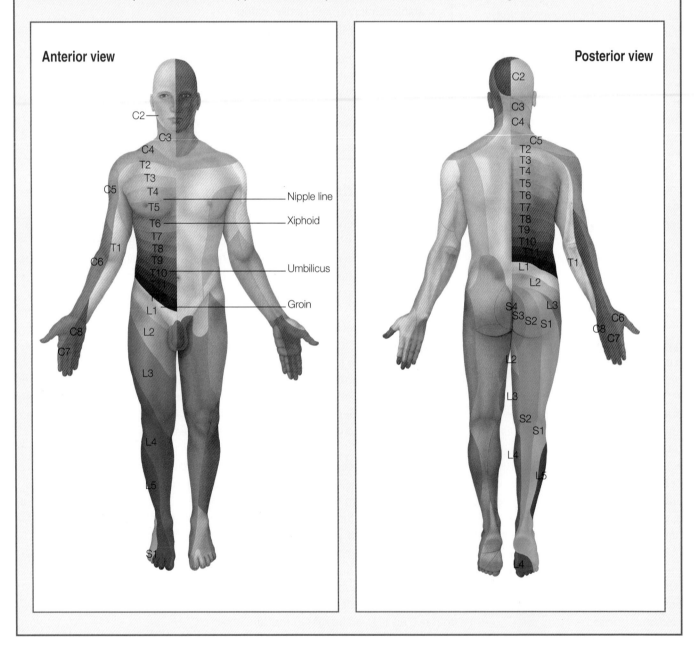

AGE FACTOR

If the patient is older, be aware of age-related changes that will alter your assessment. Monitor the patient's cardiovascular status because it can be altered by blood loss, pain, bed rest, and fluid and electrolyte imbalances. Respiratory status should also be evaluated because ventilation and oxygenation can be altered by age-related changes, smoking, or chronic disease. Monitor his level of consciousness and pain carefully because mental status changes can make pain control more difficult. Also, because drug metabolism slows with age, observe the older adult for drug reactions, toxicity, and interactions. Assess intake and output carefully, and watch for urinary tract infections due to decreased renal function and bladder capacity.

Selected references

American Society of Peri-Anesthesia Nurses. "ASPEN Pain and Comfort Clinical Guideline," *Journal of Perianesthesia Nursing* 18(4):232–36, August 2003.

Association of Perioperative Registered Nurses. *Standards, Recommended Practices, and Guidelines.* Denver: AORN, Inc., 2007.

Litusack, K. "Adjusting Postsurgical Care for Older Patients," *Nursing* 36(1):66–67, January 2006.

Schwartz., A. "Learning the Essentials of Epidural Anesthesia," *Nursing* 36(1):44–49, January 2006.

Preoperative care

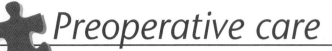

Preoperative care begins when surgery is first planned and ends with the administration of anesthesia. This phase of care includes a preoperative interview and assessment to collect baseline subjective and objective data from the patient and his family; to administer diagnostic tests, such as urinalysis, an electrocardiogram, and chest radiography; to conduct preoperative teaching; to secure informed consent from the patient; and physical preparation.

Equipment

Gloves ◆ thermometer ◆ sphygmomanometer ◆ stethoscope ◆ watch with second hand ◆ weight scale ◆ tape measure.

Implementation

▶ If the patient is having same-day surgery, make sure he knows ahead of time not to eat or drink anything for 8 hours before surgery. Confirm with him what time he's scheduled to arrive at the facility, and tell him to leave all jewelry and valuables at home. Make sure the patient has arranged for someone to accompany him home after surgery.

▶ Obtain a health history, and assess the patient's knowledge, perceptions, and expectations about his surgery. Ask about previous medical and surgical interventions. Also determine the patient's psychosocial needs; ask about occupational well-being, financial matters, support systems, mental status, and cultural beliefs. Use your facility's preoperative surgical assessment database, if available, to gather this information. Obtain a drug and anesthetic history. Ask about current prescriptions, over-the-counter medications, supplemental herbal preparations, and known allergies to foods and drugs. **JC** **AORN** **ASPN**

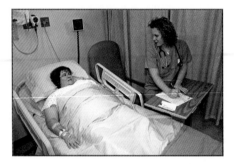

▶ Obtain the results of X-ray examinations and other preoperative tests. **ASPN**

▶ Ask the patient if he has an advance directive. If he does, make a copy and place it in his chart. If he doesn't, ask him if he wants information about advance directives. **JC**

▶ Measure the patient's height and weight and take his vital signs.

▶ Identify risk factors that may interfere with a positive expected outcome. Be sure to consider age, general health, medications, mobility, nutritional status, fluid and electrolyte disturbances, and lifestyle. Also consider the primary disorder's duration, location, and nature and the extent of the surgical procedure. **ASPN**

▶ Explain preoperative procedures to the patient. Include typical events that the patient can expect. Discuss equipment that may be used postoperatively, such as nasogastric tubes and I.V. equipment. Explain the typical incision, dressings, and staples or sutures that will be used. Preoperative teaching can help reduce postoperative anxiety and pain, increase patient compliance, hasten recovery, and decrease length of stay. **ASPN** **CS1**

▶ Discuss postoperative pain management. Teach the patient how to use your facility's pain scale. Find out his goals and expectations for pain relief. **CS2** **CS3**

▶ Talk the patient through the sequence of events from the operating room, to the postanesthesia care unit (PACU), and back to the patient's room. He may be transferred from the PACU to an intensive care unit or surgical care unit. The patient may also benefit from a tour of the areas he'll see during the perioperative events.

▶ Tell the patient that when he goes to the operating room, he may have to wait a short time in the holding area. Explain that the physicians and nurses will wear surgical dress, and even though they'll be observing him closely, they'll refrain from talking to him very much. Explain that minimal conversation will help the preoperative medication take effect.

▶ When discussing transfer procedures and techniques, describe sensations that the patient will experience. Tell him that he'll be taken to the operating room on a stretcher and transferred from the stretcher to the operating room table. For his own safety, he'll be held securely to the table with soft restraints. The operating room nurses will check his vital signs frequently.

▶ Tell the patient that the operating room may feel cool. Electrodes may be put on his chest to monitor his heart rate during surgery. Describe the drowsy floating sensation he'll feel as the anesthetic takes effect. Tell him it's important that he relax at this time.

▶ Tell the patient about exercises that he may be expected to perform after surgery, such as deep-breathing, coughing (while splinting the incision if necessary), extremity exercises, and movement and ambulation to minimize respiratory and circulatory complications. If the patient will undergo ophthalmic or neurologic surgery, he won't be asked to cough because coughing increases intracranial pressure.

▶ If the patient will have postoperative patient-controlled analgesia, explain how it works, and demonstrate the device so he'll be able to use it immediately after surgery.

▶ On the day of surgery, important interventions include giving morning care, verifying that the patient has signed an informed consent form, administering ordered preoperative medications, completing the preoperative checklist and chart, and providing support to the patient and his family.

▶ Other immediate preoperative interventions may include preparing the GI tract (restricting food and fluids for about 8 hours before surgery) to reduce vomiting and the risk of aspiration, cleaning the lower GI tract of fecal material by enemas before abdominal or GI surgery, and giving antibiotics for 2 or 3 days preoperatively to prevent contamination of the peritoneal cavity by GI bacteria.

▶ Just before the patient is moved to the surgical area, make sure he's wearing a hospital gown, has his identification band in place, and has his vital signs recorded. Check to see that hairpins, nail polish, and jewelry have been removed. Note whether dentures, contact lenses, or prosthetic devices have been removed or left in place. Verify with the patient that the correct surgical site has been marked. (See "Surgical site verification," page 502.)

Special considerations

▶ Preoperative medications must be given on time to enhance the effect of ordered anesthesia. The patient should take nothing by mouth preoperatively. Don't give oral medications unless ordered. Be sure to raise the bed's side rails immediately after giving preoperative medications. **AORN**

▶ If family members or others are present, direct them to the appropriate waiting area, and offer support as needed. **CS4**

Selected references

American Society of Peri-Anesthesia Nurses. "ASPEN Pain and Comfort Clinical Guideline," *Journal of Perianesthesia Nursing* 18(4), August 2003.

AORN Guidance Statement. "Preoperative Patient Care in the Ambulatory Surgery Setting." *AORN Journal* 81(4):871–8, April 2005.

Blay, N., and Donoghue, J. "The effect of pre-admission education on domiciliary recovery following laparoscopic cholecystectomy," Australian Journal of Advanced Nursing 22(4):14–19, June–August 2005. **CS3**

Devine, E. C and Cook, T. "A meta-analytic analysis of effects of psychoeducational interventions on length of postsurgical hospital stay," Nursing Research 32(5):267–74, September–October 1983. **CS1**

Hillier, M. "Exploring the Evidence around Pre-operative Fasting Practices," *Nursing Times* 102(28):36–38, July 2006.

Institute for Clinical Systems Improvement (ICSI). *Preoperative Evaluation.* Bloomington, Minn.: ICSI, July 2006.

Ivarsson, B., et al. "Waiting for cardiac surgery—support experienced by next of kin," European Journal of Cardiovascular Nursing 4(2):145–52, June 2005. **CS4**

Lithner, M., and Zilling, T. "Pre- and postoperative information needs," Patient Education and Counseling 40(1):29–37, April 2000. **CS2**

Preoperative skin preparation

Proper preparation of the patient's skin for surgery renders it as free as possible from microorganisms, thereby reducing the risk of infection at the incision site. **AORN** It doesn't duplicate or replace the full sterile preparation that immediately precedes surgery. Rather, it may involve a bath, shower, or local scrub with an antiseptic detergent solution, followed by hair removal. (See *Where to remove hair for surgery.*)

Hair shouldn't be removed from the area surrounding the operative site unless it's thick enough to interfere with surgery because hair removal may increase the risk of infection. If hair needs to be removed, use clippers. Clipping hair should occur immediately before an operation to decrease the risk of surgical site infection. **AORN CDC CS1** Each facility has a hair removal policy.

The area of preparation always exceeds that of the expected incision to minimize the number of microorganisms in the areas adjacent to the proposed incision and to allow surgical draping of the patient without contamination. **AORN CDC**

Equipment

Antiseptic soap solution ◆ tap water ◆ bath blanket ◆ two clean basins ◆ linen-saver pad ◆ adjustable light ◆ electric clippers ◆ scissors ◆ optional: 4″ × 4″ gauze pads, cotton-tipped applicators, acetone or nail polish remover, orangewood stick, trash bag, towel, gloves.

Implementation

▶ Check the practitioner's order, and explain the procedure to the patient, including the reason for the extensive preparations to avoid causing undue anxiety. Provide privacy, wash your hands thoroughly, and put on gloves.
▶ Place the patient in a comfortable position, drape him with the bath blanket, and expose the preparation area. For most surgeries, this area extends 12″ (30.5 cm) in each direction from the expected incision site. However, to ensure privacy and avoid chilling the patient, expose only one small area at a time while performing skin preparation.
▶ Position a linen-saver pad beneath the patient to catch spills and avoid

linen changes. Adjust the light to illuminate the preparation area.
▶ Assess the patient's skin condition in the preparation area, and report any rash, abrasion, or laceration to the physician before beginning the procedure. Any break in the skin increases the risk of infection and could cause cancellation of the planned surgery. **AORN**
▶ Have the patient remove all jewelry in or near the operative site.
▶ Put on gloves and, as ordered, begin removing hair from the preparation area by clipping any long hairs with clippers. Perform the procedure as near to the time of surgery as possible so that microorganisms will have minimal time to proliferate. **AORN CDC**
▶ Proceed with a 10-minute scrub to ensure a clean preparation area. Wash the area with a gauze pad dipped in the antiseptic soap solution. Using a circular motion, start at the expected incision site and work outward toward the periphery of the area to avoid recontaminating the clean area. Apply light friction while washing to improve the antiseptic effect of the solution. Replace the gauze pad as necessary. **AORN CDC CS2**

▶ Carefully clean skin folds and crevices because they harbor greater numbers of microorganisms. Scrub the perineal area last, if it's part of the preparation area, for the same reason. Pull loose skin taut. If necessary, use cotton-tipped applicators to clean the umbilicus and an orangewood stick to clean under nails. Be sure to remove nail polish because the anesthetist uses nail bed color to determine adequate oxygenation and may place a probe on the nail to measure oxygen saturation.
▶ Dry the area with a clean towel, and remove the linen-saver pad.
▶ Give the patient special instructions for care of the prepared area, and remind him to keep the area clean for surgery. Make sure the patient is comfortable.
▶ Properly dispose of solutions and the trash bag, and clean or dispose of soiled equipment and supplies according to your facility's policy.

Special considerations

▶ Avoid shaving facial or neck hair on women and children unless ordered. Never shave eyebrows because this disrupts normal hair growth and the new

(Text continues on page 424.)

Where to remove hair for surgery

Shoulder and upper arm

On the operative side, remove hair from the fingertips to the hairline and the center chest to the center spine, extending to the iliac crest and including the axilla.

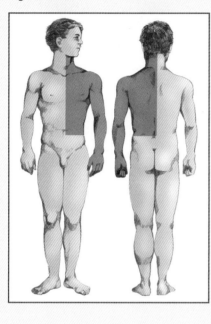

Chest

Remove hair from the chin to the iliac crest and nipple on the unaffected side to the midline of the back on the operative side (2" [5 cm] beyond the midline of the back for a thoracotomy). Include the axilla and the entire arm to the elbow on the operative side.

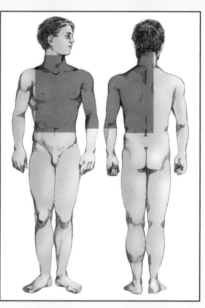

Forearm, elbow, and hand

On the operative side, remove hair from the fingertips to the shoulder. Include the axilla unless surgery is for the hand. Clean and trim fingernails.

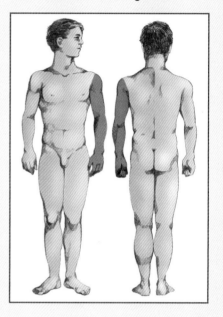

Abdomen

Remove hair from 3" (7.6 cm) above the nipples to the upper thighs, including the pubic area.

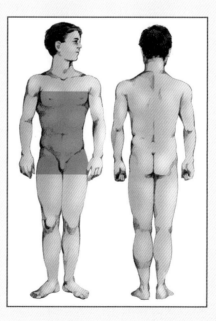

(continued)

Where to remove hair for surgery (continued)

Thigh

On the operative side, remove hair from the toes to 3″ above the umbilicus and from the midline front to the midline back, including the pubis. Clean and trim toenails.

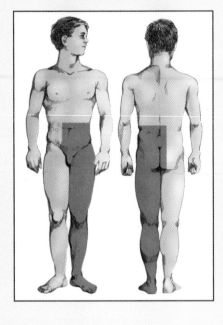

Lower abdomen

Remove hair from 2″ above the umbilicus to the midthigh, including the pubic area; for femoral ligation, to the midline of the thigh in the back; and for hernioplasty and embolectomy, to the costal margin and down to the knee.

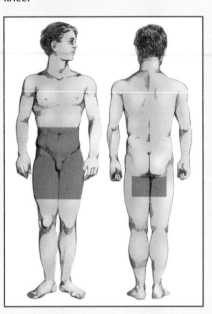

Hip

On the operative side, remove hair from the toes to the nipples and at least 3″ beyond the midline back and front, including the pubis. Clean and trim toenails.

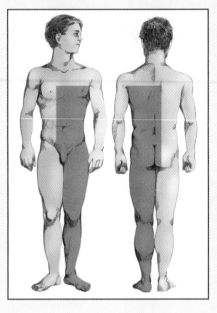

Flank

On the operative side, remove hair from the nipples to the pubis, 3″ beyond the midline in back and 2″ past the abdominal midline. Include the pubic area and, on the affected side, the upper thigh and axilla.

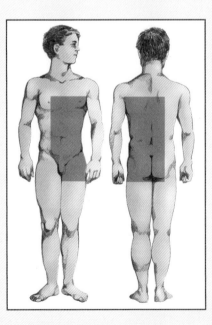

Where to remove hair for surgery (continued)

Knee and lower leg
On the operative side, remove hair from the toes to the groin. Clean and trim toenails.

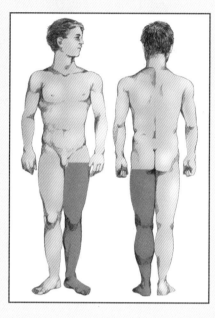

Perineum
Remove hair from the pubis, perineum, and perianal area and from the waist to at least 3" below the groin in front and at least 3" below the buttocks in back.

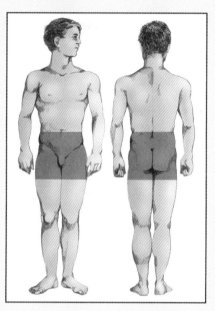

Ankle and foot
On the operative side, remove hair from the toes to 3" above the knee. Clean and trim toenails.

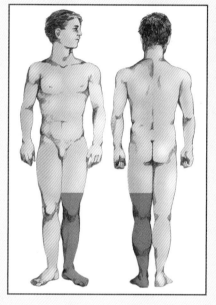

Spine
Remove hair from the entire back, including the shoulders and neck to the hairline and down to both knees. Include the axillae.

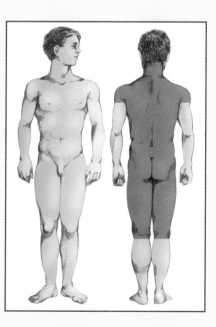

growth may prove unsightly. Scalp shaving is usually performed in the operating room, but if you're required to prepare the patient's scalp, put all hair in a plastic or paper bag, and store it with the patient's possessions.

▶ Depilatory cream can also be used to remove hair. Although this method produces clean, intact skin without risking lacerations or abrasions, it can cause skin irritation or rash, especially in the groin area. **AORN** **CDC** If possible, cut long hairs with scissors before applying the cream because removal of remaining hair then requires less cream. Use a glove to apply the cream in a layer $1/2''$ (1.3 cm) thick. After about 10 minutes, remove the cream with moist gauze pads. Next, wash the area with antiseptic soap solution, rinse, and pat dry.

Selected references

Aly, R., et al. "Comparative antibacterial efficacy of a 2-minute surgical scrub with chlorhexidine gluconate, povidone-iodine, and chloroxylenol sponge-brushes," American Journal of Infection Control 16(4):173–7, August 1988. **CS2**

Bratzler, D. W. "The Surgical Infection Prevention and Surgical Care Improvement Projects: Promises and Pitfalls," The American Surgeon 72(11):1010–1016, November 2006.

Centers for Disease Control and Prevention. Guideline for Prevention of Surgical Site Infection, 1999. Available at www.cdc.gov/ncidod/dhqp/gl_surgicalsite.html.

Odom-Forren, J. "Preventing Surgical Site Infections," Nursing 36(6):59–64, June 2006.

Olson, M. M., et al. "Preoperative hair removal with clippers does not increase infection rate in clean surgical wounds," Surgery, Gynecology, and Obstetrics 162(2):181–2. February 1986. **CS1**

Pyrek, K. M. "Preoperative Prep Should Safeguard Skin Integrity," Infection Control Today 2007. Available at www.infectioncontroltoday.com/articles/406/406_23topics.html.

Surgical Care Improvement Project Partnership. "Tips for Safer Surgery," Oklahoma Foundation for Medical Quality, 2007. Available at www.medqlc.org/scip.

Pressure dressing application

For effective control of capillary or small-vein bleeding, temporary application of pressure directly over a wound may be achieved with a bulk dressing held by a glove-protected hand, bound into place with a pressure bandage, or held under pressure by an inflated air splint. A pressure dressing requires frequent checks for wound drainage to determine its effectiveness in controlling bleeding. If the bleeding is coming from an artery, pressure will need to be held proximal to the wound to help stop the bleeding. (See *The pressure points.*)

Equipment

Two or more sterile gauze pads ◆ roller gauze ◆ adhesive tape ◆ clean disposable gloves ◆ metric ruler.

Implementation

▶ Obtain the pressure dressing quickly to avoid excessive blood loss. Use a clean cloth for the dressing if sterile gauze pads are unavailable.

▶ Quickly explain the procedure to the patient to help decrease his anxiety, and put on gloves. **CDC**

▶ Elevate the injured body part to help reduce bleeding.

▶ Place enough gauze pads over the wound to cover it. Don't clean the wound until the bleeding stops.

▶ For an extremity or a trunk wound, hold the dressing firmly over the wound and wrap the roller gauze tightly across it and around the body part to provide pressure on the wound. Secure the bandage with adhesive tape.

▶ To apply a dressing to the neck, shoulder, or another location that can't be tightly wrapped, don't use roller gauze. Instead, apply tape directly over the dressings to provide the necessary pressure at the wound site.

▶ Check the pulse, temperature, and skin condition distal to the wound site because excessive pressure can obstruct normal circulation.

▶ Check the dressing frequently to monitor wound drainage. Don't circle a potentially wet dressing with ink because this provides no permanent documentation in the medical record and may also contaminate the dressing.

▶ If the dressing becomes saturated, don't remove it because this will interfere with the pressure. Instead, apply an additional dressing over the saturat-

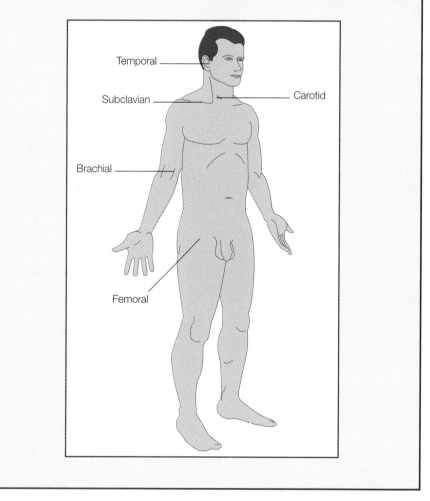

The pressure points

The illustration below shows some common pressure points for arterial bleeding.

Temporal

Subclavian

Carotid

Brachial

Femoral

ed one and continue to monitor and record drainage.

▶ Obtain additional medical care as soon as possible.

Special considerations

▶ Apply pressure directly to the wound with your gloved hand if sterile gauze pads and a clean cloth are unavailable.

▶ Avoid using an elastic bandage to bind the dressing because it can't be wrapped tightly enough to create pressure on the wound site.

Selected references

Dean, R. "Emergency First Aid for Nurses," *Nursing Standard* 20(6):57–65, October 2005.

Karabagli, Y., et al. "Industrial Foam Rubber as a Pressure Dressing," *Plastic and Reconstructive Surgery* 114(3):826, September 2004.

Kauvar, D., et al. "Impact of Hemorrhage on Trauma Outcome: An Overview of Epidemiology, Clinical Presentation, and Therapeutic Considerations," *The Journal of Trauma* 60(6 Suppl):53–61, June 2006.

Laskowski-Jones, L. "First Aid for Bleeding Wounds," *Nursing* 36(9):50–51, September 2006.

Pressure ulcer care

A pressure ulcer is a lesion caused by unrelieved pressure that results in damage to underlying tissues. Most pressure ulcers develop over bony prominences, where friction and shearing force combine with pressure to break down skin and underlying tissues. Approximately 95% of pressure ulcers occur in the lower part of the body, with the sacrum or the heel being the two most frequent sites that experience skin breakdown.

Successful pressure ulcer treatment involves relieving pressure, restoring circulation and, if possible, resolving or managing related disorders. Typically, the effectiveness and duration of treatment depend on the pressure ulcer's characteristics. Ideally, prevention is the key to avoiding extensive therapy. Preventive strategies include recognizing the risk, decreasing the effects of pressure, assessing the patient's nutritional status, avoiding excessive bed rest, and preserving skin integrity. Although many systems have been developed for the classification or "staging" of wounds, the system currently recommended by the Agency for Healthcare Research and Quality and the Wound, Ostomy, and Continence Nurses Society is a six-stage system based on the tissue layers involved. (See *Assessing pressure ulcers,* pages 428 and 429.)

The Braden scale, on the other hand, is the assessment tool of choice for determining the risk of developing pressure sores; it's also used to direct the implementation of preventive strategies. (See *Braden scale: Predicting pressure sore risk,* pages 430 and 431.)

Treatment includes methods to decrease pressure, such as frequent repositioning to shorten pressure duration, and the use of special equipment to reduce pressure intensity. Treatment may also involve special pressure-reducing devices, such as beds, mattresses, mattress overlays, and chair cushions. Other therapeutic measures include decreasing risk factors and use of topical treatments, wound cleansing, debridement, and the use of dressings to support moist wound healing.

Nurses usually perform or coordinate treatments according to your facility's policy. The detailed procedures address cleaning and dressing the pressure ulcer. Always follow the standard precautions guidelines of the Centers for Disease Control and Prevention.

Equipment

Hypoallergenic tape or elastic netting ◆ overbed table ◆ piston-type irrigating system ◆ two pairs of gloves ◆ normal saline solution as ordered ◆ sterile 4″ × 4″ gauze pads ◆ sterile cotton swab ◆ selected topical dressing ◆ linen-saver pads ◆ impervious plastic trash bag ◆ disposable wound-measuring device ◆ optional: skin sealant.

Implementation

▶ Confirm the patient's identity using two patient identifiers according to your facility's policy. **JC**
▶ Cut tape into strips for securing dressings. Loosen lids on cleaning solutions and medications for easy removal. Loosen existing dressing edges and tapes before putting on gloves. Attach an impervious plastic trash bag to the overbed table to hold used dressings and refuse.
▶ Premedicate the patient, if necessary. **WOCN**
▶ Before any dressing change, wash your hands and review the principles of standard precautions. **CDC**

Cleaning the pressure ulcer
▶ Provide privacy, and explain the procedure to the patient to allay his fears and promote cooperation.
▶ Position the patient in a way that maximizes his comfort while allowing easy access to the pressure ulcer site.

▶ Cover bed linens with a linen-saver pad to prevent soiling.
▶ Open the normal saline solution container and the piston syringe. Carefully pour normal saline solution into an irrigation container to avoid splashing. (The container may be clean or sterile, according to your facility's policy.) Put the piston syringe into the opening provided in the irrigation container. **WOCN**
▶ Open the packages of supplies.
▶ Put on gloves and remove the old dressing, exposing the pressure ulcer. Discard the soiled dressing in the impervious plastic trash bag.
▶ Inspect the wound. Note the color, amount, and odor of drainage and necrotic debris. Measure the wound

(Text continues on page 432.)

Assessing pressure ulcers

To select the most effective treatment for a pressure ulcer, you first need to assess its characteristics. The pressure ulcer staging system described here, used by the National Pressure Ulcer Advisory Panel and the Agency for Healthcare Research and Quality, reflects the anatomic depth of exposed tissue. Keep in mind that if the wound contains necrotic tissue, you won't be able to determine the stage until you can see the wound base.

Suspected deep tissue injury

Deep tissue injury is characterized by a purple or maroon localized area of intact skin or a blood-filled blister caused by damage of underlying soft tissue from pressure or shear. The injury may be preceded by tissue that's painful, firm, mushy, boggy, or warm or cool compared to adjacent tissue. Further, it may be difficult to detect in individuals with dark skin tones.

Stage I

A stage I pressure ulcer is characterized by intact skin with nonblanchable redness of a localized area, usually over a bony prominence. Darkly pigmented skin may not have visible blanching, but its color may differ from the surrounding area.

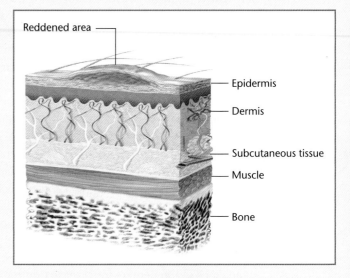

Stage II

A stage II pressure ulcer is characterized by partial-thickness loss of the dermis, presenting as a shallow, open ulcer with a red-pink wound bed without slough. It may also present as an intact or open serum-filled blister.

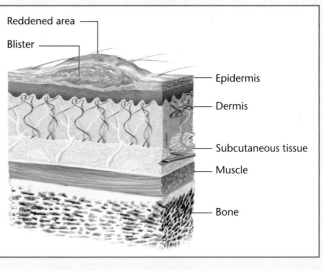

Assessing pressure ulcers (continued)

Stage III

A stage III pressure ulcer is characterized by full-thickness tissue loss. Subcutaneous fat may be visible, but bone, tendon, and muscle aren't exposed. Slough may be present but doesn't obscure the depth of tissue loss. Undermining and tunneling may be present. The depth of a stage III ulcer varies by anatomical location.

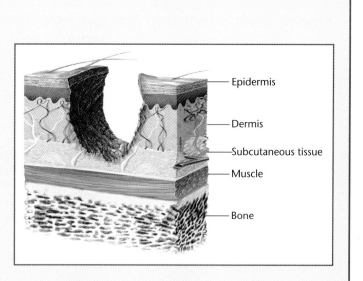

Stage IV

A stage IV pressure ulcer involves full-thickness tissue loss with exposed bone, tendon, or muscle. Slough or eschar may be present on some parts of the wound bed. Undermining and tunneling are also common. The depth of a stage IV ulcer varies by anatomical location.

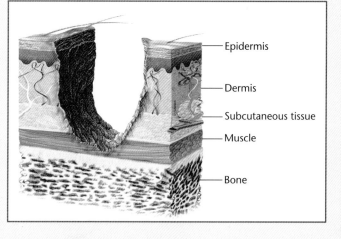

Unstageable

An unstageable ulcer is characterized by full-thickness tissue loss in which the base of the ulcer in the wound bed is covered by slough, eschar, or both. Until enough slough or eschar is removed to expose the base of the wound, the true depth, and therefore stage, can't be determined.

Braden scale: Predicting pressure sore risk

The Braden scale, shown below, is the most reliable of several instruments used to assess the risk of developing pressure sores. The numbers to the left of each description are the points to be tallied; the lower the score, the greater the risk.

Patient's name _____   Evaluator's name _____

Sensory perception Ability to respond meaningfully to pressure-related discomfort	**1. Completely limited** Patient is unresponsive (doesn't moan, flinch, or grasp in response) to painful stimuli because of diminished level of consciousness or sedation. OR Patient has a limited ability to feel pain over most of body surface.	**2. Very limited** Patient responds only to painful stimuli; can't communicate discomfort except through moaning or restlessness. OR Patient has a sensory impairment that limits ability to feel pain or discomfort over half of body.
Moisture Degree to which skin is exposed to moisture	**1. Constantly moist** Patient's skin is kept moist almost constantly by perspiration or urine; dampness is detected every time he's moved or turned.	**2. Very moist** Patient's skin is usually but not always moist; linen must be changed at least once per shift.
Activity Degree of physical activity	**1. Bedfast** Patient is confined to bed.	**2. Chairfast** Patient's ability to walk severely limited or nonexistent; can't bear own weight and must be assisted into a chair or wheelchair.
Mobility Ability to change and control body position	**1. Completely immobile** Patient doesn't make even slight changes in body or extremity position without assistance.	**2. Very limited** Patient makes occasional slight changes in body or extremity position but can't make frequent or significant changes independently.
Nutrition Usual food intake pattern	**1. Very poor** Patient never eats a complete meal; rarely eats more than one-third of any food offered; eats two servings or less of protein (meat or dairy products) per day; takes fluids poorly; doesn't take a liquid dietary supplement. OR Patient is on nothing-by-mouth status or maintained on clear liquids or I.V. fluids for more than 5 days.	**2. Probably inadequate** Patient rarely eats a complete meal and generally eats only about one-half of any food offered; protein intake includes only three servings of meat or dairy products per day; occasionally will take a dietary supplement. OR Patient receives less than optimum amount of liquid diet or tube feeding.
Friction and shear	**1. Problem** Patient requires moderate to maximum assistance in moving; complete lifting without sliding against sheets is impossible; frequently slides down in bed or chair, requiring frequent repositioning with maximum assistance; spasticity, contractures, or agitation leads to almost constant friction.	**2. Potential problem** Patient moves feebly or requires minimum assistance during a move; skin probably slides to some extent against sheets, chair restraints, or other devices; maintains relatively good position in chair or bed most of the time but occasionally slides down.

Date of Assessment _____

3. Slightly limited
Patient responds to verbal commands but can't always communicate discomfort or the need to be turned.
OR
Patient has some sensory impairment that limits ability to feel pain or discomfort in one or two extremities.

4. No impairment
Patient responds to verbal commands; has no sensory deficit that would limit ability to feel or voice pain or discomfort.

3. Occasionally moist
Patient's skin is occasionally moist; linen requires an extra change approximately once per day.

4. Rarely moist
Patient's skin is usually dry; linen requires changing only at routine intervals.

3. Walks occasionally
Patient walks occasionally during the day, but for very short distances, with or without assistance; spends majority of each shift in a bed or chair.

4. Walks frequently
Patient walks outside room at least twice per day and inside room at least once every 2 hours during waking hours.

3. Slightly limited
Patient makes frequent (although slight) changes in body or extremity position independently.

4. No limitations
Patient makes major and frequent changes in body or extremity position without assistance.

3. Adequate
Patient eats more than one-half of most meals; eats four servings of protein (meat and dairy products) per day; occasionally refuses a meal but will usually take a supplement if offered.
OR
Patient is on a tube feeding or total parenteral nutrition regimen that probably meets most nutritional needs.

4. Excellent
Patient eats most of every meal and never refuses a meal; usually eats four or more servings of meat and dairy products per day; occasionally eats between meals; doesn't require supplementation.

3. No apparent problem
Patient moves in bed and in chair independently and has sufficient muscle strength to lift up completely during move; maintains good position in bed or chair at all times.

Total Score

perimeter with the disposable wound-measuring device. **WOCN**

▶ Using the piston syringe, apply full force to irrigate the pressure ulcer to remove necrotic debris and help decrease bacteria in the wound. For nonnecrotic wounds, use gentle pressure to prevent damage to new tissue.

▶ Remove and discard your soiled gloves, and put on a fresh pair.

▶ Insert a sterile cotton swab into the wound to assess wound tunneling or undermining. Tunneling usually signals wound extension along fascial planes. **WOCN**

▶ Next, reassess the condition of the skin and the ulcer. Note the character of the clean wound bed and the surrounding skin. **WOCN**

▶ If you observe adherent necrotic material, notify a wound care specialist or a practitioner to ensure appropriate debridement.

▶ Prepare to apply the appropriate topical dressing. Directions for applying topical moist saline gauze, hydrocolloid, transparent, alginate, foam, and hydrogel dressings are detailed below. For other dressings or topical agents, follow your facility's policy or the manufacturer's instructions.

Applying a moist saline gauze dressing

▶ Irrigate the pressure ulcer with normal saline solution. Blot the surrounding skin dry with a sterile 4″ × 4″ gauze pad.

▶ Moisten the gauze dressing with normal saline solution.

▶ Gently place the dressing over the surface of the ulcer. To separate surfaces within the wound, gently place a dressing between opposing wound surfaces. To avoid damage to tissues, don't pack the gauze tightly.

▶ Change the dressing often enough to keep the wound moist. (See *Choosing a pressure ulcer dressing*.)

Applying a hydrocolloid dressing

▶ Irrigate the pressure ulcer with normal saline solution. Blot the surrounding skin dry with a sterile 4″ × 4″ gauze pad. **WOCN**

▶ Choose a clean, dry, presized dressing, or cut one to overlap the pressure ulcer by about 1″ (2.5 cm). Remove the dressing from its package, pull the release paper from the adherent side of the dressing, and apply the dressing to the wound. To minimize irritation, carefully smooth out wrinkles as you apply the dressing.

▶ If the dressing's edges need to be secured with tape, apply a skin sealant to the intact skin around the ulcer. After the area dries, tape the dressing to the skin. Avoid using tension or pressure when applying the tape.

▶ Remove your gloves and discard them in the impervious plastic trash bag. Dispose of refuse according to your facility's policy, and wash your hands.

▶ Change a hydrocolloid dressing every 2 to 7 days as necessary—for example, if the patient complains of pain, the dressing no longer adheres, or leakage occurs. Discontinue if signs of infection are present.

Applying a transparent dressing

▶ Irrigate the pressure ulcer with normal saline solution. Blot the surrounding skin dry with a sterile 4″ × 4″ gauze pad. **WOCN**

▶ Select a dressing to overlap the ulcer by 2″ (5 cm).

▶ Gently lay the dressing over the ulcer. To prevent shearing force, don't stretch the dressing. Press firmly on the edges of the dressing to promote adherence. Although this type of dressing is self-adhesive, you may have to tape the edges to prevent them from curling.

▶ If necessary, aspirate accumulated fluid with a 21G needle and syringe.

After aspirating the pocket of fluid, clean the aspiration site with an alcohol pad and cover it with another strip of transparent dressing.

▶ Change the dressing every 3 to 7 days, depending on the amount of drainage.

Applying an alginate dressing

▶ Irrigate the pressure ulcer with normal saline solution. Blot the surrounding skin dry with a sterile 4″ × 4″ gauze pad. **WOCN**

▶ Apply the alginate dressing to the ulcer surface. Cover the area with a secondary dressing (such as gauze pads), as ordered. Secure the dressing with tape or elastic netting.

▶ If the wound is draining heavily, change the dressing once or twice daily for the first 3 to 5 days. As drainage decreases, change the dressing less frequently—every 2 to 4 days or as ordered. When the drainage stops or the wound bed looks dry, stop using alginate dressing.

Applying a foam dressing

▶ Irrigate the pressure ulcer with normal saline solution. Blot the surrounding skin dry with a sterile 4″ × 4″ gauze pad. **WOCN**

▶ Gently lay the foam dressing over the ulcer.

▶ Use tape, elastic netting, or gauze to hold the dressing in place.

▶ Change the dressing when the foam no longer absorbs the exudate.

Applying a hydrogel dressing

▶ Irrigate the pressure ulcer with normal saline solution. Blot the surrounding skin dry with a sterile 4″ × 4″ gauze pad. **WOCN**

▶ Apply gel to the wound bed.

▶ Cover the area with a secondary dressing.

▶ Change the dressing daily, or as needed, to keep the wound bed moist.

Choosing a pressure ulcer dressing

Choosing the proper dressing for a wound should be guided by four questions:

▶ What does the wound need? (Does it need to be drained, protected, kept moist?)
▶ What does the dressing do?
▶ How well does the product do it?
▶ What is available and practical?

Hydrocolloid dressings

Hydrocolloid dressings are adhesive, moldable wafers that are made of a carbohydrate-based material and usually have waterproof backings. They're impermeable to oxygen, water, and water vapor and most have some absorptive properties.

Gauze dressings

Made of absorptive cotton or synthetic fabric, gauze dressings are permeable to water, water vapor, and oxygen and may be impregnated with petroleum jelly or another agent. When uncertain about which dressing to use, you may apply a gauze dressing moistened in saline solution until a wound specialist recommends definitive treatment.

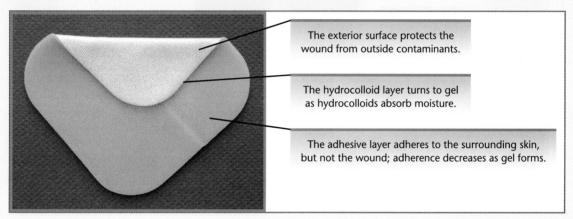

The exterior surface protects the wound from outside contaminants.

The hydrocolloid layer turns to gel as hydrocolloids absorb moisture.

The adhesive layer adheres to the surrounding skin, but not the wound; adherence decreases as gel forms.

Transparent film dressings

Transparent film dressings are clear, adherent, nonabsorptive, polymer-based dressings that are permeable to oxygen and water vapor but not to water. Their transparency allows visual inspection. Because they can't absorb drainage, these dressings are used on partial-thickness wounds with minimal exudate.

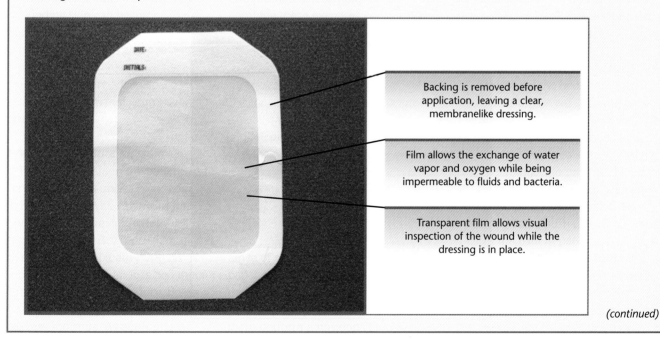

Backing is removed before application, leaving a clear, membranelike dressing.

Film allows the exchange of water vapor and oxygen while being impermeable to fluids and bacteria.

Transparent film allows visual inspection of the wound while the dressing is in place.

(continued)

However, avoid seating the patient on a rubber or plastic doughnut, which can increase localized pressure at vulnerable points. **CS4**

▶ Adjust or pad appliances, casts, or splints, as needed, to ensure proper fit and avoid increased pressure and impaired circulation.

▶ Tell the patient to avoid heat lamps and harsh soaps because they dry the skin. Applying lotion after bathing will help keep his skin moist. Also tell him to avoid vigorous massage because it can damage capillaries. **WOCN**

▶ If the patient's condition permits, recommend a diet that includes adequate calories, protein, and vitamins. Dietary therapy may involve nutritional consultation, food supplements, enteral feeding, or total parenteral nutrition. **WOCN** **CS5**

▶ If diarrhea develops or if the patient is incontinent, clean and dry soiled skin. Then apply a protective moisture barrier to prevent skin maceration. **WOCN**

▶ Make sure the patient, family members, and caregivers learn pressure ulcer prevention and treatment strategies so that they understand the importance of care, the choices that are available, the rationales for treatments, and their own role in selecting goals and shaping the care plan.

Special considerations

▶ Avoid using elbow and heel protectors that fasten with a single narrow strap. The strap may impair neurovascular function in the involved hand or foot.

▶ Avoid using artificial sheepskin. It doesn't reduce pressure, and it may create a false sense of security. **WOCN**

▶ Repair of stage III and stage IV ulcers may require surgical intervention—such as direct closure, skin grafting, and flaps—depending on the patient's needs. They may also be treated with growth factors, electrical stimulation, heat therapy, or vacuum-assisted wound closure.

Selected references

Ayello, E. A., and Baronoski, S. "Examining the Problem of Pressure Ulcers," *Advances in Skin & Wound Care* 18(4):192, May 2005.

Benbow, M. "Guidelines for the Prevention and Treatment of Pressure Ulcers," *Nursing Standard* 20(52):42–44, September 2006.

Bouza, C., et al. "Efficacy of Advanced Dressings in the Treatment of Pressure Ulcers: A Systematic Review," *Journal of Wound Care* 14(5):193–99, May 2005.

Clance, H. F. "Pressure Ulcers: Implementation of Evidence-based Nursing Practice," *Journal of Advanced Nursing* 49(6):578–90, March 2005.

Crewe, R. A. "Problems of rubber ring nursing cushions and a clinical survey of alternative cushions for ill patients," *Care Science Practice* 5(2):9–11, June 1987. **CS4**

Cullum, et al. "Support surfaces for pressure ulcer prevention," Cochrane Database of Systematic Reviews (3):CD001735, 2004. **CS2**

Fletcher, J. "Understanding Wound Dressings: Foam Dressings," *Nursing Times* 101(24):50–51, June 2005.

Kaya, A. Z., et al. "The Effectiveness of a Hydrogel Dressing Compared with Standard Management of Pressure Ulcers," *Journal of Wound Care* 14(1):42–44, January 2005.

Keast, D. H., et al. "Best Practice Recommendations for the Prevention and Treatment of Pressure Ulcers: Update 2006," *Advances in Skin & Wound Care* 20(8):447–60, August 2007.

Knox, D. M., et al. "Effects of different turn intervals on skin of healthy older adults," *Advances in Wound Care* 7(1):48–52, 54–6, January 1994. **CS3**

Lyder, C., and van Rijswijk, L. "Pressure Ulcer Prevention and Care: Preventing and Managing Pressure Ulcers in Long-term Care: An Overview of the Revised Federal Regulation," *Ostomy/Wound Management* Suppl:2–6, April 2005.

Parnell, L. K., et al. "Preliminary Use of a Hydrogel Containing Enzymes in the Treatment of Stage II and Stage III Pressure Ulcers," *Ostomy/Wound Management* 51(8):50–60, August 2005.

Stratton, R. J., et al. "Enteral nutritional support in prevention and treatment of pressure ulcers: a systematic review and meta-analysis," *Ageing Research Reviews* 4(3):422–50, August 2005. **CS5**

Vyhlidal, S. K., et al. "Mattress replacement or foam overlay? A prospective study on the incidence of pressure ulcers," *Applied Nursing Research* 10(3):111–20, August 1997. **CS1**

Wound, Ostomy, and Continence Nurses Society (WOCN). Position Statement: "Clean vs Sterile: Management of Chronic Wounds." Glenview, Ill.: WOCN, 2005.

WOCN. *Guidelines for Prevention and Management of Pressure Ulcers.* Glenview, Ill.: WOCN, 2003.

Prone positioning

Prone positioning is a therapeutic maneuver to improve oxygenation and pulmonary mechanics in patients with acute lung injury or acute respiratory distress syndrome. Also known as *proning,* the procedure involves physically turning a patient from a supine position (on the back) to a facedown position (prone position). This positioning may improve oxygenation by shifting blood flow to regions of the lung that are better ventilated. With the appropriate equipment, prone positioning may also facilitate better movement of the diaphragm by allowing the abdomen to expand more fully.

The physical challenges of proning have been a traditional barrier to its use. However, equipment innovations (such as a lightweight, cushioned frame that straps to the front of the patient before turning) have helped to minimize the risks associated with moving patients and maintaining them in the prone position for several hours at a time.

Prone positioning is contraindicated in patients whose heads can't be supported in a facedown position or in those who are unable to tolerate a head-down position. Relative contraindications include:

▶ increased intracranial pressure
▶ unstable spine, chest, or pelvis
▶ unstable bone fractures
▶ left-sided heart failure (nonpulmonary respiratory failure)
▶ shock
▶ abdominal compartment syndrome or abdominal surgery
▶ patients who are extremely obese (more than 300 lb [136 kg])
▶ pregnancy.

Hemodynamically unstable patients (systolic blood pressure less than 90 mm Hg), despite aggressive fluid resuscitation and vasopressors, should be thoroughly evaluated before being placed in the prone position.

Equipment

Vollman Prone Positioner (Hill Rom) or other prone positioning device ◆ gloves ◆ personal protective equipment as appropriate ◆ draw sheet ◆ small towel ◆ small pillow or rolled towel ◆ suction equipment as needed ◆ oral care supplies ◆ eye lubricant.

Implementation

▶ Confirm the patient's identity using two patient identifiers according to your facility's policy. **JC**
▶ Assess the patient's hemodynamic status to determine whether the patient can tolerate the prone position.
▶ Assess the patient's neurologic status before prone positioning. Generally, the patient will be heavily sedated. Although agitation isn't a contraindication for proning, it must be managed effectively.
▶ Determine whether the patient's size and weight will allow turning him on a generally narrow critical care bed. Consider obtaining a wider specialty bed, if needed.

Before turning the patient

▶ Explain the purpose and procedure of prone positioning to the patient and his family.
▶ Wash your hands, and put on gloves or other protective wear, as appropriate.
▶ Provide eye care, including lubrication and horizontal taping of the patient's eyelids, if indicated.
▶ Make sure the patient's tongue is inside his mouth; if it's edematous or protruding, insert a bite block.

▶ Secure the patient's endotracheal (ET) or tracheotomy tube to prevent dislodgment.
▶ Perform anterior body wound care and dressing changes.
▶ Empty ileostomy or colostomy drainage bags.
▶ Remove anterior chest wall electrocardiogram (ECG) monitoring leads, while ensuring the ability to monitor the patient's cardiac rate and rhythm. These leads will be repositioned onto the patient's back when he's prone.
▶ Make sure that the brake of the bed is engaged. Attach the surface of the prone positioner to the bed frame, as recommended by the manufacturer.
▶ Position staff appropriately; a minimum of three people is required: one on either side of the bed and one at the head of the bed. The staff member at

the head of the bed is responsible for monitoring the ET tube and mechanical ventilator tubing.

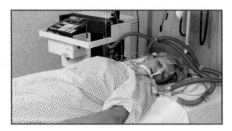

▶ Adjust all patient tubing and invasive monitoring lines to prevent dislodgment, kinking, disconnection, or contact with the patient's body during the turning procedure and while the patient remains in the prone position.

CLINICAL ALERT

Place all lines inserted in the upper torso over the right or left shoulder, with the exception of chest tubes, which are placed at the foot of the bed. All lines inserted in the lower torso are positioned at the foot of the bed.

▶ Turn the patient's face away from the ventilator, placing the ET tube on the side of the patient's face that's turned away from the ventilator. Loop the remaining tubing above the patient's head to prevent disconnection of the ventilator tubing or kinking of the ET tube during proning.

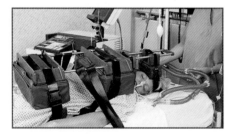

▶ Place the straps of the prone positioner under the patient's head, chest, and pelvic area.

▶ Attach the prone-positioning device to the patient by placing the frame on top of the patient.

▶ Position the nonmovable chest piece, which acts as a marker for the proper device placement, so that it's resting between the patient's clavicles and sixth ribs.

▶ Adjust the pelvic piece of the device so that it rests $1/2''$ (1.3 cm) above the iliac crest.

▶ Adjust the chin and forehead pieces of the device so that facial support is provided in either a facedown or side-lying position without interfering with the ET tube.

▶ Secure the positioning device to the patient by fastening all the soft adjustable straps on one side before tightening them on the opposite side. After it's secured, lift the positioner to ensure a secure fit.

Turning the patient

▶ Lower the side rails of the bed, and move the patient to the edge of the bed farthest away from the ventilator by using a draw sheet. The person closest to the patient maintains body contact with the bed at all times, serving as a side rail.

▶ Tuck the straps attached to the steel bar closest to the center of the bed underneath the patient. Then tuck the patient's arm and hand that are resting in the center of the bed under the buttocks. Cross the leg closest to the edge of the bed over the opposite leg at the ankle, which will help with forward motion when the turning process begins.

▶ Turn the patient toward the ventilator at a 45-degree angle.

▶ The person on the side of the bed with the ventilator grasps the upper steel bar. The person on the other side of the bed grasps the lower steel bar or turning straps of the device.

▶ Lift the patient by the frame into the prone position on the count of three.

▶ Gently move the patient's tucked arm and hand so they're parallel to his body and comfortable.

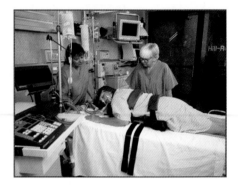

▶ Loosen the straps if the patient is clinically stable.

▶ Support the patient's feet with a pillow or towel roll to provide correct flexion while in the prone position.

▶ Monitor the patient's response to proning using vital signs, pulse oximetry, and mixed venous oxygen saturation. The patient's vital signs should return to normal within 10 minutes of being placed prone. During the initial proning, arterial blood gas values should be obtained within 30 minutes of proning and within 30 minutes before returning the patient to the supine position.

▶ Reposition the patient's head hourly while in the prone position to prevent facial breakdown. As one person lifts the patient's head, the second person moves the headpieces to provide head support in a different position.

▶ Provide range-of-motion exercise to shoulders, arms, and legs every 2 hours.

▶ Give oral care, and suction the patient as needed.

Returning the patient to the supine position

▶ Securely fasten positioning device straps.

▶ Remove the posterior chest ECG leads while ensuring the ability to monitor the patient's rate and rhythm. The leads will be replaced on the patient's chest when he's in the supine position.

▶ Position the patient on the edge of the bed closest to the ventilator.

▶ Adjust all patient tubing and monitoring lines to prevent dislodgment.

▶ Position a staff member on each side of the bed and one at the head.

▶ Straighten the patient's arms and rest them on either side. Cross the leg closest to the edge of the bed over the opposite leg.

▶ Using the steel bars of the device, turn the patient to a 45-degree angle away from the ventilator, and then roll him to the supine position.

▶ Position the patient's arms parallel to his body.

▶ Unfasten the positioning device, and remove it from the patient.

Special considerations

▶ Patients may require increased sedation during proning.

▶ The prone-positioning schedule is generally determined by the patient's ability to maintain improvements in the partial pressure of arterial oxygen while in the prone position.

▶ To reduce the risk of aspirating gastric contents during the turning procedure, turn off tube feedings 1 hour before turning the patient. The feeding can be safely restarted after the patient is positioned.

▶ Use capnography, if possible, to verify correct ET tube placement during proning.

▶ Reposition the patient every 4 to 6 hours to prevent pressure-related injury.

▶ Discontinue the procedure when the patient no longer demonstrates improved oxygenation with the position change.

Selected references

Davis, J. W., et al. "Prone Ventilation in Trauma or Surgical Patients with Acute Lung Injury and Adult Respiratory Distress Syndrome: Is it Beneficial?" *Journal of Trauma* 62(5):1201–206, May 2007.

deLeon, D. G., and Spieglern, P. "The Role of Prone Positions in the Management of Hypoxemic Acute Respiratory Failure," *Clinical Pulmonary Medicine* 12(2):128–29, March 2005.

Essat, Z. "Prone Positioning in Patients with Acute Respiratory Distress Syndrome," *Nursing Standard* 20(9):52–55, November 2005.

Lynn-McHale Wiegand, D. J., and Carlson, K. K., eds. *AACN Procedure Manual for Critical Care,* 5th ed. Philadelphia: W. B. Saunders Co., 2006.

Thomas, P. J., et al. "Positioning Practices for Ventilated Intensive Care Patients: Current Practice, Indications and Contraindications," *Australian Critical Care* 19(4):122–26, 128, 130–32, November 2006.

Vollman, K. M. "Prone Positioning in the Patient who has Acute Respiratory Distress Syndrome: The Art and Science," *Critical Care Nursing Clinics of North America* 16(3):319–36, September 2004.

Pulmonary artery pressure monitoring and PAWP monitoring

Continuous pulmonary artery pressure (PAP) and intermittent pulmonary artery wedge pressure (PAWP) measurements provide important information about left ventricular function and preload. You can use this information not only for monitoring but also for aiding diagnosis, refining your assessment, guiding interventions, and projecting patient outcomes.

Nearly all acutely ill patients are candidates for PAP monitoring—especially those who are hemodynamically unstable, who need fluid management or continuous cardiopulmonary assessment, or who are receiving multiple or frequently administered cardioactive drugs.

The original PAP monitoring catheter, which had two lumens, was invented by two physicians, Drs. Swan and Ganz. The device still bears their name (Swan-Ganz catheter) but is commonly referred to as a pulmonary artery (PA) catheter. Current versions have up to six lumens, allowing more hemodynamic information to be gathered. In addition to distal and proximal lumens used to measure pressures, a PA catheter has a balloon inflation lumen that inflates the balloon for PAWP measurement and a thermistor connector lumen that allows cardiac output measurement. Some catheters also have a pacemaker wire lumen that provides a port for pacemaker electrodes and measures continuous mixed venous oxygen saturation. (See *PA catheters: From basic to complex*.)

Fluoroscopy usually isn't required during catheter insertion because the catheter is flow directed, following venous blood flow from the right heart chambers into the pulmonary artery. Also, the pulmonary artery, right atrium, and right ventricle produce characteristic pressures and waveforms that can be observed on the monitor to help track catheter-tip location. Marks on the catheter shaft, with 10-cm graduations, assist tracking by showing how far the catheter is inserted.

The PA catheter is inserted into the heart's right side with the distal tip lying in the pulmonary artery. Left-sided pressures can be assessed indirectly.

No specific contraindications for PAP monitoring exist. However, some patients undergoing it require special precautions. These include elderly patients with pulmonary hypertension, those with left bundle-branch block, and those for whom a systemic infection would be life-threatening.

Equipment

Balloon-tipped, flow-directed PA catheter ◆ prepared pressure transducer system ◆ sterile gloves ◆ I.V. solutions ◆ alcohol pads ◆ medication-added label ◆ monitor and monitor cable ◆ I.V. pole with transducer mount ◆ emergency resuscitation equipment ◆ electrocardiogram (ECG) monitor ◆ ECG electrodes ◆ arm board (for antecubital insertion) ◆ lead aprons (if fluoroscopy is necessary) ◆ sterile marker ◆ sterile labels ◆ sutures ◆ sterile 4″ × 4″ gauze pads or dry, occlusive dressing material ◆ prepackaged introducer kit ◆ optional:

dextrose 5% in water, electric clippers (for femoral insertion site), small sterile basin, sterile water.

If a prepackaged introducer kit is unavailable, obtain the following: introducer (one size larger than the catheter) ◆ sterile tray containing instruments for procedure ◆ masks ◆ sterile gowns ◆ sterile gloves ◆ sterile drape ◆ 2% chlorhexidine solution ◆ sutures ◆ two 10-ml syringes ◆ local anesthetic (1% to 2% lidocaine) ◆ one 5-ml syringe ◆ 25G ½″ needle ◆ 1″ and 3″ tape.

Implementation

▶ To obtain reliable pressure values and clear waveforms, the pressure monitoring system and bedside monitor must be properly calibrated and zeroed. Make sure the monitor has the correct pressure modules, and then calibrate it according to the manufacturer's instructions. **MFR** (For instructions, see "Transducer system setup," page 561.)

▶ Turn the monitor on before gathering the equipment to give it time to warm up. Be sure to check the operations manual for the monitor you're

PA catheters: From basic to complex

Depending on the intended uses, pulmonary artery (PA) catheters may be simple or complex. A basic PA catheter has a distal and a proximal lumen, a thermistor, and a balloon inflation gate valve. The *distal lumen*, which exits in the pulmonary artery, monitors PA pressure. Its hub usually is marked P DISTAL or is color-coded yellow. The *proximal lumen* exits in the right atrium or vena cava, depending on the size of the patient's heart. It monitors right atrial pressure and can be used as the injected solution lumen for cardiac output determination and infusing solutions. The proximal lumen hub usually is marked PROXIMAL or is color-coded blue.

The *thermistor*, located about 1½" (3.8 cm) from the distal tip, measures temperature (aiding core temperature evaluation) and allows cardiac output measurement. The thermistor connector attaches to a cardiac output connector cable and then to a cardiac output monitor. Typically, it's red.

The *balloon inflation* gate valve is used for inflating the balloon tip with air. A stopcock connection, typically color-coded red, may be used.

Additional lumens

Complex PA catheters have additional lumens used to obtain other hemodynamic data or permit certain interventions. For instance, *a proximal infusion port*, which exits in the right atrium or vena cava, allows additional fluid administration. A *right ventricular lumen*, exiting in the right ventricle, allows fluid administration, right ventricular pressure measurement, or use of a temporary ventricular pacing lead.

Other complex PA catheters have additional right atrial and right ventricular lumens for atrioventricular pacing. A *right ventricular ejection fraction test-response thermistor*, with PA and right ventricular sensing electrodes, allows volumetric and ejection fraction measurements. Fiber-optic filaments, such as those used in pulse oximetry, exit into the pulmonary artery and permit measurement of continuous mixed venous oxygen saturation.

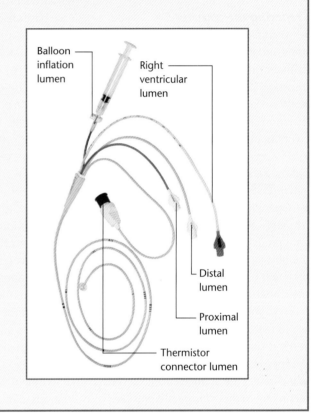

using; some older monitors may need 20 minutes to warm up.

▶ Prepare the pressure monitoring system according to policy. Your facility's guidelines may also specify whether to mount the transducer on the I.V. pole or tape it to the patient and whether to add heparin to the flush. Check the patient's chart for heparin sensitivity, which contraindicates adding heparin to the flush solution.

▶ To manage complications from catheter insertion, make sure to have emergency resuscitation equipment on hand (defibrillator, oxygen, and supplies for intubation and emergency drug administration).

▶ Prepare a sterile field for insertion of the introducer and catheter. Label all medications, medication containers, and solutions on and off the sterile field. **JC** **CDC**

▶ Confirm the patient's identity using two patient identifiers according to your facility's policy. **JC**

▶ If the patient is alert, explain the procedure to him to reduce his anxiety. Reassure him that the catheter poses little danger and rarely causes pain. Tell him that if he feels pain at the introducer insertion site, the physician will order an analgesic or a sedative.

▶ Be sure to tell the patient and his family not to be alarmed if they see the pressure waveform on the monitor "move around." Explain that the cause is usually artifact.

Positioning the patient for catheter placement

▶ Position the patient at the proper height and angle. If the physician will use a superior approach for percutaneous insertion (most commonly using the internal jugular or subclavian vein), place the patient flat or in a slight Trendelenburg position. Remove the patient's pillow to help engorge the vessel and prevent air embolism. Turn his head to the side opposite the insertion site.

Preparing the catheter

▶ Maintain sterile technique and use standard precautions throughout catheter preparation and insertion. **CDC** **AACN**

▶ Wash your hands. Then clean the insertion site with a 2% chlorhexidine solution and drape it. **CDC** **AACN**

▶ Put on a mask. Help the physician put on a sterile mask, gown, and gloves. **CDC** **AACN**

▶ Open the outer packaging of the catheter, revealing the inner sterile wrapping. Using sterile technique, the physician opens the inner wrapping and picks up the catheter. Take the catheter lumen hubs as he hands them to you.

▶ To remove air from the catheter and verify its patency, flush the catheter. In the more common flushing method, you connect the syringes using sterile technique to the appropriate pressure lines, and then flush them before insertion. This method makes pressure waveforms easier to identify on the monitor during insertion.

▶ Alternatively, you may flush the lumens after catheter insertion with sterile I.V. solution from sterile syringes attached to the lumens. Leave the filled syringes on during insertion.

▶ If the system has multiple pressure lines (such as a distal line to monitor PAP and a proximal line to monitor right atrial pressure), make sure the distal PA lumen hub is attached to the pressure line that will be observed on the monitor. Inadvertently attaching the distal PA line to the proximal lumen hub will prevent the proper waveform from appearing during insertion.

▶ To verify the integrity of the balloon, the physician inflates it with air (usually 1.5 cc) before handing you the lumens to attach to the pressure monitoring system. He then observes the balloon for symmetrical shape. He may also submerge it in a small, sterile basin filled with sterile water and observe it for bubbles, which indicate a leak.

Inserting the catheter

▶ Assist the physician as he inserts the introducer to access the vessel. He may perform a cutdown or (more commonly) insert the catheter percutaneously, as with a modified Seldinger technique.

▶ After the introducer is placed and the catheter lumens are flushed, the physician inserts the catheter through the introducer. In the internal jugular or subclavian approach, he inserts the catheter into the end of the introducer sheath with the balloon deflated, directing the curl of the catheter toward the patient's midline.

▶ As insertion begins, observe the bedside monitor for waveform variations. (See *Normal PA waveforms*.)

▶ Observe diastolic values carefully during insertion. Make sure the scale is appropriate for lower pressures. A scale of 0 to 20 mm Hg or 0 to 40 mm Hg (more common) is preferred.

▶ When the catheter exits the end of the introducer sheath and reaches the junction of the superior vena cava and right atrium (at the 15- to 20-cm mark on the catheter shaft), the monitor shows oscillations that correspond to the patient's respirations. The balloon is then inflated with the recommended volume of air to allow normal blood flow and aid catheter insertion.

▶ Using a gentle, smooth motion, the physician advances the catheter through the heart chambers, moving rapidly to the pulmonary artery because prolonged manipulation here may reduce catheter stiffness.

▶ When the mark on the catheter shaft reaches 15 to 20 cm, the catheter enters the right atrium. The waveform shows two small, upright waves; pressure is low (between 2 and 4 mm Hg). Read pressure values in the mean mode because systolic and diastolic values are similar.

▶ The physician advances the catheter into the right ventricle, working quickly to minimize irritation. The waveform now shows sharp systolic upstrokes and lower diastolic dips. Depending on the size of the patient's heart, the catheter should reach the 30- to 35-cm mark. (The smaller the heart, the shorter the catheter length needed to reach the right ventricle.) Record systolic and diastolic pressures. Systolic pressure normally ranges from 15 to 25 mm Hg; diastolic pressure, from 0 to 8 mm Hg.

▶ As the catheter floats into the pulmonary artery, note that the upstroke from right ventricular systole is smoother, and systolic pressure is nearly the same as right ventricular systolic pressure. Record systolic, diastolic, and mean pressures (typically ranging from 8 to 15 mm Hg). A dicrotic notch on the diastolic portion of the waveform indicates pulmonic valve closure.

Wedging the catheter

▶ To obtain a wedge tracing, the physician lets the inflated balloon float downstream with the blood flow to a smaller, more distal branch of the pulmonary artery. Here, the catheter lodges, or wedges, causing occlusion of right ventricular and PA diastolic pressures. The tracing resembles the right atrial tracing because the catheter tip

Normal PA waveforms

During pulmonary artery (PA) catheter insertion, the waveforms on the monitor change as the catheter advances through the heart.

Right atrium

When the catheter tip enters the right atrium, the first heart chamber on its route, a waveform like the one shown below appears on the monitor. Note the two small upright waves. The a waves represent the right ventricular end-diastolic pressure; the v waves, right atrial filling.

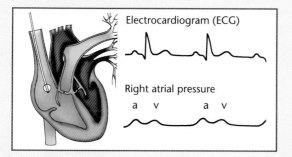

Pulmonary artery

The catheter then floats into the pulmonary artery, causing a pulmonary artery pressure (PAP) waveform such as the one shown below. Note that the upstroke is smoother than on the right ventricle waveform. The dicrotic notch indicates pulmonic valve closure.

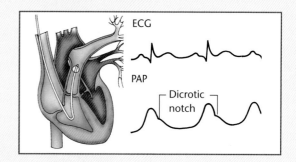

Right ventricle

As the catheter tip reaches the right ventricle, you'll see a waveform with sharp systolic upstrokes and lower diastolic dips, as shown below.

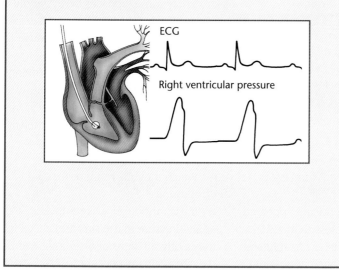

PAWP

Floating into a distal branch of the pulmonary artery, the balloon wedges where the vessel becomes too narrow for it to pass. The monitor now shows a pulmonary artery wedge pressure (PAWP) waveform, with two small upright waves, as shown below. The a wave represents left ventricular end-diastolic pressure; the v wave, left atrial filling. The balloon is then deflated, and the catheter is left in the pulmonary artery.

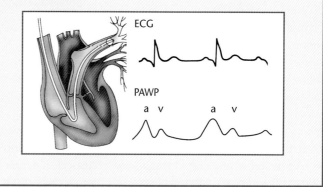

---

is recording left atrial pressure. The waveform shows two small uprises. Record PAWP in the mean mode (usually 6 to 12 mm Hg).

▶ A PAWP waveform, or wedge tracing, appears when the catheter has been inserted 45 to 50 cm. Usually, 30 to 45 seconds elapse from the time the physician inserts the introducer until the wedge tracing appears.

▶ The physician deflates the balloon, and the catheter drifts out of the wedge position and into the pulmonary artery, its normal resting place.

▶ If the appropriate waveforms don't appear at the expected times during catheter insertion, the catheter may be coiled in the right atrium and ventricle. To correct this problem, deflate the balloon. To do this, unlock the gate valve or turn the stopcock to the ON position and then detach the syringe from the balloon inflation port. Back pressure in the pulmonary artery causes the balloon to deflate on its own. (Active air withdrawal may compromise balloon integrity.) To verify balloon deflation, observe the monitor for return of the PA tracing.

▶ Typically, the physician orders a portable chest X-ray to confirm catheter position. **CDC**

▶ Apply a sterile occlusive dressing to the insertion site. **CDC** **AACN**

Obtaining intermittent PAP values

▶ After inserting the catheter and recording initial pressure readings, record subsequent PAP values and monitor waveforms. These values will be used to calculate other important hemodynamic indices. To ensure accurate values, make sure the transducer is properly leveled and zeroed at the phlebostatic axis. **AACN** **CS1** **CS2**

▶ If possible, obtain PAP values at end expiration (when the patient completely exhales). At this time, intrathoracic pressure approaches atmospheric pressure and has the least effect on PAP. If you obtain a reading during other phases of the respiratory cycle, respiratory interference may occur. For instance, during inspiration, when intrathoracic pressure drops, PAP may be false-low because the negative pressure is transmitted to the catheter. During expiration, when intrathoracic pressure rises, PAP may be false-high. **AACN** **CS2**

▶ For patients with a rapid respiratory rate and subsequent variations, you may have trouble identifying end expiration. The monitor displays an average of the digital readings obtained over time as well as those readings obtained during a full respiratory cycle. If possible, obtain a printout. Use the averaged values obtained through the full respiratory cycle. To analyze trends accurately,

be sure to record values at consistent times during the respiratory cycle.

Taking a PAWP reading

▶ PAWP is recorded by inflating the balloon and letting it float in a distal artery. Some facilities allow only physicians or specially trained nurses to take a PAWP reading because of the risk of PA rupture—a rare but life-threatening complication. If your facility permits you to perform this procedure, do so with extreme caution and make sure you're thoroughly familiar with intracardiac waveform interpretation.

▶ To begin, verify that the transducer is properly leveled and zeroed. Detach the syringe from the balloon inflation hub. Draw 1.5 cc of air into the syringe, and then reattach the syringe to the hub. Watching the monitor, inject the air through the hub slowly and smoothly. When you see a wedge tracing on the monitor, immediately stop inflating the balloon.

CLINICAL ALERT

Never inflate the balloon beyond the volume needed to obtain a wedge tracing.

▶ Take the pressure reading at end expiration. Note the amount of air needed to change the PA tracing to a wedge tracing (normally, 1.25 to 1.5 cc). If the wedge tracing appeared with the injection of less than 1.25 cc, suspect that the catheter has migrated into a more distal branch and requires repositioning. If the balloon is in a more distal branch, the tracings may move up the oscilloscope, indicating that the catheter tip is recording balloon pressure rather than PAWP. This may lead to PA rupture.

▶ Detach the syringe from the balloon inflation port and allow the balloon to

deflate on its own. Observe the waveform tracing and make sure the tracing returns from the wedge tracing to the normal PA tracing.

Removing the catheter

▶ To assist the practitioner, inspect the chest X-ray for signs of catheter kinking or knotting. (In some states, you may be permitted to remove a PA catheter yourself under an advanced collaborative standard of practice.)

▶ Obtain the patient's baseline vital signs, and note the ECG pattern.

▶ Explain the procedure to the patient. Place the head of the bed flat, unless ordered otherwise. If the catheter was inserted using a superior approach, turn the patient's head to the side opposite the insertion site. Gently remove the dressing.

▶ Remove sutures securing the catheter unless the introducer is left in place.

▶ Turn all stopcocks off to the patient. (You may turn stopcocks on to the distal port if you wish to observe waveforms. However, use caution because this may cause an air embolism.)

▶ Put on sterile gloves. After verifying that the balloon is deflated, withdraw the catheter slowly and smoothly. If you feel resistance, stop immediately, stay with the patient, and notify the practitioner.

▶ Watch the ECG monitor for arrhythmias.

▶ If the introducer was removed, apply pressure to the site, and check it frequently for signs of bleeding. Dress the site again, as necessary. If the introducer is left in place, observe the diaphragm for blood backflow, which verifies the integrity of the hemostasis valve.

▶ Return all equipment to the appropriate location. You may turn off the bedside pressure modules, but leave the ECG module on.

▶ Reassure the patient and his family that he'll be observed closely. Make sure he understands that the catheter was removed because his condition has improved and he no longer needs it.

Special considerations

▶ Advise the patient to use caution when moving about in bed to avoid dislodging the catheter.

▶ Never leave the balloon inflated because this may cause pulmonary in-farction. To determine if the balloon is inflated, check the monitor for a wedge tracing, which indicates inflation. (A PA tracing confirms balloon deflation.) (See *Troubleshooting the PAP monitoring system.*)

Troubleshooting the PAP monitoring system

When your patient has a pulmonary artery (PA) catheter, many common problems can develop. Use this table to help you recognize and resolve such problems.

ABNORMALITY	CAUSES	NURSING INTERVENTIONS
No waveform on monitor	▶ Transducer not open to catheter ▶ Transducer or monitor set up improperly ▶ Defective or cracked transducer ▶ Clotted catheter tip ▶ Large leak in the system; loose connections	▶ Check the stopcock, calibration, and scale mechanisms of the system. ▶ Tighten all connections. ▶ Rezero the setup. ▶ Replace the transducer.
Overdamped waveform	▶ Air bubble or blood clots within the catheter or tubing ▶ Catheter tip lodged in the vessel wall ▶ Kinked or knotted catheter or tubing ▶ Small leak in the system due to a loose connection	▶ Remove air bubbles observed in the catheter tubing and transducer. ▶ Restore patency to a clotted catheter by gently aspirating the clot with a syringe. (*Note:* Never irrigate the line as a first step.) ▶ Correct a lodged catheter by repositioning the patient or by having him cough and breathe deeply.
Changed waveform configuration (noisy or erratic tracings)	▶ Incorrectly positioned catheter ▶ Loose connections in the setup ▶ Faulty electrical circuitry	▶ Reposition the patient. ▶ Assist with chest X-ray to verify catheter location. ▶ Check and tighten connections in the catheter and transducer apparatus.
Ventricular irritability	▶ Irritation of the ventricular endocardium or heart valves by the catheter	▶ Notify the physician. (*Note:* The physician may prevent this problem during insertion by keeping the balloon inflated when advancing the catheter through the heart.)
Right ventricular waveform	▶ Migration of the PA catheter into the right ventricle	▶ Administer antiarrhythmics, as ordered.
Catheter fling	▶ Excessive catheter movement that may result from an arrhythmia, excessive respiratory effort, hyperdynamic circulation, excessive catheter length in the right ventricle, or location of the catheter tip near the pulmonic valve	▶ Notify the physician immediately. The catheter may need to be repositioned.
Falsely increased or decreased pulmonary artery pressure (PAP) readings	▶ System not properly leveled or zeroed ▶ Patient's body or bed repositioned without releveling or rezeroing the system	▶ Reposition the transducer level with the phlebostatic axis.

(continued)

Troubleshooting the PAP monitoring system (continued)

ABNORMALITY	CAUSES	NURSING INTERVENTIONS
Continuous pulmonary artery wedge pressure (PAWP) waveform	▶ Catheter migration ▶ Balloon still inflated	▶ Rezero the monitor. ▶ Reposition the patient or have him cough and breathe deeply. ▶ Keep the balloon inflated for no longer than two respiratory cycles or 15 seconds.
Missing PAWP waveform	▶ Malpositioned catheter ▶ Insufficient air in the balloon tip ▶ Ruptured balloon	▶ Reposition the patient. (Don't aspirate the balloon.) ▶ Reinflate the balloon adequately. (Remove the syringe from the balloon lumen, wait for the balloon to deflate passively, and then instill the correct volume of air.) ▶ Assess the balloon's competence. (Note resistance during inflation, feel how the syringe's plunger springs back after the balloon inflates, and check for blood leaking from the balloon lumen.) ▶ If the balloon has ruptured, turn the patient onto his left side, tape the balloon-inflation port, and notify the physician.

▶ Be aware that the catheter may slip back into the right ventricle. Because the tip may irritate the ventricle, check the monitor for a right ventricular waveform to detect this problem promptly.

▶ To minimize valvular trauma, make sure the balloon is deflated whenever the catheter is withdrawn from the pulmonary artery to the right ventricle or from the right ventricle to the right atrium.

▶ Change the dressing whenever it's moist, or every 48 hours for a gauze dressing, every 7 days for a transparent dressing, or according to your facility's policy. Change the pressure tubing every 48 hours and the flush solution every 24 hours. **AACN** **CDC**

▶ Perform and document the dynamic response or square wave test every 8 to 12 hours to validate the optimal waveform. **AACN** **CS3**

Selected references

American Society of Anesthesiologists. "Practice Guidelines for Pulmonary Artery Catheterization: An Updated Report by the American Society of Anesthesiologists Task Force," *Anesthesiology* 99(40):988–1014, October 2003.

Binanay, C. "Evaluation Study of Congestive Heart Failure and Pulmonary Artery Catheterization Effectiveness: The ESCAPE Trial," *JAMA* 294(13):1625–633, October 2005.

Bridges, E. J. "Pulmonary Artery Pressure Monitoring: When, How, and What Else to Use," *AACN Advanced Critical Care* 17(3):286–303, July–September 2006.

Centers for Disease Control and Prevention. "Guidelines for the Prevention of Intravascular Catheter-related Infections," *MMWR* 51(RR-10):1–26, August 2002.

Dobbin, K., et al. "Pulmonary artery pressure measurement in patients with elevated pressures: effect of backrest elevation and method of measurement," *American Journal of Critical Care* 1(2):61–9, September 1992. **CS2**

Friese, R. S., et al. "Pulmonary Artery Catheter Use Is Associated with Reduced Mortality in Severely Injured Patients: A National Trauma Data Bank Analysis of 53,312 Patients," *Critical Care Medicine* 34(6):1597–601, June 2006.

Georghiou, G. P., et al. "Knotting of a Pulmonary Artery Catheter in the Superior Vena Cava: Surgical Removal and a Word of Caution," *Heart* 90(5):e28, May 2004.

Kennedy, G. T., et al. "The effects of lateral body positioning on measurements of pulmonary artery and pulmonary artery wedge pressures," Heart & Lung 13(2):155–8, March 1984. **CS1**

Lynn-McHale Wiegand, D. J., and Carlson, K. K., eds. *AACN Procedure Manual for Critical Care,* 5th ed. Philadelphia: W. B. Saunders Co., 2005.

Quaal, S. J., "Improving the accuracy of pulmonary artery catheter measurements," Journal of Cardiovascular Nursing 15(2):71–82, January 2001. **CS3**

Shah, M. R., et al. "Impact of the Pulmonary Artery Catheter in Critically Ill Patients: Meta-analysis of Randomized Clinical Trials," *JAMA* 294(13): 1664–670, October 2005.

Task Force of the American College of Critical Care Medicine, Society of Critical Medicine. "Practice Parameters for Hemodynamic Support of Sepsis in Adult Patients: 2004 Update," *Critical Care Medicine* 32(9):1928–948, September 2004.

Pulse assessment

Blood pumped into an already-full aorta during ventricular contraction creates a fluid wave that travels from the heart to the peripheral arteries. This recurring wave—called a *pulse*—can be palpated at locations on the body where an artery crosses over bone or firm tissue. In adults and children over age 3, the radial artery in the wrist is the most common palpation site. (See *Pulse points*.) In infants and children under age 3, a stethoscope is used to listen to the heart itself rather than palpating a pulse. Because auscultation is done at the heart's apex, this is called the *apical pulse*.

An apical-radial pulse is taken by simultaneously counting apical and radial beats—the first by auscultation at the apex of the heart, the second by palpation at the radial artery. Some heartbeats detected at the apex can't be detected at peripheral sites. When this occurs, the apical pulse rate is higher than the radial; the difference is the pulse deficit.

Pulse taking involves determining the rate (number of beats per minute), rhythm (pattern or regularity of the beats), and volume (amount of blood pumped with each beat). If the pulse is faint or weak, use a Doppler ultrasound blood flow detector if available.

Equipment

Watch with a second hand ◆ stethoscope (for auscultating an apical pulse) ◆ alcohol pad ◆ Doppler ultrasound blood flow detector, if necessary.

Implementation

▶ If you aren't using your own stethoscope, disinfect the earpieces with an alcohol pad before and after use to prevent cross-contamination.
▶ Confirm the patient's identity using two patient identifiers according to your facility's policy. **JC**
▶ Wash your hands, and tell the patient that you intend to take his pulse.
▶ Make sure the patient is comfortable and relaxed because an awkward, uncomfortable position may affect the heart rate.

Taking a radial pulse

▶ Place the patient in a sitting or supine position, with his arm at his side or across his chest.
▶ Gently press your index, middle, and ring fingers on the radial artery, inside the patient's wrist, as shown at the top of the next page. You should feel a pulse with only moderate pressure;

excessive pressure may obstruct blood flow distal to the pulse site. Don't use your thumb to take the patient's pulse because your thumb's own strong pulse may be confused with the patient's pulse.

Pulse points

Shown here are anatomic locations where an artery crosses bone or firm tissue and can be palpated for a pulse.

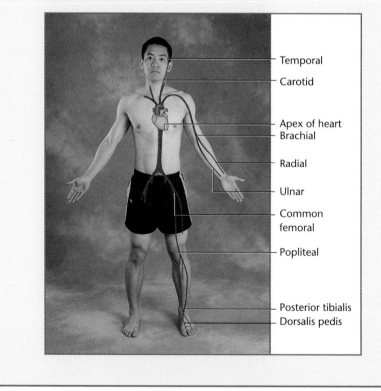

- Temporal
- Carotid
- Apex of heart
- Brachial
- Radial
- Ulnar
- Common femoral
- Popliteal
- Posterior tibialis
- Dorsalis pedis

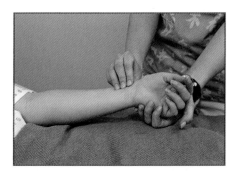

▶ After locating the pulse, count the beats for 60 seconds, or count for 30 seconds and multiply by 2. Counting for a full minute provides a more accurate picture of irregularities. While counting the rate, assess pulse rhythm and volume by noting the pattern and strength of the beats. If you detect an irregularity, repeat the count, and note whether it occurs in a pattern or ran-

domly. If you're still in doubt, take an apical pulse. (See *Identifying pulse patterns*.) **CS**

Taking an apical pulse

▶ Help the patient to a supine position, and drape him if necessary.
▶ Warm the diaphragm or bell of the stethoscope in your hand. Placing a cold stethoscope against the skin may startle the patient and momentarily increase the heart rate. Keep in mind that the bell transmits low-pitched sounds more effectively than the diaphragm.
▶ Place the diaphragm or bell of the stethoscope over the apex of the heart (normally located at the fifth intercostal space left of the midclavicular line). Then insert the earpieces into your ears. Count the beats for 30 seconds

and multiply by 2 (or count for 60 seconds if the rhythm is irregular), and note their rhythm, volume, and intensity (loudness). **CS**

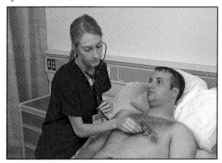

▶ Remove the stethoscope and make the patient comfortable.
▶ Clean the stethoscope with an alcohol pad to prevent cross-contamination.

Identifying pulse patterns

TYPE	RATE	RHYTHM (PER 3 SECONDS)	CAUSES AND INCIDENCE
Normal	60 to 80 beats/minute; in neonates, 120 to 140 beats/ minute	● ● ● ●	▶ Varies with such factors as age, physical activity, and gender (males usually have lower pulse rates than females)
Tachycardia	More than 100 beats/minute	●●●●●●●	▶ Accompanies stimulation of the sympathetic nervous system by emotional stress, such as anger, fear, or anxiety, or by the use of certain drugs such as caffeine ▶ May result from exercise and from certain health conditions, such as heart failure, anemia, and fever (which increases oxygen requirements and therefore the pulse rate)
Bradycardia	Less than 60 beats/minute	● ● ●	▶ Accompanies stimulation of the parasympathetic nervous system by drug use, especially cardiac glycosides, and such conditions as cerebral hemorrhage and heart block ▶ May also be present in fit athletes
Irregular	Uneven time intervals between beats (for example, periods of regular rhythm interrupted by pauses or premature beats)	●●●● ●●●	▶ May indicate cardiac irritability, hypoxia, digoxin toxicity, potassium imbalance or, sometimes, more serious arrhythmias if premature beats occur frequently ▶ Occasional premature beats normal

Taking an apical-radial pulse

▶ Two nurses work together to obtain the apical-radial pulse; one palpates the radial pulse while the other auscultates the apical pulse with a stethoscope. Both must use the same watch when counting beats.

▶ Help the patient to a supine position and drape him if necessary.

▶ Locate the apical and radial pulses.

▶ Determine a time to begin counting. Then each nurse should count beats for 60 seconds.

Special considerations

▶ When the peripheral pulse is irregular, take an apical pulse to measure the heartbeat more directly. If the pulse is faint or weak, use a Doppler ultrasound blood flow detector if available.

▶ If another nurse isn't available for an apical-radial pulse, hold the stethoscope in place with the hand that holds the watch while palpating the radial pulse with the other hand. You can then feel any discrepancies between the apical and radial pulses.

Selected references

Craven, R. F., and Hirnle, C. J. *Fundamentals of Nursing: Human Health and Function,* 5th ed. Philadelphia: Lippincott Williams & Wilkins, 2006.

Docherty, B., and Coote, S. "Monitoring the Pulse as Part of Track and Trigger," *Nursing Times* 102(43):28–29, October 2006.

Hwu, Y. J., et al. "A study of the effectiveness of different measuring times and counting methods of human radial pulse rates," Journal of Clinical Nursing 9(1):146–52, January 2000. **CS**

Thayer, J. F., et al. "Ethnic Differences in Heart Rate Variability: Does Ultralow-Frequency Heart Rate Variability Really Measure Autonomic Tone?" *American Heart Journal* 152(3):e27, September 2006.

Pulse oximetry

Performed intermittently or continuously, oximetry is a relatively simple procedure used to monitor arterial oxygen saturation noninvasively. Pulse oximeters usually denote arterial oxygen saturation values with the symbol SpO_2, whereas invasively measured arterial oxygen saturation values are denoted by the symbol SaO_2.

In this procedure, two diodes send red and infrared light through a pulsating arterial vascular bed such as the one in the fingertip. A photodetector slipped over the finger measures the transmitted light as it passes through the vascular bed, detects the relative amount of color absorbed by arterial blood, and calculates the exact mixed venous oxygen saturation without interference from surrounding venous blood, skin, connective tissue, or bone. Using the ear probe, oximetry works by monitoring the transmission of light waves through the vascular bed of a patient's earlobe. Results will be inaccurate if the patient's earlobe is poorly perfused, as from a low cardiac output. (See *How oximetry works.*)

Equipment

Oximeter ◆ finger or ear probe ◆ alcohol pads ◆ nail polish remover, if necessary.

Implementation

▶ Confirm the patient's identity using two patient identifiers according to your facility's policy. **JC**

▶ Explain the procedure to the patient.

▶ Validate pulse oximetry readings by comparing SpO_2 readings with SaO_2 values obtained by arterial blood gas (ABG) analysis. Obtain these two measurements simultaneously at the beginning of pulse oximetry monitoring, and then reevaluate periodically according to the patient's condition. **AARC**

▶ If pulse oximetry readings are being monitored continuously, set the high and low alarms according to the patient's clinical condition. **JC**

For pulse oximetry using the finger probe

▶ Select a finger for the test. Although the index finger is commonly used, a smaller finger may be selected if the

---

How oximetry works

The pulse oximeter allows noninvasive monitoring of the percentage of hemoglobin saturated by oxygen, or SpO_2, levels by measuring the absorption (amplitude) of light waves as they pass through areas of the body that are highly perfused by arterial blood. Oximetry also monitors pulse rate and amplitude.

Light-emitting diodes in a transducer (photodetector) attached to the patient's body (shown at right on the index finger) send red and infrared light beams through tissue. The photodetector records the relative amount of each color absorbed by arterial blood and transmits the data to a monitor, which displays the information with each heartbeat. If the SpO_2 level or pulse rate varies from preset limits, the monitor triggers visual and audible alarms.

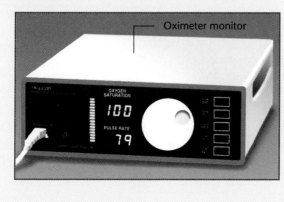

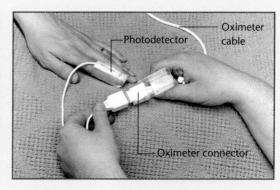

patient's fingers are too large for the equipment. Make sure the patient isn't wearing false fingernails, and remove any nail polish from the test finger. Place the transducer (photodetector) probe over the patient's finger so that light beams and sensors oppose each other. **AARC**

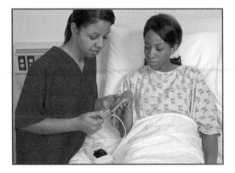

If the patient has long fingernails, position the probe perpendicular to the finger, if possible, or clip the fingernail. Always position the patient's hand at heart level to eliminate venous pulsations and to promote accurate readings.

AGE FACTOR

If you're testing a neonate or a small infant, wrap the probe around the foot so that light beams and detectors oppose each other. For a large infant, use a probe that fits on the great toe and secure it to the foot.

▶ Turn on the power switch. If the device is working properly, a beep will sound, a display will light momentarily, and the pulse searchlight will flash (as shown at top of next column). The Spo_2 and pulse rate displays will show stationary zeros. After four to six heartbeats, the Spo_2 and pulse rate displays will supply information with each beat, and the pulse amplitude indicator will begin tracking the pulse. **MFR**

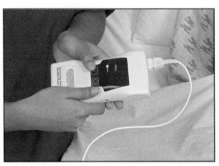

For pulse oximetry using the ear probe

▶ Using an alcohol pad, massage the patient's earlobe for 10 to 20 seconds. Mild erythema indicates adequate vascularization.

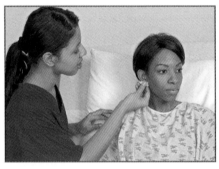

▶ Following the manufacturer's instructions, attach the ear probe to the patient's earlobe or pinna. Use the ear probe stabilizer for prolonged or exercise testing. Be sure to establish good contact on the ear; an unstable probe may set off the low-perfusion alarm. After the probe has been attached for a few seconds, a saturation reading and pulse waveform will appear on the oximeter's screen.

▶ Leave the ear probe in place for 3 or more minutes until readings stabilize at the highest point, or take three separate readings and average them. Make sure you revascularize the patient's earlobe each time.

▶ After the procedure, remove the probe, turn off and unplug the unit,

and clean the probe by gently rubbing it with an alcohol pad.

Special considerations

▶ The pulse rate on the pulse oximeter should correspond to the patient's actual pulse. If the rates don't correspond, the saturation reading can't be considered accurate. You should assess the patient, check the oximeter, and reposition the probe if necessary.

▶ Readings are typically accurate if oximetry has been performed properly; however, some factors may affect accuracy. For example, an elevated bilirubin level may falsely lower Spo_2 readings, whereas elevated carboxyhemoglobin or methemoglobin levels, such as occur in heavy smokers and urban dwellers, can cause a falsely elevated Spo_2 reading.

▶ Pulse oximetry may be used to monitor Spo_2 during respiratory arrest. Because pulse oximetry is based on perfusion, it shouldn't be used during cardiac arrest.

▶ If the patient has compromised circulation in his extremities, you can place a photodetector across the bridge of his nose.

▶ If Spo_2 is used to guide weaning the patient from forced inspiratory oxygen, obtain ABG analysis occasionally to correlate Spo_2 readings with Sao_2 levels. **AARC**

▶ If an automatic blood pressure cuff is used on the same extremity that's used for measuring Spo_2, the cuff will interfere with Spo_2 readings during inflation.

▶ If light is a problem, cover the probes; if patient movement is a problem, move the probe or select a different probe; and if ear pigment is a problem, reposition the probe, revascularize the site, or use a finger probe. **AARC**

▶ Normal SpO_2 levels for pulse oximetry are 95% to 100% for adults and 93.8% to 100% by 1 hour after birth for healthy, full-term neonates. Lower levels may indicate hypoxemia that warrants intervention. For such patients, follow your facility's policy or the practitioner's orders, which may include increasing oxygen therapy. If SaO_2 levels decrease suddenly, you may need to resuscitate the patient immediately. Notify the practitioner of any significant change in the patient's condition. `AARC`

▶ When the SaO_2 level is greater than 80%, pulse oximetry is highly accurate in healthy people. In patients on mechanical ventilation, however, accuracy is greatly reduced when the SaO_2 level is 90% or lower.

Selected references

Agashe, G. S., et al. "Forehead Pulse Oximetry: Headband Use Helps Alleviate False Low Readings Likely Related to Venous Pulsation Artifact," *Anesthesiology* 105(6):1111–116, December 2006.

Allen, K. "Principles and Limitations of Pulse Oximetry in Patient Monitoring," *Nursing Times* 100(41):34–37, October 2004.

American Association for Respiratory Care. "AARC Clinical Practice Guideline: Pulse Oximetry," *Respiratory Care* 36(12):1406–409, December 1991.

Petterson, M. T., et al. "The Effect of Motion on Pulse Oximetry and its Clinical Significance," *Anesthesia and Analgesia* 105(6 Suppl):S78–84, December 2007.

Taylor, C., et al. *Fundamentals of Nursing: The Art and Science of Nursing Care,* 6th ed. Philadelphia: Lippincott Williams & Wilkins, 2008.

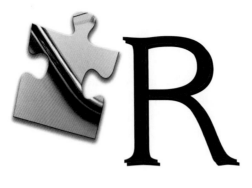

Rectal suppository and ointment

A rectal suppository is a small, solid, medicated mass, usually cone-shaped, with a cocoa butter or glycerin base. It may be inserted into the rectum to stimulate peristalsis and defecation or to relieve pain, vomiting, and local irritation. Rectal suppositories commonly contain drugs that reduce fever, induce relaxation, interact poorly with digestive enzymes, or have a taste too offensive for oral use. They melt at body temperature and are absorbed slowly.

Because insertion of a rectal suppository may stimulate the vagus nerve, this procedure is contraindicated in patients with potential cardiac arrhythmias. It may also have to be avoided in patients with recent rectal or prostate surgery because of the risk of local trauma or discomfort during insertion.

An ointment is a semisolid medication used to produce local effects. It may be applied externally to the anus or internally to the rectum. Rectal ointments commonly contain drugs that reduce inflammation or relieve pain and itching.

Equipment

Rectal suppository or tube of ointment and applicator ◆ patient's medication record and chart ◆ gloves ◆ water-soluble lubricant ◆ 4″ × 4″ gauze pads ◆ optional: bedpan.

Implementation

▶ Verify the order on the patient's medication record by checking it against the practitioner's order. **JC** **ISMP**
▶ Make sure the label on the medication package agrees with the medication order. Read the label again before you open the wrapper and again as you remove the medication. Check the expiration date. **ISMP**
▶ Wash your hands with warm water and soap.

▶ Confirm the patient's identity using two patient identifiers according to your facility's policy. **JC**
▶ If your facility uses a bar code scanning system, be sure to scan your ID badge, the patient's ID bracelet, and the medication's bar code. **JC** **ISMP**
▶ Explain the procedure and the purpose of the medication to the patient.
▶ Provide privacy.

Inserting a rectal suppository

▶ Place the patient on his left side in Sims' position. Drape him with the bedcovers to expose only the buttocks.
▶ Put on gloves. Remove the suppository from its wrapper, and lubricate it with water-soluble lubricant.

▶ Lift the patient's upper buttock with your nondominant hand to expose the anus.
▶ Instruct the patient to take several deep breaths through his mouth to help relax the anal sphincters and reduce anxiety or discomfort during insertion.
▶ Using the index finger of your dominant hand, insert the suppository—tapered end first—about 3″ (7.6 cm), until you feel it pass the internal anal sphincter. Try to direct the tapered end toward the side of the rectum so that it contacts the membranes. (See *How to administer a rectal suppository or ointment.*)

How to administer a rectal suppository or ointment

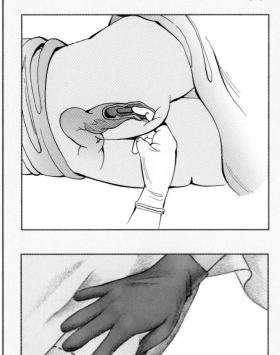

When inserting a suppository, direct its tapered end toward the side of the rectum so that it contacts the membranes to encourage absorption of the medication.

When applying a rectal ointment internally, be sure to lubricate the applicator to minimize pain on insertion. Then direct the applicator tip toward the patient's umbilicus.

▶ Ensure the patient's comfort. Encourage him to lie quietly and, if applicable, to retain the suppository for the appropriate length of time. A suppository administered to relieve constipation should be retained as long as possible (at least 20 minutes) to be effective. Press on the anus with a gauze pad if necessary until the urge to defecate passes.
▶ Remove and discard your gloves.

Applying rectal ointment
▶ Place the patient on his left side in Sims' position; then drape him to expose only the buttocks.

▶ Put on gloves.
▶ To apply externally, use gloves or a gauze pad to spread medication over the anal area.
▶ To apply internally, attach the applicator to the tube of ointment and coat the applicator with water-soluble lubricant.
▶ Expect to use about 1″ (2.5 cm) of ointment. To gauge how much pressure to use during application, squeeze a small amount from the tube before you attach the applicator.
▶ Lift the patient's upper buttock with your nondominant hand to expose the anus.

▶ Instruct the patient to take several deep breaths through his mouth to relax the anal sphincters and reduce anxiety or discomfort during insertion.
▶ Gently insert the applicator, directing it toward the umbilicus.
▶ Slowly squeeze the tube to eject the medication.
▶ Remove the applicator, and place a folded 4″ × 4″ gauze pad between the patient's buttocks to absorb excess ointment.
▶ Detach the applicator from the tube and recap the tube. Then clean the applicator thoroughly with soap and warm water.

Special considerations
▶ Because the intake of food and fluid stimulates peristalsis, a suppository for relieving constipation should be inserted about 30 minutes before mealtime to help soften the feces in the rectum and facilitate defecation. A medicated retention suppository should be inserted between meals.
▶ Instruct the patient to avoid expelling the suppository. If he has difficulty retaining it, place him on a bedpan.
▶ Make sure the patient's call button is handy, and watch for his signal because he may be unable to suppress the urge to defecate.
▶ Be sure to inform the patient that the suppository may discolor his next bowel movement.

References
The Joint Commission. *Comprehensive Accreditation Manual for Hospitals: The Official Handbook.* Standard MM.1.10. Oakbrook Terrace, Ill.: The Joint Commission, 2007.
The Joint Commission. *Comprehensive Accreditation Manual for Hospitals: The Official Handbook.* Standard MM.3.10. Oakbrook Terrace, Ill.: The Joint Commission, 2007.

The Joint Commission. *Comprehensive Accreditation Manual for Hospitals: The Official Handbook.* Standard MM.4.10. Oakbrook Terrace, Ill.: The Joint Commission, 2007.

The Joint Commission. *Comprehensive Accreditation Manual for Hospitals: The Official Handbook.* Standard MM.4.20. Oakbrook Terrace, Ill.: The Joint Commission, 2007.

The Joint Commission. *Comprehensive Accreditation Manual for Hospitals: The Official Handbook.* Standard MM.4.30. Oakbrook Terrace, Ill.: The Joint Commission, 2007.

The Joint Commission. *Comprehensive Accreditation Manual for Hospitals: The Official Handbook.* Standard MM.5.10. Oakbrook Terrace, Ill.: The Joint Commission, 2007.

The Joint Commission. *Comprehensive Accreditation Manual for Hospitals: The Official Handbook.* Standard MM.6.10. Oakbrook Terrace, Ill.: The Joint Commission, 2007.

The Joint Commission. *Comprehensive Accreditation Manual for Hospitals: The Official Handbook.* Standard MM.6.20. Oakbrook Terrace, Ill.: The Joint Commission, 2007.

The Joint Commission. *Comprehensive Accreditation Manual for Hospitals: The Official Handbook.* Standard MM.7.10. Oakbrook Terrace, Ill.: The Joint Commission, 2007.

Taylor, C., et al. *Fundamentals of Nursing: The Art and Science of Nursing Care,* 6th ed. Philadelphia: Lippincott Williams & Wilkins, 2008.

Rectal tube insertion and removal

Whether GI hypomotility simply slows the normal release of gas and feces or results in paralytic ileus, inserting a rectal tube may relieve the discomfort of distention and flatus. Decreased motility may result from various medical or surgical conditions, certain medications (such as atropine), or even swallowed air. Conditions that contraindicate using a rectal tube include recent rectal or prostate surgery, recent myocardial infarction, and diseases of the rectal mucosa.

Equipment

Stethoscope ◆ linen-saver pads ◆ drape ◆ water-soluble lubricant ◆ commercial kit or #22 to #34 French rectal tube of soft rubber or plastic ◆ container (emesis basin, plastic bag, or water bottle with vent) ◆ tape ◆ gloves.

Implementation

▶ Confirm the patient's identity using two patient identifiers according to your facility's policy. **JC**
▶ Bring all equipment to the patient's bedside, provide privacy, and wash your hands.
▶ Explain the procedure and encourage the patient to relax.
▶ Check for abdominal distention. Using a stethoscope, auscultate for bowel sounds.
▶ Place the linen-saver pads under the patient's buttocks to absorb any drainage that may leak from the tube.
▶ Position the patient in the left-lateral Sims' position.
▶ Put on gloves.
▶ Drape the patient's exposed buttocks.
▶ Lubricate the rectal tube tip with water-soluble lubricant to ease insertion and prevent rectal irritation.

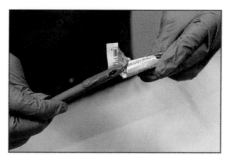

▶ Lift the patient's right buttock to expose the anus.

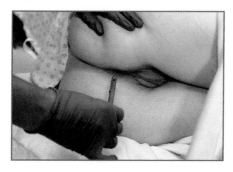

▶ Insert the rectal tube tip into the anus, advancing the tube 2″ to 4″ (5 to 10 cm) into the rectum. Direct the tube toward the umbilicus along the anatomic course of the large intestine.
▶ As you insert the tube, tell the patient to breathe slowly and deeply, or suggest that he bear down as he would for a bowel movement to relax the anal sphincter and ease insertion.
▶ Using tape, secure the rectal tube to the buttocks. Then attach the tube to the container to collect possible leakage.
▶ Remove the tube after 15 to 20 minutes. If the patient reports continued discomfort or if gas wasn't expelled, you can repeat the procedure in 2 to 3 hours if ordered.

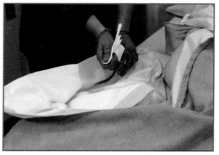

▶ Clean the patient, and replace soiled linens and the linen-saver pad. Make sure the patient feels as comfortable as possible. Again, check for abdominal distention and listen for bowel sounds.
▶ If you will reuse the equipment, clean it and store it in the bedside cabinet; otherwise, discard the tube.

Special considerations

▶ Inform the patient about each step and reassure him throughout the procedure to encourage cooperation and promote relaxation.

▶ Fastening a plastic bag (like a balloon) to the external end of the tube lets you observe gas expulsion. Leaving a rectal tube in place indefinitely does little to promote peristalsis, can reduce sphincter responsiveness, and may lead to permanent sphincter damage or pressure necrosis of the mucosa.

▶ Repeat insertion periodically to stimulate GI activity. If the tube fails to relieve distention, notify the practitioner.

References

Azpiroz, F., and Malagelada, J. R. "Abdominal Bloating," *Gastroenterology* 129(3): 1060–78, September 2005.

Craven, R. F., and Hirnle, C. J. *Fundamentals of Nursing: Human Health and Function,* 6th ed. Philadelphia: Lippincott Williams & Wilkins, 2009.

Taylor, C., et al. *Fundamentals of Nursing: The Art and Science of Nursing,* 6th ed. Philadelphia: Lippincott Williams & Wilkins, 2008.

Respiration assessment

Controlled by the respiratory center in the lateral medulla oblongata, respiration is the exchange of oxygen and carbon dioxide between the atmosphere and body cells. External respiration, or breathing, is accomplished by the diaphragm and chest muscles and delivers oxygen to the lower respiratory tract and alveoli.

Four measures of respiration—rate, rhythm, depth, and sound—reflect the body's metabolic state, diaphragm and chest-muscle condition, and airway patency. Respiratory rate is recorded as the number of cycles (with inspiration and expiration comprising one cycle) per minute; rhythm, as the regularity of these cycles; depth, as the volume of air inhaled and exhaled with each respiration; and sound, as the audible digression from normal, effortless breathing.

Equipment

Watch with second hand.

Implementation

▶ The best time to assess the patient's respirations is immediately after taking his pulse rate. Keep your fingertips over the radial artery, and don't tell the patient you're counting respirations. If you tell him, he'll become conscious of his respirations, and the rate may change.

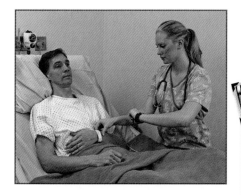

▶ Count respirations by observing the rise and fall of the patient's chest as he breathes. Alternatively, position the patient's opposite arm across his chest and count respirations by feeling its rise and fall. Consider one rise and one fall as one respiration.

▶ Count respirations for 30 seconds and multiply by 2; or, if respirations are irregular, count for 60 seconds to account for variations in respiratory rate and pattern.

▶ As you count respirations, be alert for and record such breath sounds as stertor, stridor, wheezing, and an expiratory grunt. Stertor is a snoring sound resulting from secretions in the trachea and large bronchi. Listen for it in patients with neurologic disorders and in those who are comatose. Stridor is an inspiratory crowing sound that occurs with upper airway obstruction in laryngitis, croup, or the presence of a foreign body.

AGE FACTOR

When listening for stridor in infants and children with croup, also observe for sternal, substernal, or intercostal retractions.

▶ Wheezing is caused by partial obstruction in the smaller bronchi and bronchioles. This high-pitched, musical sound is common in patients with emphysema or asthma.

AGE FACTOR

In infants, an expiratory grunt indicates imminent respiratory distress. In older patients, an expiratory grunt may result from partial airway obstruction or neuromuscular reflex.

▶ Watch the patient's chest movements, and listen to his breathing to determine the rhythm and sound of respirations. (See *Identifying respiratory patterns,* page 460.)

▶ To detect other breath sounds—such as crackles and rhonchi—or the lack of sound in the lungs, you'll need a stethoscope.

▶ Observe chest movements for depth of respirations. If the patient inhales a small volume of air, record this as shallow; if he inhales a large volume, record this as deep.

▶ Observe the patient for use of accessory muscles, such as the scalene, sternocleidomastoid, trapezius, and latissimus dorsi. Using these muscles reflects weakness of the diaphragm and the external intercostal muscles—the major muscles of respiration.

Identifying respiratory patterns

The table below shows several common types of respiratory patterns and their possible causes. It's important to assess the patient for the underlying cause and the effect on the patient.

TYPE	CHARACTERISTICS	PATTERN	POSSIBLE CAUSES
Apnea	Periodic absence of breathing	————————	▶ Mechanical airway obstruction ▶ Conditions affecting the brain's respiratory center in the lateral medulla oblongata
Apneustic	Prolonged, gasping inspiration followed by extremely short, inefficient expiration	/\/\/\/\/\/\/\/\/\/\/	▶ Lesions of the respiratory center
Bradypnea	Slow, regular respirations of equal depth	∼∼∼∼∼∼	▶ Normal pattern during sleep ▶ Conditions affecting the respiratory center: tumors, metabolic disorders, respiratory decompensation, and use of opiates or alcohol
Cheyne-Stokes	Fast, deep respirations of 30 to 170 seconds punctuated by periods of apnea lasting 20 to 60 seconds	⋀⋀__⋀⋀⋀__⋀⋀⋀__⋀	▶ Increased intracranial pressure, severe heart failure, renal failure, meningitis, drug overdose, and cerebral anoxia
Eupnea	Normal rate and rhythm	∿∿∿∿∿∿	▶ Normal respiration
Kussmaul's	Fast (more than 20 breaths/minute), deep (resembling sighs), labored respirations without pause	⋀⋀⋀⋀⋀⋀⋀⋀⋀	▶ Renal failure and metabolic acidosis, particularly diabetic ketoacidosis
Tachypnea	Rapid respirations; rate rising with body temperature—about four breaths/minute for every degree Fahrenheit above normal	∪∪∪∪∪∪∪∪∪	▶ Pneumonia, compensatory respiratory alkalosis, respiratory insufficiency, lesions of the respiratory center, and salicylate poisoning

Special considerations

▶ Respiratory rates of less than 8 or more than 40 breaths per minute are usually considered abnormal; report the sudden onset of such rates promptly. Observe the patient for signs of dyspnea, such as an anxious facial expression, flaring nostrils, a heaving chest wall, and cyanosis. To detect cyanosis, look for characteristic bluish discoloration in the nail beds or the lips, under the tongue, in the buccal mucosa, or in the conjunctiva.

▶ In assessing the patient's respiratory status, consider his personal and family history. Ask whether he smokes and, if so, for how many years and how many packs per day.

References

Aylott, M. "Observing the Sick Child: Part 2a. Respiration Assessment," *Paediatric Nursing* 18(9):38–44, November 2006.

Craven, R. F., and Hirnle, C. J. *Fundamentals of Nursing: Human Health and Function,* 6th ed. Philadelphia: Lippincott Williams & Wilkins, 2009.

Hogan, J. "Why Don't Nurses Monitor the Respiratory Rates of Patients?" *British Journal of Nursing* 15(9):489–92, May 2006.

Restraint application

Restraint is a method of physically restricting a person's freedom of movement, physical activity, or normal access to his body. This includes not only traditional restraints, such as limb restraints, but also tightly tucked sheets or the use of side rails to prevent a patient from getting out of bed.

The Joint Commission and the Centers for Medicare and Medicaid Standards (CMS) have issued standards regarding the use of restraints. According to these standards, restraints are to be limited to emergencies in which the patient is at risk for harming himself or others and when other less-restrictive measures have proved ineffective. One purpose of the standards is to reduce the use of restraints. (See *Alternatives to restraints*.) Restraints can cause numerous problems, including limited mobility, skin breakdown, impaired circulation, incontinence, psychological distress, and strangulation.

Alternatives to restraints

To reduce the need for restraints, take an individualized approach that seeks to prevent behavior problems. Look for an underlying problem that may be causing your patient's behavior—such as adverse drug effects, infection, electrolyte imbalance, or hypoxia—and take measures to correct the problem.

Look for "agenda behaviors" in which the patient's behavior may be an attempt to correct a problem, such as pain, hunger, fatigue, heat, cold, or the need for toileting.

Create an environment that's free from restraints and encourages patient mobility. This requires a unit and facility commitment because policy changes and even structural changes may be required.

If the problem behavior continues after you've identified and corrected conditions that may be the cause, consider alternatives to restraints, such as:

▶ reorienting the patient as needed
▶ providing explanations for procedures
▶ keeping the patient warm, dry, and comfortable
▶ establishing eye contact and talking to the patient
▶ listening and validating the patient's concerns
▶ determining the patient's routines and habits and trying to adhere to them
▶ wrapping elastic compression bandages around I.V. sites, other tubing, or dressings
▶ switching to a capped I.V. line if possible
▶ determining whether equipment or treatment is really necessary
▶ moving tubing or equipment out of the patient's sight
▶ using an abdominal binder to cover abdominal drains, tubes, and dressings and urinary catheters.

Equipment

Restraint (limb, vest, or mitt, as needed) ◆ padding if needed ◆ restraint flow sheet.

Implementation

▶ Follow Joint Commission and CMS standards for applying restraints. Make sure that less-restrictive measures have been tried before applying restraints. **JC CMS**

▶ When all the other methods have failed to keep the patient from harming herself or others, apply restraints for as short a time as possible. Choose a restraint that's least restrictive to the patient. **JC CMS**

▶ Tell the patient what you're about to do, and describe the restraints to her. Assure her that they're being used to protect her from injury, not to punish her.

▶ If necessary, obtain adequate assistance to restrain the patient before entering her room. Enlist the aid of several coworkers and organize their effort, giving each person a specific task; for example, one person explains the procedure to the patient and applies the restraints while the others immobilize the patient's arms and legs.

▶ When applying restraints for patient safety, inform the licensed independent practitioner within 12 hours of placing the patient in restraints and obtain a written or verbal order for the restraints. The patient must be examined by the practitioner within 24 hours of the initiation of restraints. Assess the patient every 2 hours or according to your facility's policy. **JC CMS**

▶ If the patient consented to have her family informed of her care, notify them of the use of restraints.

Applying a limb restraint

▶ Wrap the patient's wrist or ankle with a padded restraint.

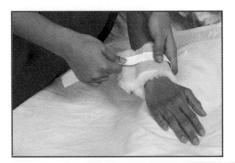

▶ Pass the strap on the narrow end of the restraint through the slot in the broad end, and adjust for a snug fit. Alternatively, fasten the buckle or Velcro cuffs to fit the restraint. You should be able to slip one or two fingers between the restraint and the patient's skin. Avoid applying the restraint too tightly because it may impair circulation distal to the restraint.

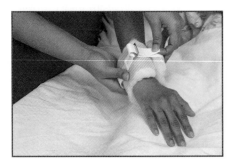

▶ Tie all restraints securely to the frame of the bed, chair, or wheelchair and out of the patient's reach. Never secure the restraint to a bedrail or other movable part of the equipment. Use a bow or a knot that can be released quickly and easily in an emergency. (See *Knots for securing soft restraints*.) Never tie a regular knot to secure the straps. Leave 1″ to 2″ (2.5 to 5 cm) of slack in the straps to allow room for movement.

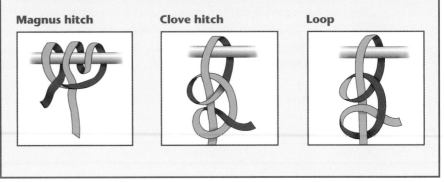

Knots for securing soft restraints

When securing soft restraints, use knots that can be released quickly and easily, like those shown below. Remember, never secure restraints to the bed's side rails.

Magnus hitch **Clove hitch** **Loop**

▶ After applying limb restraints, be alert for signs of impaired circulation, movement, or sensation in the extremity distal to the restraint. Check the patient's distal extremities for color, temperature, and pulse according to your facility's policy. If the skin appears blue or feels cold, or if the patient complains of a tingling sensation or numbness, loosen the restraint. Release the restraint every 2 hours to assess the skin, and perform range-of-motion (ROM) exercises regularly to stimulate circulation and prevent contractures and resultant loss of mobility.

Applying a vest restraint

▶ Assist the patient to a sitting position if her condition permits. Then slip the vest over her gown. Crisscross the cloth flaps at the front, placing the V-shaped opening at the patient's throat. Never crisscross the flaps in the back because this may cause the patient to choke if she tries to squirm out of the vest.

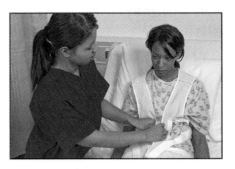

▶ Pass the tab on one flap through the slot on the opposite flap. Then adjust the vest for the patient's comfort. You should be able to slip your fist between the vest and the patient. Avoid wrapping the vest too tightly because it may restrict respiration.

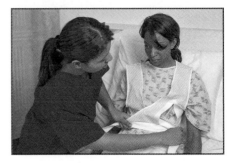

▶ Tie the restraint as shown above.

▶ After applying the vest, check the patient's respiratory rate and breath sounds regularly. Be alert for signs of respiratory distress. Also, make sure the vest hasn't tightened with the patient's movement. Loosen the vest frequently, if possible, so the patient can stretch, turn, and breathe deeply.

Applying a mitt restraint

▶ Wash and dry the patient's hands.
▶ Roll up a washcloth or gauze pad, and place it in the patient's palm. Have her form a loose fist, if possible; then pull the mitt over it and secure the closure.
▶ To restrict the patient's arm movement, attach the strap to the mitt and tie it securely, using a bow or a knot that can be released quickly and easily in an emergency.
▶ When using mitts made of transparent mesh, check hand movement and skin color frequently to assess circulation. Remove the mitts regularly to stimulate circulation, and perform passive ROM exercises to prevent contractures.

Special considerations

▶ Know the latest Joint Commission and CMS standards for restraint applications. Implement alternative strategies to reduce the need for restraints. Choose the least restrictive restraint, if necessary, for your patient. **JC CMS**
▶ Provide for continuous patient monitoring in which a designated person can directly observe the patient at all times. **JC CMS**
▶ Assess and assist the restrained patient according to your facility's policy, including injuries caused by the restraint, nutrition, hydration, circulation, ROM, vital signs, hygiene, elimination, comfort, and physical

and psychosocial status. Also assess whether the patient is ready to have restraints discontinued. **JC CMS**
▶ The condition of the restrained patient must be continually monitored, assessed, and evaluated. Release the restraints every hour; assess the patient's pulse and skin condition, and perform ROM exercises. A restraint flow sheet must be used with hourly notations. **JC CMS**
▶ When the patient is at high risk for aspiration, restrain her on her side. Never secure all four restraints to one side of the bed because the patient may fall out of bed.
▶ When loosening restraints, have a coworker on hand to assist in restraining the patient if necessary.
▶ Don't apply a limb restraint above an I.V. site because the constriction may occlude the infusion or cause infiltration into surrounding tissue.
▶ Never secure restraints to the side rails because someone might inadvertently lower the rail before noticing the attached restraint. This may jerk the patient's limb or body, causing her discomfort and trauma. Never secure restraints to the fixed frame of the bed if the patient's position is to be changed.
▶ Don't restrain a patient in the prone position. This position limits her field of vision, intensifies feelings of helplessness and vulnerability, and impairs respiration, especially if the patient has been sedated.
▶ Because the restrained patient has limited mobility, her nutrition, elimination, and positioning become your responsibility. To prevent pressure ulcers, reposition the patient every 2 hours, and massage and pad bony prominences and other vulnerable areas. **JC CMS**

References

Amato, S., et al. "Physical Restraint Reduction in the Acute Rehabilitation Setting: A Quality Improvement Study," *Rehabilitation Nursing* 31(6):235–41, November–December 2006.

The Joint Commission. *The Comprehensive Accreditation Manual for Hospitals: The Official Handbook.* Standards PC.11.10. Oakbrook Terrace, Ill.: The Joint Commission, 2007.

The Joint Commission. *The Comprehensive Accreditation Manual for Hospitals: The Official Handbook.* Standards PC.11.20. Oakbrook Terrace, Ill: The Joint Commission,. 2007.

The Joint Commission. *The Comprehensive Accreditation Manual for Hospitals: The Official Handbook.* Standards PC.11.30. Oakbrook Terrace, Ill.: The Joint Commission, 2007.

The Joint Commission. *The Comprehensive Accreditation Manual for Hospitals: The Official Handbook.* Standards PC.11.40. Oakbrook Terrace, Ill.: The Joint Commission, 2007.

The Joint Commission. *The Comprehensive Accreditation Manual for Hospitals: The Official Handbook.* Standards PC.11.50. Oakbrook Terrace, Ill.: The Joint Commission, 2007.

The Joint Commission. *The Comprehensive Accreditation Manual for Hospitals: The Official Handbook.* Standards PC.11.60. Oakbrook Terrace, Ill.: The Joint Commission, 2007.

The Joint Commission. *The Comprehensive Accreditation Manual for Hospitals: The Official Handbook.* Standards PC.11.70 Oakbrook Terrace, Ill.: The Joint Commission, 2007.

The Joint Commission. *The Comprehensive Accreditation Manual for Hospitals: The Official Handbook.* Standards PC.11.80. Oakbrook Terrace, Ill.: The Joint Commission, 2007.

The Joint Commission. *The Comprehensive Accreditation Manual for Hospitals: The Official Handbook.* Standards PC.11.90. Oakbrook Terrace, Ill.: The Joint Commission, 2007.

The Joint Commission. *The Comprehensive Accreditation Manual for Hospitals: The Official Handbook.* Standards PC.12.10. Oakbrook Terrace, Ill.: The Joint Commission, 2007.

The Joint Commission. *The Comprehensive Accreditation Manual for Hospitals: The Official Handbook.* Standards PC.12.20. Oakbrook Terrace, Ill.: The Joint Commission, 2007.

The Joint Commission. *The Comprehensive Accreditation Manual for Hospitals: The Official Handbook.* Standards PC.12.30. Oakbrook Terrace, Ill.. The Joint Commission, 2007.

The Joint Commission. *The Comprehensive Accreditation Manual for Hospitals: The Official Handbook.* Standards PC.12.40. Oakbrook Terrace, Ill.: The Joint Commission, 2007.

The Joint Commission. *The Comprehensive Accreditation Manual for Hospitals: The Official Handbook.* Standards PC.12.50. Oakbrook Terrace, Ill.: The Joint Commission, 2007.

The Joint Commission. *The Comprehensive Accreditation Manual for Hospitals: The Official Handbook.* Standards PC.12.60. Oakbrook Terrace, Ill.: The Joint Commission, 2007.

The Joint Commission. *The Comprehensive Accreditation Manual for Hospitals: The Official Handbook.* Standards PC.12.70. Oakbrook Terrace, Ill.: The Joint Commission, 2007.

The Joint Commission. *The Comprehensive Accreditation Manual for Hospitals: The Official Handbook.* Standards PC.12.80. Oakbrook Terrace, Ill.: The Joint Commission, 2007.

The Joint Commission. *The Comprehensive Accreditation Manual for Hospitals: The Official Handbook.* Standards PC.12.90. Oakbrook Terrace, Ill.: The Joint Commission, 2007.

The Joint Commission. *The Comprehensive Accreditation Manual for Hospitals: The Official Handbook.* Standards PC.12.100. Oakbrook Terrace, Ill.: The Joint Commission, 2007.

The Joint Commission. *The Comprehensive Accreditation Manual for Hospitals: The Official Handbook.* Standards PC.12.110. Oakbrook Terrace, Ill.: The Joint Commission, 2007.

The Joint Commission. *The Comprehensive Accreditation Manual for Hospitals: The Official Handbook.* Standards PC.12.120. Oakbrook Terrace, Ill.: The Joint Commission, 2007.

The Joint Commission. *The Comprehensive Accreditation Manual for Hospitals: The Official Handbook.* Standards PC.12.130. Oakbrook Terrace, Ill.: The Joint Commission, 2007.

The Joint Commission. *The Comprehensive Accreditation Manual for Hospitals: The Official Handbook.* Standards PC.12.140. Oakbrook Terrace, Ill.: The Joint Commission, 2007.

The Joint Commission. *The Comprehensive Accreditation Manual for Hospitals: The Official Handbook.* Standards PC.12.150. Oakbrook Terrace, Ill.: The Joint Commission, 2007.

The Joint Commission. *The Comprehensive Accreditation Manual for Hospitals: The Official Handbook.* Standards PC.12.160. Oakbrook Terrace, Ill.: The Joint Commission, 2007.

The Joint Commission. *The Comprehensive Accreditation Manual for Hospitals: The Official Handbook.* Standards PC.12.170. Oakbrook Terrace, Ill.: The Joint Commission, 2007.

The Joint Commission. *The Comprehensive Accreditation Manual for Hospitals: The Official Handbook.* Standards PC.12.180. Oakbrook Terrace, Ill.: The Joint Commission, 2007.

The Joint Commission. *The Comprehensive Accreditation Manual for Hospitals: The Official Handbook.* Standards PC.12.190. Oakbrook Terrace, Ill.: The Joint Commission, 2007.

Kowk, T., et al. "Does Access to Bed-Chair Pressure Sensors Reduce Physical Restraint Use in the Rehabilitative Care Setting?" *Journal of Clinical Nursing* 15(5):581–87, May 2006.

McBeth, S. "Get a Firmer Grasp on Restraints," *Nursing Management* 35(10):20, 22, October 2004.

Saulf, N. M. "Restraints Use and Falls Prevention," *Journal of Perianesthesia Nursing* 19(6):433–36, December 2004.

Suen, L. K., et al. "Use of Physical Restraints in Rehabilitation Settings: Staff Knowledge, Attitudes and Predictors," *Journal of Advanced Nursing* 55(1):20–28, July 2006.

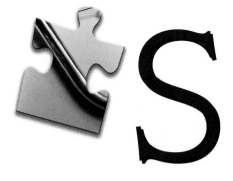

Secondary I.V. medication administration

A secondary I.V. line is a complete I.V. set—container, tubing, and microdrip or macrodrip system—connected to the lower Y-port (secondary port) of a primary line instead of to the I.V. catheter. It can be used for continuous or intermittent drug infusion. When used continuously, a secondary I.V. line permits drug infusion and titration while the primary line maintains a constant total infusion rate.

When used intermittently, a secondary I.V. line is commonly called a *piggyback set*. In this case, the primary line maintains venous access between drug doses. Typically, a piggyback set includes a small I.V. container, short tubing, and a macrodrip system. This set connects to the primary line's upper Y-port, also called a *piggyback port*. Antibiotics are most commonly administered by piggyback infusion. To make this set work, the primary I.V. container must be positioned below the piggyback container. (The manufacturer provides an extension hook for this purpose.)

Drugs can be piggybacked with a needle-free system, which consists of a blunt-tipped plastic insertion device and a rubber injection port. The port may be part of a special administration set or an adapter for existing administration sets. The rubber injection port has a preestablished slit that can open and reseal immediately. The needle-free system reduces the risk of accidental needle-stick injuries. **JC**

Equipment

Patient's medication record and chart ◆ prescribed I.V. medication ◆ prescribed I.V. solution ◆ administration set with secondary injection port ◆ needleless adapter, if needed ◆ alcohol pads ◆ 1″ adhesive tape ◆ time tape ◆ labels ◆ infusion pump ◆ extension hook and appropriate solution for intermittent, piggyback infusion ◆ optional: normal saline solution for infusion with incompatible solutions, sterile I.V. plug.

For intermittent infusion, the primary line's piggyback port has a backcheck valve that stops the flow from the primary line during drug infusion and returns to the primary flow after infusion. A volume-control set can also be used with an intermittent infusion line. (For more information, see "Volume-control sets," page 602.)

Implementation

▶ Verify the order on the patient's medication record by checking it against the practitioner's order. **JC** **ISMP**

▶ Wash your hands.

▶ Inspect the I.V. container for cracks, leaks, and contamination, and check drug compatibility with the primary solution. Verify the expiration date.

▶ Check to see whether the primary line has a secondary injection port. If it doesn't and the medication is to be given regularly, replace the I.V. set with one that has a secondary injection port.

▶ If necessary, add the drug to the secondary I.V. solution. To do so, remove any seals from the secondary container, and wipe the main port

465

with an alcohol pad. Inject the pre-scribed medication, and gently agitate the solution to mix the medication thoroughly. Properly label the I.V. mixture. **INS** **JC**

▶ Insert the administration set spike and attach the needleless adapter. Open the flow clamp and prime the line. Then close the flow clamp.

▶ Confirm the patient's identity using two patient identifiers according to your facility's policy. **JC**

▶ If your facility uses a bar code scanning system, be sure to scan your ID badge, the patient's ID bracelet, and the medication's bar code. **JC** **ISMP**

▶ Assess the patient's I.V. site for pain, redness, swelling, and patency. If the I.V. shows signs of infiltration or phlebitis, remove it and insert another I.V. catheter in a new site. **INS**

▶ If the drug is incompatible with the primary I.V. solution, replace the primary solution with a fluid that's compatible with both solutions, such as normal saline solution, and flush the line before starting the drug infusion. Many facility protocols require that the primary I.V. solution be removed and that a sterile I.V. plug be inserted into the container until it's ready to be re-hung. This maintains the sterility of the solution and prevents someone else from inadvertently restarting the incompatible solution before the line is flushed with normal saline solution.

▶ Hang the secondary set's container, and wipe the injection port of the primary line with an alcohol pad. **INS** **CDC**

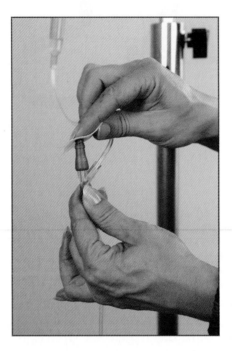

▶ Insert the needleless adapter from the secondary line into the injection port, and secure it to the primary line.

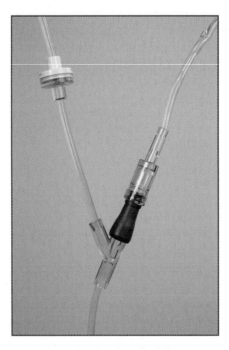

▶ To run the secondary set's container by itself, lower the primary set's container with an extension hook. To run both containers simultaneously, place them at the same height. (See *Assembling a piggyback set*.)

▶ Open the clamp and adjust the drip rate. For continuous infusion, set the secondary solution to the desired drip rate; then adjust the primary solution to achieve the desired total infusion rate.

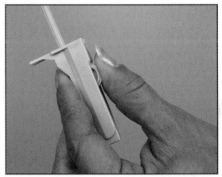

▶ For intermittent infusion, adjust the primary drip rate, as required, on completion of the secondary solution. If the secondary solution tubing is being reused, close the clamp on the tubing and follow your facility's policy: Either remove the needleless adapter and replace it with a new one, or leave it securely taped in the injection port and label it with the time it was first used. In this case, also leave the empty container in place until you replace it with a new dose of medication at the prescribed time. If the tubing won't be reused, discard it appropriately with the I.V. container.

Assembling a piggyback set

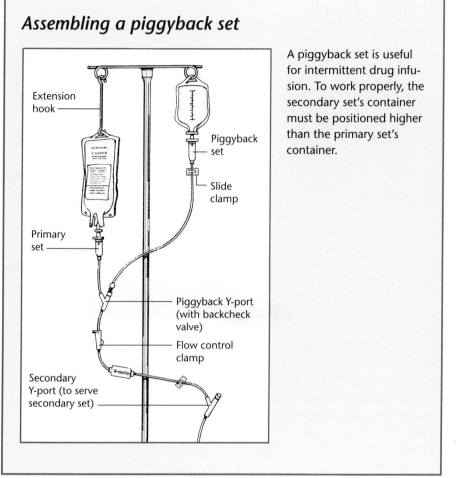

A piggyback set is useful for intermittent drug infusion. To work properly, the secondary set's container must be positioned higher than the primary set's container.

Extension hook

Piggyback set

Slide clamp

Primary set

Piggyback Y-port (with backcheck valve)

Flow control clamp

Secondary Y-port (to serve secondary set)

Special considerations

▶ If policy allows, use a pump for drug infusion. Put a time tape on the secondary container to help prevent an inaccurate administration rate.

▶ When reusing secondary tubing, change it according to your facility's policy, usually every 96 hours. Similarly, inspect the injection port for leakage with each use, and change it more often if needed. **INS CDC CS**

▶ Unless you're piggybacking lipids, don't piggyback a secondary I.V. line to a total parenteral nutrition line be-cause of the risk of contamination. Check your facility's policy for possible exceptions. **ASPEN**

References

Centers for Disease Control and Prevention. "Guidelines for the Prevention of Intravascular Device-related Infections," *MMWR* 51(RR-10):1–26, August 2002.

Fields, M., and Peterman, J. "Intravenous Medication Safety System Averts High Risk Medication Errors and Provides Actionable Data," *Nursing Administration Quarterly* 29(1):78–87, January–March 2005.

Gillies, D., et al. "Timing of Intravenous Administration Set Changes: A Systematic Review," *Infection Control and Hospital Epidemiology* 25(3):240–50, March 2004. **CS**

Infusion Nurses Society. "Standard 48I. Administration Set Change Primary and Secondary Continuous. Infusion Nursing Standards of Practice," *Journal of Infusion Nursing* 29(1s):S48, January–February 2006.

The Joint Commission. *Comprehensive Accreditation Manual for Hospitals: The Official Handbook*. Standard MM.1.10. Oakbrook Terrace, Ill.: The Joint Commission, 2007.

The Joint Commission. *Comprehensive Accreditation Manual for Hospitals: The Official Handbook*. Standard MM.3.10. Oakbrook Terrace, Ill.: The Joint Commission, 2007.

The Joint Commission. *Comprehensive Accreditation Manual for Hospitals: The Official Handbook*. Standard MM.4.10. Oakbrook Terrace, Ill.: The Joint Commission, 2007.

The Joint Commission. *Comprehensive Accreditation Manual for Hospitals: The Official Handbook*. Standard MM.4.20. Oakbrook Terrace, Ill.: The Joint Commission, 2007.

The Joint Commission. *Comprehensive Accreditation Manual for Hospitals: The Official Handbook*. Standard MM.4.30. Oakbrook Terrace, Ill.: The Joint Commission, 2007.

The Joint Commission. Comprehensive Accreditation Manual for Hospitals: The Official Handbook. Standard MM.5.10. Oakbrook Terrace, Ill.: The Joint Commission, 2007.

Self-catheterization

A patient with impaired or absent bladder function may catheterize himself for routine bladder drainage. Because clean intermittent catheterization is safer than an indwelling catheter to prevent urinary tract infections (UTIs), it's a recommended alternative by the Centers for Disease Control and Prevention. The two major advantages of self-catheterization are that patient independence is maintained and bladder control is regained. In addition, self-catheterization allows normal sexual intimacy without the fear of incontinence, decreases the chance of urinary reflux, reduces the use of aids and appliances and, in many cases, allows the patient to return to work.

Self-catheterization requires thorough and careful teaching by the nurse. The patient will probably use clean technique for self-catheterization at home, but he must use sterile technique in the hospital because of the increased risk of infection.

Equipment

Rubber catheter ◆ washcloth ◆ soap and water ◆ small packet of water-soluble lubricant ◆ plastic storage bag ◆ optional: drainage container, paper towels, rubber or plastic sheets, gooseneck lamp, catheterization record, mirror.

Implementation

▶ Tell the patient to begin by trying to urinate into the toilet or, if a toilet isn't available or he needs to measure urine quantity, to urinate into a drainage container. Then he should wash his hands thoroughly with soap and water and dry them. **CDC**

▶ Demonstrate how the patient should perform the catheterization, explaining each step clearly and carefully. Position a gooseneck lamp nearby if room lighting is inadequate to make the urinary meatus clearly visible. Arrange the patient's clothing so that it's out of the way.

Teaching the female patient

▶ Demonstrate and explain to the female patient that she should separate the vaginal folds as widely as possible with the fingers of her nondominant hand to obtain a full view of the urinary meatus. She may need to use a mirror

to visualize the meatus. Ask if she's right- or left-handed, and then tell her which is her nondominant hand. While holding her labia open with the nondominant hand, she should use the dominant hand to wash the perineal area thoroughly with a soapy washcloth, using downward strokes. Tell her to rinse the area with the washcloth, using downward strokes as well.

▶ Show her how to squeeze some lubricant onto the first 3″ (7.6 cm) of the catheter and then how to insert the catheter. (See *Teaching self-catheterization*.) **SUNA**

▶ When the urine stops draining, tell her to remove the catheter slowly, get dressed, and wash the catheter with warm, soapy water. Then she should rinse it inside and out and dry it with a paper towel.

Teaching the male patient

▶ Tell a male patient to wash and rinse the end of his penis thoroughly with soap and water, pulling back the foreskin, if appropriate. He should keep the foreskin pulled back during the procedure.

▶ Show him how to squeeze lubricant onto a paper towel and have him roll the first 7″ to 10″ (17.8 to 25 cm) of the catheter in the lubricant. Tell him that copious lubricant will make

the procedure more comfortable for him. Then show him how to insert the catheter. **SUNA**

▶ When the urine stops draining, tell him to remove the catheter slowly and, if necessary, pull the foreskin forward again. Have him get dressed and wash and dry the catheter as described previously.

Special considerations

▶ Impress upon the patient that the timing of catheterization is critical to prevent overdistention of the bladder, which can lead to infection. Self-catheterization is usually performed every 4 to 6 hours around the clock (or more often at first).

▶ Instruct the patient to keep a supply of catheters at home and to use each catheter only once before cleaning it. Advise him to wash the used catheter in warm, soapy water, rinse it inside and out, and then dry it with a clean towel and store it in a plastic bag until the next time it's needed.

▶ Advise the patient to store cleaned catheters only after they're completely dry to prevent growth of gram-negative organisms.

▶ Stress the importance of regulating fluid intake, as ordered, to prevent incontinence while maintaining ade-

Teaching self-catheterization

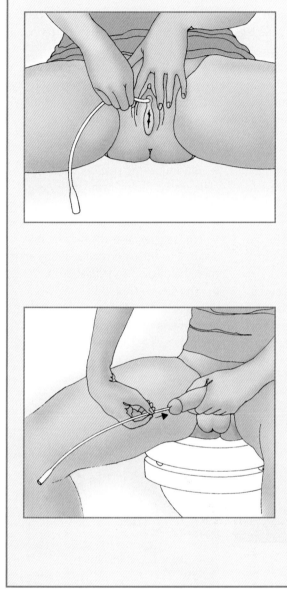

Teach a woman to hold the catheter in her dominant hand as if it were a pencil or a dart, about ½″ (1.3 cm) from its tip. Keeping the vaginal folds separated, she should slowly insert the lubricated catheter about 3″ (7.6 cm) into the urethra. Tell her to press down with her abdominal muscles to empty the bladder, allowing all urine to drain through the catheter and into the toilet or drainage container.

Teach a man to hold his penis in his nondominant hand, at a right angle to his body. He should hold the catheter in his dominant hand as if it were a pencil or a dart and slowly insert it 7″ to 10″ (17.8 to 25 cm) into the urethra until urine begins flowing. Then he should gently advance the catheter about 1″ (2.5 cm) farther, allowing all urine to drain into the toilet or drainage container.

▶ Also stress the importance of taking medications, as ordered, to increase urine retention and help prevent incontinence. Advise the patient to avoid calcium-rich and phosphorus-rich foods, as ordered, to reduce the chance of renal calculus formation.

References

Heard, L., and Buhrer, R. "How Do We Prevent UTI in People Who Perform Intermittent Catheterization?" *Rehabilitation Nursing* 30(2):44–45, 61, March–April 2005.

Robinson, J. "Intermittent Self-Catheterization Appliances for Disabled Patients," *British Journal of Community Nursing* 11(12):520–23, December 2006.

Robinson, J. "Intermittent Self-Catheterization: Principles and Practice," *British Journal of Community Nursing* 11(4):144, 146, April 2006.

Taylor, C., et al. *Fundamentals of Nursing: The Art and Science of Nursing Care,* 6th ed. Philadelphia: Lippincott Williams & Wilkins, 2008.

quate hydration. However, explain that incontinent episodes may occur occasionally. For managing incontinence, the practitioner or a home health care nurse can help develop a plan such as more frequent catheterizations. After an incontinent episode, tell the patient to wash with soap and water, pat himself dry with a towel, and expose the skin to the air for as long as possible. Bedding and furniture can be protected by covering them with rubber or plastic sheets and then covering the rubber or plastic with fabric.

Sequential compression therapy

Safe, effective, and noninvasive, sequential compression therapy helps prevent deep vein thrombosis (DVT) in surgical patients. Therapy works by massaging the legs in a wavelike, milking motion, promoting blood flow and deterring thrombosis.

Sequential compression therapy counteracts blood stasis and coagulation changes—two of the three major factors that promote DVT. It reduces stasis by increasing peak blood flow velocity, helping to empty the femoral vein's valve cusps of pooled or static blood. Also, the compressions produce an anticlotting effect by increasing fibrinolytic activity, which stimulates the release of a plasminogen activator.

Equipment

Measuring tape and sizing chart for the brand of sleeves you're using ◆ pair of compression sleeves in correct size ◆ connecting tubing ◆ compression controller.

Implementation

▶ Confirm the patient's identity using two patient identifiers according to your facility's policy. **JC**
▶ Explain the procedure to the patient to increase his cooperation.
▶ Wash your hands.

Determining proper sleeve size

▶ Before applying the compression sleeve, determine the proper size of sleeve that you need.
▶ Measure the circumference of the upper thigh while the patient rests in bed. Do this by placing the measuring tape under the thigh at the gluteal furrow.

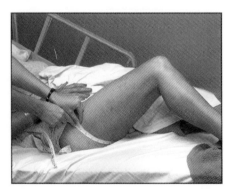

▶ Hold the tape snugly, but not tightly, around the patient's leg. Note the exact circumference.
▶ Find the patient's thigh measurement on the sizing chart, and locate the corresponding size of the compression sleeve.
▶ Remove the compression sleeves from the package and unfold them.
▶ Lay the unfolded sleeves on a flat surface with the cotton lining facing up.

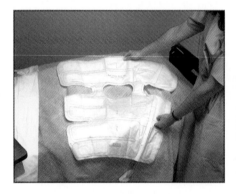

▶ Notice the markings on the lining denoting the ankle and the area behind the knee at the popliteal pulse point. Use these markings to position the sleeve at the appropriate landmarks.

Applying the sleeves

▶ Place the patient's leg on the sleeve lining. Position the back of the knee over the popliteal opening.
▶ Make sure the back of the ankle is over the ankle marking.

▶ Starting at the side opposite the clear plastic tubing, wrap the sleeve snugly around the patient's leg.
▶ Fasten the sleeve securely with the Velcro fasteners. For the best fit, first secure the ankle and calf sections and then the thigh.
▶ The sleeve should fit snugly but not tightly. Check the fit by inserting two fingers between the sleeve and the patient's leg at the knee opening. Loosen or tighten the sleeve by readjusting the Velcro fastener.
▶ Using the same procedure, apply the second sleeve.

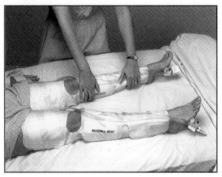

Operating the system

▶ Connect each sleeve to the tubing leading to the controller. Both sleeves must be connected to the compression controller for the system to operate. Line up the blue arrows on the sleeve connector with the arrows on the tubing connectors, and push the ends together firmly. Listen for a click, signaling a firm connection. Make sure the tubing isn't kinked.

▶ Plug the compression controller into the proper wall outlet. Turn on the power.

▶ The controller automatically sets the compression sleeve pressure at 45 mm Hg, which is the midpoint of the normal range (35 to 55 mm Hg).

▶ Observe the patient to see how well he tolerates the therapy and the controller as the system completes its first cycle.

▶ Check the AUDIBLE ALARM key. The green light should be lit, indicating that the alarm is working. `AORN`

▶ The compression sleeves should function continuously (24 hours daily) until the patient is fully ambulatory. Be sure to check the sleeves at least once each shift to ensure proper fit and inflation. `AACN` `ACCP` `AORN` `CS`

Removing the sleeves

▶ You may remove the sleeves when the patient is walking, bathing, or leaving the room for tests or other procedures. Reapply them immediately after any of these activities. To disconnect the sleeves from the tubing, press the latches on each side of the connectors, and pull the connectors apart. `AACN` `ACCP` `AORN`

▶ Store the tubing and compression controller according to facility protocol. This equipment isn't disposable.

Special considerations

▶ Remove the sleeves and assess and document skin integrity every 8 hours to avoid skin breakdown, especially in patients with decreased sensation or who are unresponsive.

▶ The compression controller also has a mechanism to help cool the patient.

▶ If you're applying only one sleeve— for example, if the patient has a cast— leave the unused sleeve folded in the plastic bag. Cut a small hole in the bag's sealed bottom edge, and pull the sleeve connector (the part that holds the connecting tubing) through the hole. Then you can join both sleeves to the compression controller.

▶ If a malfunction triggers the instrument's alarm, you'll hear beeping. The system shuts off whenever the alarm is activated.

▶ To respond to the alarm, remove the operator's card from the slot on the top of the compression controller. Follow the instructions printed on the card next to the matching code.

References

Bartley, M. "Keep Venous Thromboembolism at Bay," *Nursing* 36(10):36–41, October 2006.

Beck, D. "Venous Thromboembolism (VTE) Prophylaxis: Implications for Medical-Surgical Nurses," *Medsurg Nursing* 15(5):282–87, October 2006.

Brady, D., et al. "The Use of Knee-length Versus Thigh-length Compression Stockings and Sequential Compression Devices," *Critical Care Nursing Quarterly* 30(3):255–62, July–September 2007.

Cornwell, E. E., et al. "Compliance with Sequential Compression Device Prophylaxis in At-Risk Trauma Patients: A Prospective Analysis," *The American Surgeon* 68(5):470–3, May 2002. `CS`

"Graduated Compression Stockings: Prevention of Postoperative Venous Thromboembolism is Crucial," *AJN* 106(2):72AA-DD, February 2006.

Hirsh, J., et al. "Proceedings of the Seventh ACCP Conference on Antithrombotic and Thrombolytic Therapy: Evidence-Based Guidelines.," *Chest* 126 (3 Suppl):172S–696S, September 2004.

Lachiewicz, P. F., et al. "Two Mechanical Devices for Prophylaxis of Thromboembolism after Total Knee Arthroplasty: A Prospective, Randomized Study," *Journal of Bone and Joint Surgery* 86(8):1137–41, November 2004.

Sitz bath

A sitz bath involves immersion of the pelvic area in warm or hot water. It's used to relieve discomfort, especially after perineal or rectal surgery or childbirth. The bath promotes wound healing by cleaning the perineum and anus, increasing circulation, and reducing inflammation. It also helps relax local muscles.

To be performed correctly, the sitz bath requires frequent checks of water temperature to ensure therapeutic effects as well as correct draping of the patient during the bath and prompt dressing afterward to prevent vasoconstriction.

Equipment

Sitz tub, portable sitz bath, or regular bathtub ◆ bath mat ◆ rubber mat ◆ bath (utility) thermometer ◆ two bath blankets ◆ towels ◆ patient gown ◆ gloves, if the patient has an open lesion or has been incontinent ◆ optional: rubber ring, footstool, overbed table, I.V. pole (to hold irrigation bag), wheelchair or cart, dressing supplies.

Implementation

▶ Position the bath mat next to the bathtub, sitz tub, or commode. If you're using a tub, place a rubber mat on its surface to prevent falls. Place the rubber ring on the bottom of the tub to serve as a seat for the patient, and cover the ring with a towel for comfort.

▶ If you're using a commercial kit, open the package and familiarize yourself with the equipment.

▶ Fill the sitz tub or bathtub one-third to one-half full, so that the water will reach the seated patient's umbilicus. Use warm water (94° to 98° F [34° to 37° C]) for relaxation or wound cleaning and healing and hot water (110° to 115° F [43° to 46° C]) for heat application. Run the water slightly warmer than desired because it will cool while the patient prepares for the bath. Measure the water temperature using the bath thermometer.

▶ If you're using a commercial kit, fill the basin to the specified line with water at the prescribed temperature. Place the basin under the commode seat, clamp the irrigation tubing to block water flow, and fill the irrigation bag with water of the same temperature as that in the basin. To create flow pressure, hang the bag above the patient's head on a hook, towel rack, or I.V. pole.

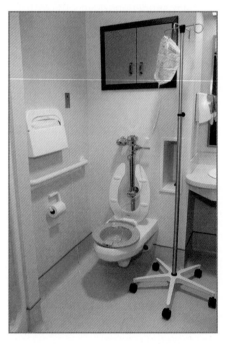

▶ Confirm the patient's identity using two patient identifiers according to your facility's policy. **JC**

▶ Check the practitioner's order, and assess the patient's condition.

▶ Explain the procedure to the patient. Wash your hands thoroughly and put on gloves.

▶ Have the patient void.

▶ Assist the patient to the bath area, provide privacy, and make sure the area is warm and free of drafts. Help the patient undress, as needed.

▶ Remove and dispose of any soiled dressings. If a dressing adheres to a wound, allow it to soak off in the tub.

▶ Assist the patient into the tub or onto the commode, as needed. Instruct him to use the safety rail for balance. Explain that the sensation may be unpleasant initially because the wound area is already tender. Assure him that this discomfort will soon be relieved by the warm water.

▶ For any apparatus except a regular bathtub, if the patient's feet don't reach the floor and the weight of his legs presses against the edge of the equipment, place a small stool under the patient's feet. This decreases pressure on local blood vessels. Also place a folded towel against the patient's lower back to prevent discomfort and promote correct body alignment.

▶ Drape the patient's shoulders and knees with bath blankets to avoid chills.

▶ If you're using the sitz bath kit, open the clamp on the irrigation tubing to allow a stream of water to flow continuously over the wound site. Refill the bag with water of the correct temperature, as needed, and encourage the patient to regulate the flow himself. Place the patient's overbed table in front of him to provide support and comfort.

▶ If you're using a tub, check the water temperature frequently with the bath thermometer. If the temperature drops significantly, add warm water. For maximum safety, first help the patient stand up slowly to prevent dizziness and loss of balance. Then, with the patient holding the safety rail for support, run warm water into the tub. Check the water temperature. When the water reaches the correct temperature, help the patient sit down again to resume the bath.

▶ If necessary, stay with the patient during the bath. If you must leave, show him how to use the call button, and ensure his privacy.

▶ Check the patient's color and general condition frequently. If he complains of feeling weak, faint, or nauseated or shows signs of cardiovascular distress, discontinue the bath, check the patient's pulse and blood pressure, and assist him back to bed. Use a wheelchair or cart to transport the patient to his room if necessary. Notify the practitioner.

▶ When the prescribed bath time has elapsed—usually 15 to 20 minutes— tell the patient to use the safety rail for balance, and help him to a standing position slowly to prevent dizziness and to allow him to regain his equilibrium.

▶ If necessary, help the patient to dry himself. Put on clean gloves, and redress the wound, as needed, and assist the patient to dress and return to bed or back to his room.

▶ Dispose of soiled materials properly. Empty, clean, and disinfect the sitz tub, bathtub, or portable sitz bath. Return the commercial kit to the patient's bedside for later use.

Special considerations

▶ Use a regular bathtub only if a special sitz tub, portable sitz bath, or commercial sitz bath kit is unavailable. Because the application of heat to the extremities causes vasodilation and draws blood away from the perineal area, a regular bathtub is less effective for local treatment than a sitz device.

▶ If the patient will be sitting in a bathtub with his extremities immersed in the hot water, check his pulse before, during, and after the bath to help detect vasodilation that could make him feel faint when he stands up.

▶ Tell the patient never to touch an open wound because of the risk of infection.

References

Albers, L. L., and Borders, N. "Minimizing Genital Tract Trauma and Related Pain Following Spontaneous Vaginal Birth," *Journal of Midwifery and Women's Health* 52(3):246–53, May–June 2007.

Craven, R. F., and Hirnle, C. J. *Fundamentals of Nursing: Human Health and Function,* 5th ed. Philadelphia: Lippincott Williams & Wilkins, 2007.

Guta, P. "Randomized, Controlled Study Comparing Sitz-Bath and No Sitz-Bath Treatments in Patients with Anal Fissures," *ANZ Journal of Surgery* 76(8):718–21, August 2006.

Taylor, C., et al. *Fundamentals of Nursing: The Art and Science of Nursing Care,* 6th ed. Philadelphia: Lippincott Williams & Wilkins, 2008.

Skin biopsy
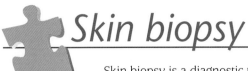

Skin biopsy is a diagnostic test in which a small piece of tissue is removed, under local anesthesia, from a lesion that's suspected of being malignant or from another dermatosis. (See *The ABCDEs of malignant melanoma*.)

One of three techniques may be used: shave biopsy, punch biopsy, or excisional biopsy. Shave biopsy cuts the lesion above the skin line, which allows further biopsy of the site. Punch biopsy removes an oval core from the center of the lesion. Excisional biopsy removes the entire lesion and is indicated for rapidly expanding lesions; for sclerotic, bullous, or atrophic lesions; and for examination of the border of a lesion surrounding normal skin.

Equipment

Gloves (sterile and clean) ◆ #15 scalpel for shave or excisional biopsy ◆ punch for punch biopsy ◆ local anesthetic ◆ specimen bottle containing 10% formaldehyde solution ◆ 4-0 sutures for punch or excisional biopsy ◆ adhesive bandage ◆ forceps ◆ laboratory specimen labels and laboratory biohazard transport bags.

Implementation

▶ Confirm the patient's identity using two patient identifiers according to your facility's policy. **JC**

▶ Describe the procedure to the patient and tell him who will perform it. Answer any questions he may have. **ASPN**

▶ Inform the patient that he need not restrict food or fluids.

▶ Tell him that he'll receive a local anesthetic for pain.

▶ Inform him that the biopsy will take about 15 minutes and that the test results are usually available within 7 days.

▶ Have the patient or an appropriate family member sign a consent form.

▶ Check the patient's history for hypersensitivity to the local anesthetic.

▶ Label all medications, medication containers, and other solutions on and off the sterile field. **JC**

▶ Position the patient comfortably, and clean the biopsy site before the local anesthetic is administered.

▶ For a shave biopsy, the protruding growth is cut off at the skin line with a #15 scalpel. The tissue is placed immediately in a properly labeled specimen bottle containing 10% formaldehyde solution. Apply pressure to the area to stop the bleeding. Apply an adhesive bandage.

▶ For a punch biopsy, the skin surrounding the lesion is pulled taut, and the punch is firmly introduced into the lesion and rotated to obtain a tissue specimen. The plug is lifted with forceps or a needle and is severed as deeply into the fat layer as possible. The specimen is placed in

---

The ABCDEs of malignant melanoma

A simple **ABCDE** rule outlines the warning signs of malignant melanoma:

A is for asymmetry: One half of a mole or birthmark doesn't match the other.

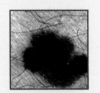

B is for border: The edges are irregular, ragged, notched, or blurred.

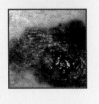

C is for color: The pigmentation isn't uniform but may have varying degrees of brown or black, or sometimes red.

D is for diameter greater than 19 (0.6 cm): Any sudden or progressive increase in size should be of concern.

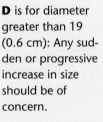

E is for elevation: If a mole is elevated, or raised from the skin, it should be considered suspicious.

a properly labeled specimen bottle containing 10% formaldehyde solution or in a sterile container if indicated. Closing the wound depends on the size of the punch: A 3-mm punch requires only an adhesive bandage, a 4-mm punch requires one suture, and a 6-mm punch requires two sutures.

▶ For an excisional biopsy, a #15 scalpel is used to excise the lesion; the incision is made as wide and as deep as necessary. The tissue specimen is removed and placed immediately in a properly labeled specimen bottle containing 10% formaldehyde solution. Apply pressure to the site to stop the bleeding. The wound is closed using a 4-0 suture. If the incision is large, a skin graft may be required.

▶ Check the biopsy site for bleeding.

▶ Label the specimen and send the specimen to the laboratory immediately in a laboratory biohazard transport bag.

▶ If the patient experiences pain, administer analgesics.

Special considerations

▶ Advise the patient going home with sutures to keep the area clean and as dry as possible. Tell him that facial sutures will be removed in 3 to 5 days and trunk sutures, in 7 to 14 days.

▶ Instruct the patient with adhesive strips to leave them in place for 14 to 21 days or until they fall off.

References

Baron, J. M., and Abazahra, F. "Evidenced-Based Staging System for Malignant Melanoma: Is Now Necessarily Better?" *Lancet* 364(9432):395–96, July–August 2004.

Maguire-Eisen, M. "Risk Assessment and Early Detection of Skin Cancers," *Seminars in Oncology Nursing* 19(1):43–51, February 2003.

Trent, J. T., et al. "Skin and Wound Biopsy: When, Why and How," *Advances in Skin and Wound Care* 16(7):372–75, December 2003.

Wahie, S., and Lawrence, C. M. "Wound Complications Following Diagnostic Skin Biopsies in Dermatology In-patients," *Archives of Dermatology* 143(10):1267–71, October 2007.

Skin medications

Topical drugs are applied directly to the skin surface. They include lotions, pastes, ointments, creams, powders, shampoos, patches, and aerosol sprays. Topical medications are absorbed through the epidermal layer into the dermis. The extent of absorption depends on the vascularity of the region.

Nitroglycerin, fentanyl, nicotine, and certain supplemental hormone replacements are used for systemic effects. Most other topical medications are used for local effects. Ointments have a fatty base, which is an ideal vehicle for drugs such as antimicrobials and antiseptics. Typically, topical medications should be applied two or three times per day to achieve their therapeutic effect.

Equipment

Patient's medication record and chart ◆ prescribed medication ◆ gloves ◆ 4″ × 4″ sterile gauze pads ◆ transparent semipermeable dressing ◆ adhesive tape ◆ solvent (such as cottonseed oil).

Implementation

▶ Verify the order on the patient's medication record by checking it against the practitioner's order on the chart. Also check the patient's medication record for allergies. **JC** **ISMP**

▶ Make sure the label on the medication agrees with the medication order. Read the label again before you open the container and as you remove the medication from the container. Check the expiration date.

▶ Confirm the patient's identity using two patient identifiers according to your facility's policy. **JC**

▶ If your facility uses a bar code scanning system, be sure to scan your ID badge, the patient's ID bracelet, and the medication's bar code. **JC** **ISMP**

▶ Provide privacy.

▶ Explain the procedure thoroughly to the patient because he may have to apply the medication by himself after discharge.

▶ Wash and glove your hands.

▶ Help the patient assume a comfortable position that provides access to the area to be treated.

▶ Expose the area to be treated. Make sure the skin or mucous membrane is intact (unless the medication has been ordered to treat a skin lesion, such as an ulcer). Applying medication to broken or abraded skin may cause unwanted systemic absorption and result in further irritation.

▶ If necessary, clean the skin of debris, including crusts, epidermal scales, and old medication. You may have to change your gloves, if they become soiled.

Applying paste, cream, or ointment

▶ Open the container. Place the lid or cap upside down to prevent contamination of the inside surface.

▶ Apply the medication to the affected area with long, smooth strokes that follow the direction of hair growth using your gloved hands. This technique avoids forcing medication into hair follicles, which can cause irritation and lead to folliculitis. Avoid excessive pressure when applying the medication because it could abrade the skin.

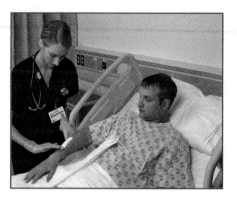

Removing ointment

▶ Wash your hands and apply gloves. Then rub solvent on them and apply it liberally to the ointment-treated area in the direction of hair growth. Alternatively, saturate a sterile gauze pad with the solvent, and use the pad to gently remove the ointment. Remove excess oil by gently wiping the area with a sterile gauze pad. Don't rub too hard to remove the medication because you could irritate the skin.

▶ Assess the patient's skin for signs of irritation, allergic reaction, or breakdown.

Special considerations

▶ To apply shampoos, follow package directions.

▶ To apply aerosol sprays, shake the container, if indicated, to completely mix the medication. Hold the container

6″ to 12″ (15 to 30 cm) from the skin, or follow the manufacturer's recommendation. Spray a thin film of the medication evenly over the treatment area.

▶ To apply powders, dry the skin surface, making sure to spread skin folds where moisture collects. Then apply a thin layer of powder over the treatment area.

▶ When applying an aerosol spray or powder, make sure to protect the patient from direct inhalation of the medication.

▶ To protect applied medications and prevent them from soiling the patients' clothes, tape an appropriate amount of sterile gauze pad or a transparent semipermeable dressing over the treated area. With certain medications, such as topical steroids, semipermeable dressings may be contraindicated.

AGE FACTOR

In children, topical medications (such as steroids) should be covered only loosely with a diaper. Don't use plastic pants.

▶ Never apply medication without first removing previous applications to prevent skin irritation from an accumulation of medication.

▶ Don't apply ointments to mucous membranes as liberally as you would to skin because mucous membranes are usually moist and absorb ointment more quickly than skin does. Also, don't apply too much ointment to any skin area because it might cause irritation and discomfort, stain clothing and bedding, and make removal difficult.

▶ Never apply ointment to the eyelids or ear canal unless ordered. The ointment might congeal and occlude the tear duct or ear canal.

▶ Inspect the treated area frequently for adverse effects, such as signs of an allergic reaction.

References

Craven, R. F., and Hirnle, C. J. *Fundamentals of Nursing: Human Health and Function,* 6th ed. Philadelphia: Lippincott Williams & Wilkins, 2009.

McCleane, G. "Topical Analgesics," *The Medical Clinics of North America* 91(1):125–39, January 2007.

McIntyre, L. J., and Courey, T. J. "Safe Medication Administration," *Journal of Nursing Care Quality* 22(1):40–42, January–March 2007.

Skin staple and clip removal

Skin staples or clips may be used instead of standard sutures to close lacerations or surgical wounds. Because they can secure a wound more quickly than sutures, they may substitute for surface sutures when cosmetic results aren't a prime consideration, such as in abdominal closure. When properly placed, staples and clips distribute tension evenly along the suture line with minimal tissue trauma and compression, facilitating healing and minimizing scarring. Because staples and clips are made from surgical stainless steel, tissue reaction to them is minimal. The practitioner usually removes skin staples and clips; however, some facilities permit qualified nurses to perform this procedure.

Equipment

Waterproof trash bag ◆ adjustable light ◆ clean gloves, if needed ◆ sterile gloves ◆ sterile gauze pads ◆ sterile staple or clip extractor ◆ antiseptic cleaning agent ◆ sterile cotton-tipped applicators ◆ optional: butterfly adhesive strips or Steri-Strips, compound benzoin tincture or other skin protectant.

Implementation

▶ If your facility allows you to remove skin staples and clips, check the practitioner's order to confirm the exact timing and details for this procedure.
▶ Assemble all equipment in the patient's room. Check the expiration date on each sterile package and inspect for tears.
▶ Open the waterproof trash bag, and place it near the patient's bed. Position the bag to avoid reaching across the sterile field or the wound when disposing of soiled articles. Form a cuff by turning down the top of the bag to provide a wide opening, then preventing contamination of instruments or gloves by touching the bag's edge.
▶ Check for patient allergies, especially to adhesive tape and povidone-iodine or other topical solutions or medications.

▶ Explain the procedure to the patient. Tell him that he may feel a slight pulling or tickling sensation but little discomfort during staple removal. Reassure him that because his incision is healing properly, removing the supporting staples or clips won't weaken the incision line.
▶ Provide privacy, and place the patient in a comfortable position that doesn't place undue tension on the incision. Because some patients experience nausea or dizziness during the procedure, have the patient recline if possible. Adjust the light to shine directly on the incision.
▶ Wash your hands thoroughly. **CDC**
▶ If the patient's wound has a dressing, put on clean gloves and carefully remove it. Discard the dressing and the gloves in the waterproof trash bag.
▶ Assess the patient's incision. Notify the practitioner of gaping, drainage, inflammation, and other signs of infection.
▶ Establish a sterile work area with all the equipment and supplies you'll need for removing staples or clips and for cleaning and dressing the incision. Open the package containing the sterile staple or clip extractor, maintaining asepsis. Put on sterile gloves.
▶ Wipe the incision gently with sterile gauze pads soaked in an antiseptic cleaning agent or with sterile cotton-

tipped applicators to remove surface encrustations.
▶ Pick up the sterile staple or clip extractor. Then, starting at one end of the incision, remove the staple or clip. (See *Removing a staple.*) Hold the extractor over the trash bag, and release the handle to discard the staple or clip.
▶ Repeat the procedure for each staple or clip until all are removed.
▶ Apply a sterile gauze dressing, if needed, to prevent infection and irritation from clothing. Then discard your gloves.
▶ Make sure the patient is comfortable. According to the practitioner's preference, inform the patient that he may shower in 1 or 2 days if the incision is dry and healing well.
▶ Properly dispose of solutions and the trash bag, and clean or dispose of soiled equipment and supplies according to your facility's policy.

Special considerations

▶ Carefully check the practitioner's order for the time and extent of staple or clip removal. The practitioner may want you to remove only alternate staples or clips initially and to leave the others in place for an additional day or two to support the incision.

Removing a staple

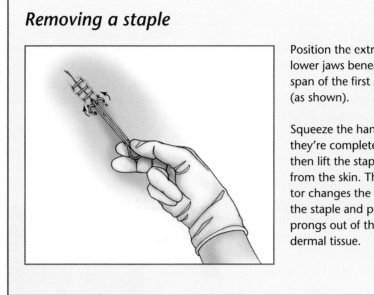

Position the extractor's lower jaws beneath the span of the first staple (as shown).

Squeeze the handles until they're completely closed; then lift the staple away from the skin. The extractor changes the shape of the staple and pulls the prongs out of the intradermal tissue.

and care for the wound. Instruct him to call the practitioner immediately if he observes wound discharge or any other abnormal change. Tell him that the redness surrounding the incision should gradually disappear and that after a few weeks, only a thin line will be visible.

References

Taylor, C., et al. *Fundamentals of Nursing: The Art and Science of Nursing Care,* 6th ed. Philadelphia: Lippincott Williams & Wilkins, 2008.

▶ When removing a staple or clip, place the extractor's jaws carefully between the patient's skin and the staple or clip to avoid patient discomfort. If extraction is difficult, notify the practitioner; staples or clips placed too deeply within the skin or left in place too long may resist removal.

▶ If the wound dehisces after staples or clips are removed, apply butterfly adhesive strips or Steri-Strips to approximate and support the edges, and call the practitioner immediately to repair the wound. (See *Types of adhesive skin closures.*)

▶ You may also apply butterfly adhesive strips or Steri-Strips after removing staples or clips, even if the wound is healing normally, to give added support to the incision and prevent lateral tension from forming a wide scar. Use a small amount of compound benzoin tincture or other skin protectant to ensure adherence. Leave the strips in place for 3 to 5 days.

▶ If the patient is being discharged, teach him how to remove the dressing

Types of adhesive skin closures

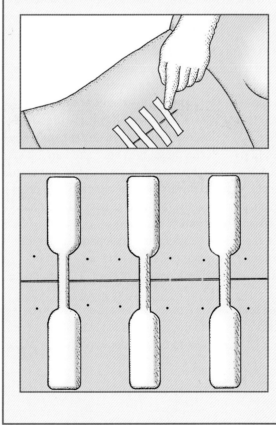

Steri-Strips are used as a primary means of keeping a wound closed after suture removal. They're made of thin strips of sterile, nonwoven, porous fabric tape.

Butterfly closures consist of sterile, waterproof adhesive strips. A narrow, nonadhesive "bridge" connects the two expanded adhesive portions. These strips are used to close small wounds and assist healing after suture removal.

Soaks

A soak involves immersion of a body part in warm water or a medicated solution. This treatment helps to soften exudates, facilitate debridement, enhance suppuration, clean wounds or burns, rehydrate wounds, apply medication to infected areas, and increase local blood supply and circulation.

Most soaks are applied with clean tap water using clean technique. Sterile solution and sterile equipment are required for treating wounds, burns, and other breaks in the skin.

Equipment

Basin or arm or foot tub ◆ bath (utility) thermometer ◆ hot tap water or prescribed solution ◆ cup ◆ pitcher ◆ linen-saver pad ◆ overbed table ◆ footstool ◆ pillows ◆ towels ◆ gauze pads and other dressing materials ◆ clean and sterile gloves, if necessary.

Implementation

▶ Confirm the patient's identity using two patient identifiers according to your facility's policy. **JC**
▶ Check the practitioner's order.
▶ Clean and disinfect the basin or tub.
▶ Run hot tap water into a pitcher, or heat the prescribed solution, as applicable. Measure the water or solution temperature with a bath thermometer. If the temperature isn't within the prescribed range (usually 105° to 110° F [40.6° to 43.3° C]), add hot or cold water or reheat or cool the solution, as needed. If you're preparing the soak outside the patient's room, heat the liquid slightly above the correct temperature to allow for cooling during transport.
▶ If the solution for a medicated soak isn't premixed, prepare the solution and heat it.

▶ Assess the patient's condition, and check for an allergy to the medicated solution.
▶ Explain the procedure to the patient. Provide privacy. Wash your hands thoroughly.
▶ If the soak basin or tub will be placed in bed, make sure the bed is flat beneath it to prevent spills. For an arm soak, have the patient sit erect. For a leg or foot soak, ask him to lie down and bend the appropriate knee. For a foot soak in the sitting position, let him sit on the edge of the bed or transfer him to a chair.
▶ Place a linen-saver pad under the treatment site and, if necessary, cover the pad with a towel.
▶ Expose the treatment site. Put on gloves before removing any dressing; dispose of the soiled dressing properly. If the dressing is encrusted and stuck to the wound, leave it in place and proceed with the soak. Remove the dressing several minutes later when it has begun to soak free.
▶ Position the soak basin under the treatment site on the bed, overbed table, footstool, or floor, as appropriate. Pour the heated liquid into the soak basin or tub. Then lower the arm or leg into the basin gradually to allow adjustment to the temperature change. Make

sure the soak solution covers the treatment site.

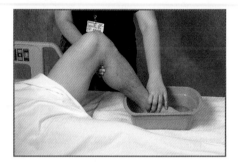

▶ Support other body parts with pillows or towels, as needed, to prevent discomfort and muscle strain. Make the patient comfortable and ensure proper body alignment.
▶ Check the temperature of the soak solution with the bath thermometer every 5 minutes. If the temperature drops below the prescribed range, remove some of the cooled solution with a cup. Then lift the patient's arm or leg from the basin, and add hot water or solution to the basin. Mix the liquid thoroughly, and then check its temperature. If the temperature is within the prescribed range, lower the patient's affected part back into the basin.
▶ Observe the patient for signs of tissue intolerance: extreme redness at the treatment site, excessive drainage, bleeding, or maceration. If such signs

develop or the patient complains of pain, discontinue the treatment, and notify the practitioner.

▶ After 15 to 20 minutes or as ordered, lift the patient's arm or leg from the basin, and remove the basin.

▶ Dry the arm or leg thoroughly with a towel. If the patient has a wound, dry the skin around it without touching the wound.

▶ While the skin is hydrated from the soak, use gauze pads to remove loose scales or crusts.

▶ Observe the treatment area for general appearance, degree of swelling, debridement, suppuration, and healing. Put on sterile gloves and re-dress the wound, if appropriate.

▶ Remove the towel and linen-saver pad, and make the patient comfortable in bed.

▶ Discard the soak solution, dispose of soiled materials properly, and clean and disinfect the basin. Remove and discard your gloves. If the treatment is to be repeated, store the equipment in the patient's room, out of his reach; otherwise, return it to the central supply department.

Special considerations

▶ To treat large areas, particularly burns, a soak may be administered in a whirlpool or Hubbard tank.

References

Craven, R. F., and Hirnle, C. J. *Fundamentals of Nursing: Human Health and Function,* 6th ed. Philadelphia: Lippincott Williams & Wilkins, 2009.

Gutman, A. B., et al. "Soak and Smear: A Standard Technique Revisited," *Archives of Dermatology* 141(12): 1556–59, December 2005.

Taylor, C., et al. *Fundamentals of Nursing: The Art and Science of Nursing Care,* 6th ed. Philadelphia: Lippincott Williams & Wilkins, 2008.

Sputum collection

Secreted by mucous membranes lining the bronchioles, bronchi, and trachea, sputum helps protect the respiratory tract from infection. When expelled from the respiratory tract, sputum carries saliva, nasal and sinus secretions, dead cells, and normal oral bacteria from the respiratory tract. Sputum specimens may be cultured for identification of respiratory pathogens.

The usual method of sputum specimen collection, expectoration, may require ultrasonic nebulization, hydration, or chest percussion and postural drainage. Less common methods include tracheal suctioning and, rarely, bronchoscopy. Tracheal suctioning is contraindicated within 1 hour of eating and in patients with esophageal varices, nausea, facial or basilar skull fractures, laryngospasm, or bronchospasm. It should be performed cautiously in patients with heart disease because it may precipitate arrhythmias.

Equipment

For expectoration: Sterile specimen container with tight-fitting cap ◆ gloves ◆ label ◆ laboratory request form and laboratory biohazard transport bag ◆ aerosol (10% sodium chloride, propylene glycol, acetylcysteine, or sterile or distilled water), as ordered ◆ facial tissues ◆ emesis basin.

For tracheal suctioning: #12 to #14 French sterile suction catheter ◆ water-soluble lubricant ◆ laboratory request form and laboratory biohazard transport bag ◆ sterile gloves ◆ mask ◆ goggles ◆ sterile in-line specimen trap (Lukens trap) ◆ normal saline solution ◆ portable suction machine, if wall unit is unavailable ◆ oxygen therapy equipment ◆ optional: nasal airway, to obtain a nasotracheal specimen with suctioning, if needed.

Commercial suction kits are available that contain the suction catheter, lubricant, sterile gloves, and specimen trap.

Implementation

▶ Confirm the patient's identity using two patient identifiers according to your facility's policy. **JC**

▶ Tell the patient that you'll collect a specimen of sputum (not saliva), and explain the procedure to promote cooperation. If possible, collect the specimen early in the morning, before breakfast, to obtain an overnight accumulation of secretions.

Collection by expectoration

▶ Instruct the patient to sit in a chair or at the edge of the bed. If he can't sit up, place him in high Fowler's position.

▶ Ask the patient to rinse his mouth with water to reduce specimen contamination. (Avoid mouthwash or toothpaste because they may affect the mobility of organisms in the sputum sample.) Then tell him to cough deeply and expectorate directly into the specimen container. Ask him to produce at least 15 ml of sputum, if possible. **CAP**

▶ Put on gloves.

▶ Cap the container and, if necessary, clean its exterior. Remove and discard your gloves, and wash your hands thoroughly.

▶ Label the container with the patient's name and room number, practitioner's name, date and time of collection, and initial diagnosis. Also include on the laboratory request form whether the patient was febrile or taking antibiotics and whether sputum was induced (because such specimens commonly appear watery and may resemble saliva). Send the specimen to the laboratory immediately in a laboratory biohazard transport bag.

Collection by tracheal suctioning

▶ If the patient can't produce an adequate specimen by coughing, prepare to suction him to obtain the specimen. Explain the suctioning procedure to him and tell him that he may cough, gag, or feel short of breath during the procedure.

▶ Check the suction machine to make sure it's functioning properly. Then place the patient in high Fowler's or semi-Fowler's position.

▶ Administer oxygen to the patient before beginning the procedure.

▶ Wash your hands thoroughly.

▶ Put on sterile gloves. Consider one hand sterile and the other hand clean to prevent cross-contamination. **AARC** **CDC**

▶ Connect the suction tubing to the male adapter of the in-line specimen trap. Attach the sterile suction catheter to the rubber tubing of the trap. (See *Attaching a specimen trap to a suction catheter.*)

Attaching a specimen trap to a suction catheter

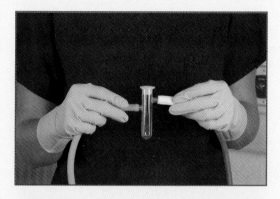

Wearing gloves, push the suction tubing onto the male adapter of the in-line trap.

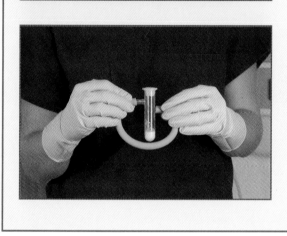

Insert the suction catheter into the rubber tubing of the trap.

After suctioning, disconnect the in-line trap from the suction tubing and catheter. To seal the container, connect the rubber tubing to the male adapter of the trap.

When collection is completed, discontinue the suction, gently remove the catheter, and administer oxygen. **AARC** **AACN**

▶ Detach the catheter from the in-line trap, gather it up in your dominant hand, and pull the glove cuff inside out and down around the used catheter to enclose it for disposal. Remove and discard the other glove and your mask and goggles.

▶ Detach the trap from the tubing connected to the suction machine. Seal the trap tightly by connecting the rubber tubing to the male adapter of the trap.

▶ Label the trap's container as an expectorated specimen, place in a laboratory biohazard transport bag, and send it to the laboratory immediately with a completed laboratory request form.

▶ Offer the patient a glass of water or mouthwash.

Special considerations

▶ If you can't obtain a sputum specimen through tracheal suctioning, perform chest percussion to loosen and mobilize secretions, and position the patient for optimal drainage. After 20 to 30 minutes, repeat the tracheal suctioning procedure.

▶ Before sending the specimen to the laboratory, examine it to make sure it's actually sputum, not saliva, because saliva will produce inaccurate test results.

▶ Because expectorated sputum is contaminated by normal mouth flora, tracheal suctioning provides a more reliable specimen for diagnosis.

▶ If the patient becomes hypoxic or cyanotic during suctioning, remove the catheter immediately and administer oxygen.

▶ If the patient has asthma or chronic bronchitis, watch for aggravated bron-

▶ Position a mask and goggles over your face. Tell the patient to tilt his head back slightly. Then lubricate the catheter with normal saline solution, and gently pass it through the patient's nostril without suction. **CDC**

▶ When the catheter reaches the larynx, the patient will cough. As he does, quickly advance the catheter into the

trachea. Tell him to take several deep breaths through his mouth to ease insertion.

▶ To obtain the specimen, apply suction for 5 to 10 seconds but never longer than 15 seconds because prolonged suction can cause hypoxia. If the procedure must be repeated, let the patient rest for four to six breaths.

chospasms with the use of more than a 10% concentration of sodium chloride or acetylcysteine in an aerosol. If he's suspected of having tuberculosis, don't use more than 20% propylene glycol with water when inducing a sputum specimen because a higher concentration inhibits growth of the pathogen and causes erroneous test results. If propylene glycol isn't available, use 10% to 20% acetylcysteine with water or sodium chloride.

▶ Patients with cardiac disease may develop arrhythmias during the procedure as a result of coughing, especially when the specimen is obtained by suctioning. Other potential complications include tracheal trauma or bleeding, vomiting, aspiration, and hypoxemia.

References

Agnes, K., and Condon, M. "Tuberculosis Guidelines and Update," *AJN* 106(6):104, June 2006.

Lynn, P. *Taylor's Clinical Nursing Skills,* 2nd ed. Philadelphia: Lippincott Williams & Wilkins, 2007.

Villarino, M., and Mazurek, G. "Tuberculosis Contact, Concerns, and Controls: What Matters for Healthcare Workers," *Infection Control and Hospital Epidemiology* 27(5):433–35, May 2006.

ST-segment monitoring

A sensitive indicator of myocardial damage, the ST segment is normally flat or isoelectric. A depressed ST segment may result from cardiac glycosides, myocardial ischemia, or a subendocardial infarction. An elevated ST segment suggests myocardial infarction.

Continuous ST-segment monitoring is helpful for patients with acute coronary syndromes and for those who have received thrombolytic therapy or have undergone coronary angioplasty or cardiac surgery. **CS1** ST-segment monitoring allows for early detection of reocclusion. It's also useful for patients who have had previous episodes of cardiac ischemia without chest pain, those who have difficulty distinguishing between cardiac pain and pain from other sources, and for those who have difficulty communicating. **CS2** ST-segment monitoring gives the practitioner the ability to identify and reverse ischemia by starting early interventions. **AHA**

Because ischemia typically occurs in a single area of the heart muscle, some electrocardiogram (ECG) leads can't detect it. Select the most appropriate lead by examining ECG tracings obtained during an ischemic episode. Use the leads that show ischemia for ST-segment monitoring. ST-segment monitoring isn't useful for patients with left- or right-bundle branch block, ventricular paced rhythm, or who are restless. **AHA**

Equipment

ECG electrodes ◆ gauze pads ◆ ECG monitor cable ◆ leadwires ◆ alcohol pads ◆ cardiac monitor programmed for ST-segment monitoring.

Implementation

▶ Confirm the patient's identity using two patient identifiers according to your facility's policy. **JC**

▶ Bring the equipment to the patient's bedside and explain the procedure to him. Provide privacy.

▶ Wash your hands. If the patient isn't already on a monitor, turn on the device and attach the cable.

▶ Select the sites for electrode placement and prepare the patient's skin for attachment as you would for continuous cardiac monitoring or a 12-lead ECG. Attach the leadwires to the electrodes and position the electrodes on the patient's skin in the appropriate positions.

▶ Activate ST-segment monitoring by pressing the MONITORING PROCEDURES key and then the ST key. Activate individual ST parameters by pressing the ON/OFF parameter key.

▶ Select the appropriate ECG for each ST channel to be monitored by pressing the PARAMETERS key and then the key labeled ECG.

▶ Identify the ECG complexes as prompted by the monitor.

▶ Adjust the ST point to 60 msec after the J point. (See *Changes in the ST segment.*) **AACN** **AHA**

▶ Set the alarm limits for each ST-segment parameter by manipulating the high and low limit keys. **JC**

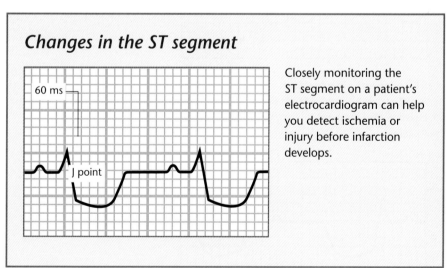

Changes in the ST segment

60 ms

J point

Closely monitoring the ST segment on a patient's electrocardiogram can help you detect ischemia or injury before infarction develops.

▶ Press the key labeled STANDARD DISPLAY to return to the display screen.

▶ Assess the waveform shown on the monitor.

Special considerations

▶ Be sure to abrade the patient's skin gently to ensure electrode adhesion and promote electrical conductivity.

▶ If monitoring only one lead, choose the lead most likely to show arrhythmias and ST-segment changes. **AACN** **AHA**

▶ Verify limit parameters for the patient with the practitioner. Typically, when a limit is surpassed for more than 1 minute, visual and audible alarms are activated.

▶ Evaluate the monitor for ST-segment depression or elevation. (See *Understanding changes in the ST segment*.)

▶ If ischemia is noted, obtain a 12-lead ECG and assess the patient for signs and symptoms of acute ischemia, such as arrhythmias, angina, and hemodynamic changes.

Understanding changes in the ST segment

Closely monitoring the ST segment can help detect ischemia or injury before infarction develops.

ST-segment elevation
An ST segment is considered elevated when it's 1 mm or more above the baseline. An elevated ST segment may indicate myocardial injury.

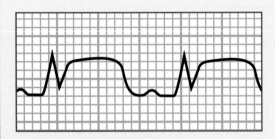

ST-segment depression
An ST segment is considered depressed when it's 0.5 mm or more below the baseline. A depressed ST segment may indicate myocardial ischemia or digoxin toxicity.

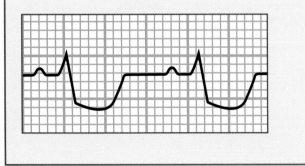

References

Drew, B. J., et al. "AHA Scientific Statement: Practice Standards for Electrocardiographic Monitoring in Hospital Settings: An American Heart Association Scientific Statement from the Councils on Cardiovascular Nursing, Clinical Cardiology, and Cardiovascular Disease in the Young: Endorsed by the International Society of Computerized Electrocardiography and the American Association of Critical Care Nurses," *Journal of Cardiovascular Nursing* 20(2):76–106, March–April 2005.

Drew, B. J., et al. "Frequency, Characteristics, and Clinical Significance of Transient ST Segment Elevation in Patients with Acute Coronary Syndromes," *European Heart Journal* 23(12):941–7, June 2002. **CS2**

Flanders, S. A. "Continuous ST-Segment Monitoring: Raising the Bar," *Critical Care Nursing Clinics of North America* 18(2):179–77, June 2006.

Flanders, S. A. "ST-segment Monitoring: Putting Standards into Practice," *AACN Advances in Critical Care Nursing* 18(3):275–84, July–September 2007.

Krucoff, M. W., et al. "Clinical Utility of Serial and Continuous ST-Segment Recovery Assessment in Patients with Acute ST-Elevation Myocardial Infarction: Assessing the Dynamics of Epicardial and Myocardial Reperfusion," *Circulation* 110(25):e533–39, December 2004.

Landesberg, G., et al. "Myocardial Ischemia, Cardiac Troponin, and Long-Term Survival of High-Cardiac Risk Critically Ill Intensive Care Unit Patients," *Critical Care Medicine* 33(6):1281–87, June 2005.

Lynn-McHale Wiegand, D. J., and Carlson, K. K., eds. *AACN Procedure Manual for Critical Care,* 5th ed. Philadelphia: W. B. Saunders Co., 2005.

Yan, A. T., et al. "Long-term Prognostic Value and Therapeutic Implications of Continuous ST-segment Monitoring in Acute Coronary Syndrome," *American Heart Journal* 153(4):500–06, April 2007. **CS1**

Standard precautions

Standard precautions were developed by the Centers for Disease Control and Prevention (CDC) to provide the widest possible protection against the transmission of infection. CDC officials recommend that health care workers handle all blood, bodily fluids (including secretions, excretions, and drainage), tissues, and contact with mucous membranes and broken skin as if they contain infectious agents, regardless of the patient's diagnosis.

Standard precautions encompass much of the isolation precautions previously recommended by the CDC for patients with known or suspected blood-borne pathogens as well as the precautions previously known as *body substance isolation*. They are to be used in conjunction with other transmission-based precautions: airborne, droplet, and contact precautions.

Airborne precautions are initiated in situations of suspected or known infections spread by the airborne route. The causative organisms are coughed, talked, or sneezed into the air by the infected person in droplets of moisture. The moisture evaporates, leaving the microorganisms suspended in the air to be breathed in by susceptible persons who enter the shared air space. Airborne precautions recommend placing the infected patient in a negative-pressure isolation room and the wearing of respiratory protection by all persons entering the patient's room.

Droplet precautions are used to protect health care workers and visitors from mucous membrane contact with oral and nasal secretions of the infected individual.

Contact precautions use barrier precautions to interrupt the transmission of specific epidemiologically important organisms by direct or indirect contact. Each institution must establish an infection control policy that lists specific barrier precautions.

Equipment

Gloves ◆ masks ◆ goggles, glasses with side pieces, or face shields ◆ gowns or aprons ◆ resuscitation bag ◆ bags for specimens ◆ Environmental Protection Agency (EPA)–registered tuberculocidal disinfectant or diluted bleach solution (diluted between 1:10 and 1:100, mixed fresh daily), or both, or EPA-registered disinfectant labeled effective against hepatitis B virus (HBV) and human immunodeficiency virus (HIV).

Implementation CDC

▶ Wash your hands immediately if they become contaminated with blood or body fluids, excretions, secretions, or drainage; also wash your hands before and after patient care and after removing gloves. Hand washing removes microorganisms from your skin. If your hands aren't visibly soiled, an alcohol-based hand rub can be used for routine decontamination.

▶ Wear gloves if you will or could come in contact with blood, specimens, tissue, body fluids, secretions or excretions, mucous membrane, broken skin, or contaminated surfaces or objects.

▶ Change your gloves and wash your hands between patient contacts to avoid cross-contamination.

▶ Wear a fluid-resistant gown, face shield, or goggles and a mask during procedures likely to generate splashing or splattering of blood or body fluids, such as surgery, endoscopic procedures, dialysis, assisting with intubation or manipulation of arterial lines, or any other procedure with the same potential.

▶ Handle used needles and other sharp instruments carefully. Don't bend, break, reinsert them into their original sheaths, remove needles from syringes, or unnecessarily handle them. (See *Recapping needles,* page 488.) Discard them intact immediately after use into a puncture-resistant disposal box. Use tools to pick up broken glass or other sharp objects. Use safety devices according to the instructions provided by the manufacturer. Activate all safety mechanisms on sharp devices immediately after use, even if the sharps disposal container is very close. Evaluate your work practices to make sure you're working safely, both for your own protection and for the protection of your patients and coworkers. These measures reduce the risk of accidental injury or infection. Always use a needleless I.V. system. JC OSHA

▶ Immediately notify your employee health care provider of all needle-stick or other sharp object injuries, mucosal splashes, or contamination of open wounds or nonintact skin with blood or body fluids to allow investigation of the incident and appropriate care and doc-

Recapping needles

If it is necessary to recap a needle, such as after withdrawing medication from a vial or ampule, use the following technique to recap the needle safely.

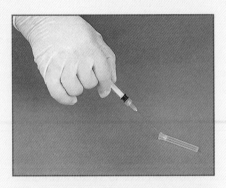

Prepare to slide the needle into the cap.

Lift the cap on to the needle

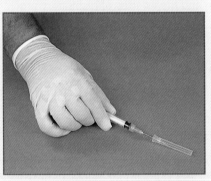

Cover the needle with the cap.

Always use extreme caution when recapping a needle. Never hold the sheath in your hand and attempt to recap the needle.

---

body fluids—such as nondisposable utensils or instruments—in a single impervious bag or container before removal from the room. Carry soiled linens in outstretched arms to avoid contaminating your uniform. Place linens and trash in single bags of sufficient thickness to contain the contents.

▶ While wearing the appropriate personal protective equipment, promptly clean all blood and body fluid spills with detergent and water followed by an EPA-registered tuberculocidal disinfectant or diluted bleach solution (diluted between 1:10 and 1:100, mixed daily), or both, or an EPA-registered disinfectant labeled effective against HBV and HIV, provided that the surface hasn't been contaminated with agents or volumes of or concentrations of agents for which higher-level disinfection is recommended.

▶ Disposable food trays and dishes aren't necessary.

▶ If you have an exudative lesion, avoid all direct patient contact until the condition has resolved, and you've been cleared by the employee health care provider.

▶ If you have dermatitis or other conditions resulting in broken skin on your hands, avoid situations where you may have contact with blood and body fluids (even though gloves could be worn) until the condition has resolved, and you've been cleared by the employee health care provider.

Special considerations

▶ Standard precautions, such as hand hygiene and appropriate use of personal protective equipment, should be routine infection control practices.

▶ Keep mouthpieces, resuscitation bags, and other ventilation devices nearby to eliminate the need for emergency mouth-to-mouth resuscitation, thus reducing the risk of exposure to body fluids.

---

umentation. Be sure to complete all follow-up screening and care as recommended by your employee health care provider. **OSHA**

▶ Properly label all specimens collected from patients, and place them in plastic bags at the collection site. Attach requisition slips to the outside of the bag.

▶ Place all items that have come in direct contact with the patient's secretions, excretions, blood, drainage, or

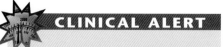

CLINICAL ALERT

Because you may not always know what organisms may be present in every clinical situation, you must use standard precautions for every contact with blood, bodily fluids, secretions, excretions, drainage, mucous membranes, and nonintact skin.

References

Boyce, J. M., et al. "Guideline for Hand Hygiene in Health-Care Settings," *MMWR* 51(RR-16):1–45, October 2002.

Centers for Disease Control and Prevention. "Guideline for Isolation Precautions: Preventing Transmission of Infections Agents in Healthcare Settings 2007." Accessed August 2007 via the Web at *www.cdc.gov/ncidod/dhqp/ gl_isolation.html.*

Chalmers, C., and Straub, M. "Standard Principles for Preventing and Controlling Infection," *Nursing Standards* 20(23):57–65, February 2006.

Department of Labor Occupational Safety and Health Administration. "29 C.F.R. Part 1920 Occupational Exposure to Bloodborne Pathogens; Needlesticks and Other Sharps Injuries; Final Rule," *Federal Register* 66(12):5318–25, January 2001.

Gardner, J. S. "Hospital Infection Control Practices Advisory Committee Guidelines for Isolation Precautions in Hospitals," *Infection Control and Hospital Epidemiology* 17:53–80, January 1996.

Houghton, D. "HAI Prevention: The Power Is in Your Hands," *Nursing Management* 37(Suppl):1–7, May 2006.

Rushing, J. "Wearing Personal Protective Gear," *Nursing* 36(10):56–57, October 2006.

Stool collection

Stool is collected to determine the presence of blood, ova and parasites, bile, fat, pathogens, or substances such as ingested drugs. Gross examination of stool characteristics, such as color, consistency, and odor, can reveal such conditions as GI bleeding and steatorrhea.

Stool specimens are collected randomly or for specific periods, such as 72 hours. Because stool specimens can't be obtained on demand, proper collection requires careful instructions to the patient to ensure an uncontaminated specimen.

Equipment

Specimen container with lid ◆ gloves ◆ two tongue blades ◆ paper towel or paper bag ◆ bedpan or portable commode ◆ two patient-care reminders (for timed specimens) ◆ laboratory request form and laboratory biohazard transport bag.

Implementation

▶ Explain the procedure to the patient and his family, if possible, to ensure their cooperation and prevent inadvertent disposal of timed stool specimens.

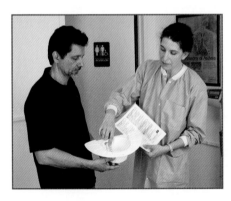

Collecting a random specimen

▶ Tell the patient to notify you when he has the urge to defecate. Have him defecate into a clean, dry bedpan or commode. Instruct him not to contaminate the specimen with urine or toilet tissue.

▶ Put on gloves.

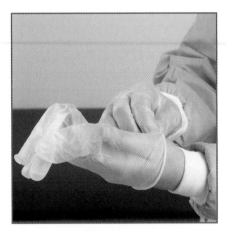

▶ Using a tongue blade, transfer the most representative stool specimen from the bedpan to the container, and cap the container. If the patient passes blood, mucus, or pus with the stool, be sure to include this with the specimen.

▶ Wrap the tongue blade in a paper towel and discard it. Remove and discard your gloves, and wash your hands thoroughly to prevent cross-contamination.

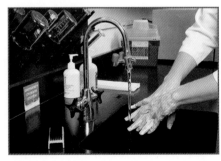

Collecting a timed specimen

▶ Place a patient-care reminder stating SAVE ALL STOOL over the patient's bed and in his bathroom.

▶ After putting on gloves, collect the first specimen, and include this in the total specimen.

▶ Obtain the timed specimen as you would a random specimen, but remember to transfer all stool to the specimen container.

▶ As ordered, send each specimen to the laboratory immediately with a laboratory request form or, if permitted, refrigerate the specimens collected during the test period, and send them when collection is complete. All specimens must be stored and transported in an approved laboratory biohazard container. Remove and discard gloves.

▶ Make sure the patient is comfortable after the procedure and that he has the opportunity to thoroughly clean his hands and perianal area. Perineal care may be necessary for some patients.

Special considerations

▶ If stool must be obtained with an enema, use only tap water or normal saline solution.

▶ Never place a stool specimen in a refrigerator that contains food or medication to prevent contamination. **JC**

▶ Notify the practitioner if the stool specimen looks unusual.

References

Fischbach, F. *A Manual of Laboratory and Diagnostic Tests,* 7th ed. Philadelphia: Lippincott Williams & Wilkins, 2004.

Kyle, G. "Bowel care. Part 3—Obtaining a Stool Sample," *Nursing Times* 103(44): 24–25, October–November 2007.

Mai, V., et al. "Timing in Collection of Stool Samples," *Science* 310(5751):1118, November 2005.

Occupational Safety and Health Administration. "Bloodborne Pathogens," 1910.1030. Accessed August 2007 via the Web at *www.osha.gov/pls/oshaweb/owadisp.show_document?p_table= STANDARDS&p_id=10051*.

Stump and prosthesis care

Patient care directly after limb amputation includes wound healing, controlling pain, reducing edema, and shaping and conditioning the stump. Postoperative care of the stump will vary slightly, depending on the amputation site (arm or leg) and the type of dressing applied to the stump (elastic bandage or plaster cast).

After the stump heals, it requires only routine daily care, such as proper hygiene and continued muscle-strengthening exercises. The prosthesis—when in use—also requires daily care. Typically, a plastic prosthesis, the most common type, must be cleaned and lubricated and checked for proper fit. As the patient recovers from the physical and psychological trauma of amputation, he will need to learn correct procedures for routine daily care of the stump and the prosthesis.

Equipment

For postoperative stump care: Pressure dressing ◆ abdominal (ABD) pad ◆ suction equipment, if ordered ◆ overhead trapeze ◆ 1″ adhesive tape, bandage clips, or safety pins ◆ sandbags or trochanter roll (for a leg) ◆ elastic stump shrinker or 4″ (10 cm) elastic bandage ◆ optional: tourniquet (as a last resort to control bleeding).

For stump and prosthesis care: Mild soap or alcohol pads ◆ stump socks or athletic tube socks ◆ two washcloths ◆ two towels ◆ appropriate lubricating oil.

Implementation

▶ Confirm the patient's identity using two patient identifiers according to your facility's policy. **JC**

▶ Perform routine postoperative care. Frequently assess respiratory status and level of consciousness, monitor vital signs and I.V. infusions, check tube patency, and provide for the patient's comfort, pain management, and safety.

Monitoring stump drainage

▶ Because gravity causes fluid to accumulate at the stump, frequently check the amount of blood and drainage on the dressing. Notify the practitioner if accumulations of drainage or blood increase rapidly. If excessive bleeding occurs, notify the practitioner immediately, and apply a pressure dressing or compress the appropriate pressure points. If this doesn't control bleeding, use a tourniquet only as a last resort. Keep a tourniquet available. **ASPN**

▶ Tape the ABD pad over the moist part of the dressing, as needed. Providing a dry area helps prevent bacterial infection.

▶ Monitor the suction drainage equipment, and note the amount and type of drainage.

Positioning the extremity

▶ Evaluate the extremity for the first 24 hours to reduce swelling and promote venous return. **ASPN**

▶ To prevent contractures, position an arm with the elbow extended and the shoulder abducted.

▶ To correctly position a leg, elevate the foot of the bed slightly and place sandbags or a trochanter roll against the hip to prevent external rotation.

✦ CLINICAL ALERT

Don't place a pillow under the thigh to flex the hip because this can cause hip flexion contracture. For the same reason, tell the patient to avoid prolonged sitting.

▶ After a below-the-knee amputation, maintain knee extension to prevent hamstring muscle contractures.

▶ After any leg amputation, place the patient on a firm surface in the prone position for at least 2 hours per day, with his legs close together and without pillows under his stomach, hips, knees, or stump, unless this position is contraindicated. This position helps prevent hip flexion, contractures, and abduction; it also stretches the flexor muscles. **ASPN**

Assisting with prescribed exercises

▶ After arm amputation, encourage the patient to exercise the remaining arm to prevent muscle contractures. Help the patient perform isometric and range-of-motion (ROM) exercises for both shoulders, as prescribed by the physical therapist, because use of the prosthesis requires both shoulders.

▶ After leg amputation, stand behind the patient and, if necessary, support him with your hands at his waist during balancing exercises.

▶ Instruct the patient to exercise the affected and unaffected limbs to maintain muscle tone and increase muscle strength. A patient with a leg amputation may perform push-ups, as ordered (in the sitting position, arms at his sides), or pull-ups on the overhead trapeze to strengthen his arms, shoulders, and back in preparation for using crutches.

Wrapping and conditioning the stump

▶ If the patient doesn't have a rigid cast, apply an elastic stump shrinker to prevent edema and shape the limb in preparation for the prosthesis. Wrap the stump so that it narrows toward the distal end. This helps to ensure comfort when the patient wears the prosthesis.

▶ Instead of using an elastic stump shrinker, you can wrap the stump in a 4″ (10cm) elastic bandage. To do this, stretch the bandage to about two-thirds its maximum length as you wrap it diagonally around the stump, with the greatest pressure distally. (Depending on the size of the leg, you may need to use two 4″ bandages.) Secure the bandage with clips, safety pins, or adhesive tape. Make sure the bandage covers all portions of the stump smoothly because wrinkles or exposed areas encourage skin breakdown. (See *Wrapping a stump*.)

▶ The use of an immediate postoperative prosthesis has proved effective in decreasing the time until final prosthetic fitting.

▶ If the patient experiences throbbing after the stump is wrapped, remove the bandage immediately and reapply it less tightly. Throbbing indicates impaired circulation.

▶ Check the bandage regularly. Rewrap it when it begins to bunch up at the end (usually about every 12 hours for a moderately active patient) or as necessary.

▶ After removing the bandage to rewrap it, massage the stump gently, always pushing toward the suture line rather than away from it. This stimu-lates circulation and prevents scar tissue from adhering to the bone.

▶ When healing begins, instruct the patient to push the stump against a pillow. Then have him progress gradually to pushing against harder surfaces, such as a padded chair, then a hard chair. These conditioning exercises will help the patient adjust to experiencing pressure and sensation in the stump.

Wrapping a stump

Proper stump care helps protect the limb, reduces swelling, and prepares the limb for a prosthesis. As you perform the procedure, teach it to the patient.

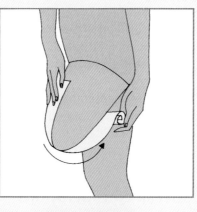

Start by obtaining two 4″ elastic bandages. Center the end of the first 4″ bandage at the top of the patient's thigh. Unroll the bandage downward over the stump and to the back of the leg.

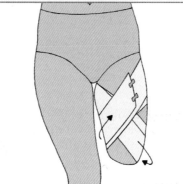

Make three figure-eight turns to adequately cover the ends of the stump. As you wrap, be sure to include the roll of flesh in the groin area. Use enough pressure to ensure that the stump narrows toward the end *so that it fits comfortably into the prosthesis.*

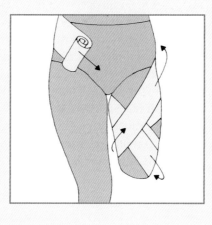

Use the second 4″ bandage to anchor the first bandage around the waist. For a below-the-knee amputation, use the knee to anchor the bandage in place. Secure the bandage with clips, safety pins, or adhesive tape. Check the stump bandage regularly, and rewrap it if it bunches at the end.

Caring for the healed stump

▶ Bathe the stump but never shave it to prevent a rash. If possible, bathe the stump at the end of the day because the warm water may cause swelling, making reapplication of the prosthesis difficult.

▶ Rub the stump with alcohol daily to toughen the skin, reducing the risk of skin breakdown. (Avoid using powders or lotions because they can soften or irritate the skin.) Because alcohol may cause severe irritation in some patients, instruct the patient to watch for and report this sign.

▶ Inspect the stump for redness, swelling, irritation, and calluses. Report any of these to the practitioner. Following the first cast change, many surgeons will have the patient begin partial weight-bearing, if the wound appears stable.

▶ Continue muscle-strengthening exercises so the patient can build the strength he'll need to control the prosthesis.

▶ Change and wash the patient's elastic bandages every day. Wash them in warm water and gentle nondetergent soap; lay them flat on a towel to dry. Machine washing or drying may shrink the elastic bandages. To shape the stump, have the patient wear an elastic bandage 24 hours per day except while bathing.

Caring for the plastic prosthesis

▶ Wipe the plastic socket of the prosthesis with a damp cloth and mild soap or alcohol to prevent bacterial accumulation.

▶ Wipe the insert (if the prosthesis has one) with a dry cloth.

▶ Dry the prosthesis thoroughly; if possible, allow it to dry overnight.

▶ Maintain and lubricate the prosthesis, as instructed by the manufacturer. **MFR**

▶ Check for malfunctions and adjust or repair the prosthesis, as necessary, to prevent further damage.

▶ Check the condition of the shoe on a foot prosthesis frequently, and change it as necessary.

Applying the prosthesis

▶ Apply a stump sock. Keep the seams away from bony prominences.

▶ If the prosthesis has an insert, remove it from the socket, place it over the stump, and insert the stump into the prosthesis.

▶ If it has no insert, merely slide the prosthesis over the stump. Secure the prosthesis onto the stump according to the manufacturer's directions.

Special considerations

▶ If a patient arrives at the hospital with a traumatic amputation, the amputated part may be saved for possible reimplantation.

▶ Teach the patient how to care for his stump and prosthesis properly. Make sure he knows signs and symptoms that indicate problems in the stump. Explain that a 10-lb (4.5-kg) change in body weight will alter his stump size and require a new prosthesis socket to ensure a correct fit.

▶ Exercise of the remaining muscles in an amputated limb must begin the day after surgery. A physical therapist will direct these exercises. For example, arm exercises progress from isometrics to assisted ROM to active ROM. Leg exercises include rising from a chair, balancing on one leg, and ROM exercises of the knees and hips.

▶ For a below-the-knee amputation, you may substitute an athletic tube sock for a stump sock by cutting off the elastic band. If the patient has a rigid plaster of Paris dressing, perform normal cast care. Check the cast frequently to make sure it doesn't slip off. If it does, apply an elastic bandage immediately and notify the practitioner because edema will develop rapidly.

▶ Complications that may develop at any time after an amputation include:
— skin breakdown or irritation from lack of ventilation
— friction from an irritant in the prosthesis
— a sebaceous cyst or boil from tight socks
— psychological problems, such as denial, depression, or withdrawal
— phantom limb pain caused by stimulation of nerves that once carried sensations from the distal part of the extremity. **ASPMN**

References

Bryant, G. "Stump Care," *AJN* 101(2):67–71, February 2001.

Goldberg, T., et al. "Postoperative Management of Lower Extremity Amputation," *Physical Medicine and Rehabilitation Clinics of North America* 11(3):559–68, August 2000.

Harker, J. "Wound Healing Complications Associated with Lower Limb Amputation." Available at: *www.worldwidewounds.com/2006/september/Harker/Wound-Healing-Complications-Limb-Amputation.html.* September 2006.

Maher, A. B., et al. *Orthopaedic Nursing,* 3rd ed. Philadelphia: W. B. Saunders Co., 2002.

Subcutaneous injection

When injected into the adipose (fatty) tissues beneath the skin, a drug moves into the bloodstream more rapidly than if given by mouth. Subcutaneous (subQ) injection allows slower, more sustained drug administration than I.M. injection; it also causes minimal tissue trauma and carries little risk of striking large blood vessels and nerves.

Absorbed mainly through the capillaries, drugs recommended for subQ injection include nonirritating aqueous solutions and suspensions contained in 0.5 to 2 ml of fluid. Heparin and insulin, for example, are usually administered subQ. (Some diabetic patients, however, may benefit from an insulin infusion pump.)

Drugs and solutions for subQ injection are injected through a relatively short needle, using meticulous sterile technique. The most common subQ injection sites are the outer aspect of the upper arm, anterior thigh, loose tissue of the lower abdomen, upper hips, buttocks, and upper back. (See *Locating subcutaneous injection sites*.) Injection is contraindicated in sites that are inflamed, edematous, scarred, or covered by a mole, birthmark, or other lesion. It may also be contraindicated in patients with impaired coagulation mechanisms.

Equipment

Prescribed medication ◆ patient's medication record and chart ◆ 25G to 27G $\frac{5}{8}''$ or $\frac{1}{2}''$ needle or insulin syringe ◆ gloves ◆ 3-ml syringe ◆ alcohol pads ◆ 2″ × 2″ gauze pad ◆ optional: antiseptic cleaning agent, filter needle.

Implementation

▶ Verify the order on the patient's medication record by checking it against the practitioner's order. Also note whether the patient has any allergies, especially before the first dose. **ISMP** **JC**

▶ Inspect the medication to make sure it isn't abnormally discolored or cloudy and doesn't contain precipitates (unless the manufacturer's instructions allow it).

▶ Wash your hands.

Locating subcutaneous injection sites

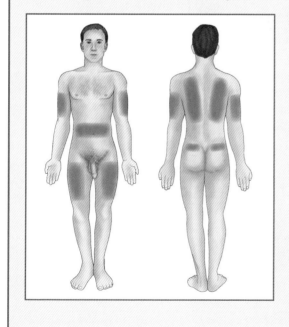

Subcutaneous (subQ) injection sites (as indicated by the colored areas in the illustration) include the fat pads on the abdomen, upper hips, upper back, and lateral upper arms and thighs. For subQ injections administered repeatedly, such as insulin, rotate sites. Choose one injection site in one area, move to a corresponding injection site in the next area, and so on.

When returning to an area, choose a new site in that area. Preferred injection sites for insulin are the arms, abdomen, thighs, and buttocks. The preferred injection site for heparin is the lower abdominal fat pad, just below the umbilicus.

▶ Check the medication label against the patient's medication record. Read the label again as you draw up the medication for injection.

▶ For a single-dose ampule, wrap an alcohol pad around the ampule's neck and snap off the top, directing the force away from your body. Attach a filter needle to the syringe and withdraw the medication, keeping the needle's bevel tip below the level of the solution. Tap the syringe to clear air from it. Cover the needle with the needle sheath. **INS**

Before discarding the ampule, check the medication label against the patient's medication record. Discard the filter needle and the ampule. Attach the appropriate needle to the syringe.

▶ For single-dose or multidose vials, reconstitute powdered drugs according to instructions. Make sure all crystals have dissolved in the solution. Warm the vial by rolling it between your palms to help the drug dissolve faster.

▶ Clean the vial's rubber stopper with an alcohol pad. Pull the syringe plunger back until the volume of air in the syringe equals the volume of drug to be withdrawn from the vial. Without inverting the vial, insert the needle into the vial. Inject the air, invert the vial, and keep the needle's bevel tip below the level of the solution as you withdraw the prescribed amount of medication. Cover the needle with the needle sheath. Tap the syringe to clear any air from it.

▶ Check the medication label against the patient's medication record before discarding the single-dose vial or returning the multidose vial to the shelf. **ISMP**

▶ Confirm the patient's identity using two patient identifiers according to your facility's policy. **JC**

▶ If your facility uses a bar code scanning system, be sure to scan your ID badge, the patient's ID bracelet, and the medication's bar code. **ISMP** **JC**

▶ Explain the procedure to the patient, and provide privacy.

▶ Select an appropriate injection site. Rotate sites according to a schedule for repeated injections, using different areas of the body unless contraindicated.

▶ Put on gloves. **CDC**

▶ Position and drape the patient if necessary.

▶ Clean the injection site with an alcohol pad, beginning at the center of the site and moving outward in a circular motion. Allow the skin to dry before injecting the drug to avoid a stinging sensation from introducing alcohol into subcutaneous tissues.

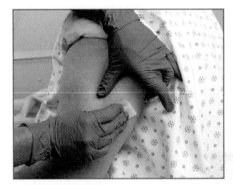

▶ Loosen the protective needle sheath.

▶ With your nondominant hand, grasp the skin around the injection site firmly to elevate the subcutaneous tissue, forming a 1″ (2.5 cm) fat fold. **CS**

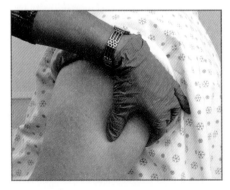

▶ Holding the syringe in your dominant hand, insert the loosened needle sheath between the fourth and fifth fingers of your other hand while still pinching the skin around the injection site. Pull back the syringe with your dominant hand to uncover the needle by grasping the syringe like a pencil. Don't touch the needle.

▶ Position the needle with its bevel up.

▶ Tell the patient he'll feel a needle prick.

▶ Insert the needle quickly in one motion at a 45- or 90-degree angle. (See *Technique for subcutaneous injection*.) Release the patient's skin to avoid injecting the drug into compressed tissue and irritating nerve fibers.

▶ Pull back the plunger slightly to check for blood return. If none appears, begin injecting the drug slowly. If blood appears on aspiration, withdraw the needle, prepare another syringe, and repeat the procedure.

▶ Don't aspirate for blood return when giving insulin or heparin. It isn't necessary with insulin and may cause a hematoma with heparin. **ADA** **CS**

▶ After injection, remove the needle gently but quickly at the same angle used for insertion.

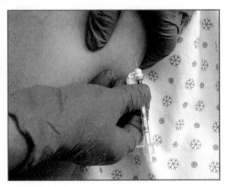

Technique for subcutaneous injection

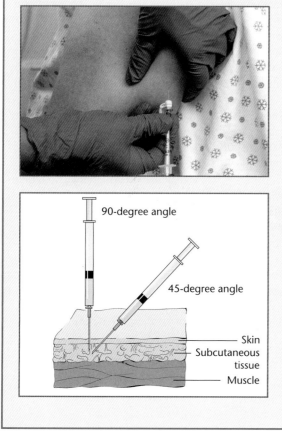

Before giving the injection, elevate the subcutaneous tissue at the site by grasping it firmly.

Insert the needle at a 45- or 90-degree angle to the skin surface, depending on needle-length and the amount of subcutaneous tissue at the site. Some medications, such as heparin, should always be injected at a 90-degree angle.

90-degree angle

45-degree angle

Skin
Subcutaneous
tissue
Muscle

▶ Cover the site with an alcohol pad or a 2″ × 2″ gauze pad and massage the site gently (unless contraindicated, as with heparin and insulin) to distribute the drug and facilitate absorption.

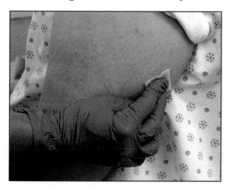

▶ Remove the alcohol pad, and check the injection site for bleeding and bruising.

▶ Dispose of injection equipment according to your facility's policy.

Special considerations

▶ When using prefilled syringes, adjust the angle and depth of insertion according to needle length.

For insulin injections

▶ To establish more consistent blood insulin levels, rotate insulin injection sites within anatomic regions. Preferred insulin injection sites are the arms, abdomen, thighs, and buttocks. **ADA**
▶ Make sure the type of insulin, unit dosage, and syringe are correct.
▶ When combining insulins in a syringe, make sure they're compatible.

Regular insulin can be mixed with all other types. Prompt insulin zinc suspension (Semilente insulin) can't be mixed with NPH insulin. Follow your facility's policy regarding which insulin to draw up first.

For heparin injections

▶ The preferred site for a heparin injection is the lower abdominal fat pad, 2″ (5 cm) beneath the umbilicus, between the right and left iliac crests. Injecting heparin into this area, which isn't involved in muscle activity, reduces the risk of local capillary bleeding. Always rotate the sites from one side to the other.
▶ Inject the drug slowly into the fat pad. Leave the needle in place for

10 seconds after injection; then with-draw it.

▶ Don't administer an injection within 2″ of a scar, a bruise, or the umbilicus.

▶ Don't aspirate to check for blood return because this can cause bleeding into the tissues at the site.

▶ Don't rub or massage the site after the injection. Rubbing can cause local-ized minute hemorrhages or bruises.

References

Annersten, M., and Willman, A. "Perform-ing Subcutaneous Injections: A Literature Review," *Worldviews on Evidence-Based Nursing* 2(3):122–30, 2005.

The Joint Commission. *Comprehensive Accreditation Manual for Hospitals: The Official Handbook.* Standard MM.1.10. Oakbrook Terrace, Ill.: The Joint Com-mission, 2007.

The Joint Commission. *Comprehensive Accreditation Manual for Hospitals: The Official Handbook.* Standard MM.3.10. Oakbrook Terrace, Ill.: The Joint Com-mission, 2007.

The Joint Commission. *Comprehensive Accreditation Manual for Hospitals: The Official Handbook.* Standard MM.4.10. Oakbrook Terrace, Ill.: The Joint Com-mission, 2007.

The Joint Commission. *Comprehensive Accreditation Manual for Hospitals: The Official Handbook.* Standard MM.4.20. Oakbrook Terrace, Ill.: The Joint Com-mission, 2007.

The Joint Commission. *Comprehensive Accreditation Manual for Hospitals: The Official Handbook.* Standard MM.4.30. Oakbrook Terrace, Ill.: The Joint Com-mission, 2007.

The Joint Commission. *Comprehensive Accreditation Manual for Hospitals: The Official Handbook.* Standard MM.5.10. Oakbrook Terrace, Ill.: The Joint Com-mission, 2007.

The Joint Commission. *Comprehensive Accreditation Manual for Hospitals: The Official Handbook.* Standard MM.6.10. Oakbrook Terrace, Ill.: The Joint Com-mission, 2007.

The Joint Commission. *Comprehensive Accreditation Manual for Hospitals: The Official Handbook.* Standard MM.6.20. Oakbrook Terrace, Ill: The Joint Com-mission,. 2007.

The Joint Commission. *Comprehensive Accreditation Manual for Hospitals: The Official Handbook.* Standard MM.7.10. Oakbrook Terrace, Ill.: The Joint Com-mission, 2007.

Rushing, J. "How to Administer a Subcu-taneous Injection," *Nursing* 34(6):32, June 2004.

Peragallo-Dittko, V. "Aspiration of the Subcutaneous Insulin Injection: Clini-cal Evaluation of Needle Size and Amount of Subcutaneous Fat," The *Diabetes Educator* 21(4):291–6, July–August 1995. **CS**

Taylor, C., et al. *Fundamentals of Nursing: The Art and Science of Nursing Care,* 6th ed. Philadelphia: Lippincott Williams & Wilkins, 2008.

Surgical attire

Surgical attire is worn in the semirestricted and restricted areas of the surgical environment to reduce microbial contamination by surgical staff. The appropriate attire varies by restriction level. The unrestricted area is a central control point where the entrance of patients, personnel, and materials can be monitored. Street clothes are permitted in this area. The semirestricted area includes the peripheral support areas of the operating room, such as the corridors leading to the restricted areas of the operating room, scrub sink areas, clean and sterile supply storage rooms, and work areas for instrument processing. Surgical scrub attire is required and all head and facial hair must be covered in this area. The restricted area includes the operating room suite, procedure rooms, and clean core. Surgical attire and hair coverings are required. Masks are required in the presence of open sterile items or scrubbed personnel.

Equipment

Two-piece scrub suit (pants and top) ◆ head covering or hood ◆ surgical mask ◆ surgical gown ◆ optional: cover gown or laboratory coat, protective eyewear or face shield, shoe covers.

Implementation

▶ Put on a surgical head cover or hood and ensure that all hair and facial hair, including sideburns, are covered to prevent hair, dandruff, and microorganisms from falling onto the sterile field. Placing the head cover first reduces the risk of contaminants falling onto the scrub clothing. **AORN** **CS1**

▶ Put on scrub pants and top that are approved and laundered by the facility before entering semirestricted and restricted areas. **AORN**

▶ Place shoe covers over foot wear if splashing or spilling of body fluid is anticipated. However, studies suggest that shoe covers don't decrease the incidence of surgical wound infections. If worn, shoe covers should be removed when leaving the semirestricted area and new ones placed upon return.

▶ Put on a surgical mask to reduce the dispersion of microbial droplets from the mouth and nasopharynx. Select a mask with microbial filtration of 95% or above to protect yourself from aerosolized particles such as laser or electrosurgical plume. **AORN**

▶ Ensure the mask covers the mouth and nose completely. Mold the malleable metal strip on the top of the mask to the nose.

▶ Remove or confine all jewelry within scrub attire to reduce the risk of transmission of microorganisms that may be on the jewelry as well as reduce the risk of jewelry falling onto the sterile field or into the wound. Wearing rings interferes with proper hand antisepsis. **AORN** **CS2**

▶ Put on protective eyewear if splashing or splattering of body fluids is likely to occur. **CDC**

Putting on a sterile gown

▶ Open the sterile gown and gloves on a flat surface away from the sterile back table.

▶ Grasp the sterile gown at the neckline, and lift up and away from the field. The exposed side of the folded gown is the inside of the gown.

▶ Step back into an area where the gown can be unfolded without the risk of contamination.

▶ Hold the gown with both hands on each side of the neckline, and allow the gown to unfold fully with the inside toward the wearer. Don't shake the gown open as this causes air currents, which could lead to contamination.

▶ Keep your arms at shoulder level and away from the body as you slide both arms into the sleeves, stopping when the hands reach the proximal edge of the cuff. Don't push the hands past the cuff, or you won't be able to perform the closed gloving technique.

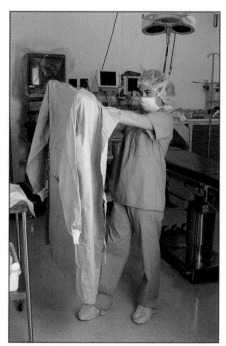

▶ Have the circulating (unsterile) nurse touch the inside of the gown shoulders and sides to bring it over the scrub person's shoulders. The scrub nurse secures the neckline of the gown and the inner gown tie at the waist. This should be done before the scrub person puts on gloves to keep the gown from flapping and becoming contaminated against a nonsterile surface.

▶ The scrub person returns to the sterile field created by the gown wrapper to put on sterile gloves.

Performing closed gloving technique

▶ Keeping hands inside the gown sleeves, open the glove wrapper. Avoid getting too close to the sterile field because the 1″ (2.5 cm) margin of the gown wrapper is considered unsterile.

▶ Pick up the glove for the dominant hand with the nondominant hand still inside the gown sleeve. Extend the forearm of your dominant hand palm side up.

▶ Place the glove for the dominant hand palm side down with the fingers facing toward the elbow. Grasp the glove cuff through the sleeve.

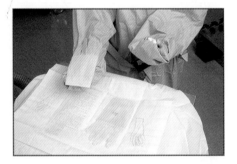

▶ Use the nondominant hand to grasp the top side of the glove cuff and stretch it over the hand, covering the wrist entirely.

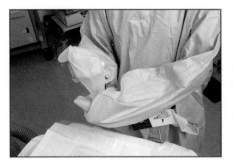

▶ Advance the gown cuff down toward the wrist, direct fingers into the glove, and adjust glove on hand.

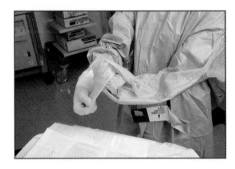

▶ Repeat the procedure for the other hand.

▶ Fold hands together and interlace fingers to help the fingers fully extend into the gloves.

▶ Hold the short tie, attached to the card in front of the gown, in your left hand. Use your right hand to release the card from the front of the gown.

▶ Hand the end of the card without the tie to another person. The person can be sterile or unsterile because the person will keep the card but never touch the tie itself.

▶ Turn to the left to wrap the gown around your back.

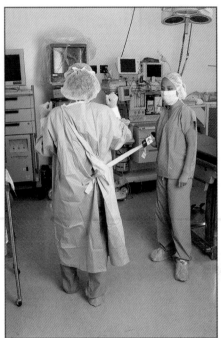

▶ While the other person holds the card securely, pull the tie out of the card without touching the card. Tie the gown in front of you.

Special considerations

▶ Sterile gowns are only sterile in front from the shoulders to the level of the sterile field. Sleeves are sterile from 2″ (5 cm) above the elbow to the cuff. The cuff itself collects moisture and is not an effective bacterial barrier and must be kept covered by sterile gloves. The neckline, shoulders, underarms, and back aren't considered sterile due to the surfaces rubbing together during head and neck movements, perspiration, and the inability to directly observe and protect these areas from contamination. Hands must be kept in front of the body at or above the waist to be considered sterile. **AORN**

▶ Choose a gown that's large enough to fully close in the back and whose cuffs don't extend beyond the glove. The cuffs of the gown are regarded as nonsterile after the hands pass through them.

▶ Surgical attire should only be worn once and then placed in the appropriate receptacle for laundering. They shouldn't be hung in a locker or worn again. Surgical attire shouldn't be laundered at home.

▶ Surgical attire that's clearly soiled or wet should be taken off and new attire put on to reduce the risk of transmission of microorganisms. **AORN**

▶ Follow your facility's policy for the use of cover gowns or laboratory coats when leaving semirestricted or restricted areas. These coverings should be removed before reentering semirestricted or restricted areas.

▶ Staff who aren't scrubbed should wear long-sleeved jackets. These jackets should be buttoned or snapped shut to reduce the risk of loose material contaminating sterile areas. Arms should be covered to decrease bacterial shedding from bare arms.

▶ Avoid hanging a face mask around the neck after use. Bacteria trapped in the mask can become dry and airborne.

▶ Keep nails in good condition, and change nail polish every 4 days because studies suggest that polish worn for longer time periods may support more bacteria. Artificial nails shouldn't be worn because they may harbor microorganisms and prevent effective hand antisepsis. **AORN** **CDC**

References

AORN Recommended Practices Committee. "Recommended Practices for Surgical Attire," *AORN Journal* 81(2): 413–20, February 2005.

Association of Perioperative Registered Nurses. *Standards, Recommended Practices, and Guidelines.* Denver: AORN, Inc., 2007.

Friberg, B., et al. "Surgical Area Contamination—Comparable Bacterial Counts Using Disposable Head and Mask and Helmet Aspirator System, but Dramatic Increase upon Omission of Head-Gear: An Experimental Study in Horizontal Laminar Air-Flow," *Journal of Hospital Infection* 47(2):110–5, February 2001. **CS1**

Trick, W. E., et al. "Impact of Ring Wearing on Hand Contamination and Comparison of Hand Hygiene Agents in a Hospital," *Clinical Infectious Disease* 36(11):1383–90, June 2003. **CS2**

Surgical site verification

Wrong-site surgery is a general term referring to a surgical procedure performed on the wrong body part or side of the body, or even the wrong patient. This error may occur in the operating room or in other settings, such as ambulatory care or interventional radiology.

Several factors may contribute to an increased risk of wrong-site surgery, including inadequate patient assessment, inadequate medical record review, inaccurate communication among health team members, multiple surgeons involved in the procedure, failure to include the patient in the site-identification process, and relying solely on the physician for site identification.

Because serious consequences may result from wrong-site surgery, the nurse must confirm that the correct site has been identified before surgery begins.

Equipment

Surgical consent ◆ medical record ◆ procedure schedule ◆ hypoallergenic, nonlatex permanent marker.

Implementation

▶ Confirm the patient's identity using two patient identifiers according to your facility's policy. **JC**
▶ Before the procedure, check the patient's chart for documentation, and compare the information using the history and physical examination form, nursing assessment, pre-procedure checklist, signed informed consent with the exact procedure site identified, procedure schedule, and the patient's verbal confirmation of the correct site.
▶ After verbally confirming the site with the patient, the person performing the procedure or another member of the surgical team who's fully informed about the patient and the intended procedure marks the site. The mark needs to be placed so that it's visible after the patient has been prepped and draped. **JC** (See *Marking the surgical site*)
▶ Make sure that the surgical team (surgeon, operating room or procedure staff, and anesthesia personnel) identifies the patient and verifies the correct procedure and correct site before beginning the surgery. **JC**

Special considerations

If the patient's condition prevents him from verifying the correct site, the surgeon will identify and mark the site

Marking the surgical site

Marking the surgical site ensures that the procedure is being carried out on the correct anatomic site. The Joint Commission requires each facility to implement a protocol for marking the exact site of any operative or invasive procedure involving:
▶ right or left distinction
▶ multiple structures, such as fingers and toes
▶ multiple levels, such as procedures involving the spine.

The site should be marked before the patient is taken to the area where the procedure will be performed. It should be marked with a marker that doesn't wash off when the site is prepared.

The Joint Commission recommends that the person who performs the procedure mark the site. The patient or whoever has authority to provide informed consent should be involved in the marking process.

The marking must be visible after the patient has been prepared and draped for the procedure.

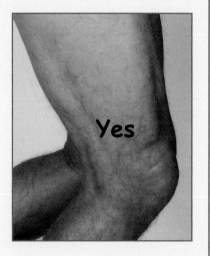

using the history and physical examination forms, signed informed consent, preprocedure verification checklist, procedure schedule, X-rays, and other imaging studies. **JC**

References

AORN. "Position Statement on Correct Site Surgery," February 2003.

The Joint Commission. "2008 Ambulatory Care and Office-Based National Patient Safety Goals," 2008.

The Joint Commission. "National Patient Safety Goals, Critical Access Hospital," 2008.

The Joint Commission. "Universal Protocol for Preventing Wrong Site, Wrong Procedure, Wrong Person Surgery," 2003.

Kwan, M. R., et al. "Incidence, Patterns, and Prevention of Wrong Site Surgery," *Archives of Surgery* 141(4):353–57, April 2006.

Surgical wound management

When caring for a surgical wound, you carry out procedures that help prevent infection by stopping pathogens from entering the wound. Besides promoting patient comfort, such procedures protect the skin surface from maceration and excoriation caused by contact with irritating drainage. They also allow you to measure wound drainage to monitor fluid and electrolyte balance.

The two primary methods used to manage a draining surgical wound are dressing and pouching. Dressing is preferred unless caustic or excessive drainage is compromising your patient's skin integrity. Usually, lightly seeping wounds with drains and wounds with minimal purulent drainage can be managed with packing and gauze dressings. Some wounds, such as those that become chronic, may require an occlusive dressing.

A wound with copious, excoriating drainage calls for pouching to protect the surrounding skin. If your patient has a surgical wound, you must monitor him and choose the appropriate dressing.

Dressing a wound calls for sterile technique and sterile supplies to prevent contamination. Be sure to change the dressing often enough to keep the skin dry.

Equipment

Waterproof trash bag ◆ clean gloves ◆ sterile gloves ◆ gown and face shield or goggles, if indicated ◆ sterile 4″ × 4″ gauze pads ◆ large absorbent dressings, if indicated ◆ sterile cotton-tipped applicators ◆ sterile dressing set ◆ antiseptic solution ◆ topical medication, if ordered ◆ adhesive or other tape ◆ soap and water ◆ optional: forceps; skin protectant; nonadherent pads; acetone-free adhesive remover; sterile normal saline solution; graduated container; and Montgomery straps, a fishnet tube elasticized dressing support, or a T-binder.

For a wound with a drain: Sterile scissors ◆ sterile 4″ × 4″ gauze pads without cotton lining ◆ sump drain ◆ ostomy pouch or another collection bag ◆ sterile precut tracheostomy pads or drain dressings ◆ adhesive tape (paper or silk tape if the patient is hypersensitive) ◆ surgical mask.

For pouching a wound: Collection pouch with drainage port ◆ sterile gloves ◆ skin protectant ◆ sterile gauze pads.

Implementation

▶ Check the practitioner's order for specific wound care and medication instructions. Note the location of surgical drains to avoid dislodging them during the procedure.

▶ Confirm the patient's identity using two patient identifiers according to your facility's policy. **JC**

▶ Assemble all equipment in the patient's room. Check the expiration date on each sterile package, and inspect for tears.

▶ Open the waterproof trash bag, and place it near the patient's bed. Position the bag to avoid reaching across the sterile field or the wound when disposing of soiled articles. Form a cuff by turning down the top of the trash bag to provide a wide opening and to prevent contamination of instruments or gloves by touching the bag's edge.

▶ Explain the procedure to the patient to allay his fears and ensure his cooperation.

Removing the old dressing

▶ Assess the patient's condition.

▶ Identify the patient's allergies, especially to adhesive tape, povidone-iodine or other topical solutions, or medications.

▶ Provide privacy, and position the patient as necessary. To avoid chilling him, expose only the wound site.

▶ Wash your hands thoroughly. Put on a gown and a face shield, if necessary. Then put on clean gloves. **CDC**

▶ Loosen the soiled dressing by holding the patient's skin and pulling the tape or dressing toward the wound. This protects the newly formed tissue and prevents stress on the incision. Moisten the tape with acetone-free adhesive remover, if necessary, to make the tape removal less painful (particularly if the skin is hairy). Don't apply solvents to the incision because they could contaminate the wound.

▶ Slowly remove the soiled dressing. If the gauze adheres to the wound, loosen the gauze by moistening it with sterile normal saline solution.

▶ Observe the dressing for the amount, type, color, and odor of drainage.

▶ Discard the dressing and gloves in the waterproof trash bag.

Caring for the wound

▶ Wash your hands. Establish a sterile field with all the equipment and supplies you'll need for suture-line care and the dressing change, including a sterile dressing set and antiseptic swabs. If the practitioner has ordered ointment, squeeze the needed amount onto the sterile field. If you're using an antiseptic cleaning agent from an un-sterile bottle, pour the antiseptic into a sterile container so you won't contaminate your gloves. Then put on sterile gloves.

▶ Saturate the sterile gauze pads with the prescribed cleaning agent. Avoid using cotton balls because they may shed fibers in the wound, causing irritation, infection, or adhesion.

▶ If ordered, obtain a wound culture; then proceed to clean the wound.

▶ Irrigate the wound, if ordered, using the specified solution.

▶ Pick up the moistened gauze pad or swab, and squeeze out the excess solution.

▶ For an open wound, clean the wound in a full or half circle, beginning in the center and working outward (as shown below). Use a new swab or pad for each circle. Clean to at least 1″ (2.5 cm) beyond the end of the new dressing or 2″ (5 cm) beyond the wound margins if you aren't applying a new dressing.

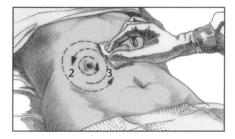

▶ For a linear incision, work from the top of the incision, wipe once to the bottom, and then discard the gauze pad. With a second moistened pad, wipe from top to bottom in a vertical path next to the incision (as shown below).

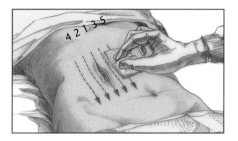

▶ Continue to work outward from the incision in lines running parallel to it. Always wipe from the clean area toward the less clean area (usually from top to bottom). Use each gauze pad or swab for only one stroke to avoid tracking wound exudate and normal body flora from surrounding skin to the clean areas.

▶ Use sterile, cotton-tipped applicators for efficient cleaning of tight-fitting wire sutures, deep and narrow wounds, and wounds with pockets.

▶ If the patient has a surgical drain, clean the drain's surface last. Because moist drainage promotes bacterial growth, the drain is considered the most contaminated area. Clean the skin around the drain by wiping in half or full circles from the drain site outward.

▶ Clean all areas of the wound to wash away debris, pus, blood, and necrotic material. Try not to disturb sutures or irritate the incision. Clean to at least 1″ beyond the end of the new dressing. If you aren't applying a new dressing, clean to at least 2″ beyond the incision.

▶ Check to make sure the edges of the incision are lined up properly, and check for signs of infection (heat, redness, swelling, induration, and odor),

dehiscence, and evisceration. If you observe such signs or if the patient reports pain at the wound site, notify the practitioner.

▶ Wash skin surrounding the wound with soap and water, and pat dry using a sterile 4″ × 4″ gauze pad. Avoid oil-based soap because it may interfere with pouch adherence. Apply any prescribed topical medication.

▶ Apply a skin protectant, if needed.

▶ If ordered, pack the wound with gauze pads or strips folded to fit, using a sterile forceps. Pack the wound, using the wet-to-damp method. Soaking the packing material in solution and wringing it out so that it's slightly moist provides a moist wound environment that absorbs debris and drainage. However, removing the packing won't disrupt new tissue. Don't pack the wound tightly; doing so will exert pressure and may damage the wound.

Applying a fresh gauze dressing

▶ Gently place sterile 4″ × 4″ gauze pads at the center of the wound, and move progressively outward to the edges of the wound site. Extend the gauze at least 1″ (2.5 cm) beyond the incision in each direction, and cover the wound evenly with enough sterile dressings (usually two or three layers) to absorb all drainage until the next dressing change. Use large absorbent dressings to form outer layers, if needed, to provide greater absorbency.

▶ Secure the dressing's edges to the patient's skin with strips of tape to

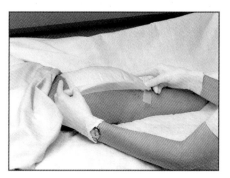

maintain the sterility of the wound site. Or, secure the dressing with a T-binder or Montgomery straps to prevent skin excoriation, which may occur with repeated tape removal necessitated by frequent dressing changes. (See *How to make Montgomery straps.*)
▶ Make sure the patient is comfortable.
▶ Properly dispose of the solutions and trash bag, and clean or discard soiled equipment and supplies according to your facility's policy.

Dressing a wound with a drain

▶ Use commercially precut gauze drain dressings or prepare a drain dressing by using sterile scissors to cut a slit in a sterile 4″ × 4″ gauze pad. Fold the pad in half; then cut inward from the center of the folded edge. Don't use a cotton-lined gauze pad because

cutting the gauze opens the lining and releases cotton fibers into the wound. Prepare a second pad the same way.
▶ Gently press one drain dressing close to the skin around the drain so that the tubing fits into the slit. Press the second drain dressing around the drain from the opposite direction so that the two dressings encircle the tubing.
▶ Layer as many uncut sterile 4″ × 4″ gauze pads or large absorbent dressings around the tubing, as needed, to absorb expected drainage. Tape the dressing in place, or use a T-binder or Montgomery straps.

Pouching a wound

▶ If your patient's wound is draining heavily or if drainage may damage surrounding skin, you'll need to apply a pouch.

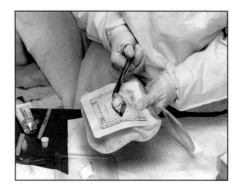

▶ Measure the wound. Cut an opening ¼″ (0.6 cm) larger than the wound in the facing of the collection pouch.
▶ Apply a skin protectant as needed. (Some protectants are incorporated within the collection pouch and also provide adhesion.)
▶ Make sure the drainage port at the bottom of the pouch is closed firmly to prevent leaks. Then gently press the contoured pouch opening around the wound, starting at its lower edge.

How to make Montgomery straps

An abdominal dressing requiring frequent changes can be secured with Montgomery straps *to promote the patient's comfort.* If ready-made straps aren't available, follow these steps to make your own:
▶ Cut four to six strips of 2″ to 3″ (5 to 7.5 cm) wide hypoallergenic tape of sufficient length to allow the tape to extend about 6″ (15 cm) beyond the wound on each side. (The length of the tape will vary according to the patient's size and the type and amount of dressing.)
▶ Fold one of each strip 2″ to 3″ back on itself (sticky sides together) to form a nonadhesive tab. Then cut a small hole in the folded tab's center, close to its top edge. Make as many pairs of straps as you'll need to snugly secure the dressing.
▶ Clean the patient's skin *to prevent irritation.* After his skin dries, apply a skin protectant. Then apply the sticky side of each tape to a skin barrier sheet composed of opaque hydrocolloidal or nonhydrocolloidal materials, and apply the sheet directly to the skin near the dressing. Next, thread a separate piece of gauze tie, umbilical tape, or twill tape (about 12″ [30.5 cm]) through each pair of holes in the

straps, and fasten each tie as you would a shoelace. Don't stress the surrounding skin by securing the ties too tightly.
▶ Repeat this procedure according to the number of Montgomery straps needed.
▶ Replace Montgomery straps every 2 or 3 days or whenever they become soiled. If skin maceration occurs, place new tapes about 1″ (2.5 cm) away from any irritation.

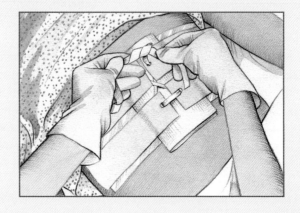

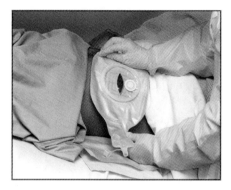

▶ To empty the pouch, put on gloves and a face shield or mask and goggles to avoid any splashing. Then insert the pouch's bottom half into a graduated biohazard container, and open the drainage port. Note the color, consistency, odor, and amount of fluid. If ordered, obtain a culture specimen, and send it to the laboratory immediately.

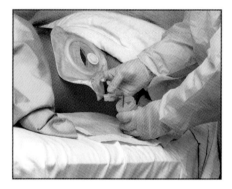

▶ Wipe the bottom of the pouch and the drainage port with a gauze pad to remove any drainage that could irritate the patient's skin or cause an odor. Then reseal the port. Change the pouch only if it leaks or fails to adhere. More frequent changes are unnecessary and only irritate the patient's skin.

Special considerations

▶ If the patient has two wounds in the same area, cover each wound separately with layers of sterile 4″ × 4″ gauze pads. Then cover each site with a large absorbent dressing secured to the patient's skin with tape. Don't use a single large absorbent dressing to cover both sites because drainage quickly saturates a pad, promoting cross-contamination.

▶ When packing a wound, don't pack it too tightly because this compresses adjacent capillaries and may prevent the wound edges from contracting. Avoid overlapping damp packing onto surrounding skin because it macerates the intact tissue.

▶ To save time when dressing a wound with a drain, use precut tracheostomy pads or drain dressings instead of custom-cutting gauze pads to fit around the drain. If your patient is sensitive to adhesive tape, use paper or silk tape because it's less likely to cause a skin reaction and peels off more easily than adhesive tape. Use a surgical mask to cradle a chin or jawline dressing; this provides a secure dressing and avoids the need to clip the patient's hair.

▶ If ordered, use a collodion spray or similar topical protectant instead of a gauze dressing. Moisture- and contaminant-proof, this covering dries in a clear, impermeable film that leaves the wound visible for observation and avoids the friction caused by a dressing.

▶ Because many practitioners prefer to change the first postoperative dressing themselves to check the incision, don't change the first dressing unless you have specific instructions to do so. If you have no such order and drainage comes through the dressings, reinforce the dressing with fresh sterile gauze. Request an order to change the dressing, or ask the practitioner to change it as soon as possible. A reinforced dressing shouldn't remain in place longer than 24 hours because it's an excellent medium for bacterial growth.

▶ For the recent postoperative patient or a patient with complications, check the dressing every 15 to 30 minutes or as ordered. For the patient with a properly healing wound, check the dressing at least once every 8 hours.

▶ If the dressing becomes wet from the outside (for example, from spilled drinking water), replace it as soon as possible to prevent wound contamination. **WOCN**

▶ If your patient will need wound care after discharge, provide appropriate teaching. If he'll be caring for the wound himself, stress the importance of using aseptic technique, and teach him how to examine the wound for signs of infection and other complications. Also show him how to change dressings, and give him written instructions for all procedures to be performed at home.

References

Baranoski, S., and Ayello, E. *Wound Care Essentials: Practice Principles,* 2nd ed. Philadelphia: Lippincott Williams & Wilkins, 2008.

Barie, P., and Eachempati, S. "Surgical Site Infections," *The Surgical Clinics of North America* 85(6):1115–35, December 2005.

Hess, C. *Clinical Guide: Skin & Wound Care,* 6th ed. Philadelphia: Lippincott Williams & Wilkins, 2008.

Schweon, S. "Stamping Out Surgical Site Infections," *RN* 69(10):12, October 2006.

Vuolo, J. "Assessment and Management of Surgical Wounds in Clinical Practice," *Nursing Standard* 20(52):46–56, September 2006.

Suture removal

The goal of this procedure is to remove skin sutures from a healed wound without damaging newly formed tissue. The timing of suture removal depends on the shape, size, and location of the sutured incision; the absence of inflammation, drainage, and infection; and the patient's general condition. Usually, for a sufficiently healed wound, sutures are removed 7 to 10 days after insertion. Techniques for removal depend on the method of suturing, but all require sterile technique to prevent contamination. Although sutures usually are removed by a physician, in many facilities, a nurse may remove them on the physician's order.

Equipment

Waterproof trash bag ♦ adjustable light ♦ clean gloves, if the wound is dressed ♦ sterile gloves ♦ sterile forceps or sterile hemostat ♦ normal saline solution ♦ sterile gauze pads ♦ antiseptic cleaning agent ♦ sterile curve-tipped suture scissors ♦ povidone-iodine pads ♦ optional: adhesive butterfly strips or Steri-Strips and compound benzoin tincture or other skin protectant.

Implementation

▶ Confirm the patient's identity using two patient identifiers according to your facility's policy. **JC**
▶ Open the waterproof trash bag, and place it near the patient's bed. Position the bag properly to avoid reaching across the sterile field or the suture line when disposing of soiled articles. Form a cuff by turning down the top of the trash bag to provide a wide opening and prevent contamination of instruments or gloves by touching the bag's edge.
▶ If your facility allows you to remove sutures, check the practitioner's order to confirm the details for this procedure.
▶ Check for patient allergies, especially to adhesive tape and povidone-iodine or other topical solutions or medications.

▶ Tell the patient that you're going to remove the stitches from his wound. Assure him that this procedure typically is painless, but that he may feel a tickling sensation as the stitches come out. Reassure him that because his wound is healing properly, removing the stitches won't weaken the incision.
▶ Provide privacy, and position the patient so he's comfortable without placing undue tension on the suture line. Because some patients experience nausea or dizziness during the procedure, have the patient recline if possible. Adjust the light to have it shine directly on the suture line.
▶ Wash your hands thoroughly. If the patient's wound has a dressing, put on clean gloves and carefully remove the dressing. Discard the dressing and the gloves in the waterproof trash bag.
▶ Observe the patient's wound for possible gaping, drainage, inflammation, signs of infection, and embedded sutures. Notify the practitioner if the wound has failed to heal properly. The absence of a healing ridge under the suture line 5 to 7 days after insertion indicates that the line needs continued support and protection during the healing process.
▶ Establish a sterile work area with all the equipment and supplies you'll need for suture removal and wound care. Open the sterile suture-removal tray,

maintaining sterility of the contents, and put on sterile gloves.
▶ Using sterile technique, clean the suture line to decrease the number of microorganisms present and reduce the risk of infection. The cleaning process should also moisten the sutures sufficiently to ease removal. Soften them further, if needed, with normal saline solution.
▶ Proceed according to the type of suture you're removing. (See *Methods for removing sutures*.) Because the visible part of a suture is exposed to skin bacteria and considered contaminated, be sure to cut sutures at the skin surface on one side of the visible part of the suture. Remove the suture by lifting and pulling the visible end off the skin to avoid drawing this contaminated portion back through subcutaneous tissue.
▶ If ordered, remove every other suture to maintain some support for the incision. Then go back and remove the remaining sutures.
▶ After removing sutures, wipe the incision gently with gauze pads soaked in an antiseptic cleaning agent or with a povidone-iodine pad. Apply a light sterile gauze dressing, if needed, to prevent infection and irritation from clothing. Then discard your gloves.
▶ Make sure the patient is comfortable. According to the practitioner's

Methods for removing sutures

Removal techniques depend on the type of sutures to be removed. The illustrations below show removal steps for four common suture types. Keep in mind that for all suture types, it's important to grasp and cut sutures in the correct place to avoid pulling the exposed (thus contaminated) suture material through subcutaneous tissue.

Plain interrupted sutures

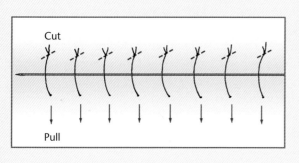

Using sterile forceps, grasp the knot of the first suture and raise it off the skin. This will expose a small portion of the suture that was below skin level. Place the rounded tip of sterile curved-tip suture scissors against the skin, and cut through the exposed portion of the suture. Then, still holding the knot with the forceps, pull the cut suture up and out of the skin in a smooth continuous motion to avoid causing the patient pain. Discard the suture. Repeat the process for every other suture, initially; if the wound doesn't gape, you can then remove the remaining sutures as ordered.

Plain continuous sutures

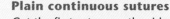

Cut the first suture on the side opposite the knot. Next, cut the same side of the next suture in line. Then lift the first suture out in the direction of the knot. Proceed along the suture line, grasping each suture where you grasped the knot on the first one.

Mattress interrupted sutures

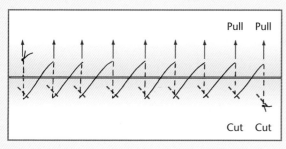

If possible, remove the small, visible portion of the suture opposite the knot by cutting it at each visible end and lifting the small piece away from the skin to prevent pulling it through and contaminating subcutaneous tissue. Then remove the rest of the suture by pulling it out in the direction of the knot. If the visible portion is too small to cut twice, cut it once, and pull the entire suture out in the opposite direction. Repeat these steps for the remaining sutures, and monitor the incision carefully for infection.

Mattress continuous sutures

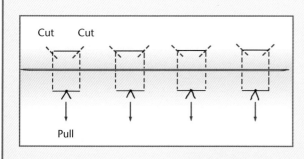

Follow the procedure for removing mattress interrupted sutures, first removing the small visible portion of the suture, if possible, to prevent pulling it through and contaminating subcutaneous tissue. Then extract the rest of the suture in the direction of the knot.

preference, inform the patient that he may shower in 1 or 2 days if the incision is dry and heals well.

▶ Properly dispose of the solutions and trash bag, and clean or dispose of soiled equipment and supplies according to your facility's policy.

Special considerations

▶ Be sure to check the practitioner's order for the time of suture removal. Usually, you'll remove sutures on the head and neck 3 to 5 days after insertion; on the chest and abdomen, 5 to 7 days after insertion; and on the lower extremities, 7 to 10 days after insertion.

▶ If the patient has interrupted sutures or an incompletely healed suture line, remove only those sutures specified by the practitioner. He may want to leave some sutures in place for an additional day or two to support the suture line.

▶ If the patient has both retention and regular sutures in place, check the practitioner's order for the sequence in which they are to be removed. Because retention sutures link underlying fat and muscle tissue and give added support to the obese or slow-healing patient, they usually remain in place for 14 to 21 days.

▶ Be particularly careful to clean the suture line before attempting to remove mattress sutures. This decreases the risk of infection when the visible, contaminated part of the stitch is too small to cut twice for sterile removal and must be pulled through tissue. After you have removed mattress sutures this way, monitor the suture line carefully for subsequent infection.

▶ If the wound dehisces during suture removal, apply butterfly adhesive strips or surgical strips to support and approximate the edges, and call the practitioner immediately to repair the wound.

▶ Apply butterfly adhesive strips or surgical strips after any suture removal, if desired, to give added support to the incision line and prevent lateral tension on the wound from forming a wide scar. Use a small amount of compound benzoin tincture or other skin protectant to ensure adherence. Leave the strips in place for 3 to 5 days, as ordered.

References

Lees, S. "The Removal of Sutures," *Nursing Times* 103(17):26–27, April 2007.

Taylor, C., et al. *Fundamentals of Nursing: The Art and Science of Nursing Care,* 6th ed. Philadelphia: Lippincott Williams & Wilkins, 2008.

Swab specimens

Correct collection and handling of swab specimens helps the laboratory staff identify pathogens accurately with a minimum of contamination from normal bacterial flora. Collection normally involves sampling inflamed tissues and exudates from the throat, nasopharynx, wounds, ear, eye, or rectum with sterile swabs of cotton or other absorbent material. The type of swab used depends on the part of the body affected. For example, collection of a nasopharyngeal specimen requires a cotton-tipped swab.

After the specimen has been collected, the swab is immediately placed in a sterile tube containing a transport medium and, in the case of sampling for anaerobes, an inert gas. Swab specimens are usually collected to identify pathogens and sometimes to identify asymptomatic carriers of certain easily transmitted disease organisms.

Equipment

For a throat specimen: Gloves ◆ tongue blade ◆ penlight ◆ sterile cotton-tipped swab ◆ sterile culture tube with transport medium (or commercial collection kit) ◆ label ◆ laboratory request form and laboratory biohazard transport bag.

For a nasopharyngeal specimen: Gloves ◆ penlight ◆ sterile, flexible cotton-tipped swab ◆ tongue blade ◆ sterile culture tube with transport medium ◆ label ◆ laboratory request form and laboratory biohazard transport bag ◆ optional: small open-ended Pyrex tube or nasal speculum.

For a wound specimen: Sterile gloves ◆ sterile forceps ◆ alcohol or povidone-iodine pads ◆ sterile swabs ◆ sterile 10-ml syringe ◆ 21G needle ◆ sterile culture tube with transport medium (or commercial collection kit for aerobic culture) ◆ labels ◆ special anaerobic culture tube containing carbon dioxide or nitrogen ◆ fresh dressings for the wound ◆ laboratory request form and laboratory biohazard transport bag ◆ optional: rubber stopper for needle.

For an ear specimen: Gloves ◆ normal saline solution ◆ two 2″ × 2″ gauze pads ◆ sterile swabs ◆ sterile culture tube with transport medium ◆ label ◆ 10-ml syringe and 22G 1″ needle (for tympanocentesis)

◆ label ◆ laboratory request form and laboratory biohazard transport bag.

For an eye specimen: Sterile gloves ◆ sterile normal saline solution ◆ two 2″ × 2″ gauze pads ◆ sterile swabs ◆ sterile wire culture loop (for corneal scraping) ◆ sterile culture tube with transport medium ◆ label ◆ laboratory request form and laboratory biohazard transport bag.

For a rectal specimen: Gloves ◆ soap and water ◆ washcloth ◆ sterile swab ◆ normal saline solution ◆ sterile culture tube with transport medium ◆ label ◆ laboratory request form and laboratory biohazard transport bag.

Implementation

▶ Confirm the patient's identity using two patient identifiers according to your facility's policy. Explain the procedure to the patient to ease his anxiety and ensure cooperation. **JC**

Collecting a throat specimen

▶ Tell the patient that he may gag during the swabbing but that the procedure will probably take less than 1 minute.

▶ Instruct the patient to sit erect at the edge of the bed or in a chair, facing you. Then wash your hands and put on gloves.

▶ Ask the patient to tilt his head back. Depress his tongue with the tongue blade, and illuminate his throat with the penlight to check for inflamed areas.

▶ If the patient starts to gag, withdraw the tongue blade and tell him to breathe deeply. After he's relaxed, reinsert the tongue blade but not as deeply as before.

▶ Using the cotton-tipped swab, wipe the tonsillar areas from side to side, including any inflamed or purulent sites. Make sure you don't touch the tongue, cheeks, or teeth with the swab to avoid contaminating it with oral bacteria.

▶ Withdraw the swab and immediately place it in the culture tube. If you're using a commercial kit, crush the ampule of culture medium at the bottom of the tube, and then push the swab into the medium to keep the swab moist.

▶ Remove and discard your gloves, and wash your hands.

▶ Label the specimen with the patient's name and identification number, the practitioner's name, and the date, time, and site of collection.

▶ On the laboratory request form, indicate whether any organism is strongly suspected, especially *Corynebacterium diphtheriae* (requires two swabs and special growth medium), *Bordetella pertussis* (requires a nasopharyngeal culture and special growth medium), and *Neisseria meningitidis* (requires enriched selective media).

▶ Place in a laboratory biohazard transport bag, and send the specimen to the laboratory immediately to prevent growth or deterioration of microbes.

Collecting a nasopharyngeal specimen

▶ Tell the patient that he may gag or feel the urge to sneeze during the swabbing but that the procedure takes less than 1 minute.

▶ Have the patient sit erect at the edge of the bed or in a chair, facing you. Then wash your hands and put on gloves.

▶ Ask the patient to blow his nose to clear his nasal passages. Then check his nostrils for patency with a penlight.

▶ Tell the patient to occlude one nostril first and then the other as he exhales. Listen for the more patent nostril because you'll insert the swab through it.

▶ Ask the patient to cough to bring organisms to the nasopharynx for a better specimen.

▶ While it's still in the package, bend the sterile swab in a curve and then open the package without contaminating the swab.

▶ Ask the patient to tilt his head back, and gently pass the swab through the more patent nostril about 3″ to 4″ (7.5 to 10 cm) into the nasopharynx, keeping the swab near the septum and floor of the nose. Rotate the swab quickly and remove it. (See *Obtaining a nasopharyngeal specimen*.)

▶ Alternatively, depress the patient's tongue with a tongue blade, and pass the bent swab up behind the uvula. Rotate the swab and withdraw it.

▶ Remove the cap from the culture tube, insert the swab, and break off the

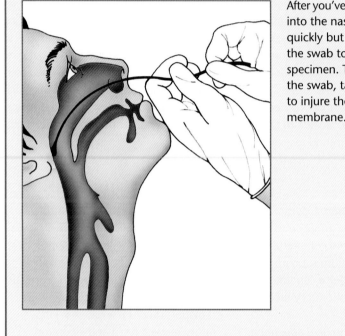

Obtaining a nasopharyngeal specimen

After you've passed the swab into the nasopharynx, quickly but gently rotate the swab to collect the specimen. Then remove the swab, taking care not to injure the nasal mucous membrane.

contaminated end. Then close the tube tightly.

▶ Remove and discard your gloves and wash your hands.

▶ Label the specimen for culture, complete a laboratory request form, and send the specimen to the laboratory immediately in a laboratory biohazard transport bag. If you're collecting a specimen to isolate a possible virus, check with the laboratory for the recommended collection technique.

Collecting a wound specimen

▶ Wash your hands, prepare a sterile field, and put on sterile gloves. With sterile forceps, remove the dressing to expose the wound. Dispose of the soiled dressings properly.

▶ Clean the area around the wound with an alcohol or a povidone-iodine pad to reduce the risk of contaminating the specimen with skin bacteria. Then allow the area to dry.

▶ For an aerobic culture, use a sterile cotton-tipped swab to collect as much exudate as possible, or insert the swab deeply into the wound and gently rotate it. Remove the swab from the wound and immediately place it in the aerobic culture tube. Send the tube to the laboratory immediately with a completed laboratory request form. Never collect exudate from the skin and then insert the same swab into the wound; this could contaminate the wound with skin bacteria.

▶ For an anaerobic culture, insert the sterile cotton-tipped swab deeply into the wound, rotate it gently, remove it, and immediately place it in the anaerobic culture tube. Or, insert a sterile 10-ml syringe, without a needle, into the wound, and aspirate 1 to 5 ml of exudate into the syringe. Then attach the 21G needle to the syringe, and immediately inject the aspirate into the anaerobic culture tube. If an anaerobic culture tube is unavailable, obtain a rubber stopper, attach the needle to the syringe, and gently push all the air out of the syringe by pressing on the plunger. Stick the needle tip into the rubber stopper, remove and discard your gloves, and send the syringe of aspirate to the laboratory immediately with a completed laboratory request form in a laboratory biohazard transport bag.

▶ Put on sterile gloves.

▶ Apply a new dressing to the wound.

Collecting an external ear specimen

▶ Wash your hands and put on gloves.

▶ Gently clean excess debris from the patient's ear with normal saline solution and gauze pads.

▶ Insert the sterile swab into the ear canal, and rotate it gently along the walls of the canal to avoid damaging the eardrum.

▶ Withdraw the swab, being careful not to touch other surfaces to avoid contaminating the specimen.

▶ Place the swab in the sterile culture tube with transport medium.

▶ Remove and discard your gloves and wash your hands.

▶ Label the specimen for culture, complete a laboratory request form, and send the specimen to the laboratory immediately in a laboratory biohazard transport bag.

Collecting a middle ear specimen

▶ Put on gloves and clean the outer ear with normal saline solution and gauze pads. Remove and discard your gloves. After the physician punctures the eardrum with a needle and aspirates fluid into the syringe, label the container, complete a laboratory request form, and send the specimen to the laboratory immediately in a laboratory biohazard transport bag.

Collecting an eye specimen

▶ Wash your hands and put on sterile gloves.

▶ Gently clean excess debris from the outside of the eye with normal saline solution and gauze pads, wiping from the inner to the outer canthus.

▶ Retract the lower eyelid to expose the conjunctival sac. Gently rub the sterile swab over the conjunctiva, being careful not to touch other surfaces. Hold the swab parallel to the eye, rather than pointed directly at it, to prevent corneal irritation or trauma due to sudden movement. (If a corneal scraping is required, this procedure is performed by a physician, using a wire culture loop.)

▶ Immediately place the swab or wire loop in the culture tube with transport medium.

▶ Remove and discard your gloves and wash your hands.

▶ Label the specimen for culture, complete a laboratory request form, and send the specimen to the laboratory immediately in a laboratory biohazard transport bag.

Collecting a rectal specimen

▶ Wash your hands and put on gloves.

▶ Clean the area around the patient's anus using a washcloth and soap and water.

▶ Insert the swab, moistened with normal saline solution or sterile broth medium, through the anus, and advance it about $3/8''$ (1 cm) for infants or $1\frac{1}{2}''$ (4 cm) for adults. While withdrawing the swab, gently rotate it against the walls of the lower rectum to sample a large area of the rectal mucosa.

▶ Place the swab in a culture tube with transport medium.

▶ Remove and discard your gloves, and wash your hands.

▶ Label the specimen for culture, complete a laboratory request form, and send the specimen to the laboratory immediately in a laboratory biohazard transport bag.

Special considerations

▶ Note recent antibiotic therapy on the laboratory request form.

▶ For a wound specimen: Although you would normally clean the area around a wound to prevent contamination by normal skin flora, don't clean a perineal wound with alcohol because this could irritate sensitive tissues. Also, make sure that antiseptic doesn't enter the wound.

▶ For an eye specimen: Don't use an antiseptic before culturing to avoid irritating the eye and inhibiting growth of organisms in the culture. If the patient is a child or an uncooperative adult, ask a coworker to restrain the patient's head to prevent eye trauma resulting from sudden movement.

References

Brook, I., and Gober, A. E. "Recovery of Potential Pathogens and Interfering Bacteria in the Nasopharynx of Smokers and Nonsmokers," *Chest* 127(6):2072–75, June 2005.

Centers for Disease Control and Prevention. "Public Health Guidance for Community-Level Preparedness and Response to Severe Acute Respiratory Syndrome (SARS)," Version 2, Supplement F: Laboratory Guidance. Accessed August 2007 via the Web at *www.cdc.gov/ncidod/sars/guidance/f/word/app4.doc.*

Clinical and Laboratory Standards Institute. "Quality Control of Microbiological Transport Systems," Approved Standard, M40, 2003.

Fischbach, F. *A Manual of Laboratory and Diagnostic Tests,* 7th ed. Philadelphia: Lippincott Williams & Wilkins, 2004.

Macfarlane, P., et al. "RSV Testing in Bronchiolitis: Which Nasal Sampling Method is Best?" *Archives of Diseases in Childhood* 90(6):634–35, June 2005.

Rushing, J. "Obtaining a Throat Culture," *Nursing* 37(3):20, 2007.

Synchronized cardioversion

Used to treat tachyarrhythmias, cardioversion delivers an electric charge to the myocardium at the peak of the R wave. This causes immediate depolarization, interrupting reentry circuits and allowing the sinoatrial node to resume control. Synchronizing the electric charge with the R wave ensures that the current won't be delivered on the vulnerable T wave and thus disrupt repolarization.

Synchronized cardioversion is the treatment of choice for arrhythmias that don't respond to vagal massage or drug therapy, such as atrial tachycardia, atrial flutter, atrial fibrillation, and symptomatic ventricular tachycardia. **AHA** (See *Monophasic energy levels for cardioversion.*)

Cardioversion may be an elective or urgent procedure, depending on how well the patient tolerates the arrhythmia. For example, if the patient is hemodynamically unstable, he would require urgent cardioversion. Remember that, when preparing for cardioversion, the patient's condition can deteriorate quickly, necessitating immediate defibrillation.

The American Heart Association recommends immediate synchronized cardioversion for treatment of symptomatic (unstable) tachycardias. If the patient is stable, a 12-lead electrocardiogram (ECG) is done to further classify the tachycardia. Unstable signs include altered mental status, shock or hypotension, and ongoing chest pain. **AHA**

Equipment

Cardioverter-defibrillator ◆ conductive medium pads ◆ anterior, posterior, or transverse paddles ◆ ECG monitor with recorder ◆ sedative ◆ oxygen therapy equipment ◆ airway ◆ hand-held resuscitation bag ◆ emergency pacing equipment ◆ emergency cardiac medications ◆ automatic blood pressure cuff (if available) ◆ pulse oximeter (if available).

Implementation

▶ Test the cardioverter-defibrillator and make sure that it works. Attach the oxygen tubing and oxygen delivery device to the oxygen source. Make sure that you have an airway and a hand-held resuscitation bag readily available for use. Also make sure that you have emergency pacing equipment available in case the patient develops asystole or bradycardia during the cardioversion.

▶ Confirm the patient's identity using two patient identifiers according to your facility's policy. **JC**

▶ Explain the procedure to the patient, and make sure he has signed a consent form.

▶ Check the patient's recent serum potassium and magnesium levels and arterial blood gas (ABG) results. Also check recent digoxin levels. Although digitalized patients may undergo cardioversion, they tend to require lower energy levels to convert. If the patient takes digoxin, withhold the dose on the day of the procedure.

▶ If possible, withhold all food and fluids for 6 to 12 hours before the procedure.

▶ Obtain a 12-lead ECG to serve as a baseline.

▶ Check to see if the practitioner has ordered administration of any cardiac drugs before the procedure. Also verify that the patient has a patent I.V. site to administer the sedative.

▶ Connect the patient to a pulse oximeter and automatic blood pressure cuff, if available.

▶ Consider administering oxygen for 5 to 10 minutes before the cardioversion to promote myocardial oxygenation. If the patient wears dentures, evaluate whether they support his airway or might cause an airway obstruction. If they might cause an obstruction, remove them.

▶ Place the patient in the supine position, and assess his vital signs, level of consciousness (LOC), cardiac rhythm, and peripheral pulses.

▶ Remove any oxygen delivery device just before cardioversion to avoid possible combustion. **AHA**

▶ Have epinephrine, lidocaine, and atropine at the patient's bedside.

▶ Administer a sedative, as ordered. The patient should be heavily sedated but still able to breathe adequately.

▶ Carefully monitor the patient's blood pressure and respiratory rate until he recovers.

▶ Press the POWER button to turn on the defibrillator. Attach ECG electrodes to the patient and attach the leadwires from the defibrillator to the electrodes. Next, push the SYNC button to synchronize the machine with the patient's QRS complexes. Make sure the SYNC button flashes with each of the pa-

Monophasic energy levels for cardioversion

When choosing an energy level for cardioversion, try the lowest energy level first. If the arrhythmia isn't corrected, repeat the procedure using the next energy level until the arrhythmia is corrected or until you reach the highest energy level.

For unstable monomorphic ventricular tachycardia with a pulse: 100 joules, 200 joules, 300 joules, 360 joules.

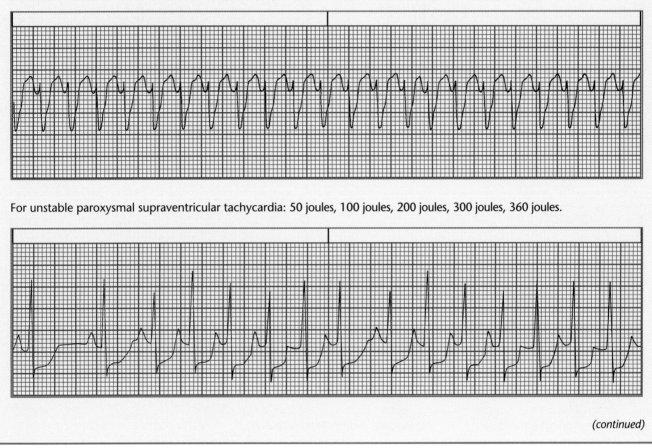

For unstable paroxysmal supraventricular tachycardia: 50 joules, 100 joules, 200 joules, 300 joules, 360 joules.

(continued)

tient's QRS complexes. You should also see a bright green flag flash on the monitor.

▶ Turn the ENERGY SELECT dial to the ordered amount of energy. Advanced cardiac life support (ACLS) protocols call for an initial shock of 50 to 100 joules for a patient with unstable supraventricular tachycardia, 100 to 200 joules for a patient with atrial fibrillation, 50 to 100 joules for a patient with atrial flutter, and 100 joules for a patient who has monomorphic ventricular tachycardia with a pulse. If there's no response with the first shock, the health care provider should increase the joules in a step-wise manner. **AHA**

▶ Remove the paddles from the machine, and prepare them as you would if you were defibrillating the patient. Place the conductive gel pads or paddles in the same positions as you would to defibrillate. **MFR**

Monophasic energy levels for cardioversion (continued)

For unstable atrial fibrilation with rapid ventricular response: 100 joules, 200 joules, 300 joules, 360 joules.

For unstable atrial flutter with rapid ventricular response: 50 joules, 100 joules, 200 joules, 300 joules, 360 joules.

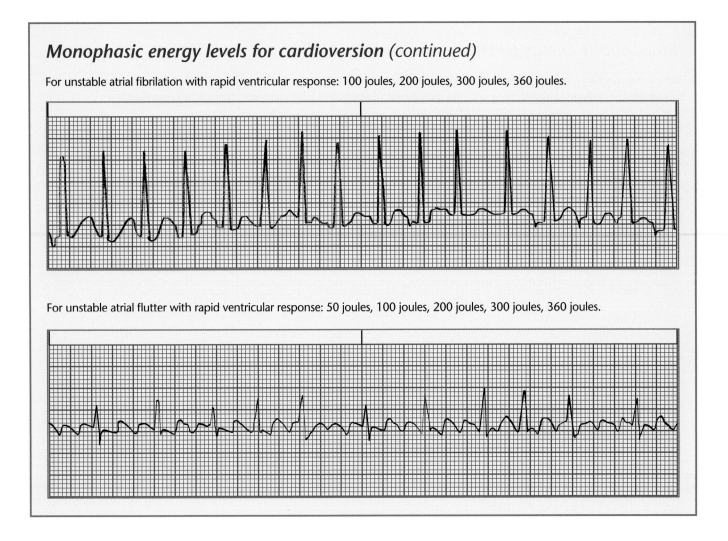

▶ Make sure everyone stands away from the bed; then push the discharge buttons. Hold the paddles in place and wait for the energy to be discharged—the machine has to synchronize the discharge with the QRS complex.

▶ Check the waveform on the monitor. If the arrhythmia fails to convert, repeat the procedure two or three more times at 3-minute intervals. Gradually increase the energy level with each additional countershock.

▶ After the cardioversion, frequently assess the patient's LOC and respiratory status, including airway patency, respiratory rate and depth, and the need for supplemental oxygen. Because the patient will be heavily sedated, he may require airway support.

▶ Record a postcardioversion 12-lead ECG, and monitor the patient's ECG rhythm for 2 hours. Check the patient's chest for electrical burns.

Special considerations

▶ If the patient is attached to a bedside or telemetry monitor, disconnect the unit before cardioversion. The electric current it generates could damage the equipment. **MFR**

▶ Be aware that improper synchronization may result if the patient's ECG tracing contains artifact-like spikes, such as peaked T waves or bundle-branch heart blocks when the R′ wave may be taller than the R wave.

▶ Although the electric shock of cardioversion won't usually damage an implanted pacemaker, avoid placing the paddles directly over the pacemaker. **MFR**

▶ Remove any patches with metallic backings such as nitroglycerin patches. This backing may cause a ring during cardioversion.

▶ Reset the synchronization mode after each cardioversion because many defibrillators automatically default back to the unsynchronized mode.

References

American Heart Association. "2005 AHA Guidelines for Cardiopulmonary Resuscitation and Emergency Cardiovascular Care: International Consensus on Science," *Circulation* 112(22Suppl): IV-1-IV-221, November 2005.

American Heart Association. "ACC/AHA/ECS 2006 Guidelines for the Management of Patients with Atrial Fibrillation," *Circulation* 114:257–54, August 2006.

Hagens, V. E., et al. "Determinants of Sudden Cardiac Death in Patients with Persistent Atrial Fibrillation in the Rate Control Versus Electrical Cardioversion (RACE) Study," *American Journal of Cardiology* 98(7):929–32, October 2006.

"Managing Atrial Fibrillation," *Harvard Women's Health Watch* 13(12):4–6, August 2006.

Tracy, C. M., et al. "American College of Cardiology/American Heart Association 2006 Update of the Clinical Competence Statement on Invasive Electrophysiology Studies, Catheter Ablation, and Cardioversion: A Report of the American College of Cardiology/American Heart Association/American College of Physicians Task Force on Clinical Competence and Training Developed in Collaboration with the Heart Rhythm Society," *American College of Cardiology* 48(7):1503–517, October 2006.

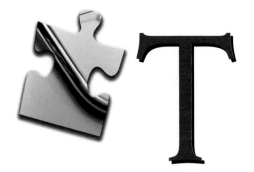

Temperature assessment

Body temperature represents the balance between heat produced by metabolism, muscular activity, and other factors and heat lost through the skin, lungs, and body wastes. A stable temperature pattern promotes proper function of cells, tissues, and organs; a change in this pattern usually signals the onset of illness.

Temperature can be measured with an electronic or a chemical-dot thermometer. A special electronic thermometer, called a *tympanic thermometer,* can be used to obtain a temperature reading from the ear canal. Oral temperature in adults normally ranges from 97° to 99.5° F (36.1° to 37.5° C); rectal temperature, the most accurate reading, is usually 1° F (0.6° C) higher; axillary temperature, the least accurate, reads 1° to 2° F (0.6° to 1.1° C) lower; and tympanic temperature reads 0.5° to 1° (0.3° to 0.6° C) higher. **CS1**

Temperature normally fluctuates with rest and activity. Lowest readings typically occur between 4 and 5 a.m.; the highest readings occur between 4 and 8 p.m. Other factors also influence temperature, including gender, age, emotional conditions, and environment. Keep the following principles in mind. Females normally have higher temperatures than males, especially during ovulation. Heightened emotions raise temperature; depressed emotions lower it. A hot external environment can raise temperature; a cold environment lowers it.

AGE FACTOR

Normal temperature is highest in neonates and lowest in elderly persons.

Equipment

Thermometer (electronic, chemical-dot, or tympanic) ◆ water-soluble lubricant or petroleum jelly (for rectal temperature) ◆ gloves (for rectal temperature) ◆ facial tissue ◆ disposable thermometer sheath or probe cover ◆ alcohol pad.

Obtain a thermometer from the nurses' station or central supply department. If you use an electronic thermometer, make sure it's been recharged. (See *Types of thermometers.*)

Implementation

▶ Confirm the patient's identity using two patient identifiers according to your facility's policy. **JC**
▶ Explain the procedure to the patient, and wash your hands. If the patient has had hot or cold liquids, chewed gum, or smoked, wait 30 minutes before taking an oral temperature. **CS2**

▶ To use a disposable sheath, disinfect the thermometer with an alcohol pad. Insert it into the disposable sheath opening; then twist to tear the seal at the dotted line. Pull it apart.

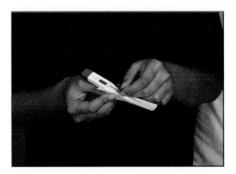

Types of thermometers

You can take an oral, rectal, or axillary temperature with such instruments as a chemical-dot device, an electronic digital thermometer, or a tympanic thermometer.

You'll usually use the oral route for adults who are awake, alert, oriented, and cooperative. For infants, young children, and confused or unconscious patients, you may need to take the temperature rectally. The tympanic route may be used on many patients.

Chemical-dot thermometer

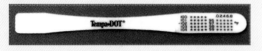

Individual electronic digital thermometer

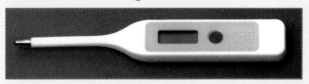

Institutional electronic digital thermometer

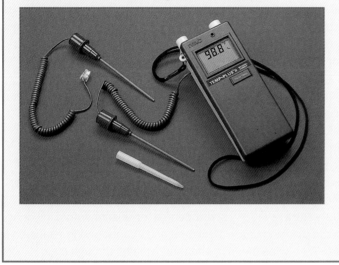

Tympanic thermometer

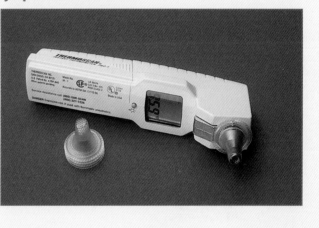

Using an electronic thermometer
▶ Insert the probe into a disposable probe cover. If taking a rectal temperature, lubricate the probe cover to reduce friction and ease insertion. Leave the probe in place until the maximum temperature appears on the digital display.

Using a chemical-dot thermometer
▶ Remove the thermometer from its protective dispenser case. Keep the thermometer sealed until use.

Using a tympanic thermometer
▶ Make sure the lens under the probe is clean and shiny. Attach a disposable probe cover.

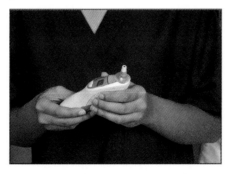

▶ Examine the patient's ears. They should be free from cerumen to obtain an accurate reading. If the patient has

any visible lesions or drainage, do not perform a tympanic temperature.
▶ Stabilize the patient's head; then gently pull the ear straight back (for children up to age 1) or up and back (for children age 1 and older to adults).

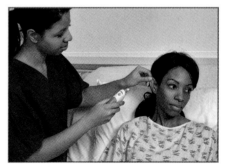

▶ Insert the thermometer until the entire ear canal is sealed. The thermometer should be inserted toward the tympanic membrane in the same way that an otoscope is inserted. Then press the activation button and hold it for 1 second. The temperature will appear on the display.

AGE FACTOR

For infants younger than age 3 months, take three readings, and use the highest.

Taking an oral temperature

▶ Position the tip of the thermometer under the patient's tongue, as far back as possible on either side of the frenulum linguae.

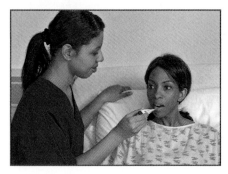

▶ Instruct the patient to close her lips but to avoid biting down with her teeth.
▶ Leave a chemical-dot thermometer in place for 45 seconds to register temperature; for an electronic thermometer, wait until the maximum temperature is displayed.
▶ For an electronic thermometer, note the temperature; then remove and discard the probe cover. For the chemical-dot thermometer, read the temperature as the last dye dot that has changed color, or fired; then discard the thermometer and its dispenser case.

Taking a rectal temperature

▶ Position the patient on her side with her top leg flexed, and drape the patient to provide privacy. Then fold back the bed linens to expose the anus.
▶ Squeeze the lubricant onto a facial tissue to prevent contamination of the lubricant supply. Put on gloves.
▶ Lubricate about ½" (1.3 cm) of the thermometer tip for an infant, 1" (2.5 cm) for a child, or about 1½" (3.8 cm) for an adult.
▶ Lift the patient's upper buttock, and ask the patient to take a slow, deep breath. This helps relax the anal sphincter to ease insertion of the thermometer. Insert the thermometer about ½" (1.3 cm) for an infant or 1½" (3.8 cm) for an adult. Gently direct the thermometer along the rectal wall toward the umbilicus.
▶ Hold the electronic thermometer in place until the maximum temperature is displayed. Holding the thermometer prevents damage to rectal tissues caused by displacement or loss of the thermometer into the rectum.
▶ Carefully remove the thermometer, wiping it as necessary. Then wipe the patient's anal area to remove any lubricant or feces. Remove and dispose of the rectal sheath. Remove and discard your gloves. Wash your hands.

Taking an axillary temperature

▶ Position the patient with the axilla exposed.
▶ Gently pat the axilla dry with a facial tissue because moisture conducts heat. Avoid harsh rubbing, which generates heat.
▶ Ask the patient to reach across her chest and grasp her opposite shoulder, lifting her elbow.
▶ Position the thermometer in the center of the axilla, with the tip pointing toward the patient's head.

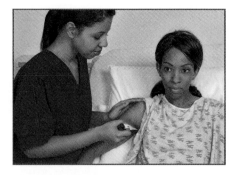

▶ Tell the patient to keep grasping her shoulder and to lower her elbow and hold it against her chest.
▶ Remove an electronic thermometer when it displays the maximum temperature. Axillary temperature takes longer to register than oral or rectal temperature because the thermometer isn't enclosed in a body cavity.
▶ Grasp the end of the thermometer and remove it from the axilla.

Special considerations

▶ Oral measurement is contraindicated in patients who are unconscious, disoriented, or seizure-prone; in young children and infants; and in patients who must breathe through their mouths. Rectal measurement is contraindicated in patients with diarrhea, recent rectal or prostate surgery or injury because it may injure inflamed tissue, or recent myocardial infarction because anal manipulation may stimulate the vagus nerve, causing bradycardia or another rhythm disturbance.
▶ Use the same thermometer for repeated temperature taking to avoid spurious variations caused by equipment differences. Store chemical-dot thermometers in a cool area because exposure to heat activates the dye dots.
▶ Don't avoid taking an oral temperature when the patient is receiving nasal oxygen because oxygen administration raises oral temperature by only about 0.3° F (0.17° C).

EVIDENCE-BASED RESEARCH

Comparing tympanic and oral temperature

Spitzer, O.P. "Comparing Tympanic Temperatures in Both Ears to Oral Temperature in the Critically Ill Adult," *Dimensions in Critical Care Nursing* 27(1):24–29, January–February 2008.

Level VI-Evidence from a single descriptive or qualitative study

Description
The most accurate method of measuring core body temperature is through using either a bladder thermometer or the thermistor on a pulmonary artery catheter. However, these methods aren't always possible. In critical care patients for whom the above methods aren't possible, the tympanic route is often used. Usually, there's a difference in the right and left ear tympanic temperature. This study compared the tympanic temperature taken in both ears to the oral temperature. Nurses used the FirsTemp Genius 3000A to take bilateral tympanic temperatures and the Dinamap PRO 100-400V2 to

measure oral temperature. The study consisted of 66 patients in two critical care units. The nurse also documented other information, such as if the patient was wearing a hearing aid, was using oxygen, or had a fan blowing as well as noted the room temperature.

Findings
The range of difference between the right and left ear using the tympanic thermometer was 0.0° F to 3.4° F. There was an average difference of 0.8° F. There was only one patient who had no difference in the readings in the left and right ear. And no consistency was found as far as one ear having a higher reading than the other ear. After statistical analysis was done on all three temperature sites, it was determined that there was no overall difference in the three measures.

Conclusion
Effective temperature measurement isn't as dependent on the site of the measurement; rather, it's associated

with *consistency* of the site used. The best site for the patient should be determined, documented, and then used on a consistent basis. This ensures that any changes in temperature are accurately tracked.

Nursing practice implications
Because the nurse is usually the one taking and evaluating the patient's temperature, it's of absolute importance that the temperature she's recording is the most accurate one possible. Here are some important nursing practice implications to keep in mind:
▶ Determine the best site to take the patient's temperature.
▶ Record the site where the temperature is taken.
▶ Continue to use the same site when taking the patient's temperature.
▶ Make sure the thermometer has been properly calibrated as recommended by the manufacturer.
▶ Use the proper technique when taking the patient's temperature.

References

Craven, R. F., and Hirnle, C. J. *Fundamentals of Nursing Human Health and Function,* 6th ed. Philadelphia: Lippincott Williams & Wilkins, 2009.

Jensen, B. N., et al. "Accuracy of Digital Tympanic, Oral, Axillary, and Rectal Thermometers Compared with Standard Rectal Mercury Thermometers,"

European Journal of Surgery 166(11):848–51, November 2000. **CS1**

Khorshid, L. "Comparing Mercury-in-Glass, Tympanic, and Disposable Thermometers in Measuring Body Temperature in Healthy Young People," *Journal of Clinical Nursing* 14(4):496–500, April 2005.

Quatrara, B., et al. "The Effect of Respiratory Rate and Ingestion of Hot and Cold Beverages on the Accuracy of Oral Temperature Measured by Electronic Thermometers," *MedSurg Nursing* 16(2):105–108, April 2007. **CS2**

"Take Care with Tympanic Temperature Readings," *Nursing* 37(4):52–53, April 2007.

Temporary pacemaker insertion and care

Usually inserted in an emergency, a temporary pacemaker consists of an external, battery-powered pulse generator and a lead or electrode system. Four types of temporary pacemakers exist: transcutaneous, transvenous, transthoracic, and epicardial.

In a life-threatening situation, when time is critical, a transcutaneous pacemaker is the best choice. This device works by sending an electrical impulse from the pulse generator to the patient's heart by way of two electrodes, which are placed on the front and back of the patient's chest. Transcutaneous pacing is quick and effective, but it's used only until the physician can institute transvenous pacing.

Transcutaneous pacing is recommended by the 2005 American Heart Association (AHA) guidelines for cardiopulmonary resuscitation (CPR) and emergency cardiovascular care for symptomatic bradycardia when a pulse is present. **AHA** If transcutaneous pacing doesn't correct the problem, transvenous pacing is indicated. Transvenous pacing involves threading an electrode catheter through a vein into the patient's right atrium or right ventricle. The electrode then attaches to an external pulse generator. As a result, the pulse generator can provide an electrical stimulus directly to the endocardium. This is the most common type of pacemaker.

However, a physician may choose to insert a transthoracic pacemaker as an elective surgical procedure or as an emergency measure during CPR. To insert this type of pacemaker, the physician performs a procedure similar to pericardiocentesis, in which he uses a cardiac needle to pass an electrode through the chest wall and into the right ventricle. This procedure carries a significant risk of coronary artery laceration and cardiac tamponade and isn't very common.

Among the contraindications to pacemaker therapy are pulseless electrical activity and ventricular fibrillation.

Equipment

For transcutaneous pacing: Transcutaneous pacing generator ◆ transcutaneous pacing electrodes ◆ cardiac monitor with ECG electrodes ◆ clippers.

For all other types of temporary pacing: Temporary pacemaker generator with new battery ◆ guide wire or introducer ◆ electrode catheter ◆ sterile gloves ◆ sterile dressings ◆ sterile marker ◆ sterile labels ◆ adhesive tape ◆ antiseptic solution ◆ emergency cardiac drugs ◆ intubation equipment ◆ defibrillator ◆ cardiac monitor with strip-chart recorder ◆ equipment to start a peripheral I.V. line, if appropriate ◆ I.V. fluids ◆ sedative ◆ electric clippers, if needed.

For transvenous pacing: All equipment listed for temporary pacing ◆ bridging cable ◆ percutaneous introducer tray or venous cutdown tray ◆ sterile gowns ◆ linen-saver pad ◆ antimicrobial soap/alcohol pads ◆ vial of 1% lidocaine ◆ 5-ml syringe ◆ fluoroscopy equipment, if necessary, including protective apron ◆ fenestrated drape ◆ prepackaged cutdown tray (for antecubital vein placement only) ◆ sutures.

For epicardial pacing: All equipment listed for temporary pacing ◆ atrial epicardial wires ◆ ventricular epicardial wires ◆ sterile rubber finger cot ◆ sterile dressing materials (if the wires won't be connected to a pulse generator).

Implementation

▶ If applicable, explain the procedure to the patient.

▶ Obtain emergency cardiac drugs and intubation equipment and have them readily available.

For transcutaneous pacing

▶ If necessary, clip the hair over the areas of electrode placement. However, don't shave the area. **CDC**

▶ Attach monitoring electrodes to the patient in lead I, II, or III position. Do this even if the patient is already on telemetry monitoring because you'll need to connect the electrodes to the pacemaker. If you select the lead II position, adjust the LL electrode placement to accommodate the anterior pacing electrode and the patient's anatomy.

▶ Plug the patient cable into the ECG input connection on the front of the pacing generator. Set the selector switch to the monitor on position.

▶ You should see the ECG waveform on the monitor. Adjust the R-wave beeper volume to a suitable level, and activate the alarm by pressing the alarm on button. Set the alarm for 10 to 20 beats lower and 20 to 30 beats higher than the intrinsic rate.

▶ Press the START/STOP button for a printout of the waveform.

▶ Now you're ready to apply the two pacing electrodes. First, make sure the patient's skin is clean and dry to ensure good skin contact.

▶ Pull off the protective strip from one electrode, and apply the electrode on the left side of the back, just below the scapula and to the left of the spine.

▶ Pull off the protective strip from the second electrode, and apply it to the skin in the anterior position—to the left side of the precordium in the usual V_2 to V_5 position. (See *Proper electrode placement*.)

▶ Now you're ready to pace the heart. After making sure the energy output in milliamperes (mA) is on 0, connect the electrode cable to the monitor output cable.

▶ Check the waveform, looking for a tall QRS complex in lead II.

▶ Next, turn the selector switch to pacer on. Tell the patient that he may feel a thumping or twitching sensation. Reassure him that you'll give him medication if he can't tolerate the discomfort.

▶ Now set the rate dial to 10 to 20 beats higher than the patient's intrinsic rhythm. Look for pacer artifact or spikes, which will appear as you increase the rate. If the patient doesn't have an intrinsic rhythm, set the rate at 60.

▶ Slowly increase the amount of energy delivered to the heart by adjusting the output mA dial. Do this until capture is achieved—you'll see a pacer spike followed by a widened QRS complex that resembles a premature ventricular contraction. This is the pacing threshold. To ensure consistent capture, increase output by 10%. Don't go any higher because you could cause the patient needless discomfort.

▶ With full capture, the patient's heart rate should be approximately the same as the pacemaker rate set on the machine. The usual pacing threshold is between 40 and 80 mA.

For transvenous pacing

▶ Check the patient's history for hypersensitivity to local anesthetics. Then attach the cardiac monitor to the patient and obtain a baseline assessment, including the patient's vital signs, skin color, level of consciousness (LOC), heart rate and rhythm, and emotional state.

▶ Insert a peripheral I.V. catheter if the patient doesn't already have one. Begin an I.V. infusion of dextrose 5% in water at a keep-vein-open rate.

▶ Insert a new battery into the external pacemaker generator, and test it to make sure it has a strong charge. **MFR** Connect the bridging cable to the generator, and align the positive and negative poles.

▶ Place the patient in the supine position. If necessary, clip the hair around the insertion site. **CDC**

▶ Open the supply tray while maintaining a sterile field. Label all medications, medication containers, and other solutions on and off the sterile field. **JC**

Proper electrode placement

MFR

Place the two pacing electrodes for a noninvasive temporary pacemaker at heart level on the patient's chest and back (as shown below). This placement ensures that the electrical stimulus must travel only a short distance to the heart.

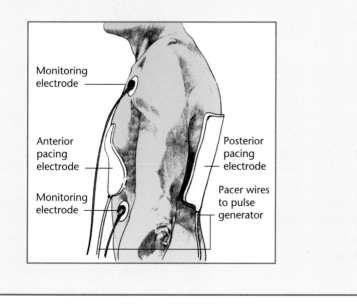

Monitoring electrode

Anterior pacing electrode

Monitoring electrode

Posterior pacing electrode

Pacer wires to pulse generator

▶ Using sterile technique, clean the insertion site with antimicrobial soap and then wipe the area with antiseptic solution. Cover the insertion site with a fenestrated drape. Because fluoroscopy may be used during the placement of leadwires, put on a protective apron.

▶ After anesthetizing the insertion site with 1% lidocaine, the physician will puncture the vein and then insert a guide wire or an introducer and advance the electrode catheter.

▶ As the catheter advances, watch the cardiac monitor. When the electrode catheter reaches the right atrium, you'll notice large P waves and small QRS complexes. Then, as the catheter reaches the right ventricle, the P waves will become smaller while the QRS complexes enlarge. When the catheter touches the right ventricular endocardium, expect to see elevated ST segments, premature ventricular contractions, or both.

▶ When the electrode catheter is in the right ventricle, it will send an impulse to the myocardium, causing depolarization. If the patient needs atrial pacing, either alone or with ventricular pacing, the physician may place an electrode in the right atrium.

▶ Meanwhile, continuously monitor the patient's cardiac status, and treat any arrhythmias, as appropriate. Also assess the patient for jaw pain and earache; these symptoms indicate that the electrode catheter has missed the superior vena cava and has moved into the neck instead.

▶ When the electrode catheter is in place, attach the catheter leads to the bridging cable, lining up the positive and negative poles.

▶ Set the pacemaker as ordered.

▶ The physician will then suture the catheter to the insertion site. Afterward, put on sterile gloves, and apply a sterile dressing to the site. Label the dressing with the date and time of application.

For epicardial pacing

▶ During your preoperative teaching, inform the patient that epicardial pacemaker wires may be placed during cardiac surgery.

▶ During cardiac surgery, the physician will hook epicardial wires into the epicardium just before the end of the surgery. Depending on the patient's condition, the physician may insert either atrial or ventricular wires, or both.

▶ If indicated, connect the electrode catheter to the generator, lining up the positive and negative poles. Set the pacemaker, as ordered.

▶ If the wires won't be connected to an external pulse generator, place them in a sterile rubber finger cot. Then cover both the wires and the insertion site with a sterile, occlusive dressing. This will help protect the patient from microshock as well as infection.

Special considerations

▶ Take care to prevent microshock. This includes warning the patient not to use any electrical equipment that isn't grounded, such as telephones, electric shavers, televisions, or lamps. **MFR**

▶ Other safety measures you'll want to take include placing a plastic cover supplied by the manufacturer over the pacemaker controls to avoid an accidental setting change. Also, insulate the pacemaker by placing the pacing unit in a dry, rubber surgical glove. If the patient needs emergency defibrillation, make sure the pacemaker can withstand the procedure. If you're unsure, disconnect the pulse generator to avoid damage.

▶ When using a transcutaneous pacemaker, don't place the electrodes over a bony area because bone conducts current poorly. With female patients, place the anterior electrode under the patient's breast but not over her diaphragm. If the physician inserts the electrode through the brachial or femoral vein, immobilize the patient's arm or leg to avoid putting stress on the pacing wires.

▶ After insertion of any temporary pacemaker, assess the patient's vital signs, skin color, LOC, and peripheral pulses to determine the effectiveness of the paced rhythm. Perform a 12-lead ECG to serve as a baseline, and then perform additional ECGs daily or with clinical changes. Also, if possible, obtain a rhythm strip before, during, and after pacemaker placement; any time that pacemaker settings are changed; and whenever the patient receives treatment because of a complication due to the pacemaker.

▶ Continuously monitor the ECG reading, noting capture, sensing, rate, intrinsic beats, and competition of paced and intrinsic rhythms. If the pacemaker is sensing correctly, the sense indicator on the pulse generator should flash with each beat. (See *When a temporary pacemaker malfunctions*.)

▶ If the patient has epicardial pacing wires in place, clean the insertion site with antiseptic solution and change the dressing daily. At the same time, monitor the site for signs of infection. Always keep the pulse generator nearby in case pacing becomes necessary.

▶ Complications associated with pacemaker therapy include microshock, equipment failure, and competitive or fatal arrhythmias. Transcutaneous pacemakers may also cause skin breakdown and muscle pain and twitching when the pacemaker fires.

When a temporary pacemaker malfunctions

Occasionally, a temporary pacemaker may fail to function appropriately. When this occurs, you'll need to take immediate action to correct the problem. Take the steps described below when your patient's pacemaker fails to pace, capture, or sense intrinsic beats.

Failure to pace

This happens when the pacemaker either doesn't fire or fires too often. The pulse generator may not be working properly, or it may not be conducting the impulse to the patient.

Nursing interventions

▶ If the pacing or sensing indicator flashes, check the connections to the cable and the position of the pacing electrode in the patient (by X-ray). The cable may have come loose, or the electrode may have been dislodged, pulled out, or broken.

▶ If the pulse generator is turned on but the indicators still aren't flashing, change the battery. If that doesn't help, use a different pulse generator.

▶ Check the settings if the pacemaker is firing too rapidly. If they're correct, or if altering them (according to your

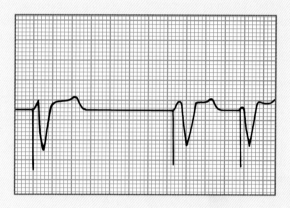

facility's policy or the physician's order) doesn't help, change the pulse generator.

Failure to capture

Here, you see pacemaker spikes but the heart isn't responding. This may be caused by changes in the pacing threshold from ischemia, an electrolyte imbalance (high or low potassium or magnesium levels), acidosis, an adverse reaction to a medication, a perforated ventricle, fibrosis, or the position of the electrode.

Nursing interventions

▶ If the patient's condition has changed, notify the physician, and ask him for new settings.

▶ If pacemaker settings have been altered by the patient (or his family members), return them to their correct positions. Then make sure the face of the pacemaker is covered with a plastic shield. Tell the patient and his family members not to touch the dials.

▶ If the heart isn't responding, try any or all of these suggestions: Carefully check all connections, making sure they're placed properly and securely; increase the

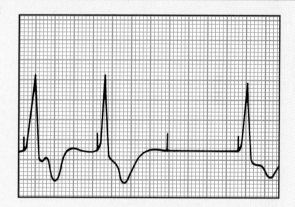

milliamperes slowly (acording to your facility's policy or the physician's order); turn the patient on his left side, then on his right (if turning him to the left didn't help); and schedule an anteroposterior or lateral chest X-ray to determine the position of the electrode.

(continued)

When a temporary pacemaker malfunctions *(continued)*

Failure to sense intrinsic beats

This could cause ventricular tachycardia or ventricular fibrillation if the pacemaker fires on the vulnerable T wave. This could be caused by the pacemaker sensing an external stimulus as a QRS complex, which could lead to asystole, or by the pacemaker not being sensitive enough, which means it could fire anywhere within the cardiac cycle.

Nursing interventions

▶ If the pacing is undersensing, turn the sensitivity control completely to the right. If it's oversensing, turn it slightly to the left.

▶ If the pacemaker isn't functioning correctly, change the battery or the pulse generator.

▶ Remove items in the room causng electromechanical interference (razors, radios, cautery devices). Check the ground wires on the bed and other equipment for obvious damage. Unplug each piece, and see if the inteference stops. When you locate the cause, notify the staff engineer, and ask him to check it.

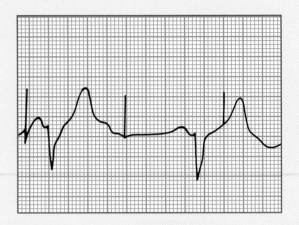

▶ If the pacemaker is still firing on the T wave and all else has failed, turn off the pacemaker. Make sure atropine is available in case the patient's heart rate drops. Be prepared to call a code and institute cardiopulmonary resuscitation if necessary.

Transvenous pacemakers may cause such complications as pneumothorax or hemothorax, cardiac perforation and tamponade, diaphragmatic stimulation, pulmonary embolism, thrombophlebitis, and infection. Also, if the physician threads the electrode through the antecubital or femoral vein, venous spasm, thrombophlebitis, or lead displacement may result. Epicardial pacemakers carry a risk of infection, cardiac arrest, and diaphragmatic stimulation.

References

American Association for Respiratory Care. "Clinical Practice Guideline. Resuscitation and Defibrillation in the Health Care Setting—2004 Revision and Update," *Respiratory Care* 89(9):1085–99, September 2004.

American Heart Association. "2005 AHA Guidelines for Cardiopulmonary Resuscitation and Emergency Cardiovascular Care: International Consensus on Science," *Circulation* 112(22Suppl): IV-1-IV-221, November 2005.

Craig, K. "How to Provide Transcutaneous Pacing," *Nursing* 35(10):52–53, October 2005.

Lynn-McHale Wiegand, D. J., and Carlson, K. K., eds. *AACN Procedure Manual for Critical Care,* 5th ed. Philadelphia: W. B. Saunders Co., 2005.

Overbay, D., and Criddle, L. "Mastering Temporary Invasive Cardiac Pacing," *Critical Care Nurse* 24(3):25–32, June 2004.

Thoracentesis

Thoracentesis involves the aspiration of fluid or air from the pleural space. It relieves pulmonary compression and respiratory distress by removing accumulated air or fluid that results from injury or such conditions as tuberculosis, cancer, or heart failure. It also provides a specimen of pleural fluid or tissue for analysis and allows instillation of chemotherapeutic agents or other medications into the pleural space. Thoracentesis is contraindicated in patients with bleeding disorders. It should be used cautiously in patients who are uncooperative, who have uncontrolled coughing, an uncertain pleural fluid location, or one functional lung, or who are on positive end-expiratory pressure ventilation.

Equipment

Most hospitals use a prepackaged thoracentesis tray that typically includes the following: sterile gloves ◆ sterile drapes ◆ antiseptic solution ◆ 1% or 2% lidocaine ◆ 5-ml syringe with 21G and 25G needles for anesthetic injection ◆ 17G thoracentesis needle for aspiration or Teflon catheter ◆ 50-ml syringe ◆ three-way stopcock and tubing ◆ sterile specimen containers ◆ sterile hemostat ◆ sterile 4″ × 4″ gauze pads.

You'll also need the following: occlusive dressing ◆ sphygmomanometer ◆ gloves ◆ stethoscope ◆ laboratory request slips ◆ drainage bottles ◆ optional: sterile marker, sterile label, clippers, biopsy needle, prescribed sedative with 3-ml syringe and 21G needle, drainage bottles if the physician expects a large amount of drainage.

Implementation

▶ Make sure the patient has signed an appropriate consent form. **JC**
▶ Note drug allergies, especially to the local anesthetic. Have the patient's chest X-rays available.
▶ Label all medications, medication containers, and other solutions on and off the sterile field. **JC**
▶ Confirm the patient's identity using two patient identifiers according to your facility's policy. **JC**

▶ Explain the procedure to the patient. Inform him that he may feel some discomfort and a sensation of pressure during the needle insertion. Provide privacy and emotional support.
▶ Wash your hands and put on gloves. **CDC**
▶ Administer the prescribed sedative as ordered.

▶ Obtain baseline vital signs, and assess respiratory function.
▶ Position the patient. Make sure he's firmly supported and comfortable. (See *Positioning for a thoracentesis*.)
▶ Remind the patient not to cough, breathe deeply, or move suddenly during the procedure to avoid puncture

Positioning for a thoracentesis

The choice of the position may vary. Usually the patient is sitting upright and leaning forward. If the patient is sitting on the edge of the bed, support his legs, and have him lean forward and rest his head and arms on a pillow on the over-bed table. If the patient can't sit, turn him on the unaffected side with the arm of the affected side raised comfortably above his head. The head of the bed may be elevated 30 to 45 degrees unless contraindicated. Recumbent thoracentesis may be performed with ultrasound guidance. Proper positioning stretches the chest or back and allows easier access to the intercostal spaces.

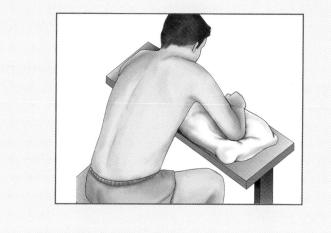

of the visceral pleura or lung. If the patient coughs, the physician will briefly halt the procedure and withdraw the needle slightly to prevent puncture.

▶ Expose the patient's entire chest or back, as appropriate.

▶ Clip the aspiration site, if needed. **CDC**

▶ Wash your hands again before touching the sterile equipment. Then using sterile technique, open the thoracentesis tray, and assist the physician, as necessary, in disinfecting the site.

▶ If an ampule of local anesthetic isn't included in the sterile tray and a multidose vial of local anesthetic is to be used, assist the physician by wiping the rubber stopper with an alcohol pad and holding the inverted vial while the physician withdraws the anesthetic solution.

▶ After draping the patient and injecting the anesthetic, the physician attaches a three-way stopcock with tubing to the aspirating needle and turns the stopcock to prevent air from entering the pleural space through the needle.

▶ Attach the other end of the tubing to the drainage bottle.

▶ The physician then inserts the needle into the pleural space and attaches a 50-ml syringe to the needle's stopcock. A hemostat may be used to hold the needle in place and prevent pleural tear or lung puncture. As an alternative, the physician may introduce a Teflon catheter into the needle, remove the needle, and attach a stopcock and syringe or drainage tubing to the catheter to reduce the risk of pleural puncture by the needle.

▶ Support the patient verbally throughout the procedure, and keep him informed of each step. Assess him for signs of anxiety, and provide reassurance, as necessary.

▶ Check vital signs regularly during the procedure. Continually observe the patient for such signs of distress as pallor, vertigo, faintness, weak and rapid pulse, decreased blood pressure, dyspnea, tachypnea, diaphoresis, chest pain, blood-tinged mucus, and excessive coughing. Alert the physician if such signs develop because they may indicate complications, such as hypovolemic shock or tension pneumothorax.

▶ Put on gloves and assist the physician, as necessary, in specimen collection, fluid drainage, and dressing the site.

▶ After the physician withdraws the needle or catheter, apply pressure to the puncture site, using a sterile 4″ × 4″ gauze pad. Then apply a new sterile gauze pad, and secure it with an occlusive dressing.

▶ Place the patient in a comfortable position, take his vital signs, and assess his respiratory status.

▶ Label the specimens properly, and send them to the laboratory.

▶ Discard disposable equipment. Clean nondisposable items, and return them for sterilization.

▶ Check the patient's vital signs and the dressing for drainage every 15 minutes for 1 hour. Then continue to assess the patient's vital signs and respiratory status, as indicated by his condition.

▶ A chest X-ray is usually done afterward to check for pneumothorax. **CS1**

Special considerations

▶ To prevent pulmonary edema and hypovolemic shock after thoracentesis, fluid is removed slowly, and no more than 1,000 ml of fluid is removed during the first 30 minutes. Removing the fluid increases the negative intrapleural pressure, which can lead to edema if the lung doesn't reexpand to fill the space. **CS2**

▶ Pleuritic or shoulder pain may indicate pleural irritation by the needle point.

▶ Pneumothorax (possibly leading to mediastinal shift and requiring chest tube insertion) can occur if the needle punctures the lung and air enters the pleural cavity. Hemoptysis may also occur if the lung is punctured.

References

Aeony, Y., et al. "Thoracentesis without Ultrasound Guidance: Infrequent Complications When Performed by an Experienced Pulmonologist," *Journal of Bronchology* 12(4):200–202, October 2005.

Feller-Kopman D., et al. "Large-Volume Thoracentesis and the Risk of Reexpansion Pulmonary Edema," *Annals of Thoracic Surgery* 84(5): 1656–61, November 2007. **CS2**

Feller-Kopman, D., et al. "The Relationship of Pleural Pressure to Symptom Development during Therapeutic Thoracentesis," *Chest* 129(6): 1556–60, June 2006.

Lynn-McHale Wiegand, D. J., and Carlson, K. K., eds. *AACN Procedure Manual for Critical Care,* 5th ed. Philadelphia: W. B. Saunders Co., 2006.

Peterson, W. G., and Zimmerman, R. "Limited Utility of Chest Radiography after Thoracentesis," *Chest* 117(4): 1038–42, April 2000. **CS1**

Rushing, J. "Assisting with Thoracentesis," *Nursing* 36(12 pt1):18, December 2006.

Thoracic drainage

Thoracic drainage uses gravity and, possibly, suction to restore negative pressure and remove any material that collects in the pleural cavity. A self-contained, disposable system combines drainage collection, a water seal, and suction into a single unit. (See *Disposable drainage systems*.)

Specifically, thoracic drainage may be ordered to remove accumulated air, fluids (blood, pus, chyle, serous fluids, gastric juices), or solids (blood clots) from the pleural cavity; to restore negative pressure in the pleural cavity; or to reexpand a partially or totally collapsed lung.

Equipment

Thoracic drainage system with tubing and connector ♦ sterile water ♦ adhesive tape ♦ two rubber-tipped Kelly clamps ♦ sterile 50-ml catheter-tip syringe ♦ suction source, if ordered.

Implementation

▶ Confirm the patient's identity using two patient identifiers according to your facility's policy. **JC**

▶ Explain the procedure to the patient, and wash your hands.

▶ Maintain sterile technique throughout the entire procedure and whenever you make changes in the system or alter any of the connections to avoid introducing pathogens into the pleural space. **CDC**

Setting up a disposable system

▶ Open the packaged system, and place it on the floor in the rack supplied by the manufacturer to avoid accidentally knocking it over or dislodging the components. After the system is prepared, it may be hung from the side of the patient's bed. **CS**

▶ Remove the plastic connector from the short tube that's attached to the water-seal chamber. Using a 50-ml catheter-tip syringe, instill sterile water into the water-seal chamber until it reaches the 2-cm mark or the mark specified by the manufacturer. Replace the plastic connector.

▶ If suction is ordered, remove the cover on the suction-control chamber to open the vent. Next, instill sterile water until it reaches the 20-cm mark or the ordered level, and recap the suction-control chamber.

▶ Using the long tube, connect the patient's chest tube to the closed drainage collection chamber. Secure the connection with tape.

▶ Connect the short tube on the drainage system to the suction source, and turn on the suction. Gentle

---

Disposable drainage systems

Commercially prepared disposable drainage systems combine drainage collection, water seal, and suction control in one unit (as shown). These systems ensure patient safety with positive- and negative-pressure relief valves and have a prominent air-leak indicator. Some systems produce no bubbling sound.

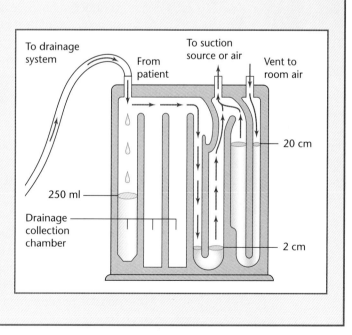

To drainage system

From patient

To suction source or air

Vent to room air

20 cm

250 ml

Drainage collection chamber

2 cm

bubbling should begin in the suction chamber, indicating that the correct suction level has been reached.

Managing closed-chest underwater seal drainage

▶ Repeatedly note the character, consistency, and amount of drainage in the drainage collection chamber.

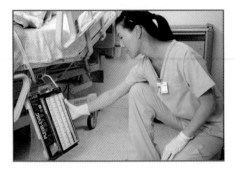

▶ Mark the drainage level in the drainage collection chamber by noting the time and date at the drainage level on the chamber every 8 hours (or more often if there's a large amount of drainage).

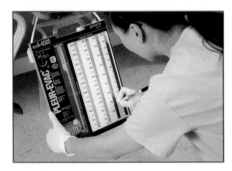

▶ Check the water level in the water-seal chamber every 8 hours. If necessary, carefully add sterile water until the level reaches the −2-cm mark indicated on the water-seal chamber of the commercial system.

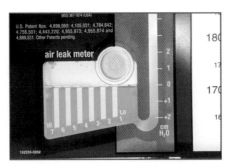

▶ Check for fluctuation in the water-seal chamber as the patient breathes. Normal fluctuations of 2″ to 4″ (5 to 10 cm) reflect pressure changes in the pleural space during respiration. To check for fluctuation when a suction system is being used, momentarily disconnect the suction system so the air vent is opened, and observe for fluctuation.

▶ Check for intermittent bubbling in the water-seal chamber. This occurs normally when the system is removing air from the pleural cavity. If bubbling isn't readily apparent during quiet breathing, have the patient take a deep breath or cough. Absence of bubbling indicates that the pleural space has sealed.

▶ Check the water level in the suction-control chamber. Detach the chamber or bottle from the suction source; when bubbling ceases, observe the water level. If necessary, add sterile water to bring the level to the −20-cm line or as ordered.

▶ Check for gentle bubbling in the suction control chamber because it indicates that the proper suction level has been reached. Vigorous bubbling in this chamber increases the rate of water evaporation.

▶ Periodically check that the air vent in the system is working properly. Occlusion of the air vent results in a buildup of pressure in the system that could cause the patient to develop a tension pneumothorax.

▶ Coil the system's tubing, and secure it to the edge of the bed. Be sure the tubing remains at the level of the patient. Avoid creating dependent loops, kinks, or pressure on the tubing. Avoid lifting the drainage system above the patient's chest because fluid may flow back into the pleural space.

▶ Be sure to keep two rubber-tipped clamps at the bedside to clamp the chest tube if system cracks or to locate an air leak in the system.

▶ Encourage the patient to cough frequently and breathe deeply to help drain the pleural space and expand the lungs.

▶ Tell him to sit upright for optimal lung expansion and to splint the insertion site while coughing to minimize pain.

▶ Check the rate and quality of the patient's respirations, and auscultate his lungs periodically to assess air exchange in the affected lung. Diminished or absent breath sounds may indicate that the lung hasn't reexpanded.

▶ Tell the patient to report breathing difficulty immediately. Notify the practitioner immediately if the patient develops cyanosis, rapid or shallow breathing, subcutaneous emphysema, chest pain, or excessive bleeding.

CLINICAL ALERT

Some facilities permit milking of tubing when clots are visible. This is a controversial procedure because it creates increased intrapleural pressure, so be sure to check your facility's policy. If permitted, gently milk the tubing in the direction of the drainage chamber when clots are visible.

▶ Check the chest tube dressing at least every 8 hours. Palpate the area surrounding the dressing for crepitus or subcutaneous emphysema, which indicates that air is leaking into the subcutaneous tissue surrounding the insertion site. Change the dressing if necessary or according to your facility's policy.

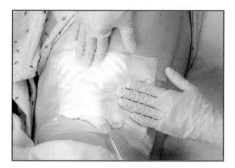

▶ Give ordered pain medication, as needed, for comfort and to help with deep-breathing, coughing, and range-of-motion exercises.

▶ Remind the ambulatory patient to keep the drainage system below chest level and to be careful not to disconnect the tubing to maintain the water seal. With a suction system, the patient must stay within range of the length of tubing attached to a wall outlet or portable pump. **CS**

Special considerations

▶ Instruct staff and visitors to avoid touching the equipment to prevent complications from separated connections.

▶ If excessive continuous bubbling is present in the water-seal chamber, especially if suction is being used, rule out a leak in the drainage system. Try to locate the leak by clamping the tube momentarily at various points along its length. Begin clamping at the tube's proximal end, and work down toward the drainage system, paying special attention to the seal around the connections. If a connection is loose, push it back together and tape it securely. The bubbling will stop when a clamp is placed between the air leak and the water seal. If you clamp along the tube's entire length and the bubbling doesn't stop, the drainage unit may be cracked and need replacement.

▶ If the drainage collection chamber fills, replace it. To do this, double-clamp the tube close to the insertion site (use two clamps facing in opposite directions), exchange the system, remove the clamps, and retape the bottle connection.

▶ If the system cracks, clamp the chest tube momentarily with the two rubber-tipped clamps at the bedside (placed there at the time of tube insertion). Place the clamps close to each other near the insertion site; they should face in opposite directions to provide a more complete seal. Observe the patient for altered respirations while the tube is clamped. Then replace the damaged equipment. (Prepare the new unit before clamping the tube.)

References

Carroll, P. "Keeping Up with Mobile Chest Drains," *RN* 68(10):26–31, October 2005.

Coughlin, A. M., and Parchinsky, C. "Go with the Flow of Chest Tube Therapy," *Nursing* 36(3):36–41, March 2006.

Lynn-McHale Wiegand, D. J., and Carlson, K. K., eds. *AACN Procedure Manual for Critical Care,* 5th ed. Philadelphia: W.B. Saunders Co., 2006.

Roman, M., and Mercado, D. "Review of Chest Tube Use," *Medsurg Nursing* 15(1):41–43, February 2006.

Schmelz, J. O., et al. "Effects of Position of Chest Drainage Tube on Volume Drained and Pressure," *American Journal of Critical Care* 8(5):319–23, September 1999. **CS**

Tracheal cuff–pressure measurement

An endotracheal (ET) or tracheostomy cuff provides a closed system for mechanical ventilation, allowing a desired tidal volume to be delivered to the patient's lungs. To function properly, the cuff must exert enough pressure on the tracheal wall to seal the airway without compromising the blood supply to the tracheal mucosa.

The ideal pressure (known as *minimal occlusive volume*) is the lowest amount needed to seal the airway. Many authorities recommend maintaining a cuff pressure lower than venous perfusion pressure—usually 20 to 25 cm H_2O. (More than 25 cm H_2O may exceed venous perfusion pressure.) **AARC** Actual cuff pressure will vary with each patient. To keep pressure within safe limits, measure minimal occlusive volume at least once each shift or as directed by your facility's policy. Cuff pressure can be measured by a respiratory therapist or by the nurse.

Equipment

10-ml syringe ◆ three-way stopcock ◆ cuff pressure manometer ◆ stethoscope ◆ suction equipment ◆ gloves.

Implementation

▶ If measuring cuff pressure with a blood pressure manometer, attach the syringe to one stopcock port; then attach the tubing from the manometer to another port of the stopcock. Turn off the stopcock port where you'll be connecting the pilot balloon cuff so that air can't escape from the cuff. Use the syringe to instill air into the manometer tubing until the pressure reading reaches 10 mm Hg. This will prevent sudden cuff deflation when you open the stopcock to the cuff and the manometer.

▶ Confirm the patient's identity using two patient identifiers according to your facility's policy. **JC**

▶ Explain the procedure to the patient.

▶ Put on gloves and suction the ET or tracheostomy tube and the patient's oropharynx to remove accumulated secretions above the cuff. **AACN** **CDC**

▶ Attach the cuff pressure manometer to the pilot balloon port.

▶ Place the diaphragm of the stethoscope over the trachea, and listen for an air leak. Keep in mind that a smooth, hollow sound indicates a sealed airway; a loud, gurgling sound indicates an air leak. **AARC**

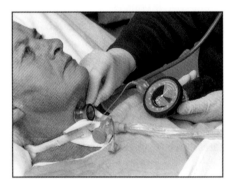

▶ If you don't hear an air leak, press the red button under the dial of the cuff pressure manometer to slowly release air from the balloon on the tracheal tube. Auscultate for an air leak.

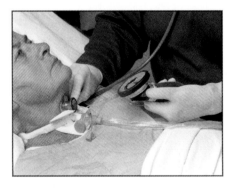

▶ As soon as you hear an air leak, release the red button, and gently squeeze the handle of the cuff pres-

sure manometer to inflate the cuff. Continue to add air to the cuff until you no longer hear an air leak.

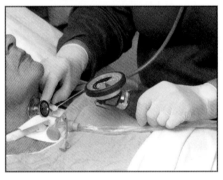

▶ When the air leak ceases, read the dial on the cuff pressure manometer. This is the minimal pressure required to effectively occlude the trachea around the tracheal tube. In many cases, this pressure will fall within the green area (20 to 25 cm H_2O) on the manometer dial.

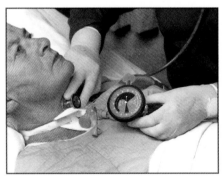

▶ Disconnect the cuff pressure manometer from the pilot balloon port. Document the pressure value.

Special considerations

▶ Measure cuff pressure at least every 8 hours. **CS**

▶ Keep in mind that some patients require less pressure, whereas others—for example, those with tracheal malacia (an abnormal softening of the tracheal tissue)—require more pressure. Maintaining the cuff pressure at the lowest possible level will minimize cuff-related problems.

▶ When measuring cuff pressure, note the volume of air needed to inflate the cuff. A gradual increase in this volume indicates tracheal dilation or erosion. A sudden increase in volume indicates rupture of the cuff and requires immediate reintubation if the patient is being ventilated.

References

Akca, O. "Endotracheal Tube Cuff Leak: Can Optimum Management of Cuff Pressure Prevent Pneumonia?" *Critical Care Medicine* 35(6):1624–26, June 2007.

Galinski, M., et al. "Intracuff Pressures of Endotracheal Tubes in the Management of Airway Emergencies: The Need for Pressure Monitoring," *Annals of Emergency Medicine* 47(6):545–47, June 2006.

Lynn-McHale Wiegand, D. J., and Carlson, K. K., eds. *AACN Procedure Manual for Critical Care,* 5th ed. Philadelphia: W.B. Saunders Co., 2006.

Tablan, O. C., et al. "Guidelines for Preventing Health-Care—Associated Pneumonia, 2003. Recommendations of CDC and the Healthcare Infection Control Practices Advisory Committee," *MMWR* 53(RR-03):1–36, March 2004.

Vyas, D., et al. "Measurement of Tracheal Tube Cuff Pressure in Critical Care," *Anaesthesia* 57(3):275–77, March 2002. **CS**

Young, P. J., et al. "A Low-Volume, Low-Pressure Tracheal Tube Cuff Reduces Pulmonary Aspiration," *Critical Care Medicine* 34(3):632–39, March 2006.

Tracheal suction

Tracheal suction involves the removal of secretions from the trachea or bronchi by means of a catheter inserted through the mouth or nose, a tracheal stoma, a tracheostomy tube, or an endotracheal (ET) tube. Besides removing secretions, tracheal suctioning also stimulates the cough reflex. This procedure helps maintain a patent airway to promote optimal exchange of oxygen and carbon dioxide and to prevent pneumonia that results from pooling of secretions. **CDC AACN** Performed as frequently as the patient's condition warrants, tracheal suction calls for strict sterile technique.

According to American Association for Respiratory Care (AARC) guidelines, before suctioning the patient, hyperoxygenate him with 100% oxygen for at least 30 seconds. Sterile technique should be employed. The duration of each suctioning should be approximately 10 to 15 seconds. Suction pressure should be set as low as possible and yet effectively clear secretions. Following suctioning, the patient should be hyperoxygenated again for 1 minute or longer by the same technique used to preoxygenate the patient. **AARC**

Perform suctioning only when necessary and when other methods of removing secretions haven't been effective. Indeed, suctioning shouldn't be performed as a routine procedure. Assess the patient for clinical signs that suctioning is necessary, such as coarse breath sounds on auscultation, noisy respirations, prolonged expiratory breath sounds, and increased or decreased heart rate, respiratory rate, or blood pressure.

Equipment

Oxygen source (mechanical ventilator, wall or portable unit, and handheld resuscitation bag with a mask, 15-mm adapter, or a positive end-expiratory pressure valve, if indicated) ◆ wall or portable suction apparatus with tubing ◆ collection container ◆ connecting tube ◆ suction catheter kit or a sterile suction catheter, one sterile glove, one clean glove, and a disposable sterile solution container ◆ 1-L bottle of sterile water or normal saline solution ◆ sterile water-soluble lubricant (for nasal insertion) ◆ syringe for deflating cuff of ET or tracheostomy tube ◆ waterproof trash bag ◆ goggles and face mask or face shield ◆ optional: sterile towel.

Implementation

▶ Choose a suction catheter of appropriate size. The diameter should be no larger than half the inside diameter of the tracheostomy or ET tube. **CS1**

▶ Place the suction apparatus on the patient's overbed table or bedside stand. Position the table or stand on your preferred side of the bed to facilitate suctioning.

▶ Attach the collection container to the suction unit and the connecting tube to the collection container.

▶ Label and date the normal saline solution or sterile water. Open the waterproof trash bag.

▶ Confirm the patient's identity using two patient identifiers according to your facility's policy. **JC**

▶ Before suctioning, determine whether your facility requires a practitioner's order, and obtain one, if necessary.

▶ Assess the patient's vital signs, breath sounds, and general appearance to establish a baseline for comparison after suctioning. Review the patient's arterial blood gas values and oxygen saturation levels if they're available. Evaluate the patient's ability to cough and deep-breathe. If you'll be performing nasotracheal suctioning, check the patient's history for a deviated septum, nasal polyps, nasal obstruction, nasal trauma, epistaxis, or mucosal swelling. **AARC**

▶ Explain the procedure to the patient even if he's unresponsive. Tell him that suctioning usually causes transient coughing or gagging but that coughing is helpful for removal of secretions. If the patient has been suctioned previously, summarize the reasons for suctioning. Continue to reassure the patient throughout the procedure to minimize anxiety, promote relaxation, and decrease oxygen demand.

▶ Unless contraindicated, place the patient in semi-Fowler's or high Fowler's position.

▶ Wash your hands. Put on personal protective equipment, as appropriate.

▶ Remove the top from the normal saline solution or water bottle.

▶ Open the package containing the sterile solution container.

► Using strict sterile technique, open the suction catheter kit, and put on the gloves. If using individual supplies, open the suction catheter and the gloves, placing the nonsterile glove on your nondominant hand and then the sterile glove on your dominant hand. **AARC** **CDC**

► Using your nondominant (nonsterile) hand, pour the normal saline solution or sterile water into the solution container.

► Place a small amount of water-soluble lubricant on the sterile area. Lubricant may be used to facilitate passage of the catheter during nasotracheal suctioning.

► Place a sterile towel over the patient's chest, if desired, to provide an additional sterile area.

► Using your dominant (sterile) hand, remove the catheter from its wrapper. Keep it coiled so it can't touch a non-sterile object. Using your other hand to manipulate the connecting tubing, attach the catheter to the tubing. **AARC**

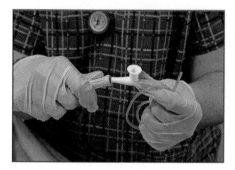

► Using your nondominant hand, set the suction pressure according to your facility's policy. Typically, pressure may be set between 100 and 150 mm Hg. Higher pressures don't enhance secretion removal and may cause traumatic injury. Occlude the suction port to assess suction pressure. **AARC**

► Dip the catheter tip in the saline solution to lubricate the outside of the catheter and reduce tissue trauma during insertion.

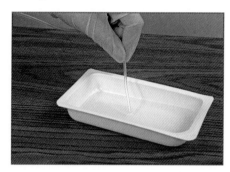

► With the catheter tip in the sterile solution, occlude the control valve with the thumb of your nondominant hand. Suction a small amount of solution through the catheter to lubricate the inside of the catheter, thus facilitating passage of secretions through it.

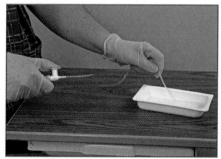

► For nasal insertion of the catheter, lubricate the tip of the catheter with the sterile, water-soluble lubricant to reduce tissue trauma during insertion. **AARC**

► If the patient isn't intubated or is intubated but isn't receiving supplemental oxygen or aerosol, instruct him to take three to six deep breaths to help minimize or prevent hypoxia during suctioning.

► If the patient isn't intubated but is receiving oxygen, evaluate his need for preoxygenation. If indicated, instruct him to take three to six deep breaths while using his supplemental oxygen.

► If the patient is being mechanically ventilated, preoxygenate him to minimize hypoxia after suctioning. Use the ventilator (rather than a handheld resuscitation bag) to hyperoxygenate and hyperinflate the lungs before suctioning. **AARC** **AACN** **CS2**

► To preoxygenate using the ventilator, first adjust the fraction of inspired oxygen (FiO_2) and tidal volume according to your facility's policy and patient need. Next, either use the sigh mode or manually deliver three to six breaths. If you have an assistant for the procedure, the assistant can manage the patient's oxygen needs while you perform the suctioning.

Nasotracheal insertion in a nonintubated patient

► Disconnect the oxygen from the patient, if applicable.

► Using your nondominant hand, raise the tip of the patient's nose to straighten the passageway and facilitate insertion of the catheter.

► Insert the catheter into the patient's nostril while gently rolling it between your fingers.

► As the patient inhales, quickly advance the catheter as far as possible. Don't apply suction during insertion. **AARC**

► If the patient coughs as the catheter passes through the larynx, briefly hold the catheter still, and then resume advancement when the patient inhales.

Insertion in an intubated patient

► If you're using a closed system, see *Closed tracheal suctioning,* page 536.

► Using your nonsterile hand, disconnect the patient from the ventilator.

► Using your sterile hand, gently insert the suction catheter into the artificial airway. Advance the catheter, without applying suction, until you

Closed tracheal suctioning

The closed tracheal suction system can ease removal of secretions and reduce patient complications. Consisting of a sterile suction catheter in a clear plastic sleeve, the system permits the patient to remain connected to the ventilator during suctioning. As a result, the patient can maintain the tidal volume, oxygen concentration, and positive end-expiratory pressure delivered by the ventilator while being suctioned. In turn, this reduces the occurrence of suction-induced hypoxemia.

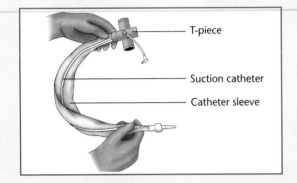

- T-piece
- Suction catheter
- Catheter sleeve

Another advantage of this system is a reduced risk of infection, even when the same catheter is used many times. **CDC** **AARC** Because the catheter remains in a protective sleeve, gloves aren't required, but are still recommended. **CDC** The caregiver doesn't need to touch the catheter, and the ventilator circuit remains closed.

Implementation

To perform the procedure, gather a closed suction control valve, a T-piece to connect the artificial airway to the ventilator breathing circuit, and a catheter sleeve that encloses the catheter and has connections at each end for the control valve and the T-piece. Put on personal protective equipment, if you haven't already done so. Then follow these steps:

▶ Remove the closed suction system from its wrapping. Attach the control valve to the connecting tubing.

▶ Depress the thumb suction control valve, and keep it depressed while setting the suction pressure to the desired level.

▶ Connect the T-piece to the ventilator breathing circuit, making sure that the irrigation port is closed; then connect the T-piece to the patient's endotracheal or tracheostomy tube (as shown above right).

▶ Hyperoxygenate the patient using the ventilator. **AARC** **AACN** **CDC**

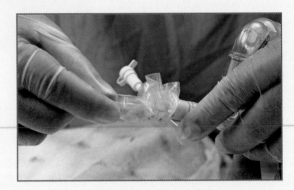

▶ With one hand keeping the T-piece parallel to the patient's chin, use the thumb and index finger of the other hand to advance the catheter through the tube and into the patient's tracheobronchial tree. It may be necessary to gently retract the catheter sleeve as you advance the catheter.

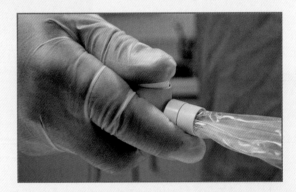

▶ While continuing to hold the T-piece and control valve, apply intermittent suction and withdraw the catheter until it reaches its fully extended length in the sleeve. Repeat the procedure, as necessary.

▶ After you've finished suctioning, flush the catheter by maintaining suction while slowly introducing normal saline solution or sterile water into the irrigation port.

▶ Place the thumb control valve in the off position.

▶ Dispose of and replace the suction equipment and supplies according to your facility's policy.

▶ Remove your gloves and wash your hands.

meet resistance. If the patient coughs, pause briefly and then resume advancement. **AARC** **AACN**

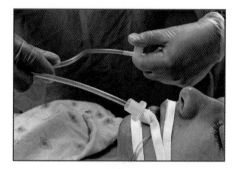

Suctioning the patient

▶ After inserting the catheter, apply suction intermittently by removing and replacing the thumb of your nondominant hand over the control valve. Simultaneously use your dominant hand to withdraw the catheter as you roll it between your thumb and forefinger. This rotating motion prevents the catheter from pulling tissue into the tube as it exits, thus avoiding tissue trauma.

▶ Never suction more than 10 to 15 seconds at a time to prevent hypoxia. Don't pass the catheter more than twice to reduce trauma to the tracheal mucosa. **AARC** **AACN**

▶ If the patient is intubated, use your nondominant hand to stabilize the tip of the ET tube as you withdraw the catheter to prevent mucous membrane irritation or accidental extubation.

▶ If applicable, resume oxygen delivery by reconnecting the source of oxygen or ventilation and hyperoxygenating the patient's lungs before continuing. **AARC** **AACN** **CS2**

▶ Observe the patient, and allow him to rest for a few minutes before the next suctioning. The timing of each suctioning and the length of each rest period depend on his tolerance of the procedure and the absence of complications. To enhance secretion removal, encourage the patient to cough between suctioning attempts.

▶ Observe the secretions. If they're thick, clear the catheter periodically by dipping the tip in the saline solution and applying suction. Normally, sputum is watery and tends to be sticky. Tenacious or thick sputum usually indicates dehydration. Watch for color variations.

▶ If the patient's heart rate and rhythm are being monitored, observe for arrhythmias. If they occur, stop suctioning and ventilate the patient.

▶ Patients who can't mobilize secretions effectively may need to perform tracheal suctioning after discharge.

After suctioning

▶ After suctioning, hyperoxygenate the patient being maintained on a ventilator by using the ventilator's sigh mode, as described earlier. **AARC** **AACN** **CS2**

▶ Readjust the FiO_2 and, for ventilated patients, the tidal volume to the ordered settings.

▶ After suctioning the lower airway, assess the patient's need for upper airway suctioning. If the cuff of the ET or tracheostomy tube is inflated, suction the upper airway before deflating the cuff with a syringe. (See "Oronasopharyngeal suction," page 362, and "Endotracheal tube care," page 177.) Always change the catheter and sterile glove before resuctioning the lower airway to avoid introducing microorganisms into the lower airway. **CDC**

▶ Discard the gloves and catheter in the waterproof trash bag. Clear the connecting tubing by aspirating the remaining saline solution or water. Discard and replace suction equipment and supplies according to your facility's policy. Wash your hands.

▶ Auscultate the lungs bilaterally and take vital signs, if indicated, to assess the procedure's effectiveness. Note the patient's skin color, breathing pattern, and respiratory rate.

Special considerations

▶ During suctioning, the catheter typically is advanced as far as the mainstem bronchi. However, because of tracheobronchial anatomy, the catheter tends to enter the right mainstem bronchi instead of the left. Using an angled catheter (such as a coudé) may help you guide the catheter into the left mainstem bronchus. Rotating the patient's head to the right seems to have a limited effect.

▶ In addition to the closed tracheal method, oxygen insufflation offers a new approach to suctioning. This method uses a double-lumen catheter that allows oxygen insufflation during the suctioning procedure.

▶ Don't allow the collection container on the suction machine to become more than three-quarters full to keep from damaging the machine.

▶ Because oxygen is removed along with secretions, the patient may experience hypoxemia and dyspnea. Anxiety may alter respiratory patterns. Cardiac arrhythmias can result from hypoxia and stimulation of the vagus nerve in the tracheobronchial tree.

▶ If the patient experiences laryngospasm or bronchospasm (rare complications) during suctioning, disconnect the suction catheter from the connecting tubing, and allow the catheter to act as an airway. Discuss with the patient's practitioner the use of bronchodilators or lidocaine to reduce the risk of this complication.

EVIDENCE-BASED RESEARCH

Pain with tracheal suctioning

Arroyo-Novoa, C.M., et al. "Pain Related to Tracheal Suctioning in Awake Acutely and Critically Ill Adults: A Descriptive Study," *Intensive and Critical Care Nursing* 24(1):20–27, February 2008.

Level VI: Evidence from a single descriptive or qualitative study

Description
Tracheal suctioning is performed on most critically ill patients and many acutely ill patients. The Centers for Disease Control and Prevention recommend tracheal suctioning as a method of decreasing ventilator-associated pneumonias. Many nurses think of tracheal suctioning as a painless procedure, which they routinely perform many times a day. This study analyzed findings from a larger pain study and looked specifically at factors that related to pain during tracheal suctioning.

A total of 755 patients had tracheal suctioning performed, with 93% of them in a critical care unit. A 0 to 10 pain rating scale, a modified McGill Pain Questionnaire-Short Form, and a behavioral observation tool were used to assess the patient's pain.

Findings
Pain intensity scores were much higher during tracheal suctioning than prior to or after the procedure. Very few patients in the study received an analgesic before the procedure. The highest pain ratings were in surgical, younger, and non-white patients. More than half the patients reported moderate-to-severe pain levels during the procedure.

Conclusion
Pain management must be tailored to the individual patient's needs as they undergo painful procedures, such as tracheal suctioning. And nurses must be mindful that procedures such as tracheal suctioning may cause the patient higher than normal levels of pain.

Nursing practice implications:
Because nurses often suction patients, they need to be aware of the patient's pain level before, during, and after tracheal suctioning. Here are some important nursing practice implications to keep in mind:
► Assess your patient's pain before and after tracheal suctioning.
► Describe the procedure to the patient so he knows what to expect.
► Administer pain medication during suctioning, as needed.
► Suction as often as needed, but don't suction the patient unnecessarily.

References

American Association for Respiratory Care. "AARC Clinical Practice Guideline: Endotracheal Suctioning of Mechanically Ventilated Adults and Children with Artificial Airways," *Respiratory Care* 38(5):500–504, May 1993.

American Association for Respiratory Care. "AARC Clinical Practice Guidelines: Suctioning of the Patient in the Home," *Respiratory Care* 44(1):99–104, January 1999.

Chluay, M. "Arterial Blood Gas Changes with a Hyperinflation and Hyperoxygenation Suctioning Intervention in Critically Ill Patients," *Heart & Lung* 17(6 Pt 1):654–61, November 1988 **CS2**

Henneman, E., et al., eds. *AACN Protocols for Practice: Care of the Mechanically Ventilated Patient Series.* Aliso Viejo, Ca.: American Association of Critical-Care Nurses, 2006.

The Joanna Briggs Institute. "Best Practice: Tracheal Suctioning of Adults with an Artificial Airway," 4(4):106, 2000. Available at *www.joannabriggs.edu.au/bpmenu/html.*

Lorente, L., et al. "Tracheal Suction by Closed System without Daily Change versus Open System," *Intensive Care Medicine* 32(4):538–44, April 2006.

Lorente, L., et al. "Ventilator-associated Pneumonia Using a Closed versus an Open Tracheal Suction System," *Critical Care Medicine* 33(1):115–19, January 2005.

Lynn-McHale Wiegand, D. J., and Carlson, K. K, eds. *AACN Procedure Manual for Critical Care,* 5th ed. Philadelphia: W. B. Saunders Co., 2006.

Shah, S., et al. "An In Vitro Evaluation of the Effectiveness of Endotracheal Suction Catheters," *Chest* 128(5): 3699–704, November 2005.

Tablan, O. C., et al. "Guidelines for Preventing Health-Care—Associated Pneumonia, 2003. Recommendations of CDC and the Healthcare Infection Control Practices Advisory Committee," *MMWR* 53(RR-03):1–36, March 2004.

Taylor, C., et al. *Fundamentals of Nursing: The Art and Science of Nursing Care,* 5th ed. Philadelphia: Lippincott Williams & Wilkins, 2008.

Vanner, R., and Bick, E. "Tracheal Pressures during Open Suctioning," *Anaesthesia* 63(3):313–15, March 2008. **CS1**

Tracheotomy

A tracheotomy involves the surgical creation of an external opening—called a *tracheostomy*—into the trachea and insertion of an indwelling tube to maintain the airway's patency. If all other attempts to establish an airway have failed, a practitioner may perform a tracheotomy at a patient's bedside. This procedure may be necessary when an airway obstruction results from laryngeal edema, foreign body obstruction, or a tumor. An emergency tracheotomy may also be performed when endotracheal intubation is contraindicated.

Use of a cuffed tracheostomy tube provides and maintains a patent airway, prevents the unconscious or paralyzed patient from aspirating food or secretions, allows removal of tracheobronchial secretions from the patient unable to cough, replaces an endotracheal tube, and permits the use of positive-pressure ventilation. Although tracheostomy tubes come in plastic and metal, plastic tubes are much more commonly used because they have a universal adapter for respiratory support equipment, such as a mechanical ventilator, and a cuff to allow positive-pressure ventilation.

Equipment

Tracheostomy tube of the proper size (usually #13 to #38 French or #00 to #9 Jackson) with obturator ◆ sterile tracheotomy tray (usually contains tracheal dilator, vein retractor, hemostats, and clamps) ◆ sutures and needles ◆ 4″ × 4″ gauze pads ◆ sterile drapes, gloves, mask, and gown ◆ sterile bowls ◆ stethoscope ◆ dressing ◆ pillow ◆ tracheostomy ties ◆ suction apparatus and tubing ◆ alcohol pad ◆ antiseptic solution ◆ sterile water ◆ 5-ml syringe with 22G needle ◆ local anesthetic such as lidocaine ◆ oxygen therapy device ◆ oxygen source ◆ syringe.

Implementation

▶ Wash your hands; then, maintaining sterile technique, open the tray. **CDC**
▶ Take the tracheostomy tube from its container, and place it on the sterile field. If necessary, set up the suction equipment, and make sure it works.
▶ When the physician opens the sterile bowls, pour in the antiseptic solution.

▶ Confirm the patient's identity using two patient identifiers according to your facility's policy. **JC**
▶ Sedate the patient, as ordered.
▶ Explain the procedure to the patient even if he's unresponsive.
▶ Assess his condition and provide privacy. Maintain ventilation until the tracheotomy is performed.
▶ Before the physician begins, place a pillow under the patient's shoulders and neck, and hyperextend his neck.
▶ Wipe the top of the local anesthetic vial with an alcohol pad. Invert the vial so that the physician can withdraw the anesthetic using the 22G needle attached to the 5-ml syringe.
▶ The physician will put on a sterile gown, gloves, and mask. **CDC**
▶ Help the physician with the tube insertion, as needed. (See *Assisting with a tracheotomy,* page 540.)
▶ When the tube is in position, attach it to the appropriate oxygen therapy device.
▶ Inject air into the distal cuff port to inflate the cuff.
▶ The physician will suture the corners of the incision.
▶ Put on sterile gloves.

▶ Apply the sterile tracheostomy dressing under the tracheostomy tube flange. Place the tracheostomy ties through the openings of the tube flanges, and tie them on the side of the patient's neck. This allows easy access and prevents pressure necrosis at the back of the neck.
▶ Clean or dispose of the used equipment according to your facility's policy. Replenish all supplies, as needed.
▶ Make sure a chest X-ray is ordered to confirm tube placement.

Special considerations

▶ Assess the patient's vital signs and respiratory status every 15 minutes for 1 hour, then every 30 minutes for 2 hours, and then every 2 hours until his condition is stable.
▶ Monitor the patient carefully for signs of infection. Ideally, the tracheotomy should be performed using sterile technique, as described. But, in an emergency, this may not be possible.

Assisting with a tracheotomy

To perform a tracheotomy, the physician will first clean the area from the chin to the nipples with antiseptic solution. Next, he'll place sterile drapes on the patient and locate the area for the incision—usually 1 to 2 cm below the cricoid cartilage. Then he'll inject a local anesthetic.

He'll make a horizontal or vertical incision in the skin. (A vertical incision helps avoid arteries, veins, and nerves on the lateral borders of the trachea.) Then he'll dissect subcutaneous fat and muscle and move the muscle aside with vein retractors to locate the tracheal rings. He'll make an incision between the second and third tracheal rings (as shown top right) and use hemostats to control bleeding.

He'll inject a local anesthetic into the tracheal lumen to suppress the cough reflex, and then he'll create a stoma in the trachea. When this is done, carefully apply suction to remove blood and secretions that may obstruct the airway or be aspirated into the lungs. The physician then inserts the tracheostomy tube and obturator into the stoma (as shown middle right). After inserting the tube, he'll remove the obturator.

Apply a sterile tracheostomy dressing, and anchor the tube with tracheostomy ties (as shown below right). Check for air movement through the tube, and auscultate the lungs to ensure proper placement.

An alternative approach

In another approach, the physician inserts the tracheostomy tube percutaneously at the bedside. Using either a series of dilators or a pair of forceps, he creates a stoma for tube insertion. Unlike the surgical technique, this method dilates rather than cuts the tissue structures.

After the skin is prepared and anesthetized, the physician makes a 1-cm midline incision. When the stoma reaches the desired size, the physician inserts the tracheostomy tube. When the tube is in place, inflate the cuff, secure the tube, and check the patient's breath sounds.

Incision site

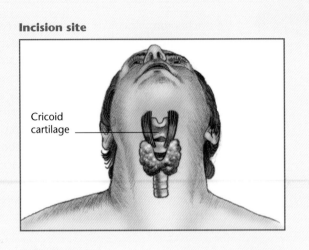

Cricoid cartilage

Tube insertion

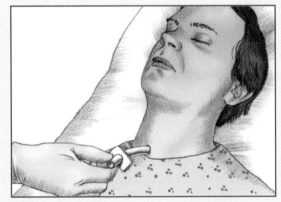

Sterile dressing

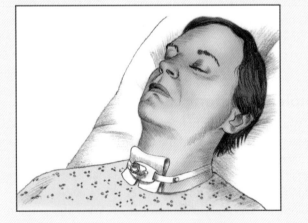

▶ Make sure the following equipment is always at the patient's bedside:

— suctioning equipment because the patient may need his airway cleared at any time

— sterile obturator used to insert the tracheostomy tube in case the tube is expelled

— sterile tracheostomy tube and obturator (the same size as the one used) in case the tube must be replaced quickly

— spare, sterile inner cannula that can be used if the cannula is expelled

— sterile tracheostomy tube and obturator one size smaller than the one used, which may be needed if the tube is expelled and the trachea begins to close

— sterile tracheal dilator or sterile hemostats to maintain an open airway before inserting a new tracheostomy tube.

▶ Review emergency first-aid measures, and always follow your facility's policy concerning an expelled or blocked tracheostomy tube. When a blocked tube can't be cleared by suctioning or withdrawing the inner cannula, policy may require you to stay with the patient while someone else calls the physician or the appropriate code. You should continue trying to ventilate the patient with whatever method works—for example, a hand-held resuscitation bag. Don't remove the tracheostomy tube entirely; doing so may close the airway completely.

▶ Use extreme caution if you try to reinsert an expelled tracheostomy tube to avoid tracheal trauma, perforation, compression, and asphyxiation.

References

Barquist, E. S., et al. "Tracheostomy in Ventilator-Dependent Trauma Patients: A Prospective, Randomized Intention-to-Treat Study," *Journal of Trauma* 60(1):90–97, January 2006.

Beiderlinden, M., et al. "Risk Factors Associated with Bleeding during and after Percutaneous Dilational Tracheostomy," *Anaesthesia* 62(4):342–46, April 2007.

Lynn-McHale Wiegand, D. J., and Carlson, K. K., eds. *AACN Procedure Manual for Critical Care,* 5th ed. Philadelphia: W. B. Saunders Co., 2006.

Miller, C. D. "Difficult Airway Society Guidelines," *Anaesthesia* 59(12): 1246–247, December 2004.

Silvester, W., et al. "Percutaneous versus Surgical Tracheostomy: A Randomized Controlled Study with Long-Term Follow-Up," *Critical Care Medicine* 34(8):2145–152, August 2006.

Tracheostomy and ventilator speaking valve

Patients with a tracheostomy tube can't speak because the cuffed tracheostomy tube that directs air into the lungs on inspiration expels air through the tracheostomy tube rather than the vocal cords, mouth, and nose. Therefore, providing a means of nonverbal communication for such patients is crucial for their physical and emotional well-being as well as that of family members and hospital personnel.

Traditional methods of communication have included writing, lip-reading, alphabet boards, and gestures. However, there's a positive-closure, one-way speaking valve that's available. The Passy-Muir Tracheostomy and Ventilator Speaking Valve (PMV) opens upon inspiration to allow the patient to inspire through the tracheostomy tube. It closes after inspiration, redirecting the exhaled air around the tube, through the vocal cords, and out the mouth, thus allowing the patient to speak. Short- and long-term adult, pediatric, and infant tracheostomy and ventilator-dependent patients may benefit from the use of a PMV. PMV use is contraindicated in patients with severe tracheal or laryngeal stenosis, laryngectomy, or excessive oral secretions and in patients who are unconscious or at risk for gross aspiration.

To function safely, the tracheostomy cuff must be completely deflated to enable the patient to exhale, or the tracheostomy tube must be cuffless. For maximum airflow around the tube, the tube should be no larger than two-thirds the size of the tracheal lumen.

The PMV 005 is most commonly used by nonventilated tracheostomy patients, but it can be used by ventilator patients with rubber, nondisposable ventilator tubing. The PMV 007 fits easily into the ventilator tubing used by medically ventilated tracheostomy patients. Both valves fit the 15-mm hub of adult, pediatric, and neonatal tracheostomy tubes and can be used by patients either on or off the ventilator.

Equipment

Appropriately sized PMV ◆ gloves ◆ suction equipment ◆ 10-ml luer-lock syringe ◆ instruction booklet.

Implementation

▶ Confirm the patient's identity using two patient identifiers according to your facility's policy. **JC**

▶ Elevate the head of the patient's bed about 45 degrees.

▶ The tracheostomy cuff must be completely deflated before the valve is placed. **MFR**

▶ Put on gloves and deflate the cuff slowly so the patient can get used to using his upper airways again. Attach a 10-ml syringe to the tracheostomy tube's pilot balloon, and remove the air until air can no longer be extracted and a vacuum is created.

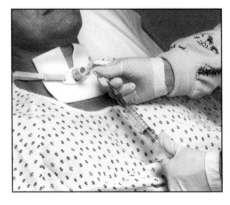

▶ Suction the trachea and oral cavity, as needed.

▶ Hold the valve between your fingers. For a patient who isn't ventilator-dependent, attach the valve to the hub of the existing tracheostomy hub with a quarter-turn twist.

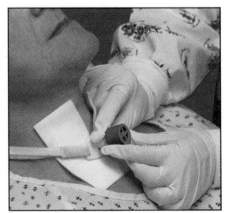

▶ After the valve is in place, encourage the patient to relax and concentrate on exhaling through his mouth and nose. Have him count aloud to 10, or speak, as he becomes comfortable breathing with the valve in place. The speech-language pathologist can facilitate voice production and speech.

▶ The aqua-colored PMV 007 is more convenient for ventilator-dependent patients because it's tapered to fit into disposable ventilator tubing. Insert the PMV into the end of the wide-mouth, short-flex tubing.

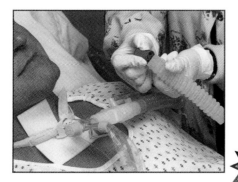

▶ Connect the other end of the short-flex tubing to the ventilator tubing. Then attach the PMV (connected to the short-flex tubing) and the ventilator tubing to the closed-suction system.

▶ The PMV can also be attached between the swivel adapter and the short-flex tubing and ventilator tubing.

▶ Post cuff-deflation warning signs in the room, and label the tracheostomy pilot balloon to remind health care providers to reinflate the pilot balloon after removing the PMV.

▶ Gently twist the PMV to remove it; restore the original setup, then return ventilator settings to original levels and reinflate the pilot balloon cuff. Always remember to reinflate the tracheostomy cuff after removing the PMV.

Special considerations

▶ For maximum airflow around the tube, the tube shouldn't be larger than two-thirds the size of the tracheal lumen.

CLINICAL ALERT

Don't place the PMV on the tracheostomy tube before deflating the cuff because the patient won't be able to breathe.

▶ The nurse and respiratory therapist are responsible for monitoring the patient's response to the PMV by evaluating blood pressure, heart rate, and respiratory status.

▶ Make sure that the patient is involved in the decision to use the ventilator speaking valve; make sure he understands how it functions and what to expect.

▶ If he's anxious, especially during cuff deflation, he may be unwilling

to use the valve; provide emotional support.

▶ If he can't tolerate the valve initially, troubleshoot to determine the cause.

▶ To correct, try repositioning the patient, using a smaller tracheostomy tube, changing to a cuffless tube, or correcting airway obstruction. Some patients have to build tolerance, wearing the valve a few minutes at a time at first.

▶ If repeated trials fail, the speech-language pathologist should assess the patient for other communication options.

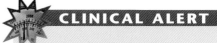

CLINICAL ALERT

Remove the PMV if the patient shows signs of distress, including significant change in blood pressure or heart rate, increased respiratory rate, dyspnea, diaphoresis, anxiety, uncontrollable coughing, or arterial oxygen saturation less than 90%. Reassess the patient before trying the valve again.

References

Hess, D. R. "Facilitating Speech in the Patient with a Tracheostomy," *Respiratory Care* 50(4):519–25, April 2005.

Hull, E. M., et al. "Tracheostomy Speaking Valves for Children: Tolerance and Clinical Benefit," *Pediatric Rehabilitation* 8(3):214–19, July–September 2005.

Tracheostomy care

Whether a tracheotomy is performed in an emergency situation or after careful preparation, as a permanent measure or as temporary therapy, tracheostomy care has identical goals: to ensure airway patency by keeping the tube free of mucus buildup, to maintain mucous membrane and skin integrity, to prevent infection, and to provide psychological support.

The patient may have one of three types of tracheostomy tube—uncuffed, cuffed, or fenestrated. Tube selection depends on the patient's condition and the practitioner's preference. (See *Types of tracheostomy tubes.*)

An uncuffed tube, which may be plastic or metal, allows air to flow freely around the tracheostomy tube and through the larynx, thus reducing the risk of tracheal damage. A cuffed tube, made of plastic, is disposable. A plastic fenestrated tube permits speech through the upper airway when the external opening is capped and the cuff is deflated. It also allows easy removal of the inner cannula for cleaning. However, a fenestrated tube may become occluded.

Tracheostomy care should be performed using aseptic technique until the stoma has healed to prevent infection. For recently performed tracheotomies—less than 7 days postoperatively—or unhealed tracheostomies, the site should be assessed at least every 4 hours, and the stoma should be cleaned and redressed every 8 hours. Tracheostomy care should be performed at least every shift on a healed tracheostomy. Sterile gloves should be worn for all manipulations at the tracheostomy site. After the stoma has healed, clean gloves may be substituted for sterile ones.

Equipment

For sterile stoma and outer-cannula care: Waterproof trash bag ◆ two sterile solution containers ◆ normal saline solution ◆ hydrogen peroxide ◆ sterile cotton-tipped applicators ◆ sterile 4″ × 4″ gauze pads ◆ sterile gloves ◆ prepackaged sterile tracheostomy dressing (or 4″ × 4″ gauze pad) ◆ equipment and supplies for suctioning and for mouth care ◆ water-soluble lubricant or topical antibiotic cream ◆ materials, as needed, for cuff procedures and for changing tracheostomy ties (see below).

For sterile inner-cannula care: All of the preceding equipment plus a prepackaged commercial tracheostomy-care set, or sterile forceps ◆ sterile nylon brush ◆ sterile 6″ (15.2-cm) pipe cleaners ◆ clean gloves ◆ a third sterile solution container ◆ disposable temporary inner cannula.

For changing tracheostomy ties: 30″ (76.2-cm) length of tracheostomy twill tape ◆ bandage scissors ◆ sterile gloves ◆ hemostat.

For emergency tracheostomy tube replacement: Sterile tracheal dilator or sterile hemostat ◆ sterile obturator that fits the tracheostomy tube in use ◆ two extra sterile tracheostomy tube and obturator in appropriate size ◆ suction equipment and supplies.

Keep these supplies in full view in the patient's room at all times for easy access in case of emergency. Consider taping an emergency sterile tracheostomy tube in a sterile wrapper to the head of the bed for easy access in an emergency.

For cuff procedures: 5- or 10-ml syringe ◆ padded hemostat ◆ stethoscope.

Implementation

▶ Wash your hands, and assemble all equipment and supplies in the patient's room. **CDC**

▶ Check the expiration date on each sterile package, and inspect the package for tears. Open the waterproof trash bag, and place it next to you.

▶ Establish a sterile field near the patient's bed (usually on the overbed table), and place equipment and supplies on it. Pour normal saline solution, hydrogen peroxide, or a mixture of equal parts of both solutions into one of the sterile solution containers; then pour normal saline solution into the second sterile container for rinsing.

Types of tracheostomy tubes

There are advantages and disadvantages to cuffed and uncuffed tracheostomy tubes. Cuffed tubes (shown below) help seal that area between the tube and trachea, decreasing the patient's risk of aspiration. However, if the cuff pressure isn't regularly monitored, it may erode the trachea. Also, if the cuff is inflated, the patient can't talk and needs an alternate means of communication.

Uncuffed tubes (shown below) allow the patient to eat and talk. However, this type of tube can't be used in a patient who's receiving mechanical ventilation because oxygen may escape from around the tube.

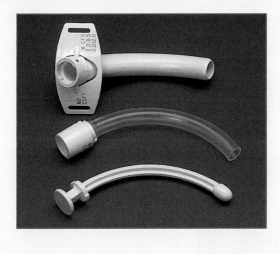

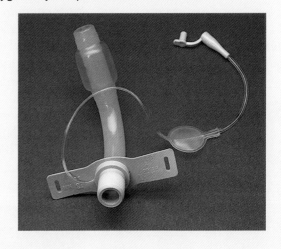

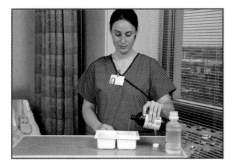

▶ For inner-cannula care, you may use a third sterile solution container to hold the gauze pads and cotton-tipped applicators saturated with cleaning solution. If you'll be replacing the disposable inner cannula, open the package containing the new inner cannula while maintaining sterile technique. Obtain or prepare new tracheostomy ties, if indicated.

▶ Confirm the patient's identity using two patient identifiers according to your facility's policy. **JC**
▶ Assess the patient's condition to determine his need for care.
▶ Explain the procedure to the patient even if he's unresponsive. Provide privacy.

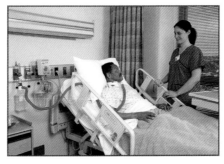

▶ Place the patient in semi-Fowler's position (unless it's contraindicated) to promote lung expansion.

▶ Remove any humidification or ventilation device.

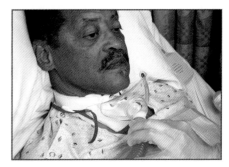

▶ If the patient is being mechanically ventilated, administer hyperoxygenation and hyperinflation using the ventilator settings. If he's breathing on his own, evaluate the need for preoxygenation and instruct him to take deep breaths. **AARC AACN**

▶ Using sterile technique, suction the entire length of the tracheostomy tube to clear the airway of any secretions that may hinder oxygenation. (See "Tracheal suction," page 534.) **AARC CDC**

▶ Reconnect the patient to the humidifier or ventilator, if necessary.

Cleaning a stoma and outer cannula

▶ Put on sterile gloves.

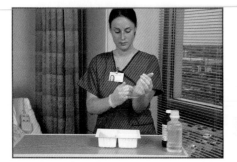

▶ With your dominant hand, saturate a sterile gauze pad with the cleaning solution. Squeeze out the excess liquid to prevent accidental aspiration. Then wipe the patient's neck under the tracheostomy tube flanges and twill tapes.

▶ Saturate a second pad, and wipe until the skin around the tracheostomy is cleaned. Use more pads or cotton-tipped applicators to clean the stoma site and the tube's flanges. Wipe only once with each pad, and then discard it to prevent contamination of a clean area with a soiled pad. **CDC**

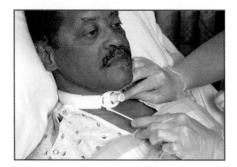

▶ Rinse debris and peroxide (if used) with one or more sterile 4″ × 4″ gauze

pads dampened in normal saline solution. Dry the area thoroughly with additional sterile gauze pads; then apply a new sterile tracheostomy dressing.

▶ Remove and discard your gloves.

Cleaning a nondisposable inner cannula

▶ Put on sterile gloves.

▶ Using your nondominant hand, remove and discard the patient's tracheostomy dressing. Then, with the same hand, disconnect the ventilator or humidification device, and unlock the tracheostomy tube's inner cannula by rotating it counterclockwise. Place the inner cannula in the container of hydrogen peroxide.

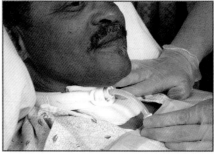

▶ Working quickly, use your dominant hand to scrub the cannula with the sterile nylon brush. If the brush doesn't slide easily into the cannula, use a sterile pipe cleaner.

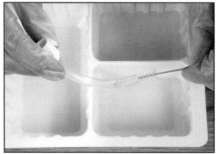

▶ Immerse the cannula in the container of normal saline solution, and agitate it for about 10 seconds to rinse it thoroughly.

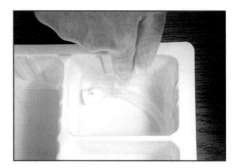

▶ Inspect the cannula for cleanliness. Repeat the cleaning process if necessary. If it's clean, tap it gently against the inside edge of the sterile container to remove excess liquid and prevent aspiration. Don't dry the outer surface because a thin film of moisture acts as a lubricant during insertion.

▶ Reinsert the inner cannula into the patient's tracheostomy tube. Lock it in place, and then gently pull on it to make sure it's positioned securely. Reconnect the mechanical ventilator. Apply a new sterile tracheostomy dressing.

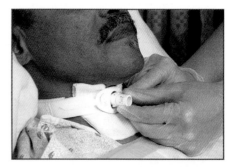

▶ If the patient can't tolerate being disconnected from the ventilator for the time it takes to clean the inner cannula, replace the existing inner cannula with a clean one, and reattach the mechanical ventilator. Then clean the cannula just removed from the patient, and store it in a sterile container the next time.

Caring for a disposable inner cannula

▶ Put on clean gloves.

▶ Using your dominant hand, remove the patient's inner cannula. After evaluating the secretions in the cannula, discard it properly.

▶ Pick up the new inner cannula, touching only the outer locking portion. Insert the cannula into the tracheostomy and, following the manufacturer's instructions, lock it securely.

Changing tracheostomy ties

▶ Change the ties as necessary and when soiled after the first change by the surgeon.

▶ Obtain assistance from another nurse or a respiratory therapist because of the risk of accidental tube expulsion during this procedure. Patient movement or coughing can dislodge the tube.

▶ Wash your hands thoroughly, and put on sterile gloves.

▶ If you aren't using commercially packaged tracheostomy ties, prepare new ties from a 30″ (76.2-cm) length of twill tape by folding one end back 1″ (2.5 cm) on itself. Then, with the bandage scissors, cut a ½″ (1.3-cm) slit down the center of the tape from the folded edge.

▶ Prepare the other end of the tape the same way.

▶ Hold both ends together and, using scissors, cut the resulting circle of tape so that one piece is approximately 10″ (25 cm) long and the other is about 20″ (51 cm) long.

▶ Help the patient into semi-Fowler's position if possible.

▶ After your assistant puts on gloves, instruct her to hold the tracheostomy tube in place to prevent its expulsion during replacement of the ties. If you must perform the procedure without

assistance, fasten the clean ties in place before removing the old ties to prevent tube expulsion.

▶ With the assistant's gloved fingers holding the tracheostomy tube in place, cut the soiled tracheostomy ties with the bandage scissors, or untie them and discard the ties. Be careful not to cut the tube of the pilot balloon.

▶ Thread the slit end of one new tie a short distance through the eye of one tracheostomy tube flange from the underside; use the hemostat, if needed, to pull the tie through. Then thread the other end of the tie completely through the slit end, and pull it taut so it loops firmly through the flange. This avoids knots that can cause throat discomfort, tissue irritation, pressure, and necrosis at the patient's throat.

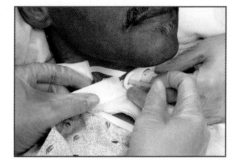

▶ Fasten the second tie to the opposite flange in the same manner.

▶ Instruct the patient to flex his neck while you bring the ties around to the side, and tie them together with a square knot. Flexion produces the same neck circumference as coughing and helps prevent an overly tight tie. Instruct your assistant to place one finger under the tapes as you tie them to ensure that they're tight enough to avoid slippage but loose enough to prevent choking or jugular vein constriction. Placing the closure on the side allows easy access and prevents pressure necrosis at the back of the neck when the patient is recumbent.

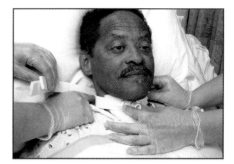

▶ After securing the ties, cut off the excess tape with the scissors, and instruct your assistant to release the tracheostomy tube.

▶ Make sure the patient is comfortable and can reach the call button easily.

▶ Check tracheostomy-tie tension often on patients with traumatic injury, radical neck dissection, or cardiac failure because neck diameter can increase from swelling and cause constriction; also check neonatal or restless patients frequently because ties can loosen and cause tube dislodgment.

Concluding tracheostomy care

▶ Replace any humidification device. `AARC`

▶ Provide oral care, as needed, because the oral cavity can become dry and malodorous or develop sores from encrusted secretions.

▶ Observe soiled dressings and any suctioned secretions for amount, color, consistency, and odor.

▶ Properly clean or dispose of all equipment, supplies, solutions, and trash according to policy.

▶ Take off and discard your gloves.

▶ Make sure the patient is comfortable and that he can easily reach the call button.

▶ Make sure all necessary supplies are readily available at the bedside.

▶ Repeat the procedure at least once every 8 hours or as needed. Change the dressing as often as necessary regardless of whether you also perform the entire cleaning procedure because a wet dressing with exudate or secretions predisposes the patient to skin excoriation, breakdown, and infection. **CDC**

Deflating and inflating a tracheostomy cuff

▶ Read the cuff manufacturer's instructions because cuff types and procedures vary widely. **MFR**

▶ Assess the patient's condition, explain the procedure to him, and reassure him. Wash your hands thoroughly.

▶ Help the patient into semi-Fowler's position, if possible, or place him in a supine position.

▶ Suction the oropharyngeal cavity to prevent pooled secretions from descending into the trachea after cuff deflation. **AARC** **CDC**

▶ Release the padded hemostat clamping the cuff inflation tubing, if a hemostat is present.

▶ Insert a 5- or 10-ml syringe into the cuff pilot balloon, and slowly withdraw all air from the cuff. Leave the syringe attached to the tubing for later reinflation of the cuff. Slow deflation allows positive lung pressure to push secretions upward from the bronchi. Cuff deflation may also stimulate the patient's cough reflex, producing additional secretions.

▶ Remove any ventilation device. Suction the lower airway through any existing tube to remove all secretions. Then reconnect the patient to the ventilation device.

▶ While the cuff is deflated, observe the patient for adequate ventilation, and suction as necessary. If the patient has difficulty breathing, reinflate the cuff immediately by depressing the syringe plunger very slowly. Inject the least amount of air necessary to achieve an adequate tracheal seal.

▶ When inflating the cuff, you may use the minimal-leak technique or the minimal occlusive volume technique to help gauge the proper inflation point. (For more information, see "Endotracheal intubation," page 170, and "Endotracheal tube care," page 177.)

▶ If you're inflating the cuff using cuff pressure measurement, be careful not to exceed 25 mm Hg. If pressure exceeds 25 mm Hg, notify the practitioner because you may need to change to a larger size tube, use higher inflation pressures, or permit a larger air leak. Recommended cuff pressure is about 18 mm Hg. **AARC**

▶ After you've inflated the cuff, if the tubing doesn't have a one-way valve at the end, clamp the inflation line with a padded hemostat (to protect the tubing), and remove the syringe.

▶ Check for a minimal-leak cuff seal. You shouldn't feel air coming from the patient's mouth, nose, or tracheostomy site, and a conscious patient shouldn't be able to speak.

▶ Be alert for air leaks from the cuff itself. Suspect a leak if injection of air fails to inflate the cuff or increase cuff pressure, if you're unable to inject the amount of air you withdrew, if the patient can speak, if ventilation fails to maintain adequate respiratory movement with pressures or volumes previously considered adequate, or if air escapes during the ventilator's inspiratory cycle.

▶ Note the exact amount of air used to inflate the cuff to detect tracheal malacia if more air is consistently needed. **AARC**

▶ Make sure the patient is comfortable and can easily reach the call button and communication aids.

▶ Properly clean or dispose of all equipment, supplies, and trash according to your facility's policy.

▶ Replenish any used supplies, and make sure all necessary emergency supplies are at the bedside.

Special considerations

▶ Keep appropriate equipment at the patient's bedside for immediate use in an emergency. (For a list, see "Tracheotomy," page 539.)

▶ Consult the practitioner about first-aid measures you can use for your tracheostomy patient should an emergency occur. Follow your facility's policy regarding procedure if a tracheostomy tube is expelled or if the outer cannula becomes blocked. Don't remove the tracheostomy tube entirely because this may allow the airway to close completely. Use extreme caution when attempting to reinsert an expelled tracheostomy tube because of the risk of tracheal trauma, perforation, compression, and asphyxiation.

▶ Refrain from changing tracheostomy ties unnecessarily during the immediate postoperative period before the stoma track is well formed (usually 4 days) to avoid accidental dislodgment and expulsion of the tube. Unless secretions or drainage is a problem, ties can be changed once per day.

▶ If the patient's neck or stoma is excoriated or infected, apply a water-soluble lubricant or topical antibiotic cream, as ordered. Remember not to use a powder or an oil-based substance on or around a stoma because aspiration can cause infection and abscess.

References

Crimslick, J. T., et al. "Standardizing Adult Tracheostomy Tube Styles: What Is the Clinical and Cost-Effective Impact?" *Dimensions of Critical Care Nursing* 25(1):35–43, January–February 2006.

Dhand, R., and Johnson, J. C. "Care of the Chronic Tracheostomy," *Respiratory Care* 51(9):984–1001, September 2006.

Dodek, P., et al. "Evidence-Based Clinical Practice Guideline for the Prevention of Ventilator-Associated Pneumonia," *Annals of Internal Medicine* 141(4): 305–13, August 2004.

Feber, T. "Tracheostomy Care for Community Nurses: Basic Principles," *British Journal of Community Nursing* 11(5): 186,188–90, 192–93, May 2006.

Lynn-McHale Wiegand, D. J., and Carlson, K. K., eds. *AACN Procedure Manual for Critical Care,* 5th ed. Philadelphia: W. B. Saunders Co., 2006.

Russel, C. "Providing the Nurse with a Guide to Tracheostomy Care and Management," *British Journal of Nursing* 14(8):428–33, April–May 2005.

Taylor, C., et al. *Fundamentals of Nursing: The Art and Science of Nursing Care,* 5th ed. Philadelphia: Lippincott Williams & Wilkins, 2008.

Transabdominal tube feeding and care

To access the stomach, duodenum, or jejunum, the physician may place a tube through the patient's abdominal wall. This procedure may be done surgically or percutaneously.

The tube may be used for feeding during the immediate postoperative period, or it may provide long-term enteral access, depending on the type of surgery. Typically, the physician will suture the tube in place to prevent gastric contents from leaking.

In contrast, a percutaneous endoscopic gastrostomy (PEG) or jejunostomy (PEJ) tube can be inserted endoscopically without the need for laparotomy or general anesthesia. Typically, the insertion is done in the endoscopy suite or at the patient's bedside. A PEG or PEJ tube may be used for nutrition, drainage, and decompression. Contraindications to endoscopic placement include obstruction (such as an esophageal stricture or duodenal blockage), previous gastric surgery, morbid obesity, and ascites. These conditions would necessitate surgical placement.

With either type of tube placement, feedings may begin after 24 hours (or when peristalsis resumes).

After a time, the tube may need replacement, and the physician may recommend a similar tube, such as an indwelling urinary catheter or a mushroom catheter, or a gastrostomy button—a skin-level feeding tube. (See "Gastrostomy feeding button care," page 219.)

Nursing care includes providing skin care at the tube site, maintaining the feeding tube, administering feeding, monitoring the patient's response to feeding, adjusting the feeding schedule, and preparing the patient for self-care after discharge.

Equipment

For feeding: Feeding formula ◆ large-bulb or catheter-tip syringe ◆ 120 ml of water ◆ 4″ × 4″ gauze pads ◆ prescribed skin cleaning solution ◆ soap ◆ skin protectant ◆ hypoallergenic tape ◆ gravity-drip administration bags ◆ mouthwash, toothpaste, or mild salt solution ◆ stethoscope ◆ gloves ◆ optional: enteral infusion pump.

For decompression: Suction apparatus with tubing and straight drainage collection set.

Implementation

▶ Place the desired amount of formula into the gavage container and purge air from the tubing. To avoid contamination, hang only a 4- to 6-hour supply of formula at a time. **ASPEN**

▶ Confirm the patient's identity using two patient identifiers according to your facility's policy. **JC**

▶ Provide privacy and wash your hands.

▶ Explain the procedure to the patient. Tell him, for example, that feedings usually start at a slow rate and increase as tolerated. After he tolerates continuous feedings, he may progress to intermittent feedings as ordered.

▶ Assess for bowel sounds with a stethoscope before feeding, and monitor for abdominal distention. **ASPEN**

▶ Ask the patient to sit, or assist him into semi-Fowler's position, for the entire feeding, if possible. This helps to prevent esophageal reflux and pulmonary aspiration of the formula. For an intermittent feeding, have him maintain this position throughout the feeding and for 1 hour afterward. **CDC** **AACN**

▶ Put on gloves. Before starting the feeding, measure residual gastric contents. Attach the syringe to the feeding tube and aspirate. If the contents measure more than twice the amount infused, hold the feeding and recheck in 1 hour. If residual contents still remain too high, notify the practitioner. Chances are the formula isn't being absorbed properly. Keep in mind that residual contents will be minimal with PEJ tube feedings.

▶ Allow 30 ml of water to flow into the feeding tube to establish patency. **ASPEN**

▶ Be sure to administer formula at room temperature. Cold formula may cause cramping.

Intermittent feedings

▶ Allow gravity to help the formula flow over 30 to 45 minutes. Faster infusions may cause bloating, cramps, or diarrhea.

▶ Begin intermittent feeding with a low volume (200 ml) daily. According to the patient's tolerance, increase the volume per feeding, as needed, to reach the desired calorie intake.

▶ When the feeding finishes, flush the feeding tube with 30 to 60 ml of water. This maintains patency and provides hydration. **ASPEN**

▶ Cap the tube to prevent leakage.

▶ Rinse the feeding administration set thoroughly with hot water to avoid contaminating subsequent feedings. Allow it to dry between feedings.

Continuous feedings

▶ Measure residual gastric contents every 4 hours.

▶ To administer the feeding with a pump, set up the equipment according to the manufacturer's guidelines, and fill the feeding bag. To administer the feeding by gravity, fill the container with formula and purge air from the tubing. **MFR**

▶ Monitor the gravity drip rate or pump infusion rate.

▶ Flush the feeding tube with 30 to 60 ml of water every 4 hours to maintain patency and to provide hydration. **ASPEN**

▶ Monitor intake and output to anticipate and detect fluid or electrolyte imbalances.

Decompression

▶ To decompress the stomach, connect the PEG port to the suction device with tubing or straight gravity drainage tubing. Jejunostomy feeding may be given simultaneously via the PEJ port of the dual-lumen tube.

Tube exit site care

▶ Provide daily skin care.

▶ Gently remove the dressing by hand. Never cut away the dressing over the catheter because you might cut the tube or the sutures holding the tube in place.

▶ At least daily and as needed, clean the skin around the tube's exit site using a 4″ × 4″ gauze pad soaked in the prescribed cleaning solution. When healed, wash the skin around the exit site daily with soap. Rinse the area with water and pat dry. Apply skin protectant, if necessary.

▶ Anchor a gastrostomy or jejunostomy tube to the skin with hypoallergenic tape to prevent peristaltic migration of the tube. This also prevents tension on the suture anchoring the tube in place.

▶ Coil the tube, if necessary, and tape it to the abdomen to prevent pulling and contamination of the tube. PEG and PEJ tubes have toggle-bolt-like internal and external bumpers that make tape anchors unnecessary. (See *Caring for a PEG or PEJ site,* page 552.)

Special considerations

▶ If the patient vomits or complains of nausea, complains of feeling too full, or regurgitates, stop the feeding immediately, and assess his condition. Flush the feeding tube, and attempt to restart the feeding in 1 hour (measure residual gastric contents first). You may have to decrease the volume or rate of feedings. If the patient develops dumping syndrome, which includes nausea, vomiting, cramps, pallor, and diarrhea, the feedings may have been given too quickly. **ASPEN**

▶ Provide oral hygiene frequently. Brush all surfaces of the teeth, gums, and tongue at least twice daily using mouthwash, toothpaste, or a mild salt solution. **CDC**

▶ You can administer most tablets and pills through the tube by crushing them and diluting as necessary. (However, don't crush enteric-coated or sustained-release drugs, which lose their effectiveness when crushed.) Medications should be in liquid form for administration.

▶ Teach the patient how to administer a syringe feeding at home. (See *Teaching the patient about syringe feeding,* page 553.)

▶ Control diarrhea resulting from dumping syndrome by using continuous pump or gravity-drip infusions, diluting the feeding formula, or adding antidiarrheal medications. Studies have shown that banana flakes are also effective at controlling diarrhea in patients receiving tube feedings. **CS**

Caring for a PEG or PEJ site

The exit site of a percutaneous endoscopic gastrostomy (PEG) or percutaneous endoscopic jejunostomy (PEJ) tube requires routine observation and care. Follow these care guidelines:

▶ Change the dressing daily while the tube is in place.
▶ After removing the dressing, carefully slide the tube's outer bumper away from the skin (as shown below) about ½″ (1 cm).
▶ Examine the skin around the tube. Look for redness and other signs of infection or erosion.

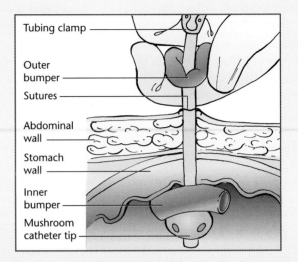

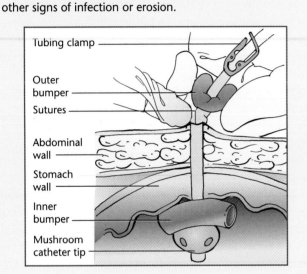

▶ Gently depress the skin surrounding the tube, and inspect for drainage (as shown above right). Expect minimal wound drainage initially after implantation. This should subside in about 1 week.

▶ Inspect the tube for wear and tear, and change if necessary.
▶ Clean the site with the prescribed cleaning solution.
▶ Rotate the outer bumper 90 degrees (to avoid repeating the same tension on the same skin area), and slide the outer bumper back over the exit site.
▶ If leakage appears at the PEG site, or if the patient risks dislodging the tube, apply a sterile gauze dressing over the site. Don't put sterile gauze underneath the outer bumper. Loosening the anchor this way allows the feeding tube free play, which could lead to wound abscess.
▶ Write the date and time of the dressing change on the tape.

Teaching the patient about syringe feeding

If the patient plans to feed himself by syringe when he returns home, you'll need to teach him how to do this before he's discharged. Here are some points to emphasize.

Initial instructions

First, show the patient how to clamp the feeding tube, remove the syringe's bulb or plunger, and place the tip of the syringe into the feeding tube (as shown below). Then tell him to instill between 30 and 60 ml of water into the feeding tube to make sure it stays open and patent.

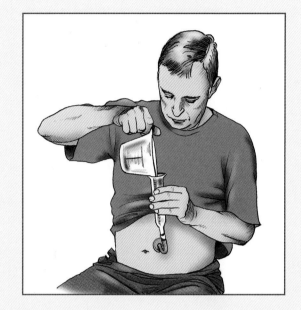

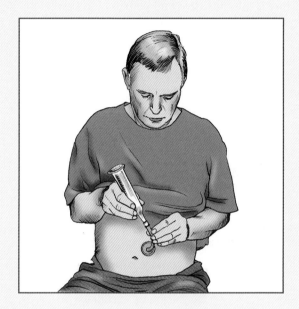

Next, tell him to pour the feeding solution into the syringe and begin the feeding (as shown above right). As the solution flows into the stomach, show him how to tilt the syringe to allow air bubbles to escape. Describe the discomfort that air bubbles may cause.

Tips for free flow

When about one-quarter of the feeding solution remains, direct the patient to refill the syringe. Caution him to avoid letting the syringe empty completely. Doing so may result in abdominal cramping and gas.

Show the patient how to increase and decrease the solution's flow rate by raising or lowering the syringe. Explain that he may need to dilute a thick solution to promote free flow.

Finishing up

Inform the patient that the feeding infusion process should take at least 15 minutes. If the process takes less than 15 minutes, dumping syndrome may result.

Show the patient the steps needed to finish the feeding, including how to flush the tube with water, clamp the tube, and clean the equipment for later use. If he's using disposable gear, urge him to discard it properly. Review instructions for storing unused feeding solution as appropriate.

References

Emery, E. A., et al. "Banana Flakes Control Diarrhea in Enterally Fed Patients," *Nutrition in Clinical Practice* 12(2):72–75, April 1997. **CS**

Reising, D. L., and Neal, R. S. "Enteral Tube Flushing: What You Think Are the Best Practices May Not Be," *AJN* 105(3):58–63, March 2005.

Scolapio, J. S. "A Review of the Trends in the Use of Enteral and Parenteral Nutrition Support," *Journal of Clinical Gastroenterology* 38(5):403–407, May–June 2004.

Taylor, C., et al. *Fundamentals of Nursing: The Art and Science of Nursing,* 6th ed. Philadelphia: Lippincott Williams & Wilkins, 2008.

Transcranial Doppler monitoring

Transcranial Doppler ultrasonography is a noninvasive, low-risk method of monitoring and assessing blood flow in the intracranial vessels, specifically the circle of Willis. This procedure is used at the patient's bedside in the intensive care unit to monitor patients who have experienced cerebrovascular disorders, such as stroke, head trauma, or subarachnoid hemorrhage. It can help detect intracranial stenosis, vasospasm, and arteriovenous malformations as well as assess collateral pathways. Because it has the advantage of monitoring a continuous waveform, it can be used in intraoperative monitoring of cerebral circulation and in tracking a patient's blood-flow velocity and trends. **AAN** **CS**

The major benefits of transcranial Doppler monitoring are that it provides instantaneous, real-time information about cerebral blood flow (CBF) and that it's noninvasive and painless for the patient. Also, the unit itself is portable and easy to use. The major disadvantage is that it relies on the ability of ultrasound waves to penetrate thin areas of the cranium; this is difficult if the patient has thickening of the temporal bone, which increases with age.

The transcranial Doppler unit should always be used with its power set at the lowest level needed to provide an adequate waveform. This procedure requires specialized training to ensure accurate vessel identification and correct interpretation of the signals.

Equipment

Transcranial Doppler unit ◆ transducer with an attachment system ◆ terry cloth headband ◆ ultrasonic coupling gel ◆ marker ◆ tissues.

Implementation

▶ Confirm the patient's identity using two patient identifiers according to your facility's policy. **JC**

▶ Explain the procedure to the patient, and answer any questions he has about the procedure as thoroughly as possible.

▶ Place him in the proper position— usually the supine position.

▶ Turn the Doppler unit on, and observe as it performs a self-test. The screen should show six parameters: PEAK (CM/S), MEAN (CM/S), DEPTH (M/M), DELTA (%), EMBOLI (AGR), and PI+.

▶ Enter the patient's name and identification number in the appropriate place on the Doppler unit. Depending on the unit you're using, you may need to enter additional information, such as the patient's diagnosis or the practitioner's name. **MFR**

▶ Indicate the vessel that you wish to monitor (usually the right or left middle cerebral artery [MCA]). You'll also need to set the approximate depth of the vessel within the skull (50 mm for the MCA).

▶ Next, use the keypad to increase the power level to 100% to initially locate the signal. You can later decrease the level, as needed, depending on the thickness of the patient's skull.

▶ Examine the temporal region of the patient's head, and mentally identify the three windows of the transtemporal access route: posterior, middle, and anterior.

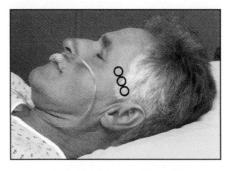

▶ Apply a generous amount of ultrasonic gel at the level of the temporal bone between the tragus of the ear and the end of the eyebrow, over the area of the three windows.

▶ Next, place the transducer on the posterior window. Angle the transducer slightly in an anterior direction, and slowly move it in a narrow circle. This movement is commonly called the "flashlighting" technique. As you hold the transducer at an angle and perform flashlighting, also begin to very slowly move the transducer forward across the temporal area. As you do this, listen for the audible signal with the highest pitch. This sound corresponds to the highest velocity signal, which corresponds to the signal of the vessel you are assessing. You can also use headphones to let you better evaluate the audible signal and provide patient privacy.

▶ After you've located the highest-pitched signal, use a marker to draw a circle around the transducer head on the patient's temple. Note the angle of the transducer so that you can duplicate it after the transducer attachment system is in place.

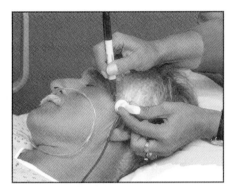

▶ Next, place the transducer system on the patient. To do this, first place the plate of the transducer attachment system over the patient's temporal area; match the circular opening in the plate exactly with the circle drawn on the patient's head. Then, holding the plate in place, encircle the patient's head with the straps attached to the system. Finally, tighten the straps so that the transducer attachment system will stay in place on the patient's head.

▶ Fill the circular opening in the plate with the ultrasonic gel.

▶ Place the transducer in the gel-filled opening in the attachment system plate. Using the plastic screws provided, loosely secure the two plates together. This will hold the transducer in place but allow it to rotate for the best angle.

▶ Adjust the position and angle of the transducer until you again hear the highest-pitched audible signal. When you hear this signal, look at the waveform on the monitor screen. You should see a clear waveform with a bright white line (called an *envelope*) at the upper edge of the waveform. The envelope exactly follows the contours of the waveform itself.

▶ If the envelope doesn't follow the waveform's contours, adjust the gain setting. If the signal is wrapping around the screen, use the scale key to increase the scale and the baseline key to drop the baseline.

▶ When you've determined that you have the strongest, highest-pitched signal and the best waveform, lock the transducer in place by tightening the plastic screws. The tightened plates will hold the transducer at the angle you've chosen. Disconnect the transducer handle.

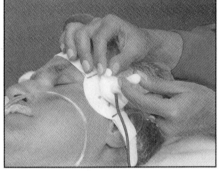

▶ Place a wide terry cloth headband over the transducer attachment system, and secure it around the patient's head to provide additional stability for the transducer. **MFR**

▶ Look at the monitor screen. You should be able to see a waveform and read the numeric values of the peak, mean velocities, and pulsatility index (PI+) above the displayed waveform. The shape of the waveform reveals more information.

Special considerations

▶ Velocity changes in the transcranial Doppler signal correlate with changes in CBF. The parameter that most clearly reflects this change is the mean velocity. First, establish a baseline for the mean velocity. Then, as the patient's velocity increases or decreases, the value (%) will change negatively or positively from the baseline.

CLINICAL ALERT

In extreme situations, such as when blood flow is reduced by a severely restricted vessel, transcranial Doppler monitoring results may not correlate with the degree of vasospasm.

▶ Emboli appear as high-intensity transients that occur randomly during the cardiac cycle. Emboli make a distinctive "clicking," "chirping," or "plunking" sound. You can set up an emboli counter to count either the total number of emboli aggregates or the number of embolic events per minute.

References

Demchuk, A. M., et al. "Transcranial Doppler in Acute Stroke," *Neuroimaging Clinics of North America* 15(3):473–80, August 2005.

Evans, D. H. "Embolus Differentiation Using Multifrequency Transcranial Doppler," *Stroke* 37(7):1641, July 2006.

Feldmann, E., et al. "The Stroke Outcomes and Neuroimaging of Intracranial Atherosclerosis (SONIA) Trial," *Neurology* 68(24):2099–106, June 2007.

Lynn-McHale Wiegand, D. J., and Carlson, K. K., eds. *AACN Procedure Manual for Critical Care,* 5th ed. Philadelphia: W. B. Saunders Co., 2005.

White, H., and Venkatesh, B. "Applications of Transcranial Doppler in the ICU: A Review," *Intensive Care Medicine* 32(7):981–94, July 2006.

Transcutaneous electrical nerve stimulation

Transcutaneous electrical nerve stimulation (TENS) is based on the gate control theory of pain, which proposes that painful impulses pass through a "gate" in the brain. TENS is performed with a portable, battery-powered device that transmits painless electrical current to peripheral nerves or directly to a painful area over relatively large nerve fibers. This treatment effectively alters the patient's perception of pain by blocking painful stimuli traveling over smaller fibers.

Used for postoperative patients and those with chronic pain, TENS reduces the need for analgesic drugs and may allow the patient to resume normal activities. **ASPMN** Typically, a course of TENS treatment lasts 3 to 5 days. Some conditions such as phantom limb pain may require continuous stimulation; other conditions such as a painful arthritic joint require shorter periods (3 to 4 hours). (See *Uses of TENS.*) TENS is contraindicated for patients with cardiac pacemakers because it can interfere with pacemaker function. **ASPMN** The procedure is also contraindicated for pregnant patients because its effect on the fetus is unknown. It's also contraindicated in patients with dementia. TENS should be used cautiously in all patients with cardiac disorders. TENS electrodes shouldn't be placed on the head or neck of patients with vascular disorders or seizure disorders.

Equipment

TENS device ◆ alcohol pads ◆ pregelled electrodes ◆ warm water and soap ◆ leadwires ◆ charged battery pack ◆ battery recharger ◆ adhesive patch or hypoallergenic tape.

Commercial TENS kits are available. They include the stimulator, leadwires, electrodes, spare battery pack, battery recharger and, occasionally, an adhesive patch.

Implementation

▶ Before beginning the procedure, always test the battery pack to make sure it's fully charged. **MFR**
▶ Confirm the patient's identity using two patient identifiers according to your facility's policy. **JC**
▶ Wash your hands and provide privacy. If the patient has never seen a TENS unit, show him the device and explain the procedure.

Before TENS treatment

▶ With an alcohol pad, thoroughly clean and dry the skin where the electrode will be applied.
▶ Place the ordered number of electrodes on the proper skin area, leaving at least 2″ (5 cm) between them. (See *Positioning TENS electrodes.*) Then secure them with the adhesive patch or hypoallergenic tape. Tape all sides evenly so that the electrodes are firmly attached to the skin.
▶ Plug the pin connectors into the electrode sockets. To protect the cords, hold the connectors—not the cords themselves—during insertion.
▶ Turn the channel controls to the OFF position or as recommended in the operator's manual.
▶ Plug the leadwires into the jacks in the control box.
▶ Turn the amplitude and rate dials slowly as the manual directs. (The patient should feel a tingling sensation.) Then adjust the controls on this device to the prescribed settings or to settings that are most comfortable.

Uses of TENS

Transcutaneous electrical nerve stimulation (TENS), which must be prescribed by a practitioner, is most successful if administered and taught to the patient by a therapist skilled in its use. TENS has been used for temporary relief of acute pain, such as postoperative pain, and for ongoing relief of chronic pain such as that associated with sciatica.

Types of pain that respond to TENS include:
▶ arthritis pain
▶ bone fracture pain
▶ bursitis pain
▶ cancer-related pain
▶ lower back pain
▶ musculoskeletal pain
▶ myofascial pain
▶ pain from neuralgias and neuropathies
▶ phantom limb pain
▶ whiplash pain.

Positioning TENS electrodes

In transcutaneous electrical nerve stimulation (TENS), electrodes placed around peripheral nerves (or an incisional site) transmit mild electrical pulses to the brain. The current is thought to block pain impulses. The patient can influence the level and frequency of his pain relief by adjusting the controls on the device.

Typically, electrode placement varies even though patients may have similar complaints. Electrodes can be placed in several ways:

▶ to cover the painful area or surround it, as with muscle tenderness or spasm or painful joints

▶ to "capture" the painful area between electrodes, as with incisional pain.

In peripheral nerve injury, electrodes should be placed proximal to the injury (between the brain and the injury site) to avoid increasing pain. Placing electrodes in a hypersensitive area also increases pain. In an area lacking sensation, electrodes should be placed on adjacent dermatomes.

These illustrations show combinations of electrode placement (red squares) and areas of nerve stimulation (shaded pink) for lower back and leg pain.

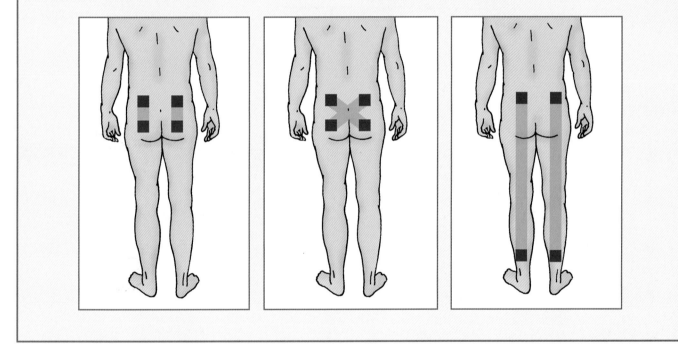

Most patients select stimulation frequencies of 60 to 100 Hz. ASPMN

▶ Attach the TENS control box to part of the patient's clothing, such as a belt, pocket, or bra.

▶ To make sure the device is working effectively, monitor the patient for signs of excessive stimulation such as muscular twitches and for signs of inadequate stimulation, signaled by the patient's inability to feel any mild tingling sensation.

After TENS treatment

▶ Turn off the controls, and unplug the electrode leadwires from the control box.

▶ If another treatment will be given soon, leave the electrodes in place; if not, remove them.

▶ Clean the patient's skin with alcohol pads. (Don't soak the electrodes in alcohol because it will damage the rubber.)

▶ Remove the battery pack from the unit, and replace it with a charged battery pack.

▶ Recharge the used battery pack so that it's always ready for use.

Special considerations

▶ If you must move the electrodes during the procedure, turn off the controls first. Follow the practitioner's orders regarding electrode placement and control settings. Incorrect placement of the electrodes will result in inappropriate pain control. Setting the controls too high can cause pain; setting them too low will fail to relieve pain.

CLINICAL ALERT

Never place the electrodes near the patient's eyes or over the nerves that innervate the carotid sinus or laryngeal or pharyngeal muscles to avoid interference with critical nerve function. **ASPMN**

▶ If TENS is used continuously for postoperative pain, remove the electrodes at least daily to check for skin irritation, provide skin care, and to rotate sites of electrode placement.

References

American Association of Neuroscience Nurses. *Core Curriculum for Neuroscience Nursing,* 4th ed. Philadelphia: W. B. Saunders Co., 2004.

Hickey, J. V. *The Clinical Practice of Neurologic and Neurosurgical Nursing,* 6th ed. Philadelphia: Lippincott Williams & Wilkins, 2009.

McLennon, S. M. *Persistent Pain Management.* Iowa City: University of Iowa Gerontological Nursing Interventions Research Center, Research Translation and Dissemination Core, August 2005.

Ottawa Panel. "Ottawa Panel Evidence-Based Clinical Practice Guidelines for Electrotherapy and Thermotherapy Interventions in the Management of Rheumatoid Arthritis in Adults," *Physical Therapy* 84(11):1016–43, November 2004.

Ying, K. N., and While, A. "Pain Relief in Osteoarthritis and Rheumatoid Arthritis: TENS," *British Journal of Community Nursing* 12(8):364–71, August 2007.

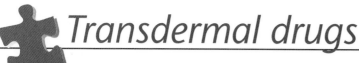

Transdermal drugs

Through an adhesive patch or a measured dose of ointment applied to the skin, transdermal drugs deliver constant, controlled medication directly into the bloodstream for a prolonged systemic effect.

Medications available in transdermal form include nitroglycerin, used to control angina; scopolamine, used to treat motion sickness; estradiol, used for postmenopausal hormone replacement; clonidine, used to treat hypertension; nicotine, used for smoking cessation; fentanyl, an opioid analgesic used to control chronic pain; and hormonal birth control. Contraindications for transdermal drug application include skin allergies or skin reactions to the drug. Transdermal drugs shouldn't be applied to broken or irritated skin because they may increase irritation or to scarred or callused skin, which might impair absorption.

Equipment

Patient's medication record and chart ◆ gloves ◆ prescribed medication (patch or ointment) ◆ application strip or measuring paper (for nitroglycerin ointment) ◆ adhesive tape ◆ plastic wrap (optional for nitroglycerin ointment) or semipermeable dressing.

Implementation

▶ Verify the order on the patient's medication record by checking it against the practitioner's order. **JC**
▶ Wash your hands and, if necessary, put on gloves.
▶ Check the label on the medication to make sure you'll be giving the correct drug in the correct dose. Note the expiration date. **JC ISMP**
▶ Confirm the patient's identity using two patient identifiers according to your facility's policy. **JC**
▶ If your facility utilizes a bar code scanning system, be sure to scan your ID badge, the patient's ID bracelet, and the medication's bar code. **JC**
▶ Explain the procedure to the patient, and provide privacy.
▶ Remove any previously applied medication.

Applying transdermal ointment
▶ Place the prescribed amount of ointment on the application strip or measuring paper, taking care not to get any on your skin. (See *Applying nitroglycerin ointment,* page 560.)
▶ Apply the strip to any dry, hairless area of the body. Don't rub the ointment into the skin.
▶ Tape the strip and ointment to the skin.
▶ If desired, cover the application strip with plastic wrap, and tape the wrap in place.

Applying a transdermal patch
▶ Open the package, and remove the patch.
▶ Without touching the adhesive surface, remove the clear plastic backing.
▶ Apply the patch to a dry, hairless area—behind the ear, for example, as with scopolamine.
▶ Write the date, time, and your initials on the dressing.

After applying transdermal medications
▶ Store the medication as ordered.
▶ Instruct the patient to keep the area around the patch or ointment as dry as possible.

▶ If you didn't wear gloves, wash your hands immediately after applying the patch or ointment to avoid absorbing the drug yourself.

Special considerations

▶ Reapply daily transdermal medications at the same time every day to ensure a continuous effect, but alternate the application sites to avoid skin irritation. Before reapplying nitroglycerin ointment, remove the plastic wrap, application strip, and any remaining ointment from the patient's skin at the previous site.
▶ When applying a scopolamine or fentanyl patch, instruct the patient not to drive or operate machinery until his response to the drug has been determined.
▶ Warn a patient using a clonidine patch to check with his practitioner before taking an over-the-counter cough preparation because such drugs may counteract clonidine's effects.

Applying nitroglycerin ointment

Unlike most topical medications, nitroglycerin ointment is used for its transdermal *systemic* effect. It's used to dilate the veins and arteries, thus improving cardiac perfusion in a patient with cardiac ischemia or angina pectoris.

To apply nitroglycerin ointment, start by taking the patient's baseline blood pressure so that you can compare it with later readings. Remove any previously applied nitroglycerin ointment. Gather your equipment. Nitroglycerin ointment, which is prescribed by the inch, comes with a rectangular piece of ruled paper to be used in applying the medication. Squeeze the prescribed amount of ointment onto the ruled paper (as shown below). Put on gloves, if desired, to avoid contact with the medication.

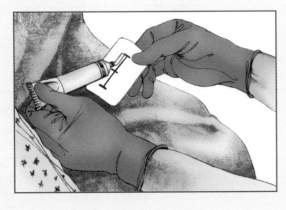

After measuring the correct amount of ointment, tape the paper—drug side down—directly to the skin (as shown below). For increased absorption, the practitioner may request that you cover the site with plastic wrap or a transparent semipermeable dressing.

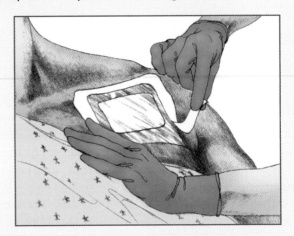

After 5 minutes, record the patient's blood pressure. If it has dropped significantly and he has a headache (from vasodilation of blood vessels in his head), notify the practitioner immediately. He may reduce the dose. If the patient's blood pressure has dropped but he's asymptomatic, instruct him to lie still until it returns to normal.

References

The Joint Commission. *Comprehensive Accreditation Manual for Hospitals: The Official Handbook*. Standard MM.1.10. Oakbrook Terrace, Ill.: The Joint Commission, 2007.

The Joint Commission. *Comprehensive Accreditation Manual for Hospitals: The Official Handbook*. Standard MM.2.10. Oakbrook Terrace, Ill.: The Joint Commission, 2007.

The Joint Commission. *Comprehensive Accreditation Manual for Hospitals: The Official Handbook*. Standard MM.3.10. Oakbrook Terrace, Ill.: The Joint Commission, 2007.

The Joint Commission. *Comprehensive Accreditation Manual for Hospitals: The Official Handbook*. Standard MM.4.10. Oakbrook Terrace, Ill.: The Joint Commission, 2007.

The Joint Commission. *Comprehensive Accreditation Manual for Hospitals: The Official Handbook*. Standard MM.4.20. Oakbrook Terrace, Ill.: The Joint Commission, 2007.

The Joint Commission. *Comprehensive Accreditation Manual for Hospitals: The Official Handbook*. Standard MM.5.10. Oakbrook Terrace, Ill.: The Joint Commission, 2007.

The Joint Commission. *Comprehensive Accreditation Manual for Hospitals: The Official Handbook*. Standard MM.6.10. Oakbrook Terrace, Ill.: The Joint Commission, 2007.

The Joint Commission. *Comprehensive Accreditation Manual for Hospitals: The Official Handbook*. Standard MM.6.20. Oakbrook Terrace, Ill.: The Joint Commission, 2007.

McErlane, K. "Keeping Track of the Patch: Transdermal Delivery in Obese Patients," *AJN* 105(6):36–37, June 2005.

Taylor, C., et al. *Fundamentals of Nursing: The Art and Science of Nursing Care,* 6th ed. Philadelphia: Lippincott Williams & Wilkins, 2008.

Transducer system setup

The exact type of transducer system used depends on the patient's needs and the practitioner's preference. Some systems monitor pressure continuously, whereas others monitor pressure intermittently. Single-pressure transducers monitor only one type of pressure—for example, pulmonary artery pressure (PAP). Multiple-pressure transducers can monitor two or more types of pressure, such as PAP and central venous pressure.

Equipment

Bag of flush solution (normal saline solution) ◆ heparin flush solution, as needed ◆ pressure infusion bag ◆ medication-added label ◆ pre-assembled disposable pressure tubing with flush device and disposable transducer ◆ monitor and monitor cable ◆ I.V. pole with transducer mount ◆ carpenter's level ◆ non-vented stopcock caps ◆ sterile gauze package.

Implementation

▶ Confirm the patient's identity using two patient identifiers according to your facility's policy. **JC**

▶ Wash your hands.

To set up and zero a single-pressure transducer system, perform the following steps:

Setting up the system

▶ Follow your facility's policy on adding heparin to the flush solution. If your patient has a history of bleeding or clotting problems, use heparin with caution. Add the ordered amount of heparin to the solution—usually, 1 to 2 units of heparin/ml of solution—and then label the bag. **CS1**

▶ Put the pressure module into the monitor, if necessary, and connect the transducer cable to the monitor.

▶ Remove the preassembled pressure tubing from the package. If necessary, connect the pressure tubing to the transducer. Tighten all tubing connections.

▶ Position all stopcocks so the flush solution flows through the entire system. Then roll the tubing's flow regulator to the off position.

▶ Spike the flush solution bag with the tubing, invert the bag, open the roller clamp, and squeeze all the air through the drip chamber. Then, compress the tubing's drip chamber, filling it no more than halfway with the flush solution.

▶ Place the flush solution bag into the pressure infuser bag. To do this, hang the pressure infuser bag on the I.V. pole, and then position the flush solution bag inside the pressure infuser bag. Don't inflate the pressure bag because priming the tubing under pressure can cause air bubbles to enter the system.

▶ Open the tubing's flow regulator, uncoil the tube if you haven't already done so, and remove the protective cap at the end of the pressure tubing. Squeeze the continuous flush device slowly to prime the entire system, including the stopcock ports, with the flush solution.

▶ As the solution nears the disposable transducer, hold the transducer at a 45-degree angle. This forces the solution to flow upward to the transducer. In doing so, the solution forces any air out of the system.

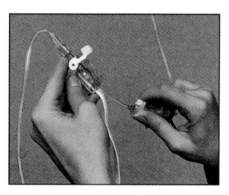

▶ When the solution nears a stopcock, open the stopcock to air, allowing the solution to flow into the stopcock. When the stopcock fills, close it to air and turn it open to the remainder of the tubing. Do this for each stopcock.

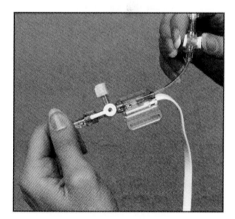

▶ After removing the air from the stopcock, replace the vented cap with a nonvented cap to prevent air from entering the system.

▶ After you've completely primed the system, replace the protective cap at the end of the tubing.

▶ Inflate the pressure infusion bag to 300 mm Hg. This bag keeps the pressure in the arterial line higher than the patient's systolic pressure, preventing blood backflow into the tubing and ensuring a continuous flow rate. When you inflate the pressure bag, take care that the drip chamber doesn't completely fill with fluid. Afterward, flush the system again to remove all air bubbles.

▶ If you're going to mount the transducer on an I.V. pole, insert the device into its holder.

Zeroing the system

▶ Now you're ready for a preliminary zeroing of the transducer. To ensure accuracy, position the patient and the transducer on the same level each time you zero the transducer or record a pressure. Typically, the patient lies flat in bed, if he can tolerate that position. **CS2**

▶ Next, use the carpenter's level to position the air-reference stopcock or the air-fluid interface of the transducer level with the phlebostatic axis (midway between the posterior chest and the sternum at the fourth intercostal space, midaxillary line). Alternatively, you may level the air-reference stopcock or the air-fluid interface to the same position as the catheter tip.

▶ After leveling the transducer, turn the stopcock next to the transducer off to the patient and open to air. Remove the cap to the stopcock port.

▶ Now zero the transducer. To do so, follow the manufacturer's directions for zeroing.

▶ When you've finished zeroing, turn the stopcock on the transducer so that it's closed to air and open to the patient. This is the monitoring position. Place a new sterile cap on the stopcock. You're then ready to attach the single-pressure transducer to the patient's catheter. Now you've assembled a single-pressure transducer system. The photograph here shows how the system will look.

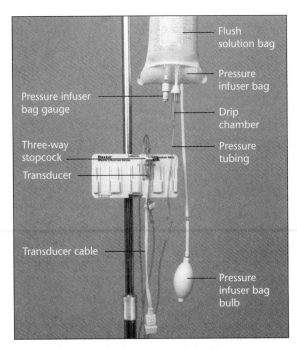

Flush solution bag
Pressure infuser bag gauge
Pressure infuser bag
Three-way stopcock
Drip chamber
Transducer
Pressure tubing
Transducer cable
Pressure infuser bag bulb

Special considerations

▶ You may use any of several methods to set up a multiple-pressure transducer system. The easiest way is to add to the single-pressure system. You'll also need another bag of heparin flush solution in a second pressure infuser bag. Then you'll prime the tubing, mount the second transducer, and connect an additional cable to the monitor. Finally, you'll zero the second transducer.

▶ Alternatively, your facility may use a Y-type tubing setup with two attached pressure transducers. This method requires only one bag of heparin flush solution. To set up the system, proceed as you would for a single transducer, with this exception: First, prime one branch of the Y-type tubing and then the other. Next, attach two cables to the monitor in the modules for each pressure that you'll be measuring. Finally, zero each transducer.

▶ Change the heparin flush bag and the tubing every 96 hours or according to your facility's policy. **CDC**

References

"Evaluation of the Effects of Heparinized and Nonheparinized Flush Solution on the Patency of Arterial Pressure Monitoring Lines: The AACN Thunder Project. By the American Association of Critical Care Nurses," *American Journal of Critical Care* 2(1):3–15, January 1993. **CS1**

Garland, J. S., et al, "The 2002 Hospital Infection Control Practices Advisory Committee Centers for Disease Control and Prevention Guideline for Prevention of Intravascular Device-Related Infections," *Pediatrics* 110(5): 1009–1013, November 2002.

Laulive, J. L. "Pulmonary Artery Pressure and Position Changes in the Critically Ill Adult," *Dimensions in Critical Care Nursing* 1(1):28–34, January–February 1982. **CS2**

Lynn-McHale Wiegand, D. J., and Carlson, K. K., eds. *AACN Procedure Manual for Critical Care*, 5th ed., Philadelphia: W. B. Saunders Co., 2005.

"Standard 48. Administration Set Change. Infusion Nursing Standards of Practice," *Journal of Infusion Nursing* 29(1S):S48–51, January–February 2006.

Transfer from bed to stretcher

Transfer from bed to stretcher, one of the most common transfers, can require the help of one or more coworkers, depending on the patient's size and condition and the primary nurse's physical abilities. Techniques for achieving this transfer include the straight lift, carry lift, lift sheet, and sliding board.

The nurse should always remember to maintain good body mechanics—a wide base of support and bent knees—when transferring a patient, to reduce the risk of injury to the patient and herself. To reduce the risk of injury to the patient during transfer, the nurse should make sure that the patient maintains proper body alignment—back straight, head in neutral position, and extremities in a functional position

In the straight (or patient-assisted) lift—used to move a child, a very light patient, or a patient who can assist transfer—the transfer team members place their hands and arms under the patient's buttocks and, if necessary, his shoulders. Other patients may require a four-person straight lift, detailed below. In the carry lift, team members roll the patient onto their upper arms and hold him against their chests. In the lift sheet transfer, they place a sheet under the patient and lift or slide him onto the stretcher. In the sliding-board transfer, two team members slide him onto the stretcher.

Equipment

Stretcher ◆ sliding board or lift sheet if necessary.

Implementation

▶ Adjust the bed to the same height as the stretcher.
▶ Tell the patient that you're going to move him from the bed to the stretcher, and place him in the supine position.
▶ Ask team members to remove watches and rings to avoid scratching the patient during transfer.

Four-person straight lift

▶ Place the stretcher parallel to the bed, and lock the wheels of both to ensure the patient's safety.
▶ Stand at the center of the stretcher, and have another team member stand at the patient's head. The two other team members should stand next to the bed, on the other side—one at the center and the other at the patient's feet.

▶ Slide your arms, palms up, beneath the patient, while the other team members do the same. In this position, you and the team member directly opposite support the patient's buttocks and hips; the team member at the head of the bed supports the patient's head and shoulders; the one at the foot supports the patient's legs and feet.
▶ On a count of three, the team members lift the patient several inches, move him onto the stretcher, and slide their arms out from under him. Keep movements smooth to minimize patient discomfort and avoid muscle strain by team members.

Four-person carry lift

▶ Place the stretcher perpendicular to the bed, with the head of the stretcher at the foot of the bed. Lock the bed and stretcher wheels to ensure the patient's safety.
▶ Raise the bed to a comfortable working height.

▶ Line up all four team members on the same side of the bed as the stretcher, with the tallest member at the patient's head and the shortest at his feet. The member at the patient's head is the leader of the team and gives the lift signals.
▶ Tell the team members to flex their knees and slide their hands, palms up, under the patient until he rests securely on their upper arms. Make sure the patient is adequately supported at the head and shoulders, buttocks and hips, and legs and feet.
▶ On a count of three, the team members straighten their knees and roll the patient onto his side, against their chests. This reduces strain on the lifters and allows them to hold the patient for several minutes if necessary.
▶ Together, the team members step back, with the member supporting the feet moving the farthest. The team members move forward to the stretcher's edge and, on a count of three, lower the patient onto the stretcher by bending at the knees and sliding their arms out from under the patient.

Four-person lift sheet transfer

▶ Position the bed, stretcher, and team members for the straight lift. Then instruct the team to hold the edges of the sheet under the patient, grasping them close to the patient to obtain a firm grip, provide stability, and spare the patient undue feelings of instability.

▶ On a count of three, the team members lift or slide the patient onto the stretcher in a smooth, continuous motion to avoid muscle strain and minimize patient discomfort.

Sliding-board transfer

▶ Place the stretcher parallel to the bed, and lock the wheels of both to ensure the patient's safety.

▶ Stand next to the bed, and instruct a coworker to stand next to the stretcher.

▶ Reach over the patient, and pull the far side of the bedsheet toward you to turn the patient slightly on his side. Your coworker then places the sliding board beneath the patient, making sure the board bridges the gap between stretcher and bed.

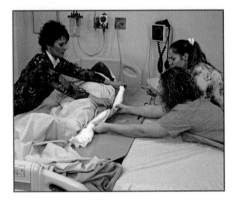

▶ Ease the patient onto the sliding board, and release the sheet. Your coworker then grasps the near side of the sheet at the patient's hips and shoulders and pulls him onto the stretcher in a smooth, continuous motion. She then reaches over the patient, grasps the far side of the sheet, and logrolls him toward her.

▶ Remove the sliding board as your coworker returns the patient to the supine position.

After all transfers

▶ Position the patient comfortably on the stretcher, apply safety straps, and raise and secure the side rails.

Special considerations

When transferring an immobile or markedly obese patient from bed to stretcher, first lift and move him, in increments, to the edge of the bed. Then rest for a few seconds, repositioning the patient if necessary, and lift him onto the stretcher. If the patient can bear weight on his arms or legs, two or three coworkers can perform this transfer: One can support the buttocks and guide the patient, another can stabilize the stretcher by leaning over it and guiding the patient into position, and a third can transfer any attached equipment. If a team member isn't available to guide equipment, move I.V. lines and other tubing first to make sure it's out of the way and not in danger of pulling loose (disconnect tubes if possible). If the patient is light, three coworkers can perform the carry lift; however, no matter how many team members are present, one must stabilize the patient's head if he can't support it himself, has cervical instability or injury, or has undergone surgery.

References

Craven, R. F., and Hirnle, C. J. *Fundamentals of Nursing Human Health and Function,* 6th ed. Philadelphia: Lippincott Williams & Wilkins, 2009.

Johnsonn, A. C., et al. "Evaluation of Nursing Students' Work Technique after Proficiency Training in Patient Transfer Methods during Undergraduate Education," *Nurse Education Today* 26(4): 322–31, May 2006.

Kjellberg, K., et al. "Patient Safety and Comfort during Transfers in Relation to Nurses' Work Technique," *Journal of Advanced Nursing* 47(3):251–59, August 2004.

Lloyd, J. D., and Baptiste, A. "Friction-Reducing Devices for Lateral Patient Transfers: A Biomechanical Evaluation," *AAOHN Journal* 54(3):113–19, March 2006.

Transfer from bed to wheelchair

For the patient with diminished or absent lower-body sensation or one-sided weakness, immobility, or injury, transfer from bed to wheelchair may require partial support to full assistance—initially by at least two nurses. Subsequent transfer of the patient with generalized weakness may be performed by one nurse. After transfer, proper positioning helps prevent excessive pressure on bony prominences, which predisposes the patient to skin breakdown.

Equipment

Wheelchair with locks (or sturdy chair) ◆ pajama bottoms (or robe) ◆ shoes or slippers with nonslip soles ◆ watch with a second hand ◆ stethoscope ◆ sphygmomanometer ◆ optional: transfer board if appropriate. (See *Teaching the patient to use a transfer board,* page 566.)

Implementation

▶ Explain the procedure to the patient and demonstrate his role.
▶ Use good body mechanics during the transfer to prevent injury.
▶ Place the wheelchair parallel to the bed and lock its wheels. Raise the wheelchair footrests to avoid interfering with the transfer. Make sure the bed wheels are also locked and the bed is in the lowest position in relation to the floor to prevent an accident.

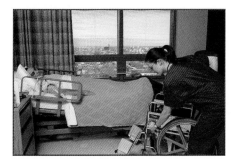

▶ Check pulse rate and blood pressure with the patient supine to obtain a baseline. Then help him put on the pa-

jama bottoms and slippers or shoes with nonslip soles to prevent falls.
▶ Raise the head of the bed, and allow the patient to rest briefly to adjust to posture changes. Then bring him to the dangling position. Don't proceed until the patient's pulse rate and blood pressure are stabilized to prevent falls.

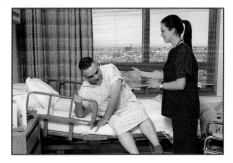

▶ Tell the patient to move toward the edge of the bed and, if possible, to place his feet flat on the floor. Stand in front of the patient, blocking his toes with your feet and his knees with yours to prevent his knees from buckling.
▶ Flex your knees slightly, place your arms around the patient's back above the level of the axilla, and tell him to place his hands on the edge of the bed. Avoid bending at your waist to prevent back strain.
▶ Ask the patient to push himself off the bed and to support as much of his own weight as possible. At the same time, straighten your knees and hips, raising the patient as you straighten your body.

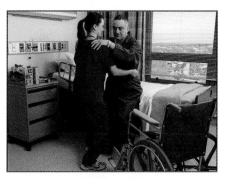

▶ Supporting the patient as needed, pivot toward the wheelchair, keeping your knees next to his. Tell the patient to grasp the farthest armrest of the wheelchair with his closest hand.

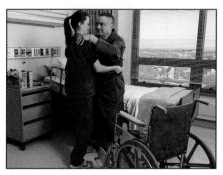

▶ Help the patient lower himself into the wheelchair by flexing your hips and knees, but not your back. Instruct him to reach back and grasp the other wheelchair armrest as he sits to avoid abrupt contact with the seat.

Teaching the patient to use a transfer board

For the patient who can't stand, a transfer board allows safe transfer from bed to wheelchair. To perform this transfer, take the following steps:

▶ First, explain and demonstrate the procedure. Eventually, the patient may become proficient enough to transfer himself independently or with supervision.

▶ Help the patient put on pajama bottoms or a robe and shoes or nonslip slippers.

▶ Lock the bed wheels.

▶ Place the wheelchair angled slightly and close to the bed. Lock the wheels, and remove the armrest closest to the patient. Make sure that the bed is flat, and adjust its height so that it's level with the wheelchair seat.

▶ Assist the patient to a sitting position on the edge of the bed, with his feet resting on the floor. Make sure that the front edge of the wheelchair seat is aligned with the back of the patient's knees (as shown below left). Although it's important that the patient have an even surface on which to transfer, he may find it easier to transfer to a slightly lower surface.

▶ Ask the patient to lean away from the wheelchair while you slide one end of the transfer board under him.

▶ Now place the other end of the transfer board on the wheelchair seat, and help the patient return to the upright position.

▶ Stand in front of the patient to prevent him from sliding forward. Tell him to push down with both arms, lifting the buttocks up and onto the transfer board. The patient then repeats this maneuver, edging along the board, until he's seated in the wheelchair. If the patient can't use his arms to assist with the transfer, stand in front of him, put your arms around him and, if he's able, have him put his arms around you. Gradually slide him across the board until he's safely in the chair (as shown below right).

▶ When the patient is in the chair, fasten a seat belt, if necessary, to prevent falls.

▶ Then remove the transfer board, replace the wheelchair armrest and footrest, and reposition the patient in the chair.

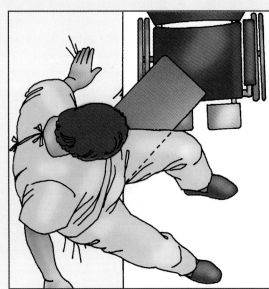

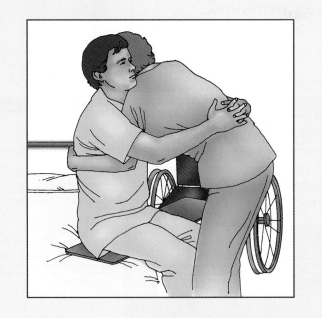

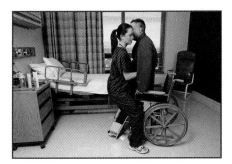

▶ Fasten the seat belt to prevent falls and, if necessary, check pulse rate and blood pressure to assess cardiovascular stability. If the pulse rate is 20 beats or more above baseline, stay with the patient and monitor him closely until it returns to normal because he's experiencing orthostatic hypotension.

▶ If the patient can't position himself correctly, help him move his buttocks against the back of the chair so that the ischial tuberosities, not the sacrum, provide the base of support.

▶ Place the patient's feet flat on the footrests, pointed straight ahead. Then position the knees and hips with the correct amount of flexion and in appropriate alignment. If appropriate, use elevating leg rests to flex the patient's hips at more than 90 degrees; this position relieves pressure on the popliteal space and places more weight on the ischial tuberosities. NPUAP

▶ Position the patient's arms on the wheelchair's armrests with shoulders abducted, elbows slightly flexed, forearms pronated, and wrists and hands in the neutral position. If necessary, support or elevate the patient's hands and forearms with a pillow to prevent dependent edema.

Special considerations

▶ If the patient starts to fall during transfer, ease him to the closest surface—bed, floor, or chair. Never stretch to finish the transfer. Doing so can cause loss of balance, falls, muscle strain, and other injuries to you and the patient.

▶ If the patient has one-sided weakness, follow the preceding steps, but place the wheelchair on the patient's unaffected side. Instruct the patient to pivot and bear as much weight as possible on the unaffected side. Support the affected side because the patient will tend to lean to this side. Use pillows to support the hemiplegic patient's affected side to prevent slumping in the wheelchair.

References

Craven, R. F., and Hirnle, C. J. *Fundamentals of Nursing Human Health and Function,* 6th ed. Philadelphia: Lippincott Williams & Wilkins, 2009.

Kirby, R. L., et al. "The Manual Wheelchair-Handling Skills of Caregivers and the Effect of Training," *Archives of Physical Medicine and Rehabilitation* 85(12):2011–119, December 2004.

Kjellberg, K., et al. "Patient Safety and Comfort during Transfers in Relation to Nurses' Work Technique," *Journal of Advanced Nursing* 47(3):251–59, August 2004.

Nelson, A. "Technology to Promote Safe Mobility in the Elderly," *The Nursing Clinics of North America* 39(3):649–71, September 2004.

Transfer with a hydraulic lift

Using a hydraulic lift to raise the immobile patient from the supine to the sitting position allows safe, comfortable transfer between bed and chair. It's indicated for the obese or immobile patient for whom manual transfer poses the potential for nurse or patient injury. Although most hydraulic lift models can be operated by one person, it's better to have two staff members present during transfer to stabilize and support the patient.

Equipment

Hydraulic lift, with sling, chains or straps, and hooks ◆ chair or wheelchair.

Implementation

▶ Because hydraulic lift models may vary in weight capacity, check the manufacturer's specifications before attempting patient transfer. **MFR**

▶ Make sure the bed and wheelchair wheels are locked before beginning the transfer.

▶ Explain the procedure to the patient, and reassure him that the hydraulic lift can safely support his weight and won't tip over.

▶ Ensure the patient's privacy.

▶ If the patient has an I.V. line or urinary drainage bag, move it first. Arrange tubing securely to prevent dangling during transfer. If the tubing of the urinary drainage bag isn't long enough to permit the transfer, clamp the tubing and drainage bag and place it on the patient's abdomen during transfer. After the transfer, place the drainage bag in a dependent position, and unclamp the tubing.

▶ Make sure the side rail opposite you is raised and secure. Then roll the patient toward you, onto his side, and raise the side rail. Walk to the opposite side of the bed and lower the side rail.

▶ Place the sling under the patient's buttocks with its lower edge below the greater trochanter. Then fanfold the far side of the sling against the back and buttocks.

▶ Roll the patient toward you onto the sling, and raise the side rail. Then lower the opposite side rail.

▶ Slide your hands under the patient, and pull the sling from beneath him, smoothing out all wrinkles. Then roll the patient onto his back and center him on the sling.

▶ Place the appropriate chair next to the head of the bed, facing the foot.

▶ Lower the side rail next to the chair, and raise the bed only until the base of the lift can extend under the bed. To avoid alarming and endangering the patient, don't raise the bed completely.

▶ Set the lift's adjustable base to its widest position to ensure optimal stability. Then move the lift so that its arm lies perpendicular to the bed, directly over the patient.

▶ Connect one end of the chains (or straps) to the side arms on the lift; connect the other hooked end to the sling. Face the hooks away from the patient to prevent them from slipping and to avoid the risk of their pointed edges injuring the patient. The patient may place his arms inside or outside the chains (or straps), or he may grasp them once the slack is gone to avoid injury. (See *Using a hydraulic lift*.)

▶ Tighten the turnscrew on the lift. Then, depending on the type of lift you're using, pump the handle or turn it clockwise until the patient has assumed a sitting position and his buttocks clear the bed surface by 1″ to 2″ (2.5 or 5 cm). Momentarily suspend him above the bed until he feels secure in the lift and sees that it can bear his weight.

▶ Steady the patient as you move the lift or, preferably, have another coworker guide the patient's body while you move the lift. Depending on the type of lift you're using, the arm should now rest in front of or to one side of the chair.

▶ Release the turnscrew. Then depress the handle or turn it counter-clockwise to lower the patient into the chair. While lowering the patient, push gently on his knees to maintain the correct sitting posture. After lowering the patient into the chair, fasten the seat belt to ensure his safety.

▶ Remove the hooks or straps from the sling, but leave the sling in place under the patient so you'll be able to transfer him back to the bed from the chair. Then move the lift away from the patient.

▶ To return the patient to bed, reverse the procedure.

Special considerations

▶ If the patient has an altered center of gravity (caused by a halo vest or a lower-extremity cast, for example), obtain help from a coworker before transferring him with a hydraulic lift.

Using a hydraulic lift

After placing the patient supine in the center of the sling, position the hydraulic lift above her (as shown below). Then attach the chains to the hooks on the sling.

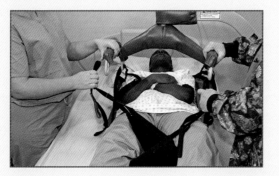

Turn the lift handle clockwise to raise the patient to the sitting position. If she's positioned properly, continue to raise her until she's suspended just above the bed.

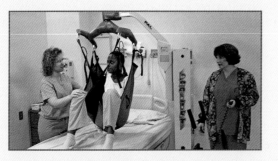

After positioning the patient above the wheelchair, turn the lift handle counter-clockwise to lower her onto the seat. When the chains become slack, stop turning and unhook the sling from the lift.

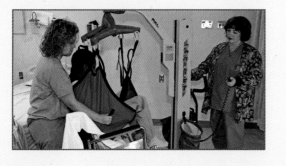

▶ If the patient will require the use of a hydraulic lift for transfers after discharge, teach his family how to use this device correctly, and allow them to practice with supervision.

References

Craven, R. F., and Hirnle, C. J. *Fundamentals of Nursing Human Health and Function,* 6th ed. Philadelphia: Lippincott Williams & Wilkins, 2009.

Kjellberg, K., et al. "Patient Safety and Comfort during Transfers in Relation to Nurses' Work Technique," *Journal of Advanced Nursing* 47(3):251–59, August 2004.

Transfusion of whole blood and packed cells

Whole blood transfusion replenishes the volume and the oxygen-carrying capacity of the circulatory system by increasing the mass of circulating red cells. Transfusion of packed red blood cells (RBCs), from which 80% of the plasma has been removed, restores only the oxygen-carrying capacity. After plasma is removed, the resulting component has a hematocrit of 65% to 80% and a usual volume of 250 to 300 ml.

Each unit of whole blood or RBCs contains enough hemoglobin to raise the hemoglobin concentration in an average-sized adult 1 g/dl. Both types of transfusion treat decreased hemoglobin level and hematocrit. Whole blood is usually used only when decreased levels result from hemorrhage; packed RBCs are used when such depressed levels accompany normal blood volume to avoid possible fluid and circulatory overload. (See *Transfusing blood and selected components*.) **CS** Whole blood and packed RBCs contain cellular debris, requiring in-line filtration during administration.

Blood and blood components should be filtered and transfused through an appropriate blood administration set. **INS** **AABB** Straight-line and Y-type blood administration sets are commonly used. Although filters come in mesh and microaggregate types, the latter type is preferred, especially when transfusing multiple units of blood. Highly effective leukocyte removal filters are available for use when transfusing blood and packed RBCs. The use of these filters can postpone sensitization to transfusion therapy. **INS**

Administer packed RBCs with a Y-type set. Using a straight-line set forces you to piggyback the tubing so you can stop the transfusion if necessary but still keep the vein open. Piggybacking increases the chance of harmful microorganisms entering the tubing as you're connecting the blood line to the established line.

Single units of whole blood or blood components should be transfused within a 4-hour period. **INS** The start of the transfusion should begin within 30 minutes from the time the blood is released from the blood bank. **INS** No medications should be added to the blood other than normal saline solution. **INS** **AABB** Patients should also be monitored 15 minutes after the start of therapy and at 15- to 30-minute intervals throughout the transfusion. **INS**

Equipment

Blood administration set (170 to 260-micron filter and tubing with drip chamber for blood, or combined set) ♦ I.V. pole ♦ gloves ♦ gown ♦ face shield ♦ multiple-lead tubing ♦ whole blood or packed RBCs ♦ 250 ml of normal saline solution ♦ venipuncture equipment, if necessary (should include 20G or larger catheter) ♦ optional: ice bag, warm compresses.

Implementation

▶ Confirm the patient's identity using two patient identifiers according to your facility's policy. **JC**
▶ Explain the procedure to the patient. Explain possible signs and symptoms of a transfusion reaction (chills, rash, fever, flank or back pain, dizziness, or blood in urine) and to report these possible signs and symptoms to the nurse. **AABB**
▶ Make sure he has signed an informed consent form before transfusion therapy is initiated. **AABB** **JC**

▶ Record the patient's baseline vital signs.
▶ Obtain whole blood or packed RBCs from the blood bank within 30 minutes of the transfusion start time. Check the expiration date on the blood bag, and observe for abnormal color, RBC clumping, gas bubbles, and extraneous material. Return outdated or abnormal blood to the blood bank. **INS**
▶ Compare the patient's confirmed identity with those on the blood bag label. Check the blood bag identification number, ABO blood group, and

(Text continues on page 573.)

Transfusing blood and selected components

BLOOD COMPONENT	INDICATIONS	COMPATIBILITY	NURSING CONSIDERATIONS
Whole blood Complete (pure) blood	▸ To restore blood volume lost from hemorrhaging, trauma, or burns ▸ Exchange transfusion in sickle cell disease	▸ ABO identical: Group A receives A; group B receives B; group AB receives AB; group O receives O ▸ Rh type must match	▸ Remember that whole blood is seldom administered. ▸ Use blood administration tubing to infuse within 4 hours. ▸ Closely monitor patient's volume status for volume overload. ▸ Warm blood if giving a large quantity. ▸ Use only with normal saline solution.
Packed red blood cells (RBCs) Same RBC mass as whole blood but with 80% of the plasma removed	▸ To restore or maintain oxygen-carrying capacity ▸ To correct anemia and surgical blood loss ▸ To increase RBC mass ▸ Red cell exchange	▸ Group A receives A or O ▸ Group B receives B or O ▸ Group AB receives AB, A, B, or O ▸ Group O receives O ▸ Rh type must match	▸ Use blood administration tubing to infuse over more than 4 hours. ▸ Use only with normal saline solution. ▸ Avoid administering packed RBCs for anemic conditions correctable by nutritional or drug therapy.
Leukocyte-poor RBCs Same as packed RBCs with about 70% of the leukocytes removed	▸ Same as packed RBCs ▸ To prevent febrile reactions from leukocyte antibodies ▸ To treat immuno-compromised patients ▸ To restore RBCs to patients who have had two or more nonhemolytic febrile reactions	▸ Same as packed RBCs ▸ Rh type must match	▸ Use blood administration tubing. ▸ May require a 40-micron filter suitable for hard-spun, leukocyte-poor RBCs. ▸ Other considerations are same as those for packed RBCs. Cells expire 24 hours after washing.
White blood cells (leukocytes) Whole blood with all the RBCs and about 80% of the plasma removed	▸ To treat sepsis that's unresponsive to antibiotics (especially if patient has positive blood cultures or a persistent fever exceeding 101° F [38.3° C]) and life-threatening granulocytopenia (granulocyte count less than 500/µl)	▸ Same as packed RBCs ▸ Compatibility with human leukocyte antigen (HLA) preferable but not necessary unless patient is sensitized to HLA from previous transfusion ▸ Rh type must match	▸ Use a blood administration set. Give 1 unit daily for 4 to 6 days or until infection resolves. ▸ As prescribed, premedicate with antihistamines, acetaminophen (Tylenol), or steroids. ▸ If fever occurs, administer an antipyretic, but don't discontinue transfusion; instead, reduce flow rate, as ordered, for patient comfort. ▸ Because reactions are common, administer slowly over 2 to 4 hours. Check patient's vital signs, and assess him every 15 minutes throughout transfusion. ▸ Give transfusion with antibiotics to treat infection.

(continued)

Transfusing blood and selected components *(continued)*

BLOOD COMPONENT	INDICATIONS	COMPATIBILITY	NURSING CONSIDERATIONS
Platelets Platelet sediment from RBCs or plasma platelets	▸ To treat bleeding caused by decreased circulating platelets or functionally abnormal platelets ▸ To improve platelet count preoperatively in a patient whose count is 50,000/μl or less	▸ ABO compatibility identical; Rh-negative recipients should receive Rh-negative platelets	▸ Use a blood filter or leukocyte-reduction filter. ▸ As prescribed, premedicate with antipyretics and antihistamines if patient's history includes a platelet transfusion reaction or to reduce chills, fever, and allergic reactions. ▸ Use single donor platelets if patient has a need for repeated transfusions. ▸ Platelets aren't used to treat autoimmune thrombocytopenia or thrombocytopenic purpura unless patient has a life-threatening hemorrhage.
Fresh frozen plasma (FFP) Uncoagulated plasma separated from RBCs and rich in coagulation factors V, VIII, and IX	▸ To treat postoperative hemorrhage ▸ To correct an undetermined coagulation factor deficiency ▸ To replace a specific factor when that factor isn't available ▸ Warfarin reversal	▸ ABO compatibility required ▸ Rh match not required	▸ Use a blood administration set, and administer infusion rapidly. ▸ Keep in mind that large-volume transfusions of FFP may require correction for hypocalcemia because citric acid in FFP binds calcium. ▸ Must be infused within 24 hours of being thawed.
Albumin 5% (buffered saline); albumin 25% (salt-poor) A small plasma protein prepared by fractionating pooled plasma	▸ To replace volume lost because of shock from burns, trauma, surgery, or infections ▸ To treat hypoproteinemia (with or without edema)	▸ Not required	▸ Use administration set supplied by manufacturer, and set rate based on patient's condition and response. ▸ Keep in mind that albumin is contraindicated in severe anemia. ▸ Administer cautiously in cardiac and pulmonary disease because heart failure may result from circulatory overload.
Factor VIII concentrate (antihemophilic factor) Cold insoluble portion of plasma recovered from FFP	▸ To treat a patient with hemophilia A ▸ To treat a patient with von Willebrand's disease	▸ ABO compatibility not required	▸ Administer by I.V. injection using a filter needle, or use administration set supplied by manufacturer.

Transfusing blood and selected components (continued)

BLOOD COMPONENT	INDICATIONS	COMPATIBILITY	NURSING CONSIDERATIONS
Cryoprecipitate Insoluble plasma portion of FFP containing fibrinogen, factor VIIIc, factor VIIvWF, factor XIII and fibronectin	▶ To treat factor VIII deficiency and fibrinogen disorders ▶ To treat significant factor XIII deficiency	▶ ABO compatibility required ▶ Rh match not required	▶ Administer with a blood administration set. ▶ Add normal saline solution to each bag of cryoprecipitate, as necessary, to facilitate infusion. ▶ Keep in mind that cryoprecipitate must be administered within 6 hours of thawing. ▶ Before administration, check laboratory studies to confirm a deficiency of one of specific clotting factors present in cryoprecipitate. ▶ Be aware that patients with hemophilia A or von Willebrand's disease should only be treated with cryoprecipitate when appropriate factor VIII concentrates aren't available.

Rh compatibility. Also, compare the patient's blood bank identification number, if present, with the number on the blood bag. Identification of blood and blood products is performed at the patient's bedside by two licensed professionals, according to the facility's policy. **INS** **AABB**

▶ Put on gloves, a gown, and a face shield.

▶ Using a blood administration set, close all the clamps on the set. Then insert the spike of the line you're using for the normal saline solution into the bag of saline solution. Next, open the port on the blood bag, and insert the spike of the line you're using to administer the blood or cellular component into the port. Hang the bag of normal saline solution and blood or cellular component on the I.V. pole, open the clamp on the line of saline solution, and squeeze the drip chamber until it's half full. Then remove the adapter cover at the tip of the blood administration set, open

the main flow clamp, and prime the tubing with saline solution.

▶ If you're administering packed RBCs with a blood administration set, you can add saline solution to the bag to dilute the cells by closing the clamp between the patient and the drip chamber and opening the clamp from the blood. Then lower the blood bag below the saline container and let 30 to 50 ml of saline solution flow into the packed cells. Finally, close the clamp to the blood bag, rehang the bag, rotate it gently to mix the cells and saline solution, and close the clamp to the saline container.

▶ If the patient doesn't have an I.V. catheter in place, perform a venipuncture, using a 20G or larger-diameter catheter. Avoid using an existing line if the catheter lumen is smaller than 20G. Central venous access devices may also be used for transfusion therapy.

▶ If you're administering whole blood, gently invert the bag several times to mix the cells.

▶ Attach the prepared blood administration set to the venipuncture device, and flush it with normal saline solution. Then close the clamp to the saline solution, and open the clamp between the blood bag and the patient. Adjust the flow rate to no greater than 5 ml/minute for the first 15 minutes of the transfusion to observe for a possible transfusion reaction. **INS** **AABB**

▶ Remain with the patient, and watch for signs of a transfusion reaction. **INS** **AABB** If such signs develop, record vital signs and stop the transfusion. Infuse saline solution at a moderately slow infusion rate, and notify the practitioner at once. If no signs of a reaction appear within 15 minutes, you'll need to adjust the flow rate to finish the transfusion within no more than 4 hours.

▶ It's undesirable for RBC preparations to remain at room temperature for more than 4 hours. If the infusion rate must be so slow that the entire unit can't be infused within 4 hours, it may be appropriate to have the blood bank divide the unit and keep one portion refrigerated until it can be administered. **AABB**

▶ Return the empty blood bag to the blood bank, if your facility's policy dictates, and discard the tubing and filter.

▶ Record the patient's vital signs.

Special considerations

▶ Although some microaggregate filters can be used for up to 10 units of blood, always replace the filter and tubing if more than 1 hour elapses between transfusions. When administering multiple units of blood under pressure, use a blood warmer to avoid hypothermia. Blood components may be warmed to no more than 107.6° F (42° C).

▶ For rapid blood replacement, you may need to use a pressure bag. Be aware that excessive pressure may develop, leading to broken blood vessels and extravasation, with hematoma and hemolysis of the infusing RBCs.

▶ If the transfusion stops, take these steps as needed:

— Check that the I.V. container is at least 3′ (1 m) above the level of the I.V. site.

— Make sure the flow clamp is open and that the blood completely covers the filter. If it doesn't, squeeze the drip chamber until it does.

— Gently rock the bag back and forth, agitating blood cells that may have settled.

— Untape the dressing over the I.V. site to check cannula placement. Reposition the cannula if necessary.

— Flush the line with saline solution, and restart the transfusion. Using a Y-type set, close the flow clamp to the patient, and lower the blood bag. Next, open the saline clamp, and allow some saline solution to flow into the blood bag. Rehang the blood bag, open the flow clamp to the patient, and reset the flow rate.

— If a hematoma develops at the I.V. site, immediately stop the infusion. Remove the I.V. cannula. Notify the practitioner, and expect to place ice on the site intermittently for 8 hours; then apply warm compresses. Follow your facility's policy.

— If the blood bag empties before the next one arrives, administer normal saline solution slowly. If you're using a Y-type set, close the blood-line clamp, open the saline clamp, and let the saline run slowly until the new blood arrives. Decrease the flow rate or clamp the line before attaching the new unit of blood.

▶ Despite improvements in cross-matching precautions, transfusion reactions can still occur. Unlike a transfusion reaction, an infectious disease transmitted during a transfusion may go undetected until days, weeks, or even months later, when it produces signs and symptoms. Measures to prevent disease transmission include laboratory testing of blood products and careful screening of potential donors, neither of which is guaranteed. (See *Guide to transfusion reactions.*)

(Text continues on page 577.)

Guide to transfusion reactions

Any patient receiving a transfusion of processed blood products risks certain complications, for example, hemosiderosis and hypothermia. The chart below describes *endogenous reactions*—those caused by an antigen-antibody reaction in the recipient, and *exogenous reactions*—those caused by external factors in administered blood.

REACTIONS AND CAUSES	SIGNS AND SYMPTOMS	NURSING INTERVENTIONS
Endogenous		
Allergic ▶ Allergen in donor blood ▶ Donor blood hypersensitive to certain drugs	▶ Anaphylaxis (chills, facial swelling, laryngeal edema, pruritus, urticaria, wheezing), fever, nausea, and vomiting	▶ Administer antihistamines as prescribed. ▶ Monitor patient for anaphylactic reaction, and administer epinephrine and corticosteroids if indicated. ▶ As prescribed, premedicate patient with diphenhydramine before subsequent transfusion. ▶ Observe patient closely for first 30 minutes of transfusion.

Guide to transfusion reactions (continued)

REACTIONS AND CAUSES	SIGNS AND SYMPTOMS	NURSING INTERVENTIONS
Endogenous *(continued)*		
Bacterial contamination ▶ Organisms that can survive cold, such as *Pseudomonas* and *Staphylococcus*	▶ Chills, fever, vomiting, abdominal cramping, diarrhea, shock, signs of renal failure	▶ Provide broad-spectrum antibiotics, corticosteroids, or epinephrine as prescribed. ▶ Maintain strict blood storage control. ▶ Change blood administration set and filter every 4 hours or after every 2 units. ▶ Infuse each unit of blood over 2 to 4 hours; stop the infusion if the time span exceeds 4 hours. ▶ Maintain sterile technique during administration. ▶ Inspect blood before transfusion for air, clots, and dark purple color.
Febrile ▶ Bacterial lipopolysaccharides ▶ Antileukocyte recipient antibodies directed against donor white blood cells	▶ Temperature up to 104° F (40° C), chills, headache, facial flushing, palpitations, cough, chest tightness, increased pulse rate, flank pain	▶ Relieve symptoms with an antipyretic, an antihistamine, or meperidine, as prescribed. ▶ If the patient requires further transfusions, use frozen RBCs, add a special leukocyte removal filter to the blood line, or premedicate him with acetaminophen, as prescribed, before starting another transfusion. ▶ Premedicate patient with an antipyretic, an antihistamine and, possibly, a steroid.
Hemolytic ▶ ABO or Rh incompatibility ▶ Intradonor incompatibility ▶ Improper cross-matching ▶ Improperly stored blood	▶ Chest pain, dyspnea, facial flushing, fever, chills, shaking, hypotension, flank pain, hemoglobinuria, oliguria, bloody oozing at the infusion site or surgical incision site, burning sensation along vein receiving blood, shock, renal failure	▶ Monitor blood pressure. ▶ Manage shock with I.V. fluids, oxygen, epinephrine, a diuretic, and a vasopressor, as prescribed. ▶ Obtain posttransfusion-reaction blood samples and urine specimens for analysis. ▶ Observe for signs of hemorrhage resulting from disseminated intravascular coagulation. ▶ Before the transfusion, check donor and recipient blood types to ensure blood compatibility.
Plasma protein incompatibility ▶ Immunoglobulin-A incompatibility	▶ Abdominal pain, diarrhea, dyspnea, chills, fever, flushing, hypotension	▶ Administer oxygen, fluids, epinephrine, or a corticosteroid, as prescribed.
Exogenous		
Bleeding tendencies ▶ Low platelet count in stored blood, causing thrombocytopenia	▶ Abnormal bleeding and oozing from a cut, a break in the skin surface, or the gums; abnormal bruising and petechiae	▶ Administer platelets, fresh frozen plasma, or cryoprecipitate, as prescribed. ▶ Monitor platelet count. ▶ Use only fresh blood (less than 7 days old) when possible.
Circulatory overload ▶ May result from infusing blood too rapidly or in large volumes	▶ Increased plasma volume, back pain, chest tightness, chills, fever, dyspnea, flushed feeling, headache, hypertension, increased central venous pressure and jugular vein pressure	▶ Monitor blood pressure. ▶ Use packed red blood cells (RBCs) instead of whole blood. ▶ Administer diuretics as prescribed. ▶ Transfuse blood slowly.

(continued)

Guide to transfusion reactions *(continued)*

REACTIONS AND CAUSES	SIGNS AND SYMPTOMS	NURSING INTERVENTIONS
Exogenous *(continued)*		
Elevated blood ammonia level ▶ Increased ammonia level in stored donor blood	▶ Confusion, forgetfulness, lethargy	▶ Monitor ammonia level in blood. ▶ Decrease the amount of protein in the patient's diet. ▶ If indicated, give neomycin.
Hemosiderosis ▶ Increased level of hemosiderin (iron-containing pigment) from RBC destruction, especially after many transfusions	▶ Iron plasma level exceeding 200 mg/dl	▶ Perform a phlebotomy to remove excess iron. ▶ Administer blood only when absolutely necessary.
Hypocalcemia ▶ Citrate toxicity occurs when citrate-treated blood is infused rapidly. Citrate binds with calcium, causing a calcium deficiency, or normal citrate metabolism becomes impeded by hepatic disease.	▶ Arrhythmias, hypotension, muscle cramps, nausea, vomiting, seizures, tingling in fingers	▶ Slow or stop the transfusion, depending on the patient's reaction. Expect a more severe reaction in hypothermic patients or patients with elevated potassium levels. ▶ Slowly administer calcium gluconate I.V., if prescribed.
Hypothermia ▶ Rapid infusion of large amounts of cold blood, which decreases body temperature	▶ Chills; shaking; hypotension; arrhythmias, especially bradycardia; cardiac arrest, if core temperature falls below 86° F (30° C)	▶ Stop the transfusion. ▶ Warm the patient with blankets. ▶ Obtain an ECG. ▶ Warm blood to 95° to 98° F (35° to 36.7° C)—especially before massive transfusions.
Increased oxygen affinity for hemoglobin ▶ Decreased level of 2,3-diphosphoglycerate in stored blood, causing an increase in the oxygen's hemoglobin affinity. When this occurs, oxygen stays in the bloodstream and isn't released into body tissues.	▶ Depressed respiratory rate, especially in patients with chronic lung disease	▶ Monitor arterial blood gas values, and provide respiratory support as needed.
Potassium intoxication ▶ An abnormally high level of potassium in stored plasma caused by hemolysis of RBCs	▶ Diarrhea, intestinal colic, flaccidity, muscle twitching, oliguria, renal failure, bradycardia progressing to cardiac arrest, electrocardiographic (ECG) changes with tall, peaked T waves	▶ Obtain an ECG. ▶ Administer sodium polystyrene sulfonate (Kayexalate) orally or by enema. ▶ Administer dextrose 50% and insulin, bicarbonate, or calcium, as prescribed, to force potassium into cells. ▶ Use fresh blood when administering massive transfusions.

References

American Association of Blood Banks. *Standards for Blood Banks and Transfusion Services,* 25th ed. Bethesda, Md.: AABB, 2008.

Gould, S., et al. "Packed Red Blood Cell Transfusion in the Intensive Care Unit: Limitations and Consequences," *American Journal of Critical Care* 16(1):39–48, January 2007. **CS**

Hainsworth, T. "Guidance for Preventing Errors in Administering Blood Transfusions," *Nursing Times* 100(27):30–31, 2004.

Rana, R. "Evidence-Based Red Cell Transfusion in the Critically Ill: Quality Improvement Using Computerized Physician Order Entry," *Critical Care Medicine* 34(7):1892–897, July 2006.

"Standard 32. Filters. Infusion Nursing Standards of Practice," *Journal of Infusion Nursing* 29(1S):S33–34, January–February 2006.

"Standard 34. Blood and Fluid Warmers. Infusion Nursing Standards of Practice," *Journal of Infusion Nursing* 29(1S):S35, January–February 2006.

"Standard 48. Administration Set Change. Infusion Nursing Standards of Practice," *Journal of Infusion Nursing* 29(1S):S48–51, January–February 2006.

"Standard 70. Transfusion Therapy. Infusion Nursing Standards of Practice," *Journal of Infusion Nursing* 29(1S):S76–77, January–February 2006.

Traumatic wound management

Traumatic wounds include abrasions, lacerations, puncture wounds, and amputations. In an abrasion, the skin is scraped, with partial loss of the skin surface. In a laceration, the skin is torn, causing jagged, irregular edges; the severity of a laceration depends on its size, depth, and location. A puncture wound occurs when a pointed object, such as a knife or glass fragment, penetrates the skin. Traumatic amputation refers to the removal of part of the body, a limb, or part of a limb.

When caring for a patient with a traumatic wound, first assess his ABCs—airway, breathing, and circulation. **AHA** It may seem natural to focus on a gruesome injury, but a patent airway and pumping heart take first priority. Once the patient's ABCs are stabilized, you can turn your attention to the traumatic wound. Initial management concentrates on controlling bleeding, usually by applying firm, direct pressure and elevating the extremity. If bleeding continues, you may need to compress a pressure point. Assess the condition of the wound. Management and cleaning technique usually depend on the specific type of wound and degree of contamination.

Equipment

Sterile basin ◆ normal saline solution ◆ sterile 4″ × 4″ gauze pads ◆ sterile gloves ◆ clean gloves ◆ sterile cotton-tipped applicators ◆ dry sterile dressing, nonadherent pad, or petroleum gauze ◆ linen-saver pad ◆ optional: clippers, towel, goggles, mask, gown, 50-ml catheter-tip syringe, surgical scrub brush, antibacterial ointment, porous tape, sterile forceps, sutures and suture set.

Implementation

▶ Place a linen-saver pad under the area to be cleaned. Remove any clothing covering the wound. If necessary, clip hair around the wound with scissors.
▶ Assemble needed equipment at the patient's bedside. Fill a sterile basin with normal saline solution. Make sure the treatment area has enough light to allow close observation of the wound. Depending on the nature and location of the wound, wear sterile or clean gloves to avoid spreading infection.
▶ Check the patient's medical history for previous tetanus immunization and, if needed and ordered, arrange for immunization. **CDC**

▶ Administer pain medication, if ordered.
▶ Wash your hands.
▶ Use appropriate protective equipment, such as a gown, a mask, and goggles, if spraying or splashing of body fluids is possible. **CDC**

For an abrasion
▶ Flush the scraped skin with normal saline solution.
▶ Remove dirt or gravel with a sterile 4″ × 4″ gauze pad moistened with normal saline solution. Rub in the opposite direction from which the dirt or gravel became embedded.
▶ If the wound is extremely dirty, you may use a surgical brush to scrub it.
▶ With a small wound, allow it to dry and form a scab. With a larger wound, you may need to cover it with a nonadherent pad or petroleum gauze and a light dressing. Apply antibacterial ointment if ordered.

For a laceration
▶ Moisten a sterile 4″ × 4″ gauze pad with normal saline solution. Clean the wound gently, working outward from its center to about 2″ (5 cm) beyond its edges. Discard the soiled gauze pad,

and use a fresh one as necessary. Continue until the wound appears clean.
▶ If the wound is dirty, you may irrigate it with a 50-ml catheter-tip syringe and normal saline solution.
▶ Assist the practitioner in suturing the wound edges using the suture kit, or apply sterile strips of porous tape.
▶ Apply the prescribed antibacterial ointment to help prevent infection.
▶ Apply a dry sterile dressing over the wound.

For a puncture wound
▶ If the wound is minor, allow it to bleed for a few minutes before cleaning it.
▶ For a larger puncture wound, you may need to irrigate it before applying a dry dressing.
▶ Stabilize any embedded foreign object until the practitioner can remove it. After he removes the object and bleeding is stabilized, clean the wound as you'd clean a laceration or deep puncture wound.

For an amputation
▶ Apply a gauze pad moistened with normal saline solution to the amputation site. Elevate the affected part, and immobilize it for surgery.

Caring for a severed body part

After traumatic amputation, a surgeon may be able to reimplant the severed body part through microsurgery. The chance of successful reimplantation is much greater if the amputated part has received proper care.

If a patient arrives at the hospital with a severed body part, first make sure that bleeding at the amputation site has been controlled. Then follow these guidelines for preserving the body part.

▶ Put on sterile gloves. Place several sterile gauze pads and an appropriate amount of sterile roller gauze in a sterile basin, and pour sterile normal saline or sterile lactated Ringer's solution over them. *Never* use another solution, and don't try to scrub or debride the part.

▶ Holding the body part in one gloved hand, carefully pat it dry with sterile gauze. Place saline-soaked gauze pads over the stump, and then wrap the whole body part with saline-soaked roller gauze. Wrap the gauze with a sterile towel, if available. Then put this package in a watertight container or bag and seal it.

▶ Fill another plastic bag with ice, and place the part, still in its watertight container, inside (as shown at right). Seal the outer bag. (Always protect the part from direct contact with ice and—*never* use dry ice—to prevent irreversible tissue damage, which would make the part unsuitable for reimplantation.) Keep this bag ice-cold until the surgeon is ready to do the reimplantation surgery.

▶ Label the bag with the patient's name, identification number, identification of the amputated part, the hospital identification number, and the date and time when cooling began.

Note: The body part must be wrapped and cooled quickly. Irreversible tissue damage occurs after only 6 hours at ambient temperature. However, hypothermic management seldom preserves tissues for more than 24 hours.

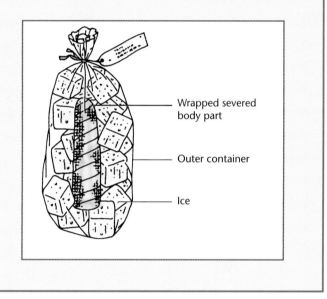

Wrapped severed body part

Outer container

Ice

▶ Recover the amputated part, and prepare it for transport to a facility where microvascular surgery is performed. (See *Caring for a severed body part.*)

Special considerations

▶ When irrigating a traumatic wound, avoid using more than 8 psi of pressure. High-pressure irrigation can seriously interfere with healing, kill cells, and allow bacteria to infiltrate the tissue.

▶ Avoid cleaning a traumatic wound with alcohol because alcohol causes pain and tissue dehydration. Also,

avoid using antiseptics for wound cleaning because they can impede healing. In addition, never use a cotton ball or cotton-filled gauze pad to clean a wound because cotton fibers left in the wound can cause contamination.

▶ After a wound has been cleaned, the practitioner may want to debride it to remove dead tissue and reduce the risk of infection and scarring. If this is necessary, pack the wound with gauze pads soaked in normal saline solution until debridement.

▶ Observe for signs and symptoms of infection, such as warm red skin at the site or purulent discharge. Be aware that infection of a traumatic wound can

delay healing, increase scar formation, and trigger systemic infection, such as septicemia.

▶ Observe all dressings. If edema is present, adjust the dressing to avoid impairing circulation to the area.

References

Day, M. W. "Traumatic Amputation," *Nursing* 36(10):88, October 2006.

Gustafsson, M., and Ahlstrom, G. "Problems Experienced during the First Year of an Acute Traumatic Hand Injury: A Prospective Study," *Journal of Clinical Nursing* 13(8):986–95, November 2004.

Khan, M. N., and Naqvi, A. H. "Antiseptics, Iodine, Povidone-Iodine and Traumatic Wound Cleansing," *Journal of Tissue Viability* 16(4):6–10, November 2006.

Laskowski-Jones, L. "First Aid for Amputation," *Nursing* 36(4):50–52, April 2006.

Pereira, C. "Policy for the Handling of Amputation Parts in Accident and Emergency Departments," *Plastic and Reconstructive Surgery* 116(1):346–47, July 2005.

Venkatramani, H., and Sabapathy, S. R. "A Simple Technique for Stabilizing Subtotal Digital Amputation during Transport," *Plastic and Reconstructive Surgery* 113(5):1527–528, April 2004.

T tube care

The T tube (or biliary drainage tube) may be placed in the common bile duct after cholecystectomy or choledochostomy. This tube facilitates biliary drainage during healing. The surgeon inserts the short end (crossbar) of the T tube in the common bile duct and draws the long end through the incision. The tube then connects to a closed gravity drainage system. (See *Understanding T tube placement*.) Postoperatively, the tube remains in place between 7 and 14 days.

Equipment

Graduated collection container ◆ small plastic bag ◆ sterile gloves ◆ clean gloves ◆ clamp ◆ sterile 4″ × 4″ gauze pads ◆ transparent dressings ◆ rubber band ◆ normal saline solution ◆ sterile cleaning solution ◆ two sterile basins ◆ antimicrobial swab ◆ sterile precut drain dressings ◆ hypoallergenic paper tape ◆ skin protectant, such as petroleum jelly, zinc oxide, or aluminum-based gel ◆ optional: Montgomery straps.

Implementation

▶ Place one sterile 4″ × 4″ gauze pad in each sterile basin. Using sterile technique, pour 50 ml of cleaning solution into one basin and 50 ml of normal saline solution into the other basin. Tape a small plastic bag on the table to use for refuse.

▶ Confirm the patient's identity using two patient identifiers according to your facility's policy. **JC**

▶ Provide privacy and explain the procedure to the patient.

▶ Wash your hands thoroughly. **CDC**

Emptying drainage

▶ Put on clean gloves.

▶ Place the graduated collection container under the outlet valve of the drainage bag. Without contaminating the clamp, valve, or outlet valve, empty the bag's contents completely into the container and reseal the outlet valve. Carefully measure and record the character, color, and amount of drainage.

▶ Discard your gloves.

Re-dressing the T tube

▶ Wash your hands thoroughly. Put on clean gloves. **CDC**

Understanding T tube placement

The T tube is placed in the common bile duct, anchored to the abdominal wall, and connected to a closed drainage system.

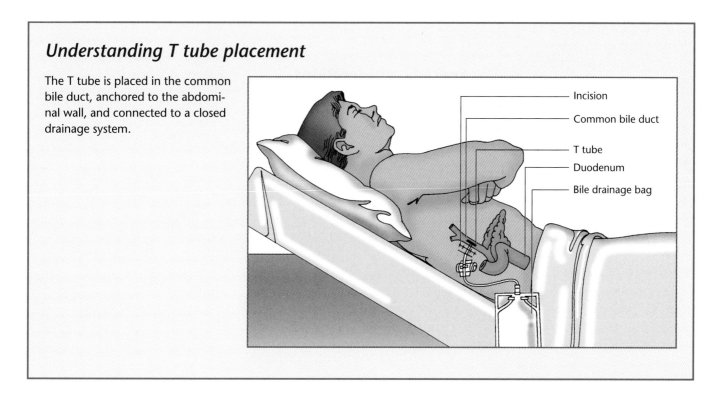

► Without dislodging the T tube, remove old dressings, and dispose of them in the small plastic bag. Remove the clean gloves.

► Wash your hands again, and put on sterile gloves. From this point on, follow sterile technique to prevent bacterial contamination of the incision. **CDC**

► Inspect the incision and tube site for signs of infection, including redness, edema, warmth, tenderness, induration, skin excoriation, or drainage. Assess for wound dehiscence or evisceration.

► Use sterile cleaning solution, as prescribed, to clean and remove dried matter or drainage from around the tube. Always start at the tube site, and gently wipe outward in a continuous motion to prevent recontamination of the incision.

► Use normal saline solution to rinse off the prescribed cleaning solution. Dry the area with a sterile 4″ × 4″ gauze pad, and discard all used materials.

► Using an antimicrobial swab, wipe the incision site in a circular motion. Allow the area to dry thoroughly.

► Lightly apply a skin protectant, such as petroleum jelly, zinc oxide, or aluminum-based gel, to protect the skin from injury caused by draining bile.

► Apply a sterile precut drain dressing on each side of the T tube to absorb drainage.

► Apply a sterile 4″ × 4″ gauze pad or transparent dressing over the T tube and the drain dressings. Be careful not to kink the tubing, which might block the drainage. Also avoid putting the dressing over the open end of the T tube because this end connects to the closed drainage system.

► Secure the dressings with the hypoallergenic paper tape or Montgomery straps, if necessary.

Clamping the T tube

► As ordered, occlude the tube lightly with a clamp, or wrap a rubber band around the end. Clamping the tube 1 hour before and after meals diverts bile back to the duodenum to aid digestion.

► Monitor the patient's response to clamping.

► To ensure patient comfort and safety, check bile drainage amounts regularly. Be alert for such signs of obstructed bile flow as chills, fever, tachycardia, nausea, right-upper-quadrant fullness and pain, jaundice, dark foamy urine, and clay-colored stools. Report them immediately.

Special considerations

► Normal daily bile drainage ranges from 500 to 1,000 ml of viscous, green-brown liquid. The T tube usually drains 300 to 500 ml of blood-tinged bile in the first 24 hours after surgery. Report drainage that exceeds 500 ml in the first 24 hours after surgery. This

amount typically declines to 200 ml or less after 4 days. Monitor fluid, electrolyte, and acid-base status carefully.

► To prevent excessive bile loss (over 500 ml in first 24 hours) or backflow contamination, secure the T tube drainage system at abdominal level. Bile will flow into the bag only when biliary pressure increases. As ordered, return excessive bile drainage (between 1,000 and 1,500 ml daily) to the patient mixed with chilled fruit juice or, if possible, through a nasogastric tube.

► Provide meticulous skin care and frequent dressing changes. Observe for bile leakage, which may indicate obstruction. Assess tube patency and site condition hourly for the first 8 hours and then every 4 hours until the physician removes the tube. Protect the skin edges and avoid excessive taping to prevent shearing the skin.

► Monitor all urine and stools for color changes. Assess for icteric skin and sclera, which may signal jaundice.

References

Craven, R. F., and Hirnle, C. J. *Fundamentals of Nursing: Human Health and Function,* 6th ed. Philadelphia: Lippincott Williams & Wilkins, 2009.

Taylor, C., et al. *Fundamentals of Nursing: The Art and Science of Nursing,* 6th ed. Philadelphia: Lippincott Williams & Wilkins, 2008.

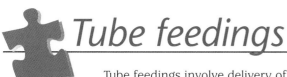

Tube feedings

Tube feedings involve delivery of a liquid feeding formula directly to the stomach (known as *gastric gavage*), duodenum, or jejunum. Gastric gavage typically is indicated for a patient who can't eat normally because of dysphagia or oral or esophageal obstruction or injury. Gastric feedings also may be given to an unconscious or intubated patient or to a patient recovering from GI tract surgery who can't ingest food orally.

According to the American Gastroenterological Association, nutrition support should be initiated after 1 to 2 weeks without nutrient intake. Enteral feeding is preferable to parenteral therapy provided there are no contraindications, access can be safely attained, and oral intake isn't possible. For short-term (less than 30-day) feeding, nasogastric or nasoenteric tubes are preferable to gastrostomy or jejunostomy tubes. Tube feeding is contraindicated in patients who have no bowel sounds or a suspected intestinal obstruction.

Equipment

For gastric feedings: Feeding formula ♦ graduated container ♦ 120 ml of water ♦ gavage bag with tubing and flow regulator clamp ♦ towel or linen-saver pad, if needed ♦ 60-ml syringe ♦ pH test strip ♦ optional: infusion pump, tubing set (for continuous administration), adapter to connect gavage tubing to feeding tube.

For duodenal or jejunal feedings: Feeding formula ♦ enteral administration set containing a gavage container, drip chamber, roller clamp or flow regulator, and tube connector ♦ I.V. pole ♦ 60-ml syringe with adapter tip ♦ water ♦ optional: pump administration set (for an enteral infusion pump), Y connector.

For nasal and oral care: Cotton-tipped applicators ♦ water-soluble lubricant ♦ sponge-tipped swabs ♦ petroleum jelly.

A bulb syringe or large catheter-tip syringe may be substituted for a gavage bag after the patient demonstrates tolerance for a gravity drip infusion.

Implementation

▶ Be sure to refrigerate formulas prepared in the dietary department or pharmacy. Pour 60 ml of water into the graduated container. After closing the flow clamp on the administration set, pour the appropriate amount of formula into the gavage bag. Hang no more than a 4- to 6-hour supply at one time to prevent bacterial growth. **ASPEN** Open the flow clamp on the administration set to remove air from the lines.

▶ Confirm the patient's identity using two patient identifiers according to your facility's policy. **JC**

▶ Provide privacy and wash your hands.

▶ Inform the patient that he'll receive nourishment through the tube, and explain the procedure to him. If possible, give him a schedule of subsequent feedings.

▶ If the patient has a nasal or oral tube, cover his chest with a towel or linen-saver pad to protect him and the bed linens from spills.

▶ Assess the patient's abdomen for bowel sounds and distention. **ASPEN**

Delivering a gastric feeding

▶ To limit the risk of aspiration and reflux, raise the head of the patient's bed 30 to 45 degrees during feeding and for 1 hour after feeding. Use intermittent or continuous feeding regimens rather than the rapid bolus method. **ASPEN**

▶ Check placement of the feeding tube to be sure it hasn't slipped out since the last feeding.

▶ To check tube patency and position, remove the cap or plug from the feeding tube, and use the syringe to aspirate stomach contents. Examine the aspirate, and place a small amount on the pH test strip. The probability of gastric placement is increased if the aspirate has a gastric fluid appearance (grassy-green, clear and colorless with mucus shreds, or brown) and a pH less than or equal to 5.0.

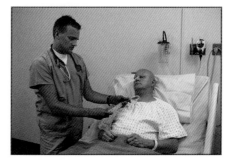

▶ If there's no gastric secretion return, the tube may be in the esophagus. You'll need to advance the tube and recheck placement before continuing.

▶ To assess gastric emptying, aspirate and measure residual gastric contents. Hold feedings if residual volume is greater then the predetermined amount specified in the practitioner's order (usually 50 to 100 ml). Reinstill any aspirate obtained. **ASPEN**

▶ Connect the gavage bag tubing to the feeding tube. Depending on the type of tube used, you may need to use an adapter to connect the two.

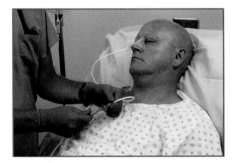

▶ If you're using a bulb or catheter-tip syringe, remove the bulb or plunger and attach the syringe to the pinched-off feeding tube to prevent excess air from entering the patient's stomach, causing distention. If you're using an infusion pump, thread the tube from the formula container through the pump according to the manufacturer's directions. Purge the tubing of air, and attach it to the feeding tube.

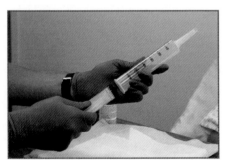

▶ Open the regulator clamp on the gavage bag tubing, and adjust the flow rate appropriately. When using a bulb syringe, fill the syringe with formula, and release the feeding tube to allow formula to flow through it. The height at which you hold the syringe will determine the flow rate. When the syringe is three-quarters empty, pour more formula into it.

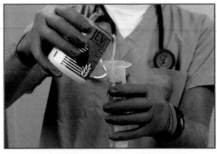

▶ To prevent air from entering the tube and the patient's stomach, never allow the syringe to empty completely. If you're using an infusion pump, set the flow rate according to the manufacturer's directions. Always administer a tube feeding slowly—typically 200 to 350 ml over 15 to 30 minutes, depending on the patient's tolerance and the practitioner's order—to prevent sudden stomach distention, which can cause nausea, vomiting, cramps, or diarrhea.

▶ After administering the appropriate amount of formula, flush the tubing by adding about 60 ml of water to the gavage bag or bulb syringe, or manually flush it using a barrel syringe. This maintains the tube's patency by removing excess formula, which could occlude the tube. **ASPEN**

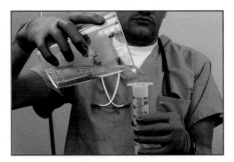

▶ If you're administering a continuous feeding, flush the feeding tube every 4 hours to help prevent tube occlusion. Monitor gastric emptying every 4 hours. **ASPEN**

▶ To discontinue gastric feeding (depending on the equipment you're using), close the regulator clamp on the gavage bag tubing, disconnect the syringe from the feeding tube, or turn off the infusion pump.

▶ Cover the end of the feeding tube with its plug or cap to prevent leakage and contamination of the tube.

▶ Leave the patient in semi-Fowler's or high Fowler's position for at least 1 hour. **ASPEN** **AACN**

▶ Rinse all reusable equipment with warm water. Dry it and store it in a convenient place for the next feeding. Change equipment every 24 hours or according to your facility's policy.

Delivering a duodenal or jejunal feeding

▶ Elevate the head of the bed, and place the patient in low Fowler's position.

▶ Open the enteral administration set, and hang the gavage container on the I.V. pole.

▶ If you're using a nasoduodenal tube, measure its length to check tube placement. Remember that you may not get any residual when you aspirate the tube.

▶ Open the flow clamp, and regulate the flow to the desired rate. To regulate the rate using a volumetric infusion pump, follow the manufacturer's directions for setting up the equipment. Most patients receive small amounts initially, with volumes increasing gradually once tolerance is established.

▶ Flush the tube every 4 hours with water to maintain patency and provide hydration. **ASPEN**

▶ Change equipment every 24 hours or according to your facility's policy.

Special considerations

▶ If the feeding solution doesn't initially flow through a bulb syringe, attach the bulb and squeeze it gently to start the flow. Then remove the bulb. Never use the bulb to force the formula through the tube.

▶ If the patient becomes nauseated or vomits, stop the feeding immediately. The patient may vomit if the stomach becomes distended from overfeeding or delayed gastric emptying.

▶ To reduce oropharyngeal discomfort from the tube, allow the patient to brush his teeth or care for his dentures regularly, and encourage frequent gargling. If the patient is unconscious, administer oral care with sponge-tipped swabs every 4 hours. Use petroleum jelly on dry, cracked lips. (*Note:* Dry mucous membranes may indicate dehydration, which requires increased fluid intake.) Clean the patient's nostrils with cotton-tipped applicators, apply lubricant along the mucosa, and assess the skin for signs of breakdown. **CDC**

▶ During continuous feedings, assess the patient frequently for abdominal distention. Flush the tubing by adding about 50 ml of water to the gavage bag or bulb syringe. This maintains the tube's patency by removing excess formula, which could occlude the tube. **ASPEN**

▶ If the patient develops diarrhea, administer small, frequent, less concentrated feedings, or administer bolus feedings over a longer time. Also, make sure the formula isn't cold and that proper storage and sanitation practices have been followed. The loose stools associated with tube feedings make extra perineal and skin care necessary. Changing to a formula with more fiber may eliminate liquid stools. Studies have shown that banana flakes are also effective at controlling diarrhea in patients receiving tube feedings. **CS**

▶ If the patient becomes constipated, the practitioner may increase the fruit, vegetable, or sugar content of the formula. Assess the patient's hydration status because dehydration may produce constipation. Increase fluid intake as necessary.

▶ Drugs can be administered through the feeding tube. Except for enteric-coated drugs or sustained-release medications, crush tablets or open and dilute capsules in water before administering them. Be sure to flush the tubing afterward to ensure full instillation of medication.

▶ For duodenal or jejunal feeding, most patients tolerate a continuous drip better than bolus feedings. Bolus feedings can cause such complications as hyperglycemia, glycosuria, and diarrhea.

▶ Until the patient acquires a tolerance for the formula, you may need to dilute it to half or three-quarters strength to start, and increase it gradually. Patients under stress or who are receiving steroids may experience a pseudodiabetic state. Assess such patients frequently to determine the need for insulin.

▶ Check your facility's policy regarding the frequency of changing feeding tubes to prevent complications. (See *Managing tube feeding problems,* page 586.)

▶ Using the gastric route, frequent or large-volume feedings can cause bloating and retention. Dehydration, diarrhea, and vomiting can cause metabolic disturbances. Cramping and abdominal distention usually indicate intolerance.

▶ Using the duodenal or jejunal route, clogging of the feeding tube is common. The patient may experience metabolic, fluid, and electrolyte abnormalities including hyperglycemia, hyperosmolar dehydration, coma, edema, hypernatremia, and essential fatty acid deficiency.

▶ The patient also may experience dumping syndrome, in which a large amount of hyperosmotic solution in the duodenum causes excessive diffusion of fluid through the semipermeable membrane and results in diarrhea. In a patient with low serum albumin levels, these symptoms may result from low oncotic pressure in the duodenal mucosa.

Managing tube feeding problems

COMPLICATION	NURSING INTERVENTIONS
Aspiration of gastric secretions	▶ Discontinue feeding immediately. ▶ Perform tracheal suction of aspirated contents, if possible. ▶ Notify the practitioner. Prophylactic antibiotics and chest physiotherapy may be ordered. ▶ Check tube placement before feeding to prevent complication.
Tube obstruction	▶ Flush the tube with warm water. If necessary, replace the tube. ▶ Flush the tube with 50 ml of water after each feeding to remove excess sticky formula, which could occlude the tube. ▶ When possible, use liquid forms of medications. Otherwise, and if not contraindicated, crush well.
Oral, nasal, or pharyngeal irritation or necrosis	▶ Provide frequent oral hygiene using mouthwash or sponge-tipped swabs. Use petroleum jelly on cracked lips. ▶ Change the tube's position. If necessary, replace the tube.
Vomiting, bloating, diarrhea, or cramps	▶ Reduce the flow rate. ▶ Verify tube placement. ▶ Administer metoclopramide to increase GI motility. ▶ Warm the formula to prevent GI distress. ▶ For 30 minutes after feeding, position the patient on his right side with his head elevated to facilitate gastric emptying. ▶ Notify the practitioner. He may want to reduce the amount of formula being given during each feeding.
Constipation	▶ Provide additional fluids if the patient can tolerate them. ▶ Have the patient participate in an exercise program, if possible. ▶ Administer a bulk-forming laxative. ▶ Review medications. Discontinue medications that have a tendency to cause constipation. ▶ Increase fruit, vegetable, or sugar content of the feeding.
Electrolyte imbalance	▶ Monitor serum electrolyte levels. ▶ Notify the practitioner. He may want to adjust the formula content to correct the deficiency.
Hyperglycemia	▶ Monitor blood glucose levels. ▶ Notify the practitioner of elevated levels. ▶ Administer insulin, if ordered. ▶ The practitioner may adjust the sugar content of the formula.

References

American Society for Parenteral and Enteral Nutrition. "Access for Administration of Nutrition Support," *Journal of Parenteral Enteral Nutrition* 26(Suppl 1): 33SA–41SA, January–February 2002.

Bowman, A., et al. "Implementation of an Evidence-Based Feeding Protocol and Aspiration Risk Reduction Algorithm," *Critical Care Nursing Quarterly* 28(4):324–33, October–December 2005.

Ellett, M. L. "Important Facts about Intestinal Feeding Tube Placement," *Gastroenterology Nursing* 29(2):112–24, March–April 2006.

Emery, E. A., et al. "Banana Flakes Control Diarrhea in Enterally Fed Patients," *Nutrition in Clinical Practice* 12(2):72–75, April 1997. **CS**

Guenter, P., and Silkroski, M. *Tube Feeding: Practical Guidelines and Nursing Protocols.* Gaithersburg, Md.: Aspen Pubs., Inc., 2001.

Metheny, N. A. "Preventing Respiratory Complications of Tube Feedings: Evidence-Based Practice," *American Journal of Critical Care* 15(4):360–69, July 2006.

Metheny, N. A., et al. "Indicators of Tubesite during Feedings," *Journal of Neuroscience Nursing* 37(6):320–25, December 2005.

Taylor, C., et al. *Fundamentals of Nursing: The Art and Science of Nursing Care,* 6th ed. Philadelphia: Lippincott Williams & Wilkins, 2008.

U

Urine collection

A random urine specimen, usually collected as part of the physical examination or at various times during hospitalization, permits laboratory screening for urinary and systemic disorders as well as for drug screening. A clean-catch midstream specimen is replacing random collection because it provides a virtually uncontaminated specimen without the need for catheterization.

An indwelling catheter specimen—obtained either by clamping the drainage tube and emptying the accumulated urine into a container or by aspirating a specimen with a syringe—requires sterile collection technique to prevent catheter contamination and urinary tract infection. This method is contraindicated after genitourinary surgery.

Equipment

For a random specimen: Bedpan or urinal with cover, if necessary ◆ gloves ◆ graduated container ◆ specimen container with lid ◆ label ◆ laboratory request form and laboratory biohazard transport bag.

For a clean-catch midstream specimen: Soap and water ◆ gloves ◆ graduated container ◆ three sterile 2″ × 2″ gauze pads ◆ antiseptic solution ◆ sterile specimen container with lid ◆ label ◆ bedpan or urinal, if necessary ◆ laboratory request form and laboratory biohazard transport bag. (Commercial clean-catch kits containing antiseptic towelettes, sterile specimen container with lid and label, and instructions for use in several languages are widely used.)

For an indwelling catheter specimen: Gloves ◆ antiseptic pad ◆ 10-ml syringe ◆ blunt needle if needleless access port isn't available ◆ tube clamp ◆ sterile specimen container with lid ◆ label ◆ laboratory request form and laboratory biohazard transport bag.

Implementation

▶ Verify the order for the urine specimen.

▶ Confirm the patient's identity using two patient identifiers according to your facility's policy. **JC**

▶ Tell the patient that you need a urine specimen for laboratory analysis. Explain the procedure to him and his family, if necessary, to promote cooperation and prevent accidental disposal of specimens.

Collecting a random specimen

▶ Provide privacy. Instruct the patient on bed rest to void into a clean bedpan or urinal, or ask the ambulatory patient to void into either one in the bathroom.

▶ Put on gloves. Then pour at least 120 ml of urine into the specimen container, and cap the container securely. If the patient's urine output must be measured and recorded, pour the remaining urine into the graduated container. Otherwise, discard the remaining urine. If you inadvertently spill urine on the outside of the container, clean and dry it to prevent cross-contamination.

▶ After you label the specimen container with the patient's name and identification number and the date and time of collection, attach the laboratory request form, place it in the laboratory biohazard transport bag, and send it the laboratory immediately. Delayed transport of the specimen may alter test results.

▶ Clean the graduated container and urinal or bedpan, and return them to their proper storage area. Discard disposable items.

▶ Wash your hands thoroughly. Offer the patient a washcloth and soap and water to wash his hands.

Collecting a clean-catch midstream specimen

▶ Because the goal is a virtually uncontaminated specimen, explain the procedure to the patient carefully. Provide illustrations to emphasize the correct collection technique, if possible.

▶ Tell the male patient to remove all clothing from the waist down and to stand in front of the toilet as for urination or, if female, to sit far back on the toilet seat and spread her legs. Then have the patient clean the periurethral area (tip of the penis or labial folds, vulva, and urinary meatus) with soap and water and wipe the area three times, each time with a fresh $2'' \times 2''$ gauze pad soaked in antiseptic solution or with the wipes provided in a commercial kit. Instruct the female patient to separate her labial folds with the thumb and forefinger. Tell her to wipe down one side with the first pad and discard it, to wipe the other side with the second pad and discard it and, finally, to wipe down the center over the urinary meatus with the third pad and discard it. Stress the importance of cleaning from front to back to avoid contaminating the genital area with fecal matter. For the uncircumcised male patient, emphasize the need to retract his foreskin to effectively clean the meatus and to keep it retracted during voiding.

▶ Tell the female patient to straddle the bedpan or toilet to allow labial spreading and to keep her labia separated while voiding.

▶ Instruct the patient to begin voiding into the bedpan, urinal, or toilet. Then, without stopping the urine stream, the patient should move the collection container into the stream, collecting 30 to 50 ml at the midstream portion of the voiding. He can then finish voiding into the bedpan, urinal, or toilet.

▶ Put on gloves before discarding the first and last portions of the voiding, and measure the remaining urine in a graduated container for intake and output records, if necessary. Be sure to include the amount in the specimen container when recording the total amount voided.

▶ Take the sterile container from the patient, and cap it securely. Avoid touching the inside of the container or the lid. If the outside of the container is soiled, clean it and wipe it dry. Remove gloves and discard them properly.

▶ Wash your hands thoroughly. Tell the patient to wash his hands also.

▶ Label the container with the patient's name and identification number, name of test, type of specimen, collection time, and suspected diagnosis, if known. If a urine culture has been ordered, note any current antibiotic therapy on the laboratory request form. Place the specimen in a laboratory biohazard transport bag, and send the container to the laboratory immediately or place it on ice to prevent specimen deterioration and altered test results.

Collecting an indwelling catheter specimen

▶ About 30 minutes before collecting the specimen, clamp the drainage tube to allow urine to accumulate.

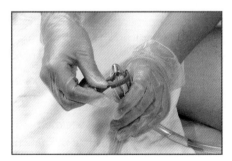

▶ Put on gloves. Wipe the aspiration port with an alcohol pad. Attach the syringe to the needleless aspiration port, and withdraw the sample. If the aspiration port is not needleless, attach the blunt needle to the syringe, insert the needle into the aspiration port, and withdraw the sample. **CDC**

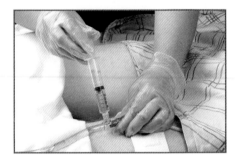

▶ Transfer the specimen to a sterile container, label it, and send it to the laboratory immediately in a laboratory biohazard transport bag, or place it on ice. If a urine culture is to be performed, be sure to list any current antibiotic therapy on the laboratory request form.

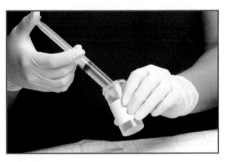

Special considerations

▶ To avoid contaminating the specimen, don't touch the inside of the container.

▶ If the specimen is to be collected by the patient at home, instruct the patient to collect the specimen in a clean container with a tight-fitting lid and to keep it on ice or in the refrigerator (separate from food items) for up to 24 hours.

References

Craven, R. F., and Hirnle, C. J. *Fundamentals of Nursing: Human Health and Function,* 6th ed. Philadelphia: Lippincott Williams & Wilkins, 2009.

Davis, K. "Need Urine from a Catheter System? Forget the Needle," *Nursing* 34(12):64, December 2004.

Fernandez, R. S., et al. "Clamping Short-Term Indwelling Catheters: A Systematic Review of the Evidence," *Journal of Wound, Ostomy, and Continence Nursing* 32(5):329–36, September–October, 2005.

Fischbach, F. A. *Manual of Laboratory and Diagnostic Tests,* 7th ed. Philadelphia: Lippincott Williams & Wilkins, 2004.

Occupational Safety and Health Administration. "Bloodborne Pathogens," 1910.1030. Available at *www.osha.gov/pls/oshaweb/owadisp.show_document?p_table=STANDARDS&p_id=10051.*

Ribby, K. J. "Decreasing Urinary Tract Infections through Staff Development, Outcomes, and Nursing Process," *Journal of Nursing Quality Care* 21(2):194–198, April–June, 2006.

U.S. Department of Health and Human Services Division of Workplace Program. "Drug Testing Specimen Collection." Available at *http://www.workplace.samhsa.gov/DrugTesting/SpecimenCollection/index.html.*

Wilson, L. A. "Urinalysis," *Nursing Standard* 19(35):51–54, May 2005.

V

Vacuum-assisted closure therapy

Vacuum-assisted closure (VAC) therapy, also known as *negative pressure wound therapy,* is used to enhance delayed or impaired wound healing. The VAC device applies localized subatmospheric pressure to draw the edges of the wound toward the center. It's applied after a special dressing is placed in the wound or over a graft or flap; this wound packing removes fluids from the wound and stimulates growth of healthy granulation tissue. (See *Understanding vacuum-assisted closure therapy*.)

VAC therapy is indicated for acute and traumatic wounds, pressure ulcers, and chronic open wounds, such as diabetic ulcers, meshed grafts, and skin flaps. It's contraindicated for fistulas that involve organs or body cavities, necrotic tissue with eschar, untreated osteomyelitis, malignant wounds, and wounds with exposed arteries and veins. This therapy should be used cautiously in patients with active bleeding, in those taking anticoagulants, and when achieving wound hemostasis has been difficult.

Equipment

Waterproof trash bag ◆ goggles ◆ gown, if indicated ◆ emesis basin ◆ sterile irrigating solution ◆ normal saline solution ◆ clean gloves ◆ sterile gloves ◆ sterile scissors ◆ linen-saver pad ◆ irrigating syringe ◆ reticulated foam ◆ fenestrated tubing ◆ evacuation tubing ◆ skin protectant wipe ◆ transparent occlusive air-permeable drape ◆ evacuation canister ◆ vacuum unit.

Implementation

▶ Assemble the VAC device at the bedside per the manufacturer's instructions. Set negative pressure according to the practitioner's order (25 to 200 mm Hg). **MFR**

▶ Warm the irrigating solution to 90° to 95° F to reduce discomfort.

▶ Confirm the patient's identity using two patient identifiers according to your facility's policy. **JC**

▶ Assess the patient's condition.

▶ Explain the procedure to the patient, provide privacy, and wash your hands. Put on goggles—and a gown, if necessary. **CDC**

▶ Place a linen-saver pad under the patient to catch any spills and avoid linen changes. Position the patient to allow maximum wound exposure. Place the emesis basin under the wound to collect any drainage.

▶ Use sterile technique, and prepare a sterile field with all your supplies. **CDC**

▶ Put on clean gloves. Remove the soiled dressing, and discard it in the waterproof trash bag. Remove your gloves.

▶ Put on sterile gloves, and irrigate the wound thoroughly using the normal saline solution and the irrigating syringe.

▶ Clean the area around the wound with normal saline solution; wipe intact skin with a skin protectant wipe, and allow it to dry well. Remove and discard your gloves. **MFR**

▶ If your sterile gloves are contaminated, remove them and put on a new pair. Using sterile scissors, cut the foam to the shape and measurement of the wound. More than one piece of foam may be necessary if the first piece is cut too small. Carefully place the foam in the wound. **MFR**

Understanding vacuum-assisted closure therapy

Vacuum-assisted closure (VAC) therapy, also called *negative pressure wound therapy,* is an option to consider when a wound fails to heal in a timely manner. VAC therapy encourages healing by applying localized subatmospheric pressure at the site of the wound. This reduces edema and bacterial colonization and stimulates the formation of granulation tissue.

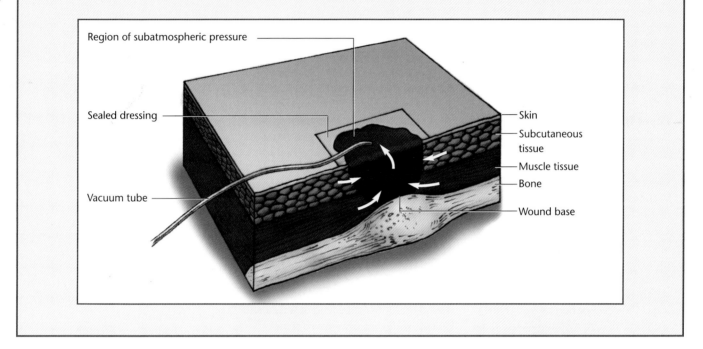

▶ Next, place the fenestrated tubing into the center of the foam. The fenestrated tubing, embedded into the foam, delivers negative pressure to the wound. Make sure there's foam between the tubing and the base of the wound and over the top of the tubing.

▶ Place the transparent occlusive air permeable drape over the foam, enclosing both the foam and the tubing. Leave at least a 2″ (5-cm) margin around the wound of intact skin covered by the dressing. **MFR**

▶ Connect the free end of the fenestrated tubing to the evacuation tubing connected to the evacuation canister. Make sure the tubing isn't located over any bony prominences. **MFR**

▶ Remove and discard your gloves.

▶ Turn on the vacuum unit. Make sure the transparent dressing shrinks to the foam and the skin. This confirms a good seal is present.

▶ Make sure the patient is comfortable.

▶ Properly dispose of drainage, solution, linen-saver pad, and trash bag. **CDC**

Special considerations

▶ Change the dressing every 48 to 72 hours. Try to coordinate dressing change with the practitioner's visit so he can inspect the wound.

▶ Measure the amount of drainage every shift.

▶ Adjust the negative pressure setting according to the practitioner's orders.

▶ Audible and visual alarms alert you if the unit is tipped greater than 45 degrees, the canister is full, the dressing has an air leak, or the canister becomes dislodged. **MFR**

▶ Change the canister once a week or according to your facility's policy.

▶ To obtain optimal therapy, the unit must be applied at least 22 out of 24 hours.

EVIDENCE-BASED RESEARCH

Cost-effectiveness of VAC therapy

Braakenburg, A., et al. "The Clinical Efficacy and Cost-Effectiveness of the Vacuum-Assisted Closure Technique in the Management of Acute and Chronic Wound: A Randomized Controlled Trial," *Plastic and Reconstructive Surgery* 118(2):390–97, August 2006.

Level II
Evidence obtained from at least one well-designed randomized controlled trial

Description
Vacuum-assisted closure (VAC) therapy is used to facilitate wound-healing capacity. This study investigated the effect of VAC therapy on wound healing, (decrease in) bacterial concentration, pain, time, and total costs compared to traditional wound dressings. Sixty-five patients—with either a chronic or acute wound—were randomized to initial treatment with VAC therapy or traditional wound dressings. The endpoint for the study was a granulated wound or a wound that was ready for skin grafting or healing by secondary intention.

Findings
There was no significant decrease in the time to the endpoint, with the exception of patients with cardiovascular disease or diabetes. VAC therapy didn't decrease bacterial concentration or the wound surface. However, there was a significant increase in patient comfort, compared with traditional wound dressings. The amount of time the staff was involved was also significantly lower with the VAC therapy. However, the costs of VAC therapy and traditional wound dressings were similar.

Conclusion
VAC therapy is as effective as traditional wound dressings for healing of wounds. Patients with cardiovascular disease and diabetes have improved healing times with the use of VAC therapy. VAC therapy should always be considered as an option for patients.

Nursing practice implications
Nurses are the ones who are usually responsible for wound care duties. Using VAC therapy is not only more comfortable for their patients, but also decreases the time spent performing wound care. Here are some important nursing practice implications:
▶ Discuss the use of VAC therapy for your patient with the practitioner, especially if the patient has cardiovascular disease or diabetes.
▶ Document wound care carefully, noting the characteristics of the wound.
▶ Medicate the patient for pain before beginning any wound care routine.
▶ Educate the staff on the proper use of VAC therapy.
▶ Actively learn how to use VAC therapy and equipment properly.
▶ Perform wound care according to the practitioner's orders.

References

Andros, G., et al. "Consensus Statement on Negative Pressure Wound Therapy (V.A.C. Therapy) for the Management of Diabetic Foot Wounds," *Ostomy/ Wound Management* Suppl:1–32, June 2006.

Attinger, C. E., et al. "Clinical Approach to Wounds: Debridement and Wound Bed Preparation Including the Use of Dressing and Wound-Healing Adjuvants,"

Plastic and Reconstructive Surgery 117 (7 Suppl):72S–109S, June 2006.

Llanos, S., et al. "Effectiveness of Negative Pressure Closure in the Integration of Split Thickness Skin Grafts: A Randomized, Double-Masked, Controlled Trial," *Annals of Surgery* 244(5):700–705, November 2006.

Morris, G. H., et al. "Negative Pressure Wound Therapy Achieved By Vacuum-Assisted Closure: Evaluating the

Assumption," *Ostomy/Wound Management* 53(1):52–57, January 2007.

Pham, C. T., et al. "The Safety and Efficacy of Topical Negative Pressure in Non-Healing Wounds: A Systematic Review," *Journal of Wound Care* 15(6):240–50, June 2006.

Vagal maneuvers

When a patient suffers sinus, atrial, or junctional tachyarrhythmias, vagal maneuvers—Valsalva's maneuver and carotid sinus massage—can slow his heart rate. These maneuvers work by stimulating nerve endings, which respond as they would to an increase in blood pressure. They send this message to the brain stem, which in turn stimulates the autonomic nervous system to increase vagal tone and decrease the heart rate.

In Valsalva's maneuver, the patient holds his breath and bears down, raising his intrathoracic pressure. When this pressure increase is transmitted to the heart and great vessels, venous return, stroke volume, and systolic blood pressure decrease. Within seconds, the baroreceptors respond to these changes by increasing the heart rate and causing peripheral vasoconstriction.

When the patient exhales at the end of the maneuver, his blood pressure rises to its previous level. This increase, combined with the peripheral vasoconstriction caused by bearing down, stimulates the vagus nerve, decreasing the heart rate.

In carotid sinus massage, manual pressure applied to the left or right carotid sinus slows the heart rate. This method is used both to diagnose and treat tachyarrhythmias. The patient's response to carotid sinus massage depends on the type of arrhythmia. If he has sinus tachycardia, his heart rate will slow gradually during the procedure and speed up again after it. If he has atrial tachycardia, the arrhythmia may stop and the heart rate may remain slow because the procedure increases atrioventricular (AV) block. With atrial fibrillation or flutter, the ventricular rate may not change; AV block may even worsen. With paroxysmal atrial tachycardia, reversion to sinus rhythm occurs only 20% of the time. Nonparoxysmal tachycardia and ventricular tachycardia won't respond. **AHA**

Vagal maneuvers are contraindicated for patients with severe coronary artery disease, acute myocardial infarction, or hypovolemia. Carotid sinus massage is contraindicated for patients with cardiac glycoside toxicity or cerebrovascular disease and for patients who have had carotid surgery.

Although usually performed by a physician, vagal maneuvers may also be done by a specially prepared nurse under a physician's supervision.

AGE FACTOR

Because older patients commonly have undiagnosed atherosclerosis, and carotid bruits aren't always present even with significant atherosclerosis, most experts avoid carotid sinus massage in elderly and late middle-age patients. In these patients, experts agree that Valsalva's maneuver should be used.

Equipment

Crash cart with emergency medications and airway equipment ◆ electrocardiogram (ECG) monitor and electrodes ◆ I.V. catheter ◆ insertion supplies ◆ dextrose 5% in water (D_5W) ◆ optional: clippers, if needed, cardiotonic drugs.

Implementation

▶ Confirm the patient's identity using two patient identifiers according to your facility's policy. **JC**
▶ Explain the procedure to the patient to ease his fears and promote cooperation. Ask him to let you know if he feels light-headed.
▶ Place the patient in a supine position. Insert an I.V. line, if necessary. Then administer D_5W at a keep-vein-open rate, as ordered. This line will be used if emergency drugs become necessary.
▶ Prepare the patient's skin, including clipping the hair if necessary, and attach ECG electrodes. Adjust the size of the ECG complexes on the monitor so that you can see the arrhythmia clearly.

Valsalva's maneuver

▶ Ask the patient to take a deep breath and bear down, as if he were trying to defecate. If he doesn't feel light-headed or dizzy, and if no new arrhythmias occur, have him hold his breath and bear down for 10 seconds. **AHA**
▶ If he does feel dizzy or light-headed, or if you see a new arrhythmia on the monitor—asystole for more than 6 seconds, frequent premature ventricular contractions (PVCs), or ventricular

tachycardia or ventricular fibrillation—allow him to exhale and stop bearing down.

▶ After 10 seconds, ask him to exhale and breathe quietly. If the maneuver was successful, the monitor will show his heart rate slowing before he exhales.

Carotid sinus massage

▶ Begin by obtaining a rhythm strip, using the lead that shows the strongest P waves.

▶ Auscultate both carotid sinuses. If you detect bruits, inform the practitioner, and don't perform carotid sinus massage. If you don't detect bruits, proceed as ordered. (See *Location and technique for carotid sinus massage*.)

▶ Monitor the ECG throughout the procedure. Stop massaging when the ventricular rate slows sufficiently to permit diagnosis of the rhythm. Or, stop as soon as any evidence of a rhythm change appears. Have the crash cart handy to give emergency treatment if a dangerous arrhythmia occurs. **AHA**

▶ If the procedure has no effect within 5 seconds, stop massaging the right carotid sinus and begin to massage the left. If this also fails, administer cardiotonic drugs, as ordered.

Special considerations

▶ Remember that a brief period of asystole—from 3 to 6 seconds—and several PVCs may precede conversion to normal sinus rhythm.

▶ If the vagal maneuver succeeded in slowing the patient's heart rate and converting the arrhythmia, continue monitoring him for several hours.

▶ Vagal maneuvers can occasionally cause bradycardia or complete heart block, so monitor the patient's cardiac rhythm closely.

References

American Association of Critical Care Nurses Standards. Available at *www.aacn.org/AACN/practice.nsf/Files/acstds/$file/130300StdsAcute.pdf.*

American Heart Association. "2005 AHA Guidelines for Cardiopulmonary Resuscitation and Emergency Cardiovascular Care: International Consensus on Science," *Circulation* 112 (22Suppl):IV-1-IV-221, November 2005.

Deepak, S. M., et al. "Ventricular Fibrillation Induced by Carotid Sinus Massage without Preceding Bradycardia," *Europace* 7(6):638–40, November 2005.

Farwell, D. J., and Sulke, A. N. "A Randomized Prospective Comparison of Three Protocols for Head-Up Tilt Testing and Carotid Sinus Massage," *International Journal of Cardiology* 105(3):241–49, February 2006.

Felker, G. M., et al. "The Valsalva Maneuver: A Bedside 'Biomarker' for Heart Failure," *American Journal of Medicine* 119(2):117–22, February 2006.

Location and technique for carotid sinus massage

Before applying manual pressure to the patient's right carotid sinus, locate the bifurcation of the carotid artery on the right side of the neck. Turn the patient's head slightly to the left, and hyperextend the neck. This brings the carotid artery closer to the skin and moves the sternocleidomastoid muscle away from the carotid artery.

Then using a circular motion, gently massage the right carotid sinus between your fingers and the transverse processes of the spine for 3 to 5 seconds. Don't massage for more than 5 seconds to avoid risking life-threatening complications.

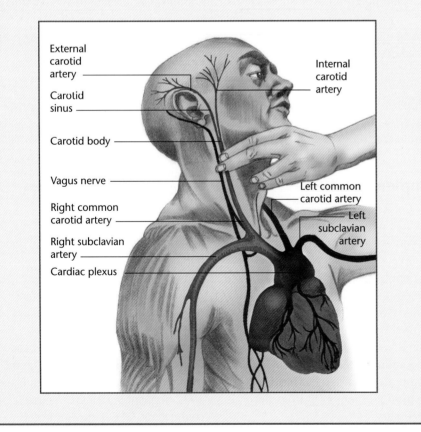

External carotid artery

Carotid sinus

Carotid body

Vagus nerve

Right common carotid artery

Right subclavian artery

Cardiac plexus

Internal carotid artery

Left common carotid artery

Left subclavian artery

Vaginal medications

Vaginal medications include suppositories, creams, gels, and ointments. These medications can be inserted as topical treatments for infection or inflammation or as a contraceptive. Suppositories melt when they contact the vaginal mucosa, and their medication diffuses topically (as effectively as creams, gels, and ointments).

Vaginal medications usually come with a disposable applicator that enables placement of medication in the anterior and posterior fornices. Vaginal administration is most effective when the patient can remain lying down afterward to retain the medication.

Equipment

Patient's medication record and chart ◆ prescribed medication and applicator, if necessary ◆ water-soluble lubricant ◆ gloves ◆ small sanitary pad.

Implementation

▶ If possible, plan to insert vaginal medications at bedtime, when the patient is recumbent.
▶ Verify the order on the patient's medication record by checking it against the practitioner's order. **JC** **ISMP**
▶ Confirm the patient's identity using two patient identifiers according to your facility's policy. **JC**
▶ If your facility utilizes a bar code scanning system, be sure to scan your ID badge, the patient's ID bracelet, and the medication's bar code. **JC** **ISMP**
▶ Wash your hands, explain the procedure to the patient, and provide privacy.
▶ Ask the patient to void.
▶ Ask the patient if she would rather insert the medication herself. If so, provide appropriate instructions. If not, proceed with the following steps.
▶ Help her into the lithotomy position.
▶ Expose only the perineum.

Inserting a suppository
▶ Remove the suppository from the wrapper, and lubricate it with water-soluble lubricant.

▶ Put on gloves, and expose the vagina by spreading the labia.
▶ With an applicator or the forefinger of your free hand, insert the suppository about 2″ (5 cm) into the vagina.

Inserting ointments, creams, or gels
▶ Insert the plunger into the applicator. Then attach the applicator to the tube of medication.
▶ Gently squeeze the tube to fill the applicator with the prescribed amount of medication. Detach the applicator

from the tube, and lubricate the applicator.
▶ Put on gloves, and expose the vagina by spreading the labia.
▶ Insert the applicator as you would a small suppository, and administer the medication by depressing the plunger on the applicator. (See *How to insert vaginal cream.*)

After vaginal insertion
▶ Remove and discard your gloves.
▶ Wash the applicator with soap and warm water and store it, unless it's

How to insert vaginal cream

Fill the applicator with the prescribed amount of medication. Then lubricate the applicator, hold it by the cylinder, and insert it into the vagina. To ensure the patient's comfort, direct the applicator down initially, toward the spine, and then up and back, toward the cervix (as shown).

Administer the medication by depressing the plunger. Remove the applicator while the plunger is still depressed.

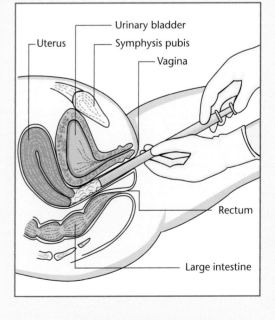

disposable. If the applicator can be used again, label it so that it will be used only for the same patient.

▶ To prevent the medication from soiling the patient's clothing and bedding, provide a sanitary pad.

▶ Help the patient return to a comfortable position, and advise her to remain in bed as much as possible for the next several hours.

▶ Wash your hands thoroughly.

Special considerations

▶ Refrigerate vaginal suppositories that melt at room temperature.

▶ If possible, teach the patient how to insert the vaginal medication because she may have to administer it herself after discharge. Give her a patient-teaching sheet if one is available.

▶ Instruct the patient not to wear a tampon after inserting vaginal medication because it would absorb the medication and decrease its effectiveness.

▶ Instruct the patient to avoid sexual intercourse during treatment.

References

The Joint Commission. *Comprehensive Accreditation Manual for Hospitals: The Official Handbook.* Standard MM.1.10. Oakbrook Terrace, Ill.: The Joint Commission, 2007.

The Joint Commission. *Comprehensive Accreditation Manual for Hospitals: The Official Handbook.* Standard MM.2.10. Oakbrook Terrace, Ill.: The Joint Commission, 2007.

The Joint Commission. *Comprehensive Accreditation Manual for Hospitals: The Official Handbook.* Standard MM.3.10. Oakbrook Terrace, Ill.: The Joint Commission, 2007.

The Joint Commission. *Comprehensive Accreditation Manual for Hospitals: The Official Handbook.* Standard MM.4.10. Oakbrook Terrace, Ill.: The Joint Commission, 2007.

The Joint Commission. *Comprehensive Accreditation Manual for Hospitals: The Official Handbook.* Standard MM.4.20. Oakbrook Terrace, Ill.: The Joint Commission, 2007.

The Joint Commission. *Comprehensive Accreditation Manual for Hospitals: The Official Handbook.* Standard MM.5.10. Oakbrook Terrace, Ill.: The Joint Commission, 2007.

The Joint Commission. *Comprehensive Accreditation Manual for Hospitals: The Official Handbook.* Standard MM.6.10. Oakbrook Terrace, Ill.: The Joint Commission, 2007.

The Joint Commission. *Comprehensive Accreditation Manual for Hospitals: The Official Handbook.* Standard MM.6.20. Oakbrook Terrace, Ill.: The Joint Commission, 2007.

Taylor, C., et al. *Fundamentals of Nursing: The Art and Science of Nursing Care,* 6th ed. Philadelphia: Lippincott Williams & Wilkins, 2008.

Venipuncture

Performed to obtain a venous blood sample, venipuncture involves piercing a vein with a needle and collecting blood in a syringe or evacuated tube. Typically, venipuncture is performed using the antecubital fossa. If necessary, however, it can be performed on a vein in the dorsal forearm, the dorsum of the hand or foot, or another accessible location. The inner wrist shouldn't be used because of the high risk of damage to underlying structures. Although laboratory personnel usually perform this procedure in the hospital setting, you may perform it. You should also determine if special conditions exist before venipuncture, such as anticoagulant therapy, low platelet count, bleeding disorders, and other abnormalities that increase the risk of bleeding and hematoma formation.

Equipment

Tourniquet ◆ gloves ◆ syringe or evacuated tubes and needle holder ◆ chlorhexidine sponge ◆ 20G or 21G needle for the forearm or 25G needle for the wrist, hand, and ankle, and for children ◆ color-coded collection tubes containing appropriate additives ◆ labels ◆ laboratory request form and laboratory biohazard transportation bag ◆ 2″ × 2″ gauze pads ◆ adhesive bandage. (See *Guide to color-top collection tubes.*)

Implementation

▶ If you're using evacuated tubes, open the needle packet, attach the needle to its holder, and select the appropriate tubes. If you're using a syringe, attach the appropriate needle to it. Be sure to choose a syringe large enough to hold all the blood required for the test.

▶ Label all collection tubes clearly with the patient's name and room number, the practitioner's name, the date and time of collection, and initials of the person performing the venipuncture. **JC**

▶ Wash your hands thoroughly and put on gloves. **CDC**

▶ Confirm the patient's identity using two patient identifiers according to your facility's policy.

▶ Tell him that you're about to collect a blood sample, and explain the procedure to ease his anxiety and ensure his cooperation. Ask him if he has ever felt faint, sweaty, or nauseated when having blood drawn.

Guide to color-top collection tubes

TUBE COLOR	DRAW VOLUME	ADDITIVE	PURPOSE
Red	2 to 20 ml	None	Serum studies
Lavender	2 to 10 ml	EDTA	Whole-blood studies
Green	2 to 15 ml	Heparin (sodium, lithium, or ammonium)	Plasma studies
Blue	2.7 or 4.5 ml	Sodium citrate and citric acid	Coagulation studies on plasma
Black	2.7 or 4.5 ml	Sodium oxalate	Coagulation studies on plasma
Gray	3 to 10 ml	Glycolytic inhibitor, such as sodium fluoride, powdered oxalate, or glycolytic-microbial inhibitor	Glucose determinations on serum or plasma
Yellow	12 ml	Acid-citrate-dextrose	Whole-blood studies

▶ If the patient is on bed rest, ask him to lie in a supine position, with his head slightly elevated and his arms at his sides. Ask the ambulatory patient to sit in a chair and support his arm securely on an armrest or a table.

▶ Assess the patient's veins to determine the best puncture site. (See *Common venipuncture sites*.) Observe the skin for the vein's blue color, or palpate the vein for a firm rebound sensation.

▶ Tie a tourniquet 2″ (5 cm) proximal to the area chosen. If arterial perfusion remains adequate, you'll be able to feel the radial pulse. (If the tourniquet fails to dilate the vein, have the patient open and close his fist a few times. Then ask him to close his fist as you

insert the needle and to open it again when the needle is in place.)

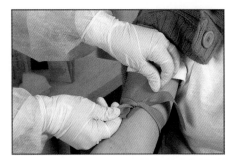

Common venipuncture sites

These illustrations show the anatomic locations of veins commonly used for venipuncture. The most commonly used sites are on the forearm, followed by those on the hand.

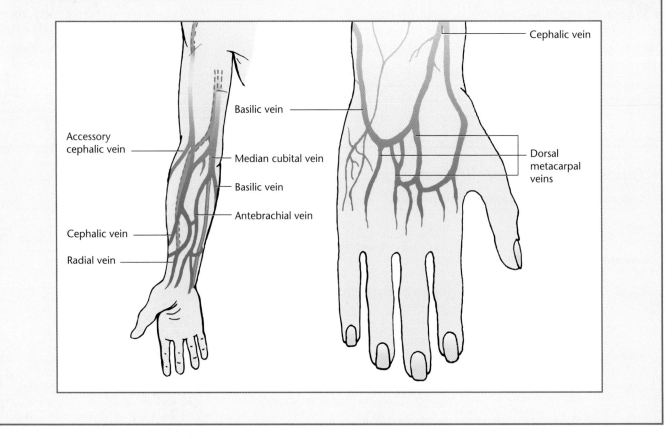

▶ Clean the venipuncture site using a chlorhexidine sponge with a back and forth motion. Allow the skin to dry before performing venipuncture. **CDC** **INS**

▶ Immobilize the vein by pressing just below the venipuncture site with your thumb and drawing the skin taut.

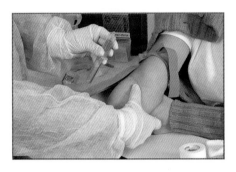

▶ Position the needle holder or syringe with the needle bevel up and the shaft parallel to the path of the vein and at a 30-degree angle to the arm. Insert the needle into the vein. If you're using a syringe, venous blood will appear in the hub; withdraw the blood slowly, pulling the plunger of the syringe gently to create steady suction until you obtain the required sample. Pulling the plunger too forcibly may collapse the vein. If you're using a needle holder and an evacuated tube, grasp the holder securely to stabilize it in the vein, and push down on the collection tube until the needle punctures the rubber stopper. Blood will flow into the tube automatically.

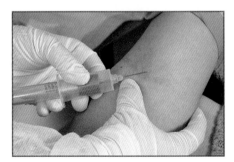

▶ Remove the tourniquet as soon as blood flows adequately to prevent stasis and hemoconcentration, which can impair test results. If the flow is sluggish, leave the tourniquet in place longer, but always remove it before withdrawing the needle. Don't leave the tourniquet on for more than 3 minutes.

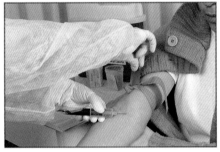

▶ Continue to fill the required tubes, removing one and inserting another. Gently rotate each tube as you remove it to help mix the additive with the sample.

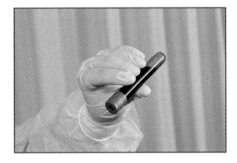

▶ After you've drawn the sample, place a gauze pad over the puncture site, and slowly and gently remove the needle from the vein. When using an evacuated tube, remove it from the needle holder to release the vacuum before withdrawing the needle from the vein.

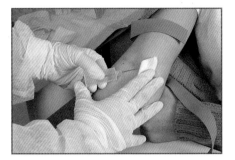

▶ Apply gentle pressure to the puncture site for 2 to 3 minutes or until bleeding stops. **INS**

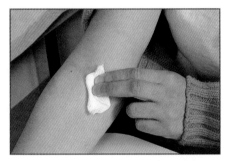

▶ After bleeding stops, apply an adhesive bandage.

▶ If you've used a syringe, transfer the sample to a collection tube. Place the specimen tubes inside the biohazard transport bag.

▶ Finally, check the venipuncture site to see if a hematoma has developed. If it has, apply pressure until you're sure bleeding has stopped (about 5 minutes), after which you may apply warm soaks to the site.

▶ Discard syringes, needles, and used gloves in the appropriate containers. **CDC**

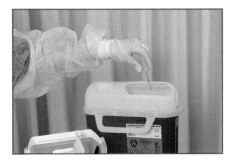

Special considerations

▶ Many manufacturers make safety-engineered blood collection sets; their use is recommended to prevent needle sticks. `JC` `OSHA` `CDC`

▶ Never collect a venous sample from an arm or a leg that's already being used for I.V. therapy or blood administration because this may affect test results. Don't collect a venous sample from an infection site because this may introduce pathogens into the vascular system. Likewise, avoid collecting blood from edematous areas, arteriovenous shunts, an upper extremity on the same side as a previous lymph node dissection, and sites of previous hematomas or vascular injury. `INS`

▶ If the patient has large, distended, highly visible veins, perform venipuncture without a tourniquet to minimize the risk of hematoma formation. `CDC` If the patient has a clotting disorder or is receiving anticoagulant therapy, maintain firm pressure on the venipuncture site for at least 5 minutes after withdrawing the needle to prevent hematoma formation.

▶ Avoid using veins in the patient's legs for venipuncture, if possible, because this increases the risk of thrombophlebitis. Some facilities require a practitioner's order to collect blood from a leg or foot vein. Check your facility's policy and procedure.

EVIDENCE-BASED RESEARCH

Drawing blood in anticoagulation therapy

Zengin, N., and EnÇ, N. "Comparison of Two Blood Sampling Methods in Anticoagulation Therapy: Venipuncture and Peripheral Venous Catheter," *Journal of Clinical Nursing* 17(3):386–93, February 2008.

Level VI
Evidence from a single descriptive or qualitative study

Description
Patients who are on anticoagulation therapy need to have frequent blood draws in order to monitor their coagulation status. This study examined if there was a difference in the prothrombin time (PT) and activated partial thromboplastin time (PTT) in samples that were drawn by direct venipuncture and from a peripheral venous catheter. A 21G needle was used in the direct venipuncture method and 18G, 20G, and 22G needles were used for the peripheral venous catheter

method. The amount of blood drawn for both methods was 1.8 ml.

Findings
There was no significant difference in the PT and activated PTT samples.

Conclusions
Patients who are receiving anticoagulant therapy are at an increased risk for bleeding due to their coagulation status and require frequent blood draws; therefore, this study recommends using peripheral venous catheters for drawing blood in these patients.

Nursing practice implications
Nurses may prefer to use peripheral venous catheters rather than venipuncture for both the comfort of the patient and the prevention of risks related to venipuncture. Using a peripheral venous catheter decreases the risk of bleeding, pain, and anxiety caused by venipuncture. However, the

Infusion Nurses Society (INS) and Centers for Disease Control and Prevention (CDC) both recommend avoiding the use of peripheral venous catheters for blood collection unless no other venous access is possible in order to decrease the risk of intravascular-related complications. Here are some important nursing practice implications:

▶ Assess the patient's vascular status and determine the best method of collecting a blood sample.

▶ Disinfect the collection hub of a peripheral venous catheter with alcohol before drawing blood.

▶ Monitor the patient's PT and activated PTT when he is receiving anticoagulants.

▶ Monitor the patient receiving anticoagulants for complications after a venipuncture.

▶ Follow the INS and CDC recommendations for venipuncture in order to decrease the patient's risk of intravascular infection.

References

Centers for Disease Control and Prevention. Hospital Infection Control Practices Advisory Committee. "Guideline for Prevention of Intravascular Device-related Infections." Available at: *www.cdc.gov/ncidod/dhqp/g1_intra vascular.html.*

Occupational Safety and Health Administration. "Bloodborne Pathogens," 1910.1030. Available at: *www.osha.gov/ pls/oshaweb/owadisp.show_document?p_ table=STANDARDS&p_id=10051.*

Rosenthal, K., "Tips for Venipuncture in Children," *Nursing* 35(12):31, December 2005.

"Standard 71. Phlebotomy. Infusion Nursing Standards of Practice," *Journal of Intravenous Nursing* 29(15):571–72. January–February 2006.

Volume-control sets

A volume-control set—an I.V. line with a graduated chamber—delivers precise amounts of fluid and shuts off when the fluid is exhausted, preventing air from entering the I.V. line. It may be used as a secondary line in adults for intermittent infusion of medication.

AGE FACTOR

A volume-control set is used as a primary line in children for continuous infusion of fluids or medication.

Equipment

Volume-control set ◆ I.V. pole (for setting up a primary I.V. line) ◆ I.V. solution ◆ alcohol pad ◆ medication in labeled syringe ◆ tape ◆ label.

Although various models of volume-control sets are available, each one consists of a graduated fluid chamber (120 to 250 ml) with a spike and a filtered air line on top and administration tubing underneath. Floating-valve sets have a valve at the bottom that closes when the chamber empties; membrane-filter sets have a rigid filter at the bottom that, when wet, prevents the passage of air.

Implementation

▶ Confirm the patient's identity using two patient identifiers according to your facility's policy. **JC**
▶ Wash your hands, and explain the procedure to the patient.
▶ If an I.V. line is already in place, observe its insertion site for signs of infiltration and infection. **JC**
▶ Remove the volume-control set from its box, and close all the clamps.
▶ Remove the protective cap from the volume-control set spike, insert the

spike into the I.V. solution container, and hang the container on the I.V. pole.
▶ Open the air vent clamp, and close the upper slide clamp. Then open the lower clamp on the I.V. tubing, slide it upward until it's slightly below the drip chamber, and close the clamp.
▶ Open the upper clamp until the fluid chamber fills with about 30 ml of solution. Then close the clamp, and carefully squeeze the drip chamber until it's half full.
▶ Keeping the drip chamber flat, close the lower clamp. Now release the drip chamber so that it fills halfway.
▶ Open the lower clamp, prime the tubing, and close the clamp. To use the set as a primary line, insert the distal end of the tubing into the catheter or needle hub.

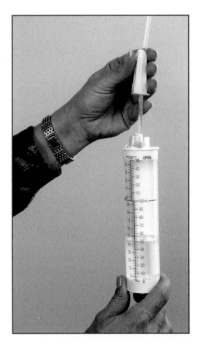

▶ To use the set as a secondary line, wipe the Y-port of the primary tubing with an alcohol pad, and attach the distal end of the tubing to the Y-port of the primary tubing, following the manufacturer's instructions.
▶ To add medication, wipe the injection port on the volume-control set with an alcohol pad and inject the medication.
▶ Place a label on the chamber, indicating the drug, dose, and date. Don't write directly on the chamber because the plastic absorbs ink.
▶ Open the upper clamp, fill the fluid chamber with the prescribed amount of solution, and close the clamp. Gently rotate the chamber to mix the medication.
▶ Turn off the primary solution (if present), or lower the drip rate to maintain an open line.
▶ Open the lower clamp on the volume-control set, and adjust the drip rate as ordered. After completion of the infusion, open the upper clamp, and let 10 ml of I.V. solution flow into the chamber and through the tubing to flush them.
▶ If you're using the volume-control set as a secondary I.V. line, close the lower clamp and reset the flow rate of the primary line. If you're using the set as a primary I.V. line, close the lower clamp, refill the chamber to the prescribed amount, and begin the infusion again.

Special considerations

▶ Always check compatibility of the medication and the I.V. solution. If you're using a membrane-filter set, avoid administering suspensions, lipid emulsions, blood, or blood components through it. **INS**

▶ The diaphragm may stick after repeated use. If it does, close the air vent and upper clamp, invert the drip chamber, and squeeze it. If the diaphragm opens, reopen the clamp and continue to use the set.

▶ If the drip chamber overfills, immediately close the upper clamp and air vent, invert the chamber, and squeeze the excess fluid from the drip chamber back into the graduated fluid chamber.

References

"Standard 15. Product Evaluation, Integrity, and Defect Report. Infusion Nursing Standards of Practice," *Journal of Infusion Nursing* 29(1S):S23, January–February 2006.

"Standard 48. Administration Set Change. Infusion Nursing Standards of Practice," *Journal of Infusion Nursing* 29(1S): S48–51, January–February 2006.

"Standard 68. Parenteral Medication and Solution Administration. Infusion Nursing Standards of Practice," *Journal of Infusion Nursing* 29(1S):S74–75, January–February 2006.

Weinstein, S. M. *Plumer's Principles and Practices of Intravenous Therapy,* 8th ed. Philadelphia: Lippincott Williams & Wilkins, 2007.

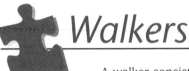

W xy

Walkers

A walker consists of a metal frame with handgrips and four legs that buttresses the patient on three sides; one side remains open. Because this device provides greater stability and security than other ambulatory aids, it's recommended for the patient with insufficient strength and balance to use crutches or a cane or with weakness requiring frequent rest periods.

Attachments for standard walkers and modified walkers help meet special needs. For example, a walker may have a platform added to support an injured arm.

Equipment

Walker ◆ platform or wheel attachments, as necessary.

Implementation

▶ Obtain the appropriate walker with the advice of a physical therapist, and adjust it to the patient's height: His elbows should be flexed at a 15- to 30-degree angle when standing comfortably within the walker with his hands on the grips. To adjust the walker, turn it upside down, and change the leg length by pushing in the button on each shaft and releasing it when the leg is in the correct position. Make sure the walker is level before the patient attempts to use it.

▶ Help the patient stand within the walker, and instruct him to hold the handgrips firmly and equally. Stand behind him, closer to the involved leg.

▶ If the patient has one-sided leg weakness, tell him to advance the walker 6″ to 8″ (15 to 20 cm) and to step forward with the involved leg and follow with the uninvolved leg, supporting himself on his arms. Encourage him to take equal strides. If he has equal strength in both legs, instruct him to advance the walker 6″ to 8″ and to step forward with either leg. If he can't use one leg, tell him to advance the walker 6″ to 8″ and to swing onto it, supporting his weight on his arms.

▶ If the patient is using a reciprocal walker, teach him the two-point gait. Instruct the patient to stand with his weight evenly distributed between his legs and the walker. Stand behind him, slightly to one side. Tell him to simultaneously advance the walker's right side and his left foot. Then have the patient advance the walker's left side and his right foot.

▶ If the patient is using a reciprocal walker, you may also teach him the four-point gait. Instruct the patient to evenly distribute his weight between his legs and the walker. Stand behind him and slightly to one side. Have him move the right side of the walker forward. Then have the patient move his left foot forward. Next, instruct him to move the left side of the walker forward. Finally, have him move his right foot forward.

▶ If the patient is using a wheeled or stair walker, reinforce the physical therapist's instructions. Stress the need for caution when using a stair walker.

▶ Teach the patient how to sit down and get up from a chair safely. (See *Teaching safe use of a walker*.)

Teaching safe use of a walker

Sitting down

▶ First, tell the patient to stand with the back of his stronger leg against the front of the chair, his weaker leg slightly off the floor, and the walker directly in front.

▶ Tell him to grasp the armrests on the chair one arm at a time while supporting most of his weight on the stronger leg. (In the illustrations, the patient has left leg weakness.)

▶ Tell the patient to lower himself into the chair and slide backward. After he's seated, he should place the walker beside the chair.

Getting up

▶ After bringing the walker to the front of his chair, tell the patient to slide forward in the chair. Placing the back of his stronger leg against the seat, he should then advance the weaker leg.

▶ Next, with both hands on the armrests, the patient can push himself to a standing position. Supporting himself with the stronger leg and the opposite hand, the patient should grasp the walker's handgrip with his free hand.

▶ Then the patient should grasp the free handgrip with his other hand.

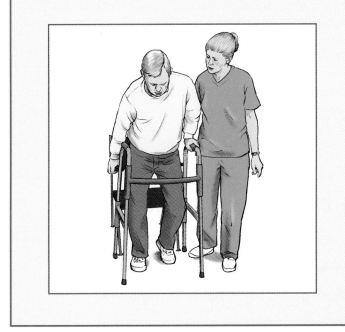

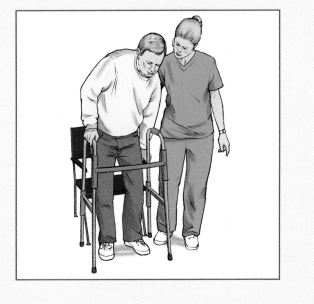

Special considerations

If the patient starts to fall, support his hips and shoulders to help him maintain an upright position if possible. If unsuccessful, ease him slowly to the closest surface—bed, floor, or chair.

References

Craven, R. F., and Hirnle, C. J. *Fundamentals of Nursing Human Health and Function,* 6th ed. Philadelphia: Lippincott Williams & Wilkins, 2009.

Haubert, L. L., et al. "A Comparison of Shoulder Joint Forces during Ambulation with Crutches versus a Walker in Persons with Incomplete Spinal Cord Injury," *Archives of Physical Medicine and Rehabilitation* 87(1):63–70, January 2006.

Wound dehiscence and evisceration management

Although surgical wounds typically heal without incident, occasionally the edges of a wound may fail to join or may separate even after they seem to be healing normally. This development, called *wound dehiscence,* may lead to an even more serious complication: evisceration, in which a portion of the viscera (usually a bowel loop) protrudes through the incision. Evisceration, in turn, can lead to peritonitis and septic shock. (See *Recognizing dehiscence and evisceration.*)

Dehiscence and evisceration are most likely to occur 6 to 7 days after surgery. By then, sutures may have been removed, and the patient can cough easily and breathe deeply—both of which strain the incision. Some wound dehiscence may be managed conservatively using a medical approach, such as sterile dressing application and wound monitoring.

Several factors can contribute to these complications. Poor nutrition—either from inadequate intake or a condition such as diabetes mellitus—may hinder wound healing. Chronic pulmonary or cardiac disease can also slow healing because the injured tissue doesn't get needed nutrients and oxygen. Localized wound infection may limit closure, delay healing, and weaken the incision. Also, stress on the incision from coughing or vomiting may cause abdominal distention or severe stretching. A midline abdominal incision, for instance, poses a high risk of wound dehiscence.

Equipment

Two sterile towels ◆ 1 L of sterile normal saline solution ◆ sterile irrigation set, including a basin, solution container, and 50-ml catheter-tip syringe ◆ several large abdominal dressings ◆ sterile, waterproof drape ◆ linen-saver pads ◆ sterile gloves.

If the patient will return to the operating room, also gather the following equipment: I.V. administration set and I.V. fluids ◆ equipment for nasogastric (NG) intubation ◆ sedative, as ordered ◆ suction apparatus.

Implementation

▶ Provide reassurance and support to ease the patient's anxiety. Tell him to stay in bed. If possible, stay with him while someone else notifies the practitioner and collects the necessary equipment.

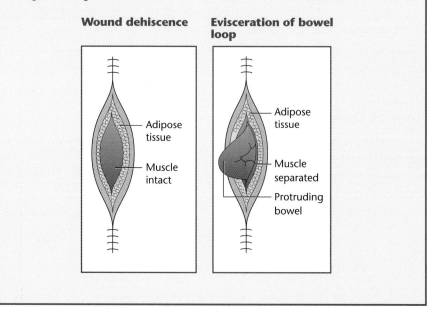

Recognizing dehiscence and evisceration

In wound dehiscence (below left), the layers of the surgical wound separate. In evisceration (below right), the viscera (in this case, a bowel loop) protrude through the surgical incision.

Wound dehiscence

— Adipose tissue

— Muscle intact

Evisceration of bowel loop

— Adipose tissue

— Muscle separated

— Protruding bowel

▶ Place a linen-saver pad under the patient.

▶ Using sterile technique, unfold a sterile towel to create a sterile field. Open the package containing the irrigation set, and place the basin, solution container, and 50-ml syringe on the sterile field. **CDC**

▶ Open the bottle of normal saline solution, and pour about 400 ml into the solution container. Also pour about 200 ml into the sterile basin.

▶ Open several large abdominal dressings, and place them on the sterile field.

▶ Put on the sterile gloves, and place one or two of the large abdominal dressings into the basin to saturate them with saline solution.

▶ Place the moistened dressings over the exposed viscera. Then place a sterile, waterproof drape over the dressings to prevent the sheets from getting wet.

▶ Moisten the dressings every hour by withdrawing saline solution from the container through the syringe and then gently squirting the solution on the dressings.

▶ When you moisten the dressings, inspect the color of the viscera. If it appears dusky or black, notify the practitioner immediately. With its blood supply interrupted, a protruding organ may become ischemic and necrotic.

▶ Keep the patient on absolute bed rest in low Fowler's position (no more than 20-degrees elevation) with his knees flexed. This prevents injury and reduces stress on an abdominal incision.

▶ Don't allow the patient to have anything by mouth to decrease the risk of aspiration during surgery.

▶ Monitor the patient's pulse, respirations, blood pressure, and temperature every 15 minutes to detect shock.

▶ If necessary, prepare the patient to return to the operating room. After gathering the appropriate equipment, start an I.V. infusion, as ordered.

▶ Insert an NG tube, and connect it to continuous or intermittent low suction, as ordered.

▶ Continue to reassure the patient while you prepare him for surgery. Make sure he has signed a consent form and that the operating room staff has been informed about the procedure.

▶ Administer preoperative medications to the patient, as ordered.

Special considerations

▶ Depending on the circumstances, some of these procedures may not be done at the bedside. For instance, NG intubation may make the patient gag or vomit, causing further evisceration. For this reason, the physician may choose to have the NG tube inserted in the operating room with the patient under anesthesia.

▶ The best treatment is prevention. If you're caring for a postoperative patient who's at risk for poor healing, make sure he receives an adequate supply of protein, vitamins, and calories. Monitor his dietary deficiencies, and discuss any problems with the practitioner and the dietitian.

▶ When changing wound dressings, always use sterile technique. Inspect the incision with each dressing change, and if you recognize the early signs of infection, start treatment before dehiscence or evisceration can occur. If local infection develops, clean the wound as necessary to eliminate a buildup of purulent drainage. Make sure bandages aren't so tight that they limit blood supply to the wound.

References

Banwell, P. E., et al. "Treatment of Dehisced and Infected Wounds," *Journal of Wound Care* 14(3):110, March 2005.

Doughty, D. B. "Preventing and Managing Surgical Wound Dehiscence," *Home Healthcare Nurse* 22(6):364–67, June 2004.

Hahler, B. "Surgical Wound Dehiscence," *Medsurg Nursing* 15(5):296–300; quiz 301, October 2006.

Wilson, J. A., and Clark, J. J. "Obesity: Impediment to Postsurgical Wound Healing," *Advances in Skin & Wound Care* 17(8):426–35, October 2004.

Wound irrigation

Irrigation cleans tissues and flushes cell debris and drainage from an open wound. Irrigation with a commercial wound cleaner helps the wound heal properly from the inside tissue layers outward to the skin surface; it also helps prevent premature surface healing over an abscess pocket or infected tract. Performed properly, wound irrigation requires strict sterile technique. After irrigation, open wounds usually are packed to absorb additional drainage.

Equipment

Waterproof trash bag ◆ linen-saver pad ◆ emesis basin ◆ clean gloves ◆ sterile gloves ◆ goggles, if indicated ◆ gown, if indicated ◆ prescribed irrigant such as sterile normal saline solution ◆ sterile water or normal saline solution ◆ sterile irrigating syringe ◆ sterile container ◆ materials, as needed, for wound care ◆ sterile dressing ◆ commercial wound cleaner ◆ 35-ml piston syringe with 19G catheter ◆ skin protectant wipe ◆ gauze pad.

Implementation

▶ Using aseptic technique, dilute the prescribed irrigant to the correct proportions with sterile water or normal saline solution, if necessary. Let the solution stand until it reaches room temperature, or warm it to 90° to 95° F (32.2° to 35° C). **CS**

▶ Open the waterproof trash bag, and place it near the patient's bed. Position the bag to avoid reaching across the sterile field or the wound when disposing of soiled articles.

▶ Confirm the patient's identity using two patient identifiers according to your facility's policy. **JC**

▶ Check the practitioner's order.

▶ Assess the patient's condition. Identify the patient's allergies, especially to povidone-iodine or other topical solutions or medications.

▶ Explain the procedure to the patient, provide privacy, and position the patient correctly for the procedure.

▶ Place the linen-saver pad under the patient to catch any spills and avoid linen changes. Place the emesis basin below the wound so that the irrigating solution flows from the wound into the basin and so that the irrigating solution will drain from the clean to the dirty end of the wound.

▶ Wash your hands thoroughly. If necessary, put on a gown and goggles to protect your clothing from wound drainage and contamination. Put on clean gloves. **CDC**

▶ Remove the soiled dressing; then discard the dressing and gloves in the trash bag.

▶ Assess the wound and surrounding tissue for information about the healing process or presence of infection.

▶ Establish a sterile field with all the equipment and supplies you'll need for irrigation and wound care. Pour the prescribed amount of irrigating solution into a sterile container so you won't contaminate your sterile gloves later by picking up unsterile containers. **CDC**

▶ Put on sterile gloves, gown, and goggles, if indicated. **CDC**

▶ Fill the syringe with the irrigating solution.

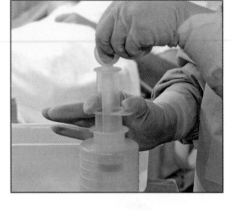

▶ Position the irrigation syringe above the wound. Make sure the solution flows from the clean to the dirty area of the wound to prevent contamination of clean tissue by exudate.

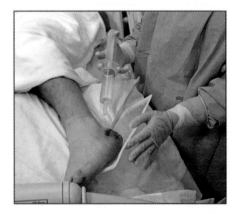

▶ Gently instill a slow, steady stream of irrigating solution into the wound until the syringe empties. Also make sure the solution reaches all areas of the wound.

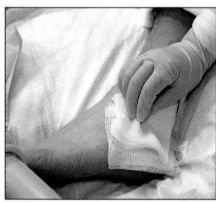

▶ Refill the syringe and repeat the irrigation.

▶ Continue to irrigate the wound until you've administered the prescribed amount of solution or until the solution returns clear. Note the amount of solution administered. Then discard the syringe in the waterproof trash bag. **CS2**

▶ Keep the patient positioned to allow further wound drainage into the basin.

▶ Dry intact skin with a sterile gauze pad, apply with a skin protectant wipe, and allow it to dry well to help prevent skin breakdown and infection.

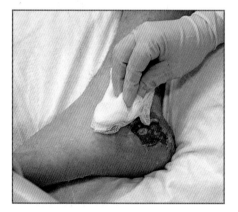

▶ Pack the wound, if ordered, and apply a sterile dressing. Remove and discard your gloves and gown.

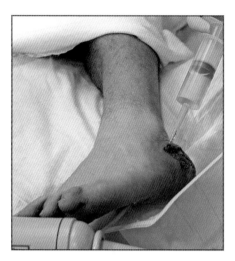

▶ Make sure the patient is comfortable.

▶ Properly dispose of drainage, solutions, and trash bag, and clean or dispose of soiled equipment and supplies according to your facility's policy and Centers for Disease Control and Prevention guidelines. To prevent contamination of other equipment, don't return unopened sterile supplies to the sterile supply cabinet.

Special considerations

▶ Try to coordinate wound irrigation with the practitioner's visit so that he can inspect the wound.

▶ Irrigate with a bulb syringe if the wound is small or not particularly deep or if a piston syringe is unavailable. However, use a bulb syringe cautiously because this type of syringe doesn't deliver enough pressure to adequately clean the wound.

▶ Never use a larger syringe or a small needle because this would result in more than 13 psi of pressure, which may damage the wound. **CS1** **CS2**

▶ If the procedure is likely to cause the patient pain, premedicate him before beginning irrigation, as ordered.

References

Fernandez, R., et al. "The Effectiveness of Solutions, Techniques, and Pressure in Wound Cleansing." *The Joanna Briggs Institute for Evidence-Based Nursing and Midwifery* Available at *http://www.joannabriggs.edu.au/pdf/EXwoundclen.pdf.* **CS2**

Fernandez, R., and Griffiths, R. "Water for Wound Cleansing." *Cochrane Database of Systematic Reviews* 2002, Issue 4. Art. No.: CD003861. DOI: 10.1002/14651858.CD003861.pub2. **CS1**

Hassinger, H. M., et al. "High-Pressure Pulsatile Lavage Propagates Bacteria into Soft Tissue," *Clinical Orthopaedics and Related Research* 439:27–31, October 2005.

Svoboda, S. J., et al. "Comparison of Bulb Syringe and Pulsed Lavage Irrigation with Use of a Bioluminescent Musculoskeletal Wound Model," *The Journal of Bone and Joint Surgery* 88(10): 2167–174, October 2006.

Willcox, M. "Cleaning Simple Wounds: Healing by Secondary Intention," *Nursing Times* 100(46):57, November 2004.

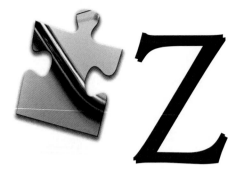

Z-track injection

The Z-track method of I.M. injection prevents leakage, or tracking, into the subcutaneous tissue. It's typically used to administer drugs that irritate and discolor subcutaneous tissue, primarily iron preparations such as iron dextran. It may also be used in elderly patients who have decreased muscle mass. Lateral displacement of the skin during the injection helps to seal the drug in the muscle.

This procedure requires careful attention to technique because leakage into subcutaneous tissue can cause patient discomfort and may permanently stain some tissues.

Equipment

Patient's medication record and chart ◆ two 20G 1¼″ to 2″ needles ◆ prescribed medication ◆ gloves ◆ 3- or 5-ml syringe ◆ two alcohol pads.

Implementation

▶ Verify the order on the patient's medication record by checking it against the practitioner's order. **JC** **ISMP**

▶ Wash your hands. **CDC**

▶ Make sure the needle you're using is long enough to reach the muscle. As a rule of thumb, a 200-lb (90.7-kg) patient requires a 2″ needle; a 100-lb (45-kg) patient, a 1¼″ to a 1½″ needle.

▶ Attach one needle to the syringe, and draw up the prescribed medication. Remove the first needle and attach the second to prevent tracking the medication through the subcutaneous tissue as the needle is inserted. Draw up 0.2 to 0.3 cc of air into the syringe. **CS**

▶ Confirm the patient's identity using two patient identifiers according to your facility's policy. **JC**

▶ If your facility utilizes a bar code scanning system, be sure to scan your ID badge, the patient's ID bracelet, and the medication's bar code. **JC** **ISMP**

▶ Explain the procedure, and provide privacy.

▶ Place the patient in the lateral position, exposing the gluteal muscle to be used as the injection site. The patient may also be placed in the prone position.

▶ Clean an area on the upper outer quadrant of the patient's buttock with an alcohol pad.

▶ Put on gloves. Then displace the skin laterally by pulling it away from the injection site. (See *Displacing the skin for Z-track injection.*)

▶ Insert the needle into the muscle at a 90-degree angle.

▶ Aspirate for blood return; if none appears, inject the drug slowly, followed by the air. Injecting air after the drug helps clear the needle and prevents tracking the medication through subcutaneous tissues as the needle is withdrawn.

▶ Wait 10 seconds before withdrawing the needle to ensure dispersion of the medication.

▶ Withdraw the needle slowly. Then release the displaced skin and subcutaneous tissue to seal the needle track. Don't massage the injection site or allow the patient to wear a tight-fitting garment over the site because it could force the medication into subcutaneous tissue.

▶ Encourage the patient to walk or move about in bed to facilitate absorption of the drug from the injection site.

▶ Discard the needles and syringe in an appropriate sharps container. Don't recap needles to avoid needle-stick injuries. **JC** **CDC** **ISMP**

▶ Remove and discard your gloves.

Displacing the skin for Z-track injection

By blocking the needle pathway after an injection, the Z-track technique allows I.M. injection while minimizing the risk of subcutaneous irritation and staining from such drugs as iron dextran. The illustrations here show you how to perform a Z-track injection.

Before the procedure begins, the skin, subcutaneous fat, and muscle lie in their normal positions.

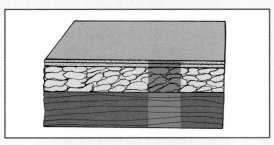

To begin, place your finger on the skin surface, and pull the skin and subcutaneous layers out of alignment with the underlying muscle. You should move the skin about ½″ (1 cm).

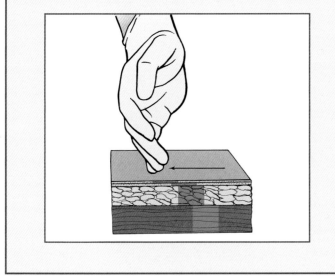

Insert the needle at a 90-degree angle at the site where you initially placed your finger. Inject the drug and withdraw the needle.

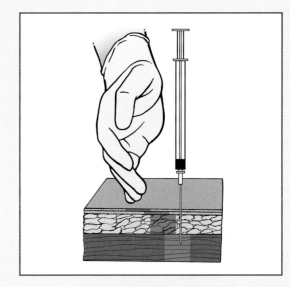

Finally, remove your finger from the skin surface, allowing the layers to return to their normal positions. The needle track is now broken at the junction of each tissue layer, trapping the drug in the muscle.

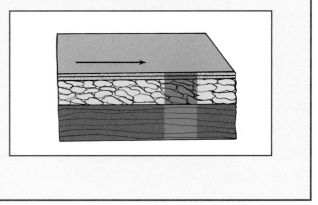

Special considerations

▶ Never inject more than 5 ml of solution into a single site using the Z-track method. Alternate gluteal sites for repeat injections.

▶ Always encourage the patient to relax the muscle you'll be injecting because injections into tense muscle are more painful than usual and may bleed more readily.

▶ If the patient is on bed rest, encourage active range-of-motion (ROM) exercises or perform passive ROM exercises to facilitate absorption from the injection site.

▶ I.M. injections can damage local muscle cells, causing elevated serum enzyme levels (for example, of creatine kinase) that can be confused with the elevated enzyme levels resulting from damage to cardiac muscle, as in myocardial infarction. If measuring enzyme levels is important, suggest that the practitioner switch to I.V. administration, and adjust dosages accordingly.

References

"Administering Medication by the Z-Track Method," *Nursing* 35(7):24, July 2005.

Donaldson, D., and Green, J. "Using the Ventrogluteal Site for Intramuscular Injections," *Nursing Times* 101(16):36–38, April 2005.

"I.M. Injections: Pick Your Site," *Nursing* 36(6):34, June 2006.

The Joint Commission. *Comprehensive Accreditation Manual for Hospitals: The Official Handbook.* Standard MM.1.10. Oakbrook Terrace, Ill.: The Joint Commission, 2007.

The Joint Commission. *Comprehensive Accreditation Manual for Hospitals: The Official Handbook.* Standard MM.2.10. Oakbrook Terrace, Ill.: The Joint Commission, 2007.

The Joint Commission. *Comprehensive Accreditation Manual for Hospitals: The Official Handbook.* Standard MM.3.10. Oakbrook Terrace, Ill.: The Joint Commission, 2007.

The Joint Commission. *Comprehensive Accreditation Manual for Hospitals: The Official Handbook.* Standard MM.4.10. Oakbrook Terrace, Ill.: The Joint Commission, 2007.

The Joint Commission. *Comprehensive Accreditation Manual for Hospitals: The Official Handbook.* Standard MM.4.20. Oakbrook Terrace, Ill.: The Joint Commission, 2007.

The Joint Commission. *Comprehensive Accreditation Manual for Hospitals: The Official Handbook.* Standard MM.5.10. Oakbrook Terrace, Ill.: The Joint Commission, 2007.

The Joint Commission. *Comprehensive Accreditation Manual for Hospitals: The Official Handbook.* Standard MM.6.10. Oakbrook Terrace, Ill.: The Joint Commission, 2007.

The Joint Commission. *Comprehensive Accreditation Manual for Hospitals: The Official Handbook.* Standard MM.6.20. Oakbrook Terrace, Ill.: The Joint Commission, 2007.

Quartermaine, S., and Taylor, R. "A Comparative Study of Depot Injection Techniques," *Nursing Times* 91(30):36–39, August–July 1995.

Taylor, C., et al. *Fundamentals of Nursing: The Art and Science of Nursing Care,* 6th ed. Philadelphia: Lippincott Williams & Wilkins, 2008.

Wynaden, D., et al. "Establishing Best Practice Guidelines for Administration of Intramuscular Injections in the Adult: A Systematic Review of the Literature," *Contemporary Nurse* 20(2):267–77, December 2005.

INDEX

t refers to a table.

t refers to a table.

t refers to a table.